Textbook of Orthopaedics

Textbook of
Orthopaedics

Binoti Sheth
Associate Professor and Head of the Unit
Department of Orthopaedics
Lokmanya Tilak Municipal Medical College and Hospital
Sion, Mumbai

Muqtadeer Ansari
Associate Professor
Department of Orthopaedics
Government Medical College
Aurangabad

Atul Kantilal Patil
Associate Professor
Department of Orthopaedics
Terna Medical College, Navi Mumbai

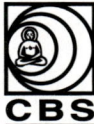

CBS

CBS Publishers & Distributors Pvt Ltd

New Delhi • Bengaluru • Chennai • Kochi • Kolkata • Mumbai
Hyderabad • Jharkhand • Nagpur • Patna • Pune • Uttarakhand

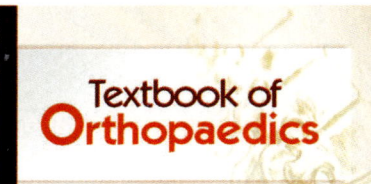

ISBN: 978-93-86478-15-3

Copyright © Authors and Publisher

First Edition 2018

Published by Satish Kumar Jain and Produced by Varun Jain for

CBS Publishers & Distributors Pvt Ltd

4819/XI Prahlad Street, 24 Ansari Road, Daryaganj, New Delhi 110 002, India.
Ph: 23289259, 23266861, 23266867   Fax: 011-23243014   Website: www.cbspd.com
                                                                                    e-mail: delhi@cbspd.com; cbspubs@airtelmail.in.

Corporate Office: 204 FIE, Industrial Area, Patparganj, Delhi 110 092, India
Ph: 4934 4934   Fax: 4934 4935   e-mail: publishing@cbspd.com; publicity@cbspd.com

Branches

- **Bengaluru:** Seema House 2975, 17th Cross, K.R. Road,
  Banasankari 2nd Stage, Bengaluru 560 070, Karnataka, India
  Ph: +91-80-26771678/79   Fax: +91-80-26771680   e-mail: bangalore@cbspd.com
- **Chennai:** 7, Subbaraya Street, Shenoy Nagar, Chennai 600 030, Tamil Nadu, India
  Ph: +91-44-26260666, 26208620   Fax: +91-44-42032115   e-mail: chennai@cbspd.com
- **Kochi:** Ashana House, No. 39/1904, AM Thomas Road, Valanjambalam, Ernakulam 682 016, Kochi, Kerala, India
  Ph: +91-484-4059061-65   Fax: +91-484-4059065   e-mail: kochi@cbspd.com
- **Kolkata:** No. 6/B, Ground Floor, Rameswar Shaw Road, Kolkata-700014 (West Bengal), India
  Ph: +91-33-2289-1126, 2289-1127, 2289-1128   e-mail: kolkata@cbspd.com
- **Mumbai:** 83-C, Dr E Moses Road, Worli, Mumbai-400018, Maharashtra, India
  Ph: +91-22-24902340/41   Fax: +91-22-24902342   e-mail: mumbai@cbspd.com

Representatives

- **Hyderabad** 0-9885175004
- **Jharkhand** 0-9811541605
- **Nagpur** 0-9021734563
- **Patna** 0-9334159340
- **Pune** 0-9623451994
- **Uttarakhand** 0-9000660880

Printed at: Nutech Print Services - India

Foreword

It gives me immense pleasure to comment on this basic yet extremely important textbook authored by Dr Binoti Sheth, Dr Atul Patil and Dr Muqtadeer Ansari. This book has been written keeping in mind the fast pace of changes in medical technology, the treatment and the protocols that have evolved in this new era. The work has been painstakingly completed and documented into print format as a textbook and is targeted for the benefit of the undergraduate medical and therapy students and junior postgraduate students.

I appreciate the efforts of the authors in undertaking this enormous work of compiling the orthopaedic work for the benefit of academic community at large. All aspects of orthopaedic disorders are touched upon in a precise and clear way, using artistic diagrams, X-rays and clinical pictures. I take great pride in writing the Foreword to this book and wish the authors a great success. I am sure this textbook will go a long way in helping the students master the subject of orthopaedics and help them pass with flying colours.

AB Goregaonkar
Professor and Head
Department of Orthopaedics
Lokmanya Tilak Municipal Medical College
Mumbai

Preface

It gives me immense pleasure to present the first edition of Textbook of Orthopaedics to medical students. Orthopaedic surgery has progressed from an immature limited speciality to a vast field of various orthopaedic subspecialities. Having worked in the field of medical education for the past 20 years, I felt the need for a concise textbook that the students would enjoy reading and which would enable them to thoroughly grasp important concepts required for exams and clinical practice. This book is prepared to serve as a textbook for undergraduate and junior postgraduate medical students as well as physiotherapy, occupational therapy and nursing students.

We have endeavoured to make the text simple and easy to understand. The text has been supplemented by relevant simple line diagrams, radiographs and clinical pictures, wherever necessary for better understanding of the subject. The section on clinical examination provides a systematic approach to case presentations for practical examination.

I am thankful to my seniors, colleagues and family members for their constant support and encouragement. I also thank Dr Mohan Desai and Dr Dinshaw Pardiwala for their contribution to the section on clinical examination, Dr Rahul Jagtap for excellent diagrams work, and Dr Aditya Pathak, Dr Chetan Anchan and Dr Kshitij Chaudhary for their contribution to clinical photographs.

Finally, I am highly indebted to the dedicated team of Rajesh Bhalani of Bhalani Publishers and CBS Publisher & Distributors Pvt Ltd for their constant guidance and advice in the preparation of this book. I wish the students happy reading and great success in their examinations.

Binoti A Sheth

Contents

Section IV: Spine

Section V: Tumours

Section VI: Paediatric Orthopeadics

Section VII: Other Orthopaedic Disorders and Special Subjects

Section VIII: Orthopaedic Clinical Examinations

Section IX: Orthopaedic Implants, Radiology and Orthotics

Abbreviations

ABC	Aneurysmal bone cyst	EDQ	Extensor digiti quinti
ACL	Anterior cruciate ligament	EIP	Extensor indicis proprius
AFO	Ankle foot orthosis	EMG	Electromyography
AK	Above knee	EPB	Extensor pollicis brevis
AKT	Anti-Koch's treatment	EPL	Extensor pollicis longus
ALL	Anterior longitudinal ligament	FCR	Flexor carpi radialis
AMC	Arthrogryposis multiplex congenita	FDL	Flexor digitorum longus
AMP	Austin Moore prosthesis	FDP	Flexor digitorum profundus
AP	Anteroposterior	FDS	Flexor digitorum superficialis
APB	Abductor pollicis brevis	FFD	Fixed flexion deformity
APL	Abductor pollicis longus	FHL	Flexor hallucis longus
AS	Ankylosing spondylitis	FPB	Flexor pollicis brevis
ASH	Anterior spinal hyperextension	GCT	Giant cell tumour
ASIS	Anterior superior iliac spine	HKAFO	Hip knee ankle foot orthosis
AVN	Avascular necrosis	HNP	Herniated nucleus pulposus
BB	Bohler Braun	HTO	High tibial osteotomy
BK	Below knee	IP	Interphalangeal
BMD	Bone mineral density	JESS	Joshi's external stabilisation system
CDK	Congenital dislocation of knee	KAFO	Knee ankle foot orthosis
CNS	Central nervous system	LCL	Lateral collateral ligament
CP	Cerebral palsy	LCPD	Legg-Calvé-Perthes disease
CPK	Creatine phosphokinase	LCS	Lumbar canal stenosis
CPPD	Calcium pyrophosphate deposition	MCC	Multiple congenital contracture
CPT	Congenital pseudoarthrosis of tibia	MCL	Medial collateral ligament
CRIF	Closed reduction internal fixation	MCP	Metacarpophalangeal
CRP	C-reative protein	MCP	Metacarpophalangeal
CRPS	Complex regional pain syndrome	MIPPO	Minimally invasive percutaneous plate osteosynthesis
CTEV	Congenital talipes equinovarus		
DCP	Dynamic compression plate	MMC	Meningomyelocele
DD	Differential diagnosis	MTP	Metatarsophalangeal
DDH	Developmental dysplasia of hip	MUGA	Manipulation under general anaesthesia
DIP	Distal interphalangeal	NCV	Nerve conduction velocity
DMARD	Disease modifying anti-rheumatic drugs	NSAID	Non-steroidal anti-inflammatory drugs
DMD	Duchenne's muscular dystrophy	OA	Osteoarthritis
DRUJ	Distal radio-ulnar joint	OGS	Osteogenic sarcoma
DVT	Deep vein thrombosis	OI	Osteogenesis imperfecta
ECRB	Extensor carpi radialis brevis	ORIF	Open reduction internal fixation
ECRL	Extensor carpi radialis longus	PA	Posterior anterior
ECU	Extensor carpi ulnaris	PBH	Pelvis both hips
EDC	Extensor digitorum communis	PCL	Posterior cruciate ligament

PID	Prolapsed intervertebral disc
PIP	Proximal interphalangeal
PL	Palmaris longus
POP	Plaster of Paris
PPRP	Post polio residual paralysis
PQ	Pronator quadratus
PSIS	Posterosuperior iliac spine
PT	Pronator teres
PTB	Patellar tendon bearing
RA	Rheumatoid arthritis
ROM	Range of motion
RSD	Reflex sympathetic dystrophy
SCFE	Slipped capital femoral epiphysis

SI	Sacroiliac
SLE	Systemic lupus erthematosus
SLR	Straight leg raising
SWD	Short vlave diathermy
TBW	Tension band wiring
TENS	• Titanium elastic nailing system
	• Trascutaneous electric nerve stimulation
TFCC	Triangular fibrocartilaginous complex
THR	Total hip replacement
TKR	Total knee replacement
TNF	Tumour necrosis factor
UBC	Unicameral bone cyst
USG	Ultrasonography
VDRO	Varus derotation osteotomy

Introduction

Introduction to Orthopaedics

Orthopaedics evolved as a speciality in 18th century. In the year 1741, Nicholas Andry (Fig. 1.1), a French physician coined the term 'Orthopaedics' from two Greek words, 'Ortho' meaning straight and 'Paedia' meaning child (Fig. 1.2). Today 'Orthopaedics' deals with not just correcting childhood deformities but offers specialized treatment options in various aspects of trauma, infection, tumours, degenerative, metabolic and congenital disorders.

Change in lifestyle, rise in the number of vehicular accidents and newer diagnostic modalities have contributed to tremendous surge in various orthopaedic ailments. Synthetic casts, newer methods of fixation like the AO system, minimally invasive surgeries, advances in arthroplasty, arthroscopy, use of bone substitutes are some of the recent advances in orthopaedics. But it is important not to forget the basics and understand the pathology clearly. It is also important to have a systematic approach to any orthopaedic condition. Through this book, we wish to present various orthopaedic pathologies in a simple and

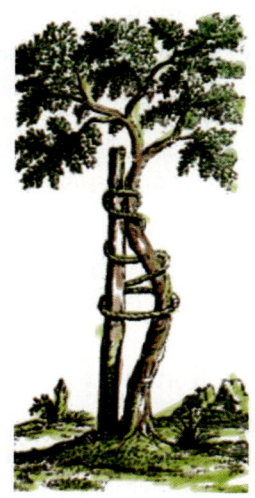

Fig. 1.2: Frontispiece of orthopaedia

systematic way, along with useful illustrations, to help the students understand and reproduce well in the exam.

COMMON ORTHOPAEDIC TERMINOLOGIES

Abduction: Motion within the coronal plane of the body where the limb moves away from the midline.

Adduction: Motion within the coronal plane of the body where the limb moves towards the midline.

Active motion: Joint motion carried out by the patient.

Ankylosis: Pathological or non-intentional fusion of a joint.

Arthrodesis: Intentional fusion of a joint done to relieve pain. The two bones forming a joint are joined together so that the resulting fused joint loses flexibility. However, a fused joint can bear weight better, is more stable, and is no longer painful.

Arthrogram: A specific X-ray to view bone structures following an injection of a contrast fluid into a joint

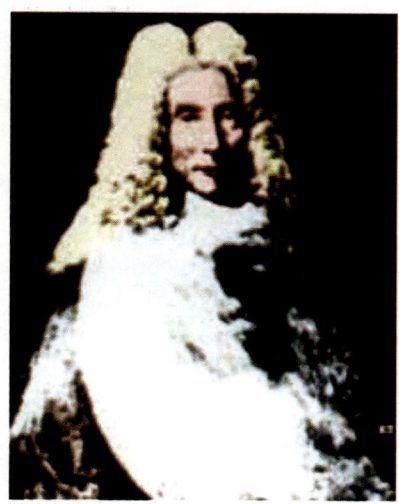

Fig. 1.1: Nicholas Andry

area. When the fluid leaks into an area that it does not belong, disease or injury may be considered as a leak would provide evidence of a tear, opening, or blockage.

Bunion: A bunion is a localised painful swelling at the base of the big toe (the great toe). The joint is enlarged (due to new bone formation) and the toe is often malaligned. It is frequently associated with inflammation. It can be related to inflammation of the nearby bursa (bursitis) or degenerative joint disease (osteoarthritis).

Bursa: A closed fluid-filled sac that functions to provide a gliding surface to reduce friction between tissues of the body.

Bursitis: Bursitis is inflammation of a bursa.

Computed tomography scan (CT scan): Pictures of structures within the body created by a computer that takes the data from multiple X-ray images and turns them into pictures on a screen. The CT scan can reveal some soft tissues and other structures that cannot even be seen in conventional X-rays.

Closed reduction: The reduction of a displaced part (e.g. a fractured bone) by manipulation without opening fracture site.

Distal: Means away from the trunk.

Dorsal: Relating to the back or posterior of a structure. Some of the dorsal surfaces of the body are the back, buttocks, calves, and the knuckle side of the hand.

Electromyogram (EMG): A test used to record the electrical activity of muscles. When muscles are active, they produce an electrical current that is usually proportional to the level of muscle activity.

Extension: The process of straightening or the state of being straight.

Flexion: The process of bending or the state of being bent.

Greenstick fracture: A fracture in which one side of a bone is broken while the other is bent.

Internal fixation: A surgical procedure that stabilises and joins the ends of fractured (broken) bones by mechanical devices such as metal plates, pins, rods, wires or screws.

Lateral: The side of the body or a body part that is farther from the middle or centre of the body. Typically, lateral refers to the outer side of the body part, but it is also used to refer to the side of a body part. For example, when referring to the knee, lateral refers to the side of the knee farthest from the opposite knee. The opposite of lateral is medial.

Medial: Pertaining to the middle; in or toward the middle; nearer the middle of the body. For example, the medial side of the knee is the side closest to the other knee. The opposite of medial is lateral.

MRI (magnetic resonance imaging): A special radiology technique designed to image internal structures of the body using magnetism, radio waves, and a computer to produce the images of body structures. The image and resolution is quite detailed and can detect tiny changes of structures within the body, particularly in the soft tissue, brain and spinal cord, abdomen and joints.

Muscular dystrophy: A group of degenerative disorders of muscle resulting in atrophy and weakness.

Myelogram: A specific X-ray study that uses an injection of a dye or contrast material into the spinal canal to allow careful evaluation of the spinal canal and nerve roots.

Open reduction: Realignment of a fractured bone after incision into the fracture site.

Proximal: Means closer to the trunk.

Passive motion: Movement of a patient's joint by a person who is examining or treating the patient.

Pronation: A movement of the forearm and hand such that the palm faces downward.

Spinal fusions: A surgical procedure in which two or more of the vertebrae in the spine are united together so that motion no longer occurs between them.

Supination: A movement of the forearm and hand such that the palm faces upward.

It is opposite of pronation.

Prosthetics: The art and science of developing artificial replacements for body parts.

Scoliosis: Three-dimensional deformity of the vertebral column in which lateral deviation in coronal plane is associated with rotation of the vertebrae.

Scoliotic list: Lateral deviation of the vertebral column in coronal plane due to muscle spasm.

Spina bifida: A birth defect (a congenital malformation) in which there is a bony defect in the vertebral column so that part of the spinal cord, which is normally protected within the vertebral column, is exposed.

Varus: The two limb segments create an angle that points away from the midline.

Valgus: The two limb segments create an angle that points toward the midline.

Trauma

Trauma: General Principles

Trauma is the leading cause of death for people of age group 1 to 34 years of all races and socio-economic levels and the third leading cause of death for all age groups.

ORTHOPAEDIC ASSESSMENT AND MANAGEMENT OF POLYTRAUMA PATIENTS

Polytrauma is defined as injury to at least two organ systems with a potential life-threatening condition of the patient.

The ABCs of Trauma Care

A systematic approach is required in all cases. The patient is assessed and treatment priorities are established according to the type of injury, stability of vital signs, and mechanism of injury. In a severely injured patient, treatment priorities are dictated by the patient's overall condition, with the first goal being to save life and preserve the major functions of the body. Assessment consists of four overlapping phases:

1. Primary survey **(ABCDE)**
2. Resuscitation
3. Secondary survey (head-to-toe evaluation and history)
4. Definitive care

Primary Survey

* **A**irway maintenance (with cervical spine protection)
* **B**reathing and ventilation
* **C**irculation (with haemorrhage control)
* **D**isability (neurological status)
* **E**xposure and environmental control (undress the patient for complete evaluation).

Airway

Great care should be taken while assessing the airway. The cervical spine should be carefully protected at all times and not be hyperextended, hyperflexed, or rotated to obtain a patent airway. The airway should be rapidly assessed for signs of obstruction, foreign bodies and facial or mandibular fractures. A chin lift or jaw thrust manoeuvre (Figs 2.1 and 2.2) should be used to establish an airway.

A Glasgow Coma Scale of 8 or less is an indication for placement of definitive airway, i.e. endotracheal intubation (Table 2.1).

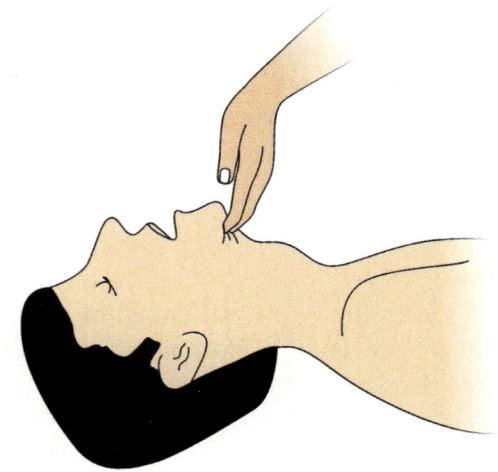

Fig. 2.1: Chin lift manoeuvre

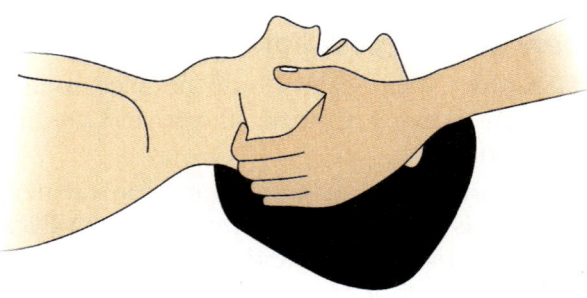

Fig. 2.2: Jaw thrust manoeuvre

Table 2.1: The Glasgow Coma Scale and score

Feature	Scale resposes	Score notation
Eye opening	Spontaneous	4
	To speech	3
	To pain	2
	None	1
Verbal response	Oriented	5
	Confused conversation	4
	Words (inappropriate)	3
	Sounds (incomprehensible)	2
	None	1
Best motor response	Obey commands	6
	Localise pain	5
	Flexion	
	Normal	4
	Abnormal	3
	Extension	2
	None	1
Total Coma 'Score'		**3/15–15/15**

Breathing

The trauma surgeon should evaluate the patient's chest. The following conditions, if present, must be addressed as an emergency:

1. Tension pneumothorax
2. Flail chest with pulmonary contusion
3. Open pneumothorax
4. Massive haemothorax

Circulation

Haemorrhage is the principal cause of post injury deaths that are preventable. Post injury hypotension is considered hypovolemic in origin until proved otherwise. Level of consciousness, skin colour and pulse are simple to assess and reliably indicate the haemodynamic status of the patient, especially if recorded serially. Fractures of the femur or the pelvis can cause major blood loss, which can severely compromise the ultimate survival of the patient.

Disability (Neurological Status)

The Glasgow Coma Scale should be used to assess neurological status; it is quick, simple, and predictive of patient outcome.

An even simpler way to monitor central neurological status is to remember the mnemonic **AVPU** and check if the patient is *Alert* and oriented, responds to *vocal* stimuli, responds only to *painful* stimuli, is *unresponsive*.

Exposure and Environmental Control

Recognition of lacerations, contusions, abrasions, swelling and deformity can only be accomplished in the completely exposed patient. The safest way to achieve this is to cut off all clothing. This permits complete examination of the patient, prevents further displacement of fractures and minimizes the risk of overlooking significant problems. Sterile dressings should be applied to any wounds and wound exploration in the emergency department should be avoided to prevent further contamination.

Care of Patient before Hospitalization

The diagnosis and treatment of musculoskeletal injuries in polytrauma patients should be initiated in the field by the paramedics. Recognition and appropriate splinting of major fractures, adequate immobilization of the cervical spine, and proper handling of the injured patient are essential to prevent further damage to the neurovascular elements and limit haemorrhage. In many cases, proper care at this stage will prevent or limit shock as well as avoid catastrophic damage to the spinal cord.

The old saying "splint them where they lie" remains especially true when the exact nature and extent of the fractures remain obscure. As a general rule, the following measures should be taken:

1. The joints above and below the fracture should be immobilized.
2. Splints can be improvised with pillows, blankets, or clothing.
3. Immobilization does not need to be absolutely rigid.
4. Apply gentle in-line traction to realign the extremity in severe angulation.
5. Overt bleeding should be tamponaded with available dressings and firm pressure.
6. Tourniquets should be avoided, unless it is obvious that the patient's life is in danger.

ORTHOPAEDIC EXAMINATION

History

Injury mechanism: An adequate assessment of the conditions in which the injury was sustained is crucial. Obtain the following information according to injury mechanism:

1. **Motor vehicular accident (MVA):** Speed; direction; patient location in the vehicle, impact location, post-impact location of the patient (if ejection, determine distance); internal and external damage to the vehicle; restraint use and type.
2. **Falls:** Distance of the fall; landing position, e.g. in case of fall from significant height on feet, one should suspect calcaneal and vertebral body fractures.

3. **Crush:** Weight of the object, site of the injury, duration of weight application.
4. **Explosion:** Blast magnitude; patient distance from the blast; primary blast injury (force of the blast wave); secondary blast injury (projectiles).

General Examination

The clinical orthopaedic examination requires assessment of the axial skeleton, pelvis, and extremities. Swelling, haematomas, and open wounds are assessed visually in the undressed patient. It is obligatory to palpate the entire spine, pelvis, and each joint. Examination soon after trauma may precede telltale swelling in joint or long bone injuries. In the unresponsive patient, only crepitation and false motion may be discerned. Patients with a better mental status, however, can provide feedback regarding pain resulting from palpation. The pelvis is examined by gentle compression of the iliac wings in a mediolateral, anterior–posterior direction and palpation of the pubis.

Neurological Examination

The neurological examination of the extremities should be documented to the fullest extent possible, in light of the patient's mental status, as it is central to subsequent decision making. This examination includes delineation of sensory function in the major nerves and dermatomes in the upper and lower extremities. Perianal sensation is also important in cases of spinal injuries.

Muscle Examination

Motor examination can be difficult because of pain or impaired mental status, but even in such cases, useful and relatively complete information can be obtained. Particularly important in the face of spinal cord injury and suspected injury are the reflexes of the anal "wink" and bulbocavernosus muscle.

Imaging Studies

Radiological assessment follows the same general hierarchy as the clinical assessment.

1. **First level:** The severely injured polytrauma patient requires plain films of the chest, abdomen, and pelvis to indicate sources of respiratory and circulatory compromise.
2. **Second level:** Requires the cervical spine cross-table lateral view. The information obtained from this film dictates treatment and the need for any further evaluation of the cervical spine.
3. **Third level:** Subsequent evaluation is dependent on clinical findings. Any long bone or joint with a laceration, haematoma, angulation, or swelling must

undergo X-ray evaluation. Any long bone fracture requires complete evaluation of the joints proximal and distal to the fracture. At the minimum, two views of the extremities are needed, usually the anteroposterior and lateral views.

"CLEARING" THE CERVICAL SPINE

In the evaluation of the trauma patient, an important consideration is the status of the cervical spine. The cervical spine is easily injured because of the large mass of the head relative to the neck, especially in motor vehicle accidents involving rapid acceleration or deceleration. Consequently, the cervical spine can receive significant force and suffer injury. In the conscious and responsive patient, swelling or tenderness on physical examination of the cervical spine is readily apparent. In the unconscious patient, cervical spine injuries can go undetected, and a careful physical examination must be performed with heavy reliance upon radiographic evaluation.

The essential radiographs for evaluation of the cervical spine include anterior–posterior (AP) views, lateral views, and an open-mouth odontoid view (Fig. 2.3). It is essential to be able to see to the top of T1 (first thoracic vertebra).

Immediate Management of Musculoskeletal Trauma

The orthopaedic injuries in the polytrauma patient are seldom truly emergency situations, except for those involving neural or vascular compromise.

For example, fracture-dislocation of the ankle or knee resulting in distal ischaemia justifies immediate attempts at reduction to minimize the sequelae of ischaemia. A more subtle situation requiring emergent treatment would be dislocation of the hip in which vascular compromise of the femoral head may result. Arterial bleeding from an open fracture should be treated immediately with pressure to minimize blood loss. Other bone and joint injuries, although urgent, may be approached in a more deliberate manner.

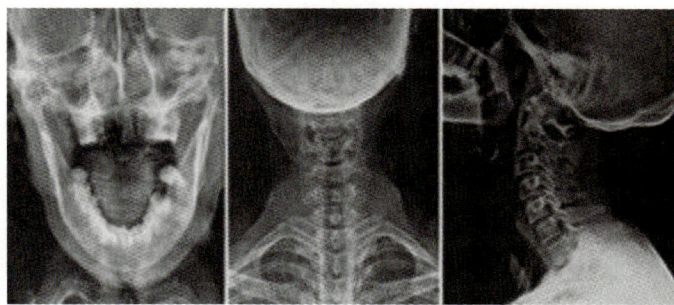

Fig. 2.3: Open mouth, AP and lateral views of cervical spine

General Principles of Fracture

DEFINITION

A break in structural continuity of the bone is known as fracture.

CLASSIFICATION

Fractures can be described, categorized, and presented in a number of ways. No one system of classification is all-encompassing, and orthopaedicians must be aware of the terminology to better understand and convey information to colleagues.

1. Based on Direction of Fracture Lines (Fig. 3.1)

Transverse: A transverse fracture runs perpendicular or at an angle less than 30 degrees to the long axis of bone. This occurs due to bending force on the bone.

Oblique: An oblique fracture is similar to transverse in that there is no torsional appearance to the fracture. The fracture line usually runs across the bone at an angle of 45 to 60°.

Spiral: The fracture line curves around the bone in a spiral manner. A spiral fracture has a torsional component as it occurs due to twisting force.

Comminuted: A comminuted fracture is any fracture in which there are more than two fragments noted. Other examples of comminuted fractures are the segmental and butterfly fractures.

Impacted: An impacted fracture is one where the fractured ends are compressed together. These are usually very stable fractures.

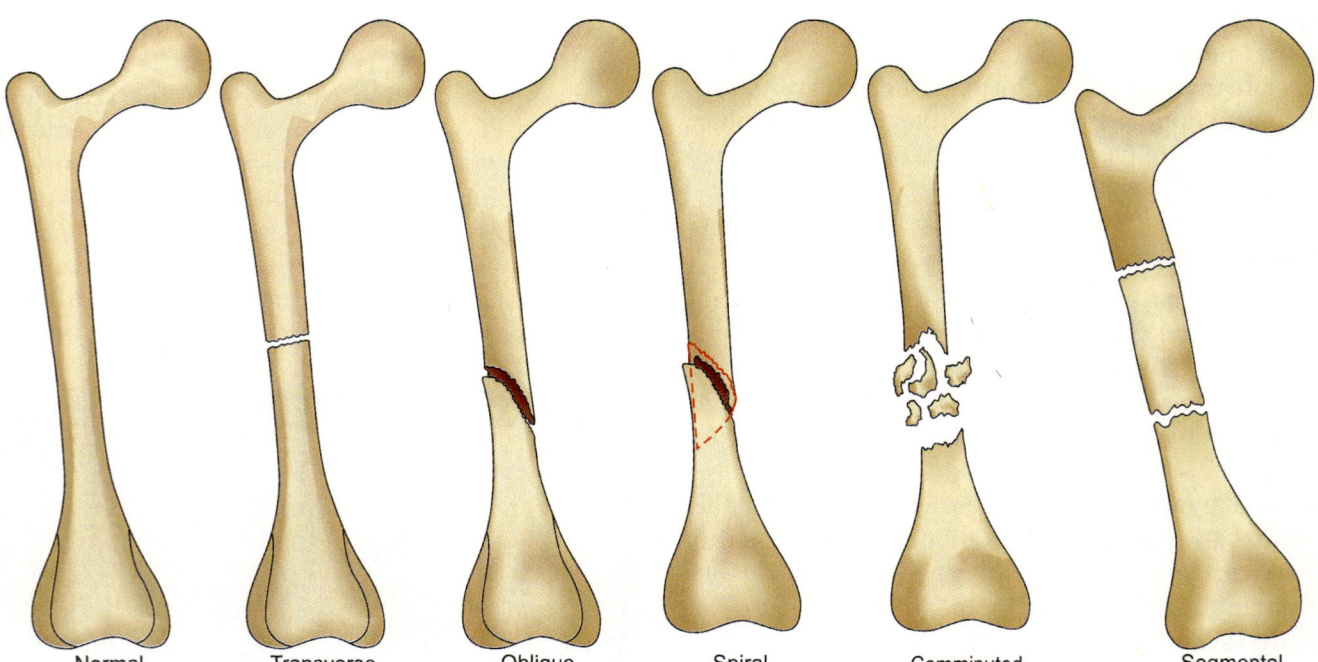

| Normal | Transverse | Oblique | Spiral | Comminuted | Segmental |

Fig. 3.1: Classification based on orientation of fracture line

Segmental: In segmental fracture, the bone is broken in more than one place.

2. Based on Anatomical Location

Fractures are usually categorized as being in either the proximal, middle, or distal thirds of a long bone.

Other anatomic terms used to describe the location of a fracture are head, shaft, and base (e.g. metacarpal and metatarsal fractures). In paediatrics, fractures are described in relation to the growth plate (physis). Fractures that occur between the joint and the growth plate are epiphyseal fractures. Fractures of the diaphysis refer to the shaft of the bone. The zone of growth between the epiphysis and diaphysis during development of a bone is the metaphysis (Fig. 3.2).

3. Intra-articular/Extra-articular

If the fracture extends into the joint space it is described as intra-articular. Fractures that do not involve the joint are extra-articular (Fig. 3.3).

4. Alignment

Alignment is the relationship of the axes of the fragments of a long bone. Alignment is described in degrees of angulation of the distal fragment in relation to the proximal fragment.

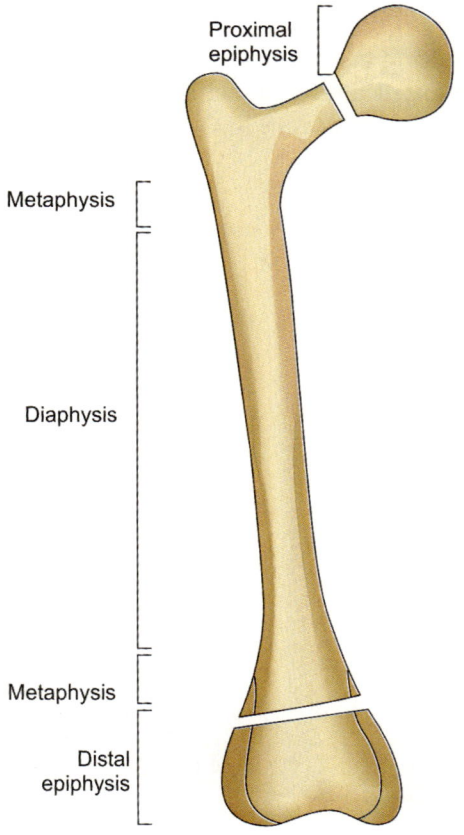

Fig. 3.2: Different regions of bone

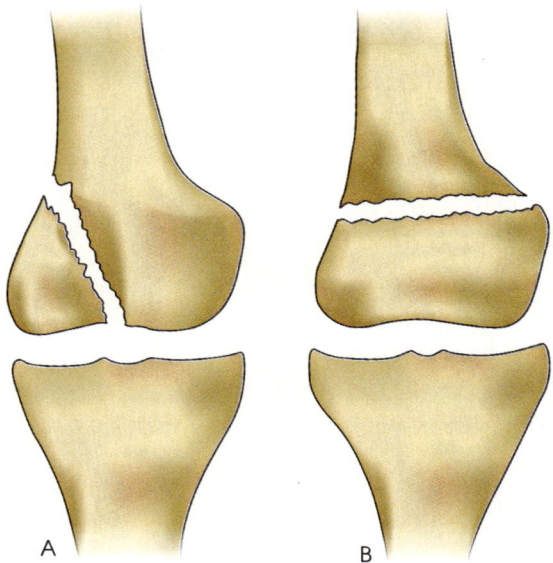

Fig. 3.3A and B: Intra- and extra-articular supracondylar femur fracture

5. Displacement

This term is used to describe movement of fracture fragments from their usual position in a direction perpendicular to the long axes of the bone. Displacement is described as a percentage of the bone's width. The direction of displacement is described based on the movement of the distal fragment in relation to the proximal fragment (Fig. 3.4).

Apposition describes the contact of the fracture surfaces. If the fragments are not only 100% displaced but also overlapping, the term commonly used is *bayonet apposition*. Bayonet apposition is the relationship of two fracture fragments that lie next to each other rather than in end-to-end contact. This is frequently seen in femoral shaft and humeral fractures (Fig. 3.5).

When the displacement is in the longitudinal axis of the bone, the term distraction is used.

6. Associated Soft-tissue Injury

Closed: A fracture in which the overlying skin and soft tissue remains intact.

Open: A fracture in which the fractured bone or its haematoma is communicating with exterior is known as an open or compound fracture.

7. Depending on Stability

Stable fracture: A fracture that does not have a tendency to displace after reduction.

Unstable fracture: A fracture that tends to displace after reduction.

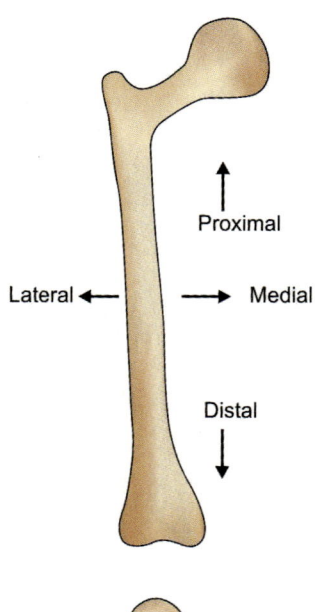

Proximal

Lateral ← → Medial

Distal

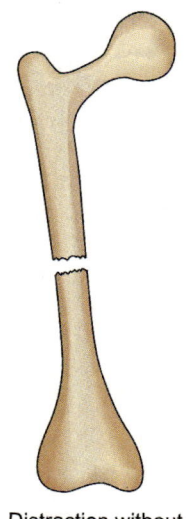

Distraction without
displacement or
angulation

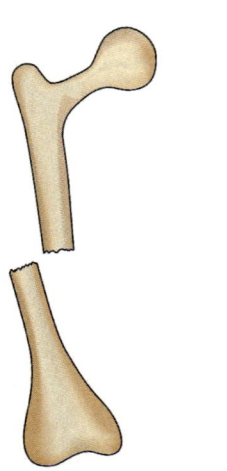

Complete (100%)
lateral displacement
with shortening
without angulation

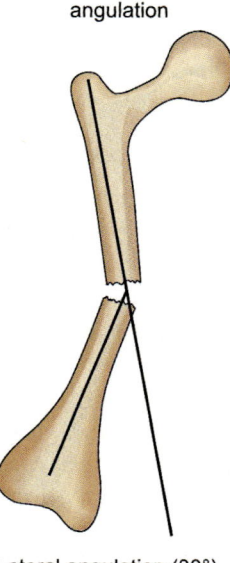

Lateral angulation (30°)
without displacement

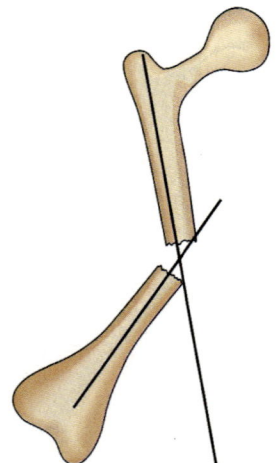

Lateral displacement (about 50%)
Lateral angulation (about 45°)

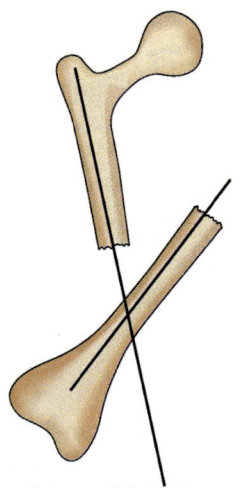

Complete medial displacement
with shortening and lateral
angulation (about 45°)

Fig. 3.4: Displacement of fracture fragments

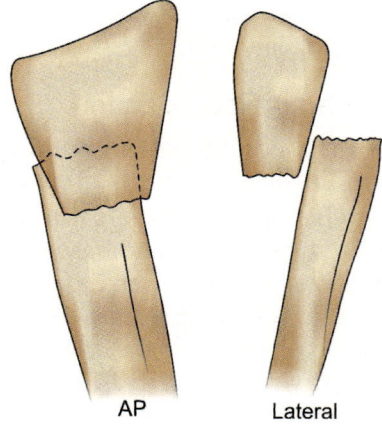

AP   Lateral

Fig. 3.5: Bayonet apposition

8. Based on Aetiology

Traumatic

Mechanism of injury

- Direct forces cause a fracture that will usually be transverse, oblique, or comminuted. An example of a direct force causing a fracture is the *nightstick* fracture caused by a direct blow to the ulna. A comminuted fracture resulting from a crush injury or a fracture from a high-velocity bullet is also caused by direct impact.
- Indirect forces may also induce a fracture by transmitting energy to the fracture site. Traction on a ligament or tendon attached to a bone can result in an avulsion fracture (Fig. 3.6).

Pathological Fracture

This is the fracture in a bone weakened due to some pathology, e.g. bone cyst.

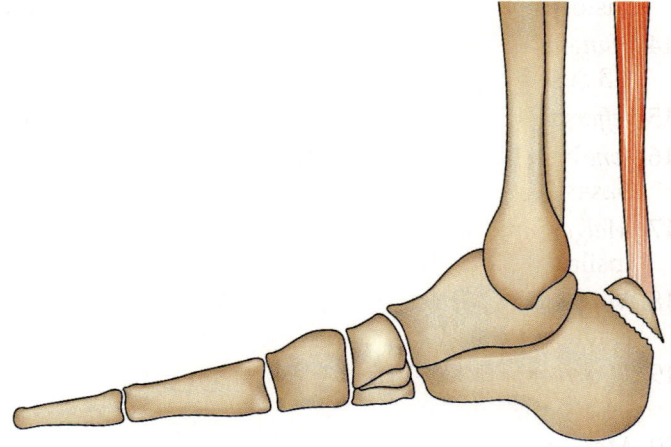

Fig. 3.6: Calcaneal avulsion fracture: Indirect injury

Stress Fracture/Fatigue Fracture

It occurs due to repetitive direct or indirect stress on bone, e.g. March fracture.

FRACTURES WITH EPONYMS

1. *Aviator's fracture:* Fracture neck of talus.
2. *Barton's fracture:* Intra-articular marginal distal end radius fracture displaced in either volar or dorsal direction along with carpals.
3. *Bennett's fracture dislocation:* Oblique intra-articular fracture of the base of first metacarpal with subluxation of 1st carpometacarpal joint.
4. *Bumper's fracture:* Comminuted and depressed fracture of tibial lateral condyle.
5. *Burst fracture:* Comminuted fracture of vertebral body.
6. *Chauffeur's fracture:* Intra-articular fracture of radial styloid process.
7. *Chance fracture/seat belt injury:* Horizontal fracture of vertebral body extending into posterior elements.
8. *Chopart's fracture dislocation:* Fracture dislocation through intertarsal joint.
9. *Clay–shoveler's fracture:* Avulsion fracture of spinous process of lower cervical or upper thoracic vertebra.
10. *Colles' fracture:* Distal end radius fracture at cortico-cancellous junction with dorsal and lateral displacement.
11. *Cotton's fracture:* Trimalleolar ankle fracture (medial, lateral and posterior malleolus).
12. *Dashboard fracture:* Posterior lip of acetabulum fracture may be associated with posterior knee dislocation or posterior cruciate ligament injury.
13. *Galeazzi fracture dislocation:* Fracture of radius with dislocation of distal radio-ulnar joint.
14. *Hangman's fracture dislocation:* C2 fracture with C2-C3 subluxation.
15. *Jefferson's fracture:* Fracture of C1.
16. *Jones' fracture:* Avulsion fracture of 5th metatarsal base.
17. *Malgaigne's fracture:* Fracture of pubic rami with ipsilateral ilium fracture or sacroiliac joint injury.
18. *Mallet finger:* Injury (avulsion or rupture) of extensor tendon at the base of distal phalanx.
19. *March fracture:* Stress fracture of the shaft of 2nd or 3rd metatarsal.
20. *Maisonneuve's fracture:* Ankle fracture with associated fibula neck fracture.
21. *Monteggia fracture dislocation:* Fracture of ulna with radial head dislocation.
22. *Night stick fracture:* Isolated fracture of ulna shaft sustained while trying to wardoff a stick blow.
23. *Pott's fracture:* Bimalleolar ankle fracture (medial and lateral malleolus).
24. *Rolando's fracture:* Comminuted intra-articular fracture of the base of first metacarpal.
25. *Sideswipe fracture:* Elbow injury sustained when one's elbow projecting out of car is sideswept by other vehicle. Usually lower end humerus and upper end radius ulna are fractured.
26. *Straddle fracture:* Bilateral superior and inferior pubic rami fracture, usually sustained when one leg slips into manhole.
27. *Whiplash injury:* Cervical spine injury where sudden flexion followed by sudden extension leads to neurological deficit without any bony injury.

ANATOMY OF BONE AND FRACTURE HEALING

Anatomy of Bone

The strength and stiffness of bone combined with its light weight gives vertebrates their mobility, dexterity, and strength.

Gross Structure

Bone Shapes

Bones assume a remarkable variety of shapes and sizes. The variety of shapes allows them to be classified into three groups: Long bones, short bones, and flat bones. Long bones like the femur, tibia, or humerus have an expanded metaphysis and epiphysis at either end with thick walled tubular diaphysis. The thick cortical walls of the diaphysis become thinner and increase in diameter as they form the metaphysis, and articular cartilage covers the epiphysis where they form synovial joints (Fig. 3.2).

Cortical and Cancellous Bone

Examination of the cut surface of a bone shows that the tissue assumes two forms: The outer cortical or compact bone and the inner cancellous or trabecular bone. Cortical bone forms about 80% of the skeleton and surrounds the thin bars or plates of cancellous bone with compact lamellae. In long bones, dense cortical bone forms the cylindrical diaphysis that surrounds a marrow cavity containing little or no trabecular bone. In the metaphysis of long bones, the cortical bone thins and trabecular bone fills the medullary cavity. Short and flat bones usually have thinner cortices than the diaphysis of long bones and contain cancellous bone.

Microscopic Structure

During skeletal growth and bone remodelling, osteoblasts form seams of un-mineralized bone organic matrix, called osteoid, on the surface of mineralized bone matrix. Normally, osteoid mineralizes soon after it appears. Therefore, normal bone contains only small amounts of un-mineralized matrix.

Mineralized bone exists in two forms: Woven (immature, primary) bone and lamellar (mature, secondary) bone. Woven bone forms the embryonic skeleton and the new bone formed in the metaphyseal parts of growth plates. Mature bone replaces this woven bone as the skeleton develops and during skeletal growth.

The basic structural unit of a lamellar bone is an Osteon. It consists of a series of concentric laminations surrounding a central canal, called haversian canal. These channels run longitudinally and are connected to each others with perpendicularly oriented Volkmann's canals. The later run from endosteal to periosteal surfaces of the bone (Fig. 3.7).

STRUCTURAL COMPOSITION OF BONE

Bone consists of following two basic components.

1. Bone Cells

a. *Osteoblasts:* They lie on bone surfaces where, when stimulated, they form new bone organic matrix and participate in controlling matrix mineralization. Their cytoplasmic processes extend through the osteoid to contact osteocytes within mineralized matrix. Once they are actively engaged in synthesizing new matrix, they can follow one of two courses. They can decrease their synthetic activity, remain on the bone surface, and assume the flatter form of a bone surface lining cell or they can surround themselves with matrix and become osteocytes.

b. *Osteocytes:* Contribute more than 90% of the cells of the mature skeleton. Combined with the periosteal and endosteal cells, they cover the bone matrix surfaces.

c. *Osteoclasts:* They are bone resorbing cells. They usually lie directly against the bone matrix on endosteal, periosteal, and haversian system bone surfaces, but unlike osteocytes, and presumably osteoblasts, they can move from one site of bone resorption to another. Osteoclasts appear to form by fusion of multiple bone-marrow-derived mononuclear cells. When they have finished their bone resorbing activity, they may divide to reform multiple mononuclear cells.

2. Bone Matrix

Bone matrix consists of the organic macromolecules, the inorganic mineral, and the matrix fluid. The inorganic matrix component contributes approximately 70% of wet bone weight and consists mainly of Hydroxyapatite, i.e. $Ca_{10} (PO_4)_6 (OH)_2$. The organic macromolecules contribute about 20% of the bone weight and water contributes 8 to 10%. The organic matrix gives bone, its form and provides its tensile strength; the mineral component gives bone strength in compression.

BLOOD SUPPLY OF LONG BONE

Long bone diaphyses and metaphyses have three sources of blood supply: Nutrient arteries, epiphyseal and metaphyseal penetrating arteries, and periosteal arteries (Fig. 3.8).

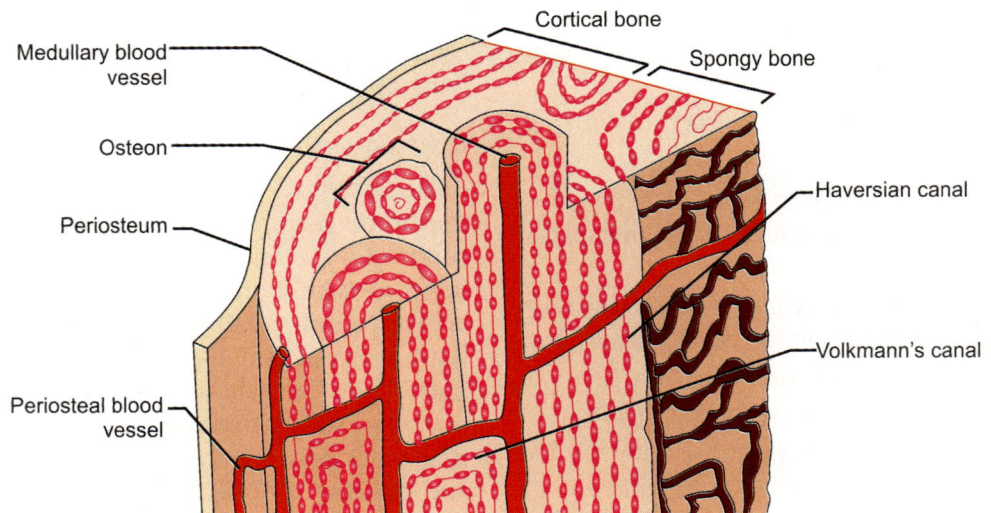

Fig. 3.7: Blood supply of the long bone

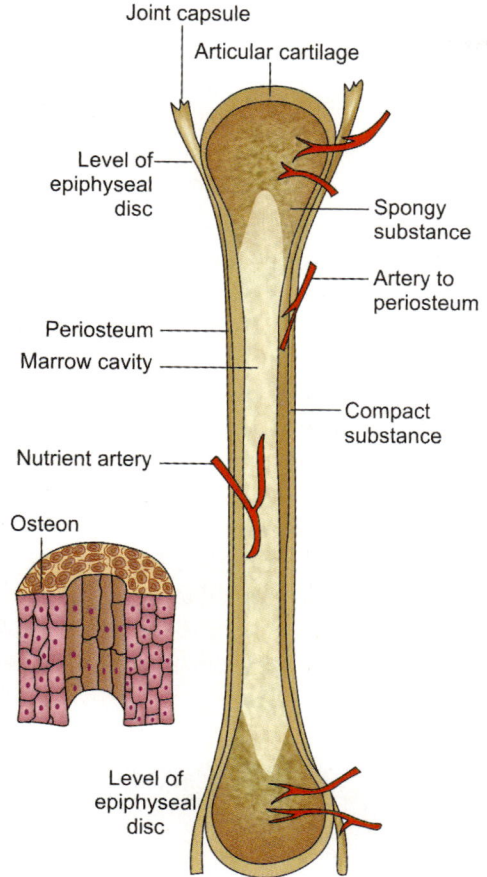

Fig. 3.8: Blood supply of the long bone

The nutrient arteries pass through the diaphyseal cortex and branch proximally and distally forming the medullary arterial system that supplies the diaphysis. The proximal and distal branches of the nutrient arteries join multiple fine branches of periosteal and metaphyseal arteries that contribute to the medullary vascular system.

Under normal circumstances this medullary vascular system supplies most of periosteum covered bone, therefore, the primary direction of blood flow through the cortex is centrifugal. In regions of dense fascial insertions into bone, such as muscle insertions or interosseous membrane insertions, periosteal or insertion site vessels usually supply the outer third of the bone cortex. Before closure of the physis, medullary vessels rarely cross the growth plate, and epiphysis depend on penetrating epiphyseal vessels for their blood supply. With closure of the physis, interosseous anastomoses develop between the penetrating epiphyseal arteries and the medullary arteries.

FRACTURE HEALING

Fracture healing can be divided into five overlapping phases (Fig. 3.9).

1. *Haematoma (up to 7 days):* After a fracture occurs, haematoma forms at the site between the fracture ends and rapidly organizes to form a clot. Damage to the blood vessels of the bone deprives the osteocytes at the fracture site of their nutrition and they die. With this necrotic tissue, an intense inflammatory response results, accompanied by vasodilatation, edema formation, and the release of inflammatory mediators. In addition, polymorphonuclear leukocytes, macrophages, and osteoclasts migrate to the area to resorb the necrotic tissue.

2. *Granulation tissue (2–3 weeks):* Begins with the migration of mesenchymal cells from the periosteum. These cells function to form the earliest bone. Osteoblasts from the endosteal surface also form bone. Granulation tissue invades from surrounding vessels and replaces the haematoma. Most healing occurs around the capillary buds that invade the fracture site. Osteoblasts are responsible for collagen formation, which is then followed by mineral deposition of calcium hydroxyapatite crystals.

3. *Callus (4–12 weeks):* Soon the scaffolding of fibrous tissue starts getting mineralized, thus forming callus and the first signs of clinical as well as radiological union are noted.

4. *Remodelling (1–2 years):* The healing fracture gains strength. As the process of healing continues, the bone organizes into trabeculae. Osteoclastic activity is first seen resorbing poorly formed trabeculae. New bone is then formed corresponding to the lines of force or stress.

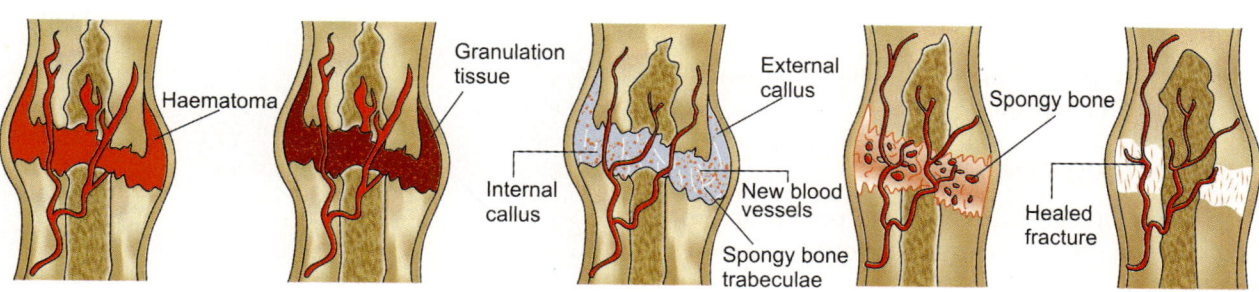

Fig. 3.9: Stages of fracture healing

5. *Modelling (continues over many years):* This is a slow process in which the united bone tries to become like the natural bone. This phase is more marked in children than in adults.

Factors Affecting Fracture Healing

Patient Related Factors

1. Age—children have better bone healing as compared to adults due to thicker periosteum. They also have better remodelling potential.
2. Nutrition—anaemia, protein deficiency, etc. delay fracture healing.
3. Systemic diseases like thyroid disorders, Cushing's syndrome, etc. affect union adversely.
4. Smoking delays union.
5. Exercise increases the rate of repair and this should be encouraged, particularly isometric exercise around an immobilized joint.

Fracture Related Factors

1. Level of fracture—metaphyseal fractures heal faster than diaphyseal fractures due to more blood supply and cellularity.
2. The healing of intra-articular fractures is inhibited by exposure to synovial fluid. The synovial fluid contains fibrinolysins that retard the initial stage of fracture healing due to lysis of the clot.
3. Blood supply—a few areas are known for precarious blood supply, e.g. distal third tibia; thus delaying union.
4. Comminution encourages union due to more surface area available for union.
5. Segmental fracures, fractures associated with bone loss affect healing adversely.
6. Infection—diverts blood required for healing for control of infection, thus delaying union.
7. Open fractures delay healing due to many reasons. First it strips away soft tissue thus impairing blood supply. Haematoma necessary for healing is drained away. There may be bone loss through wound. Lastly, there is more chance of infection with open fractures.
8. Soft tissue interposition and distraction at fracture adversely affect healing.

FRACTURES IN CHILDREN

Immature skeleton has some unique properties that make fractures in children different from adults.
- Increased resilience to stress.
- Thicker periosteum and better periosteal healing

- Increased potential to remodel
- Shorter healing time
- Presence of physes, hence complications of growth disturbance

Specific Fractures in Children

1. **Plastic deformation:** Immature bone is weaker in bending strength but absorbs more energy prior to fracture, because of the ability to undergo plastic deformation (Fig. 3.10). It occurs especially in forearm (Ulna). Remodelling to some extent is possible. Reduction of fracture is indicated if there is clinically evident deformity, especially >20° angulation with limitation of forearm rotation in children >4 years of age.
2. **Torus (buckle) fracture:** As a result of compression injury, complete or incomplete fracture occurs at the transition zone between metaphyseal woven bone and lamellar diaphyseal bone. It leads to buckling at the metaphyseal-diaphyseal junction, called torus fracture (Fig. 3.11).

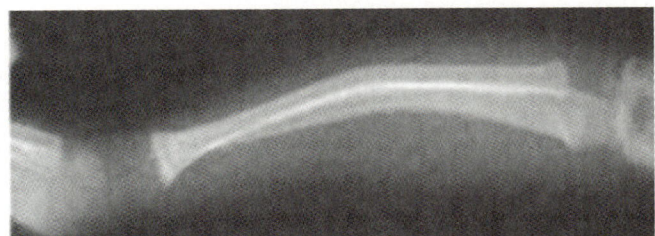

Fig. 3.10: Plastic deformation of radius and ulna

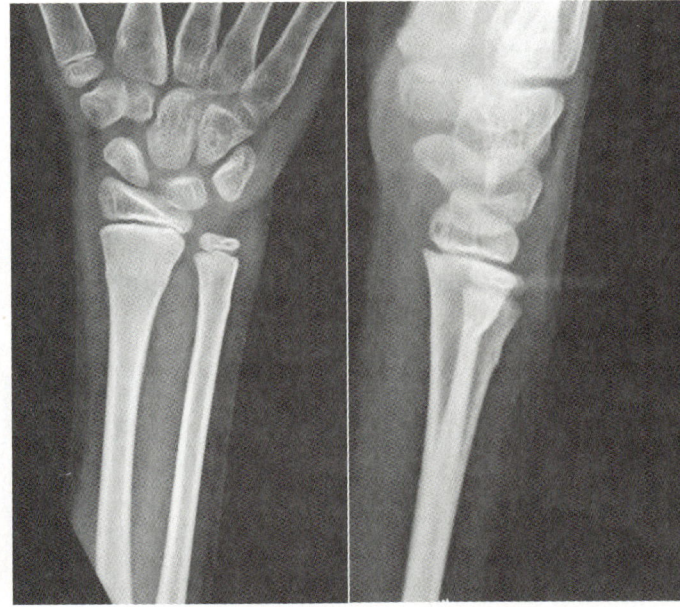

Fig. 3.11: Torus fracture of distal radius and ulna

Reduction may be required if the fracture is displaced or associated with complications.

3. **Greenstick fracture:** Immature bone is more flexible and has thicker periosteum. As a result of bending/ tensile force, sometimes cortex on the tension side breaks but on the compression side remains intact or undergoes plastic deformation. This type of fracture is called greenstick fracture (Fig. 3.12). It is necessary to unlock the impacted fragment while attempting reduction. There is increased chance of refracture.

Physeal Injuries

The physis has traditionally been divided into four zones:

- Resting or germinal zone
- Proliferative zone
- Zone of hypertrophy
- Zone of enchondral ossification, which is continuous with metaphysis

The first two zones have an abundant extracellular matrix and consequently, good mechanical integrity, particularly in response to shear force. The third zone of hypertrophy contains scant extracellular matrix and is weaker. On the metaphyseal side of hypertrophic zone, there is an area of provisional calcification leading to the zone of endochondral ossification. The calcification in this area provides additional resistance to shear. Hence, the area of the hypertrophic zone just above the area of provisional calcification is the weakest area of the physis, where usually injuries occur.

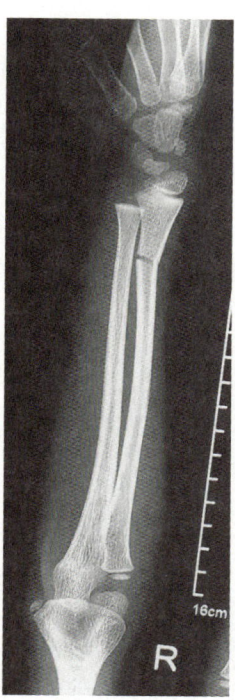

Fig. 3.12: Greenstick fracture of distal radius

Classification of Physeal Injuries

The most widely used classification system is that of Salter and Harris (Fig. 3.13).

Type I

- Separation of the epiphysis from the metaphysis that occurs entirely through the physis.
- As the germinal layer remains with epiphysis, growth is not disturbed unless the blood supply is interrupted.

Type II

- The fracture extends along the hypertrophic zone of physis and at some point exits through the metaphysis.
- The epiphyseal fragment contains the entire germinal layer as well as a metaphyseal fragment of varying size. This fragment is known as the 'Thurston Holland sign'.
- Growth disturbance is rare because the germinal layer remains intact.

Type III

- The fracture extends along the hypertrophic zone until it exits through the epiphysis.
- The fracture crosses the germinal layer and is usually intra-articular.

Type IV

- The fracture extends from the metaphysis across the physis and into the epiphysis.

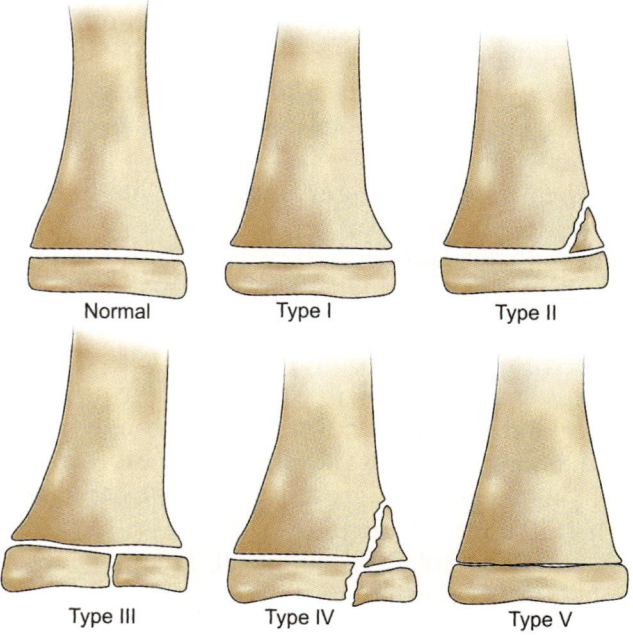

Fig. 3.13: Salter Harris classification of physeal injuries

- The fracture crosses the germinal layer and is intra-articular.
  Types III and IV, if displaced require anatomic reduction, which may require open reduction.

Type V

- It is a crushing injury to the physis from a pure compression force.
- Though rare, it has poor prognosis with almost universal growth disturbance.
  Mercer Rang has described type VI as an injury to the perichondrial ring.

Treatment of Physeal Injuries

The goal of treatment of physeal injuries is to achieve and maintain an acceptable reduction without subjecting the germinal layer of the physis to any further damage. This can be achieved by closed or open reduction. Reduction can be maitained with cast, pins, internal fixation or some combination of these.

Unique Complications of Physeal Injuries

1. *Growh distrubance:* Seen in 1 to 10% of physeal injuries. It is usually the result of development of a bony bridge or bar across the physeal cartilage. Salter-Harris types III, IV and V are more likely to be associated with growth arrest.
2. *Angular deformity:* If the physeal injury slows the growth of a portion of the physis or creates a partial bony bar, it leads to angular deformity.

Remodelling Potentials of Fractures

Paediatric fractures have increased chance of remodelling as compared to adults. Remodelling potential depends on:
1. *Amount of growth remaining:* If more growth is remaining before skeletal maturity, higher chance of remodelling.
2. *Skeletal age:* Younger children have better remodelling potential
3. *Proximity to physis and growth potential of that physis:* In the upper limb, 80% growth occurs from the physis around shoulder and wrist, whereas 20% growth occurs from physis around elbow. In the lower limb, 65% growth occurs from physis around knee and 35% growth from physis around hip and ankle. Fractures close to physis and especially the physis with more growth potential have better chance of remodelling.
4. *Plane of deformity:* Fractures with angulation in the plane of motion of the adjacent joint have better remodelling potential. There is no correction of rotational deformity.

FRACTURES OF NECESSITY

They are the fractures for which surgery is almost always necessary.
1. Lateral humeral condyle.
2. Femoral neck.
3. Distal tibial epiphysis.

PATHOLOGICAL FRACTURE

A fracture occurring in a bone weakened by some pathological process is known as pathological fracture (Fig. 3.14). Usually history is of trivial fall or minor twisting injury. At times these may occur spontaneously.

Causes of Pathological Fracture

Congenital

- Osteogenesis imperfecta
- Osteopetrosis
- Chondrodysplasia

Infective

- Pyogenic osteomyelitis (usually subacute)
- Tuberculous osteomyelitis

Neoplastic

- *Benign tumor:* Simple bone cyst
- Aneurysmal bone cyst
- Giant cell tumor
- Enchondroma
- *Malignant tumor:* Primary like multiple myeloma, osteosarcoma
- *Secondary from:* Prostate, lung and kidney in males; breast, lung and cervix in females. Usually these fractures occur in vertebrae and peritrochanteric region of femur.

Metabolic

Osteomalacia, rickets, scurvy, Paget's disease.

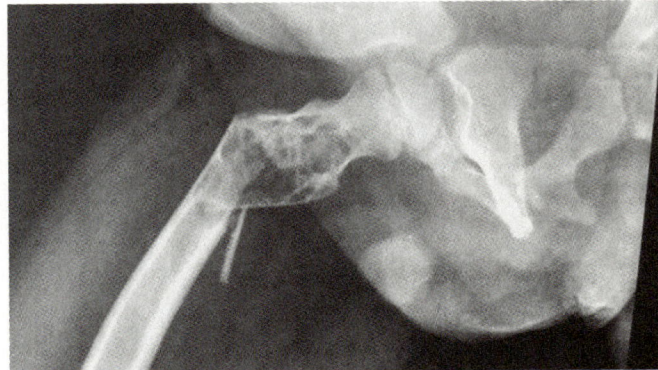

Fig. 3.14: Pathological fracture of proximal femur

Senile osteoporosis is probably the commonest cause of pathological fracture. Commonly involves Colles' fracture, vertebral body fracture and femoral neck fracture.

Miscellaneous

Eosinophilic granuloma, fibrous dysplasia.

Diagnosis

Whenever a fracture occurs without history of significant trauma, pathological fracture should be suspected.

Detailed history may reveal repeated fractures in past or history of being treated for some malignancy.

If such history is not there, detailed examination and investigations of other systems is mandatory.

Treatment

The most important point in these cases is to determine union potential of the bone. Usually in generalized disorders of bone like Paget's disease, osteoporosis or osteogenesis imperfecta union is expected with standard modalities of fracture management.

Localized pathologies like bone cysts may require more than usual time for union.

Metastasis to the bones usually don't heal and usually require augmentation using bone cement.

If the life expectancy of patient with pathological intertrochanteric fracture is only a few months, then immediate mobilization of patient should be priority. Replacement arthroplasty in such cases should be preferred over fixation.

STRESS FRACTURE

Under normal conditions of strain, bone hypertrophies. A stress fracture results when repetitive loading of the bone overwhelms the reparative ability of the skeletal system. People in poor physical condition who begin a strenuous fitness program are at a greater risk of developing a stress fracture. Alternatively, a conditioned athlete can develop a stress fracture after a recent increase in activity level. The diagnosis requires a thorough clinical examination with a high index of suspicion.

A number of possible factors may predispose a person to stress fractures.

1. The type of surface (i.e. hard surface) may cause a stress fracture, as could a change in the intensity, speed, or distance at which a patient is doing exercise.
2. Inappropriate shoes can result in stress fractures.
3. Mechanical problems such as a leg length discrepancy, increased knee valgus, foot disorders, or decreased tibial bone width.

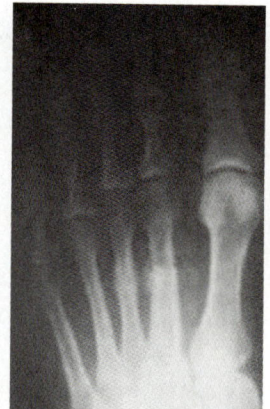

Fig. 3.15: Stress fracture 2nd and 3rd metatarsals

The most common sites for stress fractures are metatarsal shaft especially 2nd and 3rd (Fig. 3.15). Other sites are tarsals and femoral neck. Stress fractures can occur in the upper extremities, but are much less common. Stress fractures are more common in women.

Diagnosis

In early stage X-rays may not reveal fracture. So in athlete if there is point tenderness and X-ray is normal, other investigations like bone scan should be done.

Treatment

Rest to the limb for 4 to 6 weeks is needed.

JOINT INJURY

Joint dissociations can be categorized into three groups depending on degree and type of joint involved (Fig. 3.16).

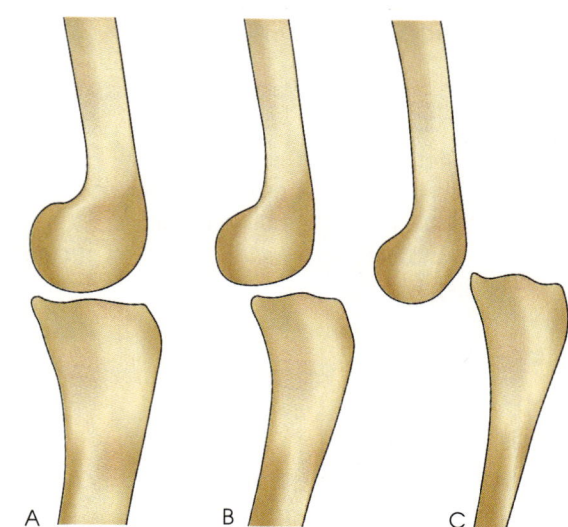

Fig. 3.16A to C: Different grades of joint injuries. (A) Normal Joint; (B) Subluxation; (C) Dislocation

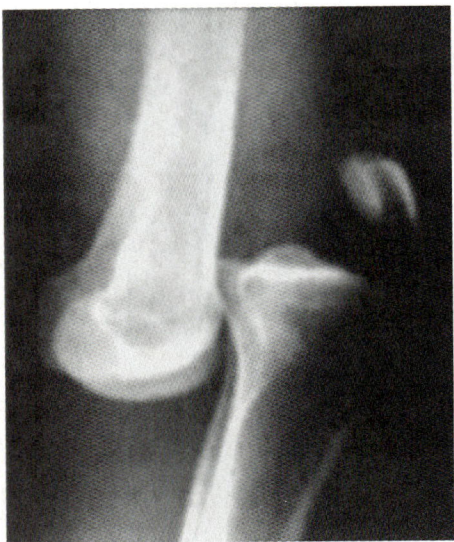

Fig. 3.17: Knee dislocation

- *Dislocation:* A dislocation is a total disruption of the joint surface with loss of normal contact between the two bony ends (Fig. 3.17).
- *Subluxation:* A subluxation is a partial disruption of a joint with partial contact remaining between the two bones that make up the joint.
- *Diastasis:* Certain bones come together in a syndesmotic articulation in which there is little motion. An interosseous membrane that traverses the area between the two bones interconnects these joints. Two syndesmotic joints occur in humans between the radius and ulna and between the fibula and tibia. A disruption of the interosseous membrane connecting these two joints is called a diastasis.

Common Dislocations at Different Joints (Table 3.1)

Table 3.1		
Joint	*Direction*	*Cause*
Hip	Posterior	Dash board injury
Shoulder	Anterior	Common due to intrinsic instability
	Posterior	Seen in epileptics
	Luxatio erecta	Inferior dislocation of shoulder
Elbow	Posterior	
Knee	Posterior	Dashboard injury
Patella	Lateral	

Diagnosis

Usually dislocations can be diagnosed easily on clinical examination due to following features

1. Pain—dislocations are very painful
2. Deformity (Table 3.2)

Table 3.2: Common deformities of various joint dislocations

Shoulder anterior dislocation	Abduction deformity, loss of contour of shoulder
Elbow posterior dislocation	Flexion, bow stringing of triceps
Hip posterior dislocation	Flexion, adduction, internal rotation
Hip anterior dislocation	Abduction, external rotation
Knee posterior dislocation	Flexion, external rotation

However, sometimes deformity is not evident clinically, e.g. posterior dislocation of shoulder.
3. Shortening of the limb
4. Loss of movements
5. Telescopy test is positive but may be difficult to elicit in acute dislocations.

Treatment

1. *Acute dislocation:* It requires urgent reduction by closed or open method. Most of the times closed methods succeed.
2. *Old unreduced dislocations:* Usually require open reduction.
3. Recurrent dislocations need additional reconstructive procedures, e.g. Bankart's repair for recurrent anterior dislocation of shoulder.

LIGAMENT INJURY

An injury to a ligament is called a sprain.

Classification of Sprain

1. *First degree sprain:* It occurs when only a few fibres are torn.
   - Little pain and swelling.
   - No disability or instability.
2. *Second degree sprain:* It occurs when significant number of fibres are torn.
   - Significant pain and swelling.
   - Inability to use the joint.
   - Significant pain on stress test.
3. *Third degree sprain:* It occurs when all the fibres are torn.
   - Significant pain and swelling
   - Significant instability in using the limb.
   - Opening up of the joint on stress test (Fig. 3.18)

Diagnosis

History of injury followed by pain, swelling and ecchymosis is typical. Usually haemarthrosis is noticed

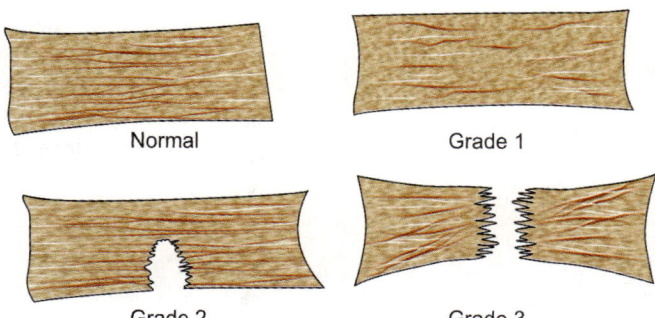

Fig. 3.18: Grades of sprain

in 2nd and 3rd degree sprain within 2 hrs. It may be delayed when ligaments are covered with synovium.

Importance of Stress Test

It is an important test to diagnose sprain clinically and to judge its severity. The ligament to be tested is stressed, e.g. if lateral collateral ligament is suspected to be sprained then the knee is flexed to 30 degrees and varus force is applied so as to stress the lateral collateral ligament (Fig. 3.19).

In first degree sprain there is little pain and in second degree sprain there is significant pain on stress test.

In third degree sprain, pain may not be significant but there is opening of the joint on the same side.

This can be documented by taking stress X-rays (Fig. 3.20).

Investigation

Plain X-rays may reveal soft tissue swelling. Stress X-rays can be helpful in diagnosing third degree sprain with opening of the joint.

MRI is the investigation of choice for confirmation of diagnosis.

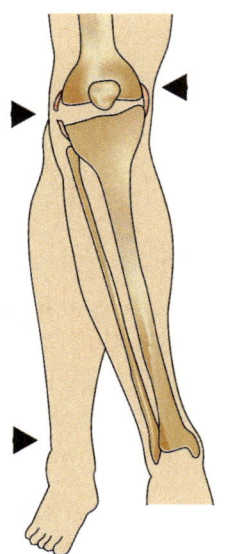

Fig. 3.19: Varus stress test

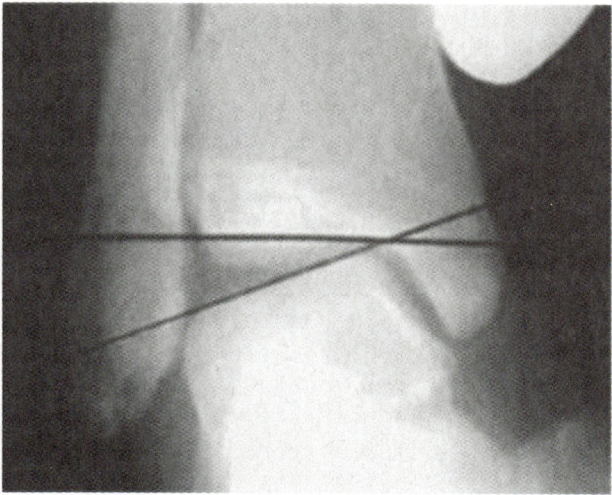

Fig. 3.20: Stress X-ray of ankle: Adduction stress view

Treatment

First degree sprain usually require symptomatic treatment in the form of rest, ice application and anti-inflammatory drugs.

Second degree sprain requires immobilization in appropriate position for 4 to 6 weeks.

Third degree sprain needs surgical repair in most cases.

MUSCLE AND TENDON INJURIES

Muscle injury is called strain and is seen commonly in young patients. On the contrary, elderly patients usually tend to have tendon ruptures. Usual cause of injury is stretching force applied on contracting muscles. Cut by sharp objects is also common.

Common Sites of Tendon Rupture

1. Supraspinatous tendon
2. Achilles tendon
3. Long head of biceps brachii
4. Extensor pollicis longus

A few conditions in which tendon degeneration and subsequent tear is commonly seen are as follows:

1. Rheumatoid arthritis
2. SLE (systemic lupus erythematosis)
3. Diabetes mellitus
4. Steroid injection in tendon
5. Age related wear and tear especially around shoulder

Treatment

Acute ruptures usually require end to end repair. Elderly patients with minimum functional disability from tendon rupture may not require any treatment.

Fracture: Management

Correct diagnosis of fracture is important before starting treatment.

CLINICAL DIAGNOSIS

With history of trauma, most of the fractures can be diagnosed clinically.

Clinical Features of Fracture

1. *Pain:* It is the most common presenting complaint of a fracture. The pain is usually well localised to the fracture site but can be more diffuse if there is significant associated soft-tissue injury.
2. *Tenderness:* It is the commonest sign of fracture. One should always try to elicit point tenderness as this may be the only sign of fracture in a few cases, e.g. stress fractures.
3. *Swelling:* Fracture of bone leads to haematoma formation. This haematoma along with associated soft tissue injury leads to swelling.
4. *Deformity:* If the fracture is displaced, there is obvious deformity, e.g. Colles' fracture leads to dinner fork deformity.
5. Abnormal mobility at fracture site.
6. Crepitus is felt at fracture site on palpation due to rubbing of the irregular fracture fragments.
7. Loss of transmitted movements, e.g. in case of radius shaft fracture if one rotates forearm at wrist, the rotatory movement is not transmitted to radial head.
8. Symptoms and signs of the complication of fracture, e.g. absent distal pulsation or peripheral nerve injury.

RADIOLOGICAL DIAGNOSIS

Once patient is suspected to have fracture on clinical examination, after resuscitation he should be evaluated with X-rays.

1. To confirm diagnosis
2. To see the fracture pattern, so that definitive treatment can be planned.
3. For documentation for medico-legal purpose.

At least two views perpendicular to each other should be taken. AP (anteroposterior) and lateral views are sufficient in most of the cases. Additional special views are helpful in a few fractures (Table 4.1).

Table 4.1: Special radiological views for fractures	
Judet's views	Acetabulum fracture
Scaphoid view	Scaphoid fracture
Mortise view	Ankle fracture
Broden's view	Talus fracture

Rarely it may happen that fracture is strongly suspected clinically but is not visible on X-rays. In such situation comparison with opposite side X-ray or CT scan can be helpful.

TREATMENT OF FRACTURE

This is divided in three phases
Phase 1: Emergency care in field
Phase 2: Definitive care
Phase 3: Rehabilitation

Phase 1

Pre-hospital Management

An unstable fracture must be stabilized by some form of external splinting or traction before movement of the patient. The purposes of emergency splinting are:

1. To prevent further soft-tissue injury by the fracture fragments
2. To reduce pain
3. To lower the incidence of fat embolism and hypovolemic shock
4. To make transportation easy

A neurovascular examination should be performed both prior to splinting and immediately afterwards.

Before splinting a fracture, remove all the circumferentially constricting things such as bangles. Any available object can be used for splinting such as cardboard, umbrella, bamboo, metal rod, wooden plank, etc. Perhaps the oldest known lower extremity traction splint is the Thomas splint.

Trauma Ward Management

As soon as the patient reaches hospital he should be assessed according to ABCs of basic life support. A thorough examination of the patient should be done. The splints should be checked as they may be excessively tight.

Phase 2

Definitive Management of the Fracture

The aim of management of fracture is to regain preinjury function at the earliest. In order to achieve this, three fundamental principles to be followed are:

1. *Reduction:* Reduce the fracture, i.e. to set the fracture fragments in proper alignment.
2. *Immobilisation:* Immobilise the fracture so as to maintain reduction and allow union in that position
3. *Rehabilitation:* Mobilise patient at the earliest so that he is back to his preinjury function.

It is not that all the patients need to go through all 3 phases. The treatment of each type of fracture is different and needs to be individualized.

Various Modalities of Fracture Treatment

1. Immobilisation, e.g. fracture of scapula may be treated by immobilization for 1–2 weeks till pain relief.
2. Closed reduction and external immobilization in cast or brace: Commonly used modality so as to maintain alignment and length of the limb, e.g. shaft humerus fracture.
3. Closed reduction and internal fixation is commonly used in paediatric fractures, e.g. supracondylar humerus fracture.
4. Open reduction and internal fixation is done where anatomy needs to be restored perfectly, e.g. intra-articular fractures.

Methods of Reduction

1. *Closed reduction:* It consists of realigning the fracture fragments by palpating them through soft tissues. It should be done under anaesthesia and preferably under C-arm imaging (Fig. 4.1).

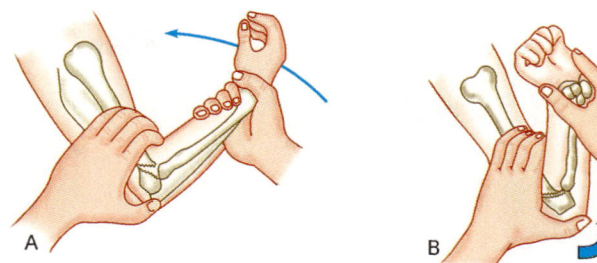

Fig. 4.1A and B: Closed reduction

2. *Continuous traction:* It is used when strong muscle forces do not allow fracture reduction. In such cases reduction is achieved and maintained with the help of traction to overcome muscle forces, e.g. fracture shaft femur in infants is treated by Gallow's traction (Fig. 4.2).

3. *Open reduction*

Indications

Absolute indications:
- Displaced intra-articular fractures
- Failure of closed reduction
- Avulsion fractures
- Nonunion

Relative indications:
- Delayed union
- Pathological fractures
- Where closed reduction is known to be ineffective, e.g. fracture neck femur
- Other associated injuries requiring opening, e.g. vascular injury.

Methods of Immobilization

Non-operative methods

1. *Strapping:* Fractured part is strapped to adjacent part of body, e.g. phalanx fracture (Fig. 4.3).
2. *Sling:* When relative immobilization is necessary as in fracture proximal humerus in elderly patients (Fig. 4.4).
3. *Plaster of paris:* POP is the commonest material used for fracture immobilization. It can be used in the form of a slab or cast. A slab supports the limb only from one side while cast is applied circumferentially.
4. *Splints* like Thomas splint can be used in case of fracture of shaft femur in children. This method of immobilization is not practical in adults.
5. *Traction:* Skeletal traction applied through steinmann pin can be used as definitive treatment for few fractures like minimally displaced tibial condyle fractures.

These nonoperative methods of fracture immobilization are discussed in detail in Chapter 39.

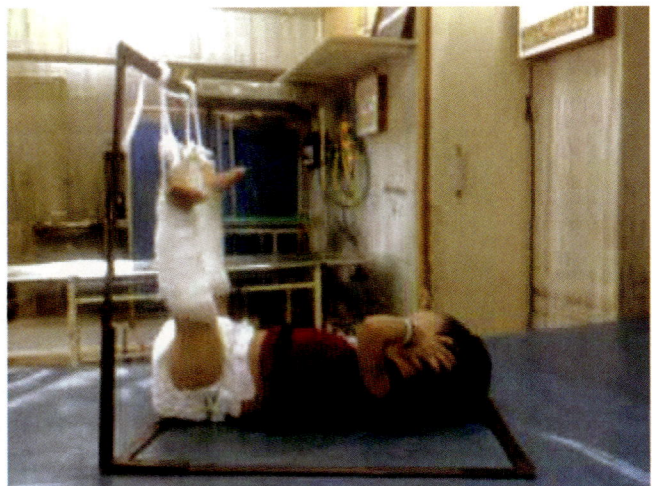

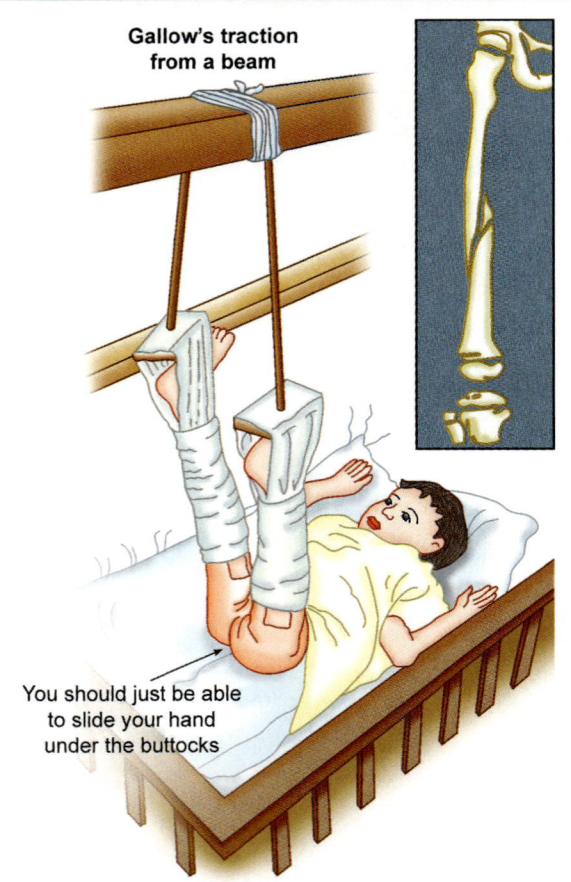

Gallow's traction from a beam

You should just be able to slide your hand under the buttocks

Fig. 4.2: Gallow's traction

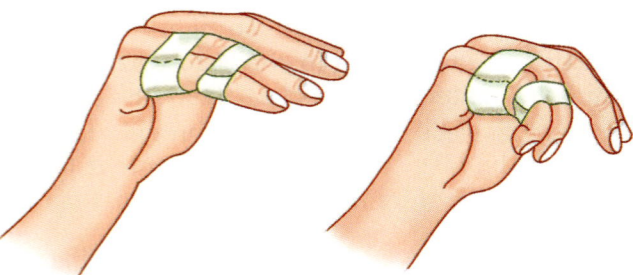

Fig. 4.3: Buddy strapping

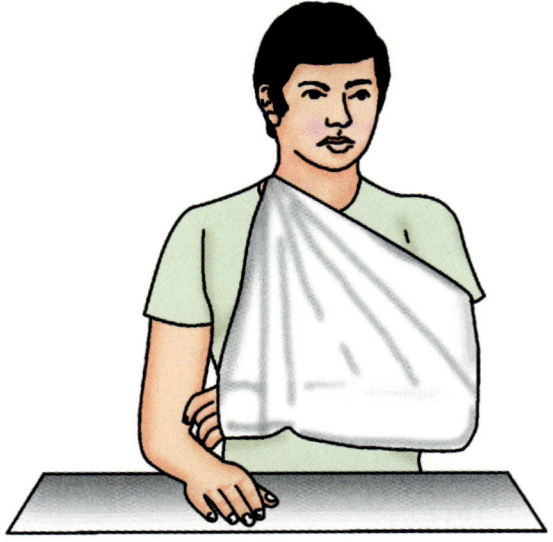

Fig. 4.4: Sling

Operative methods of immobilization: This can be divided into internal fixation and external fixation.

Internal fixation: After open reduction of fracture the reduction is maintained using various implants like K-wires, intra-medullary nails or plates and screws. The advantage of this method is that fixation is rigid, so immediate mobilization is possible.

External fixation: A device in which the fracture is kept in its alignment through a frame placed external to body is known as external fixator. The wires are placed percutaneously and connected to the frame placed externally. It is used when internal fixation is not possible due to severe comminution or due to threat of infection as in open fractures (Fig. 4.5).

Phase 3

Rehabilitation: This phase starts as early as fracture is reduced and fixed. It basically consists of maintaining motion of the adjacent joints and power of the muscles.

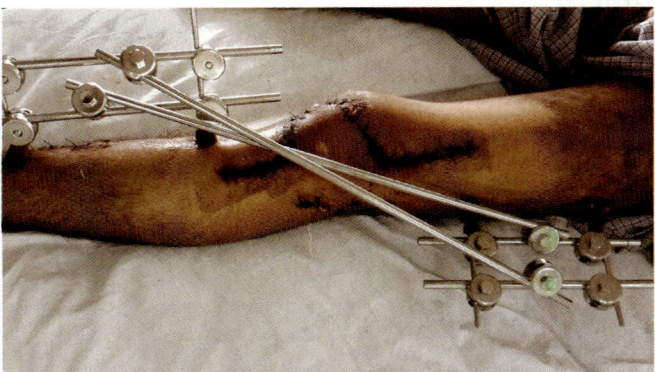

Fig. 4.5: External fixator for lower limb

Open Fractures

DEFINITION

An open fracture is the one in which fracture fragments or its haematoma communicates with exterior due to breach in the overlying soft tissue and skin. The breach of the skin may be because of injury force causing fracture (external compounding) or the fractured end of the bone poking through the overlying skin (internal compounding).

CLASSIFICATION

Gustilo and Anderson have classified open fractures by the severity of associated soft-tissue damage and degree of wound contamination (Fig. 5.1 and Table 5.1).

Table 5.1: Gustilo Anderson classification of open fracture

Classification	Description
Type I	Puncture wound of less than or equal to 1 cm with minimal soft tissue injury Minimal wound contamination or muscle crushing
Type II	Wound is greater than 1 cm in length Moderate soft-tissue injury Soft tissue coverage of the bone is adequate Comminution is minimal
Type IIIa	Extensive soft tissue damage Includes massively contaminated, severely comminuted, or segmental fractures Soft tissue coverage of the bone is adequate
Type IIIb	Extensive soft tissue damage with periosteal stripping and bone exposure Usually severely contaminated and comminuted Flap coverage is required to provide soft tissue coverage
Type IIIc	Associated with an arterial injury requiring repair for limb salvage

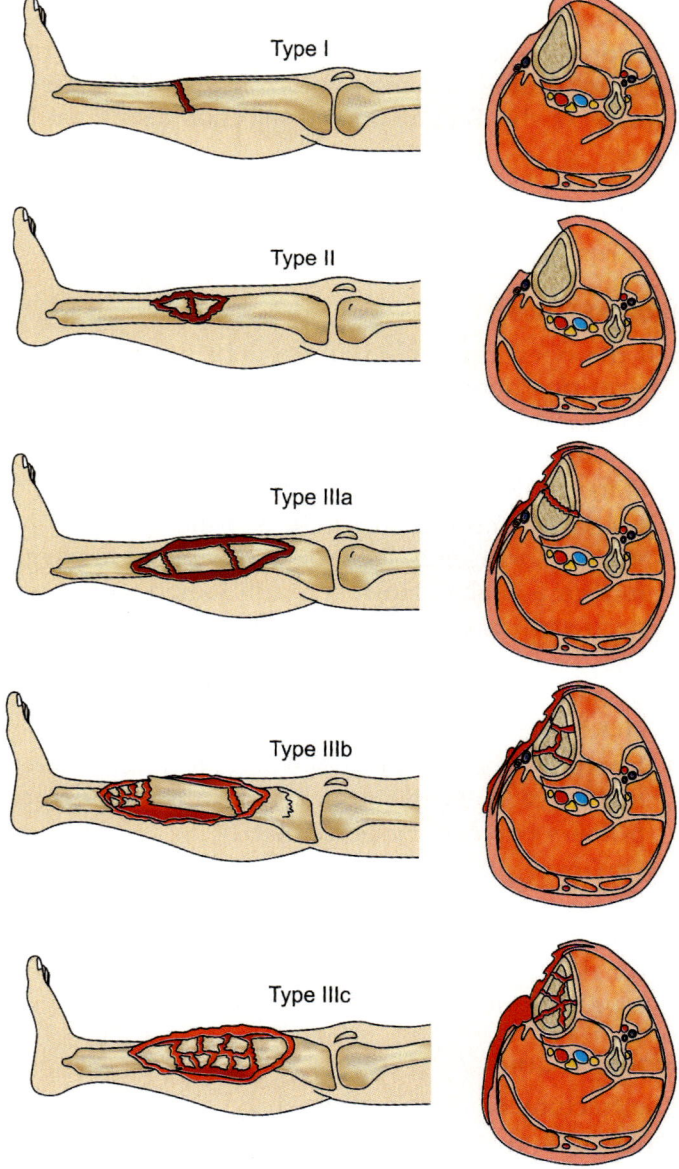

Fig. 5.1: Grades of open fracture

Management of Open Wound

The basic principle is to convert open fracture into closed fracture by meticulous wound care.

Pre-hospitalization Care

Bleeding from the bone can be controlled by applying firm pressure by clean cloth on the wound. If there is gross contamination, it can be irrigated with clean water.

In Trauma Ward

In the emergency department, foreign bodies or obvious debris should be removed in a sterile way either manually or with forceps. Loose pieces of bone without any soft tissue attached to it should be removed.

The wound should be irrigated with at least 6 litres of normal saline.

Prophylactic antibiotics usually cephalosporin, aminoglycoside and metronidazole should be given intravenously. Tetanus toxoid injection also must be given.

Definitive Care

This consists of wound care and fracture care.

Wound Care

All the open fractures require debridement in the operation theatre under anaesthesia. Following principles should be observed during debridement of the wound:

1. Skin should be debrided conservatively.
2. Fascia and muscles should be debrided generously. A pink looking muscle contracting after holding with forceps is viable. However, dull looking and non-contractile muscle should be debrided.
3. Only bone pieces with soft tissue attached to it should be preserved. Loose pieces without soft tissue attachment should be discarded.
4. If complete debridement of wound is done within 6 to 8 hrs of injury then primary closure of wound or primary flap cover is permitted.
5. However, if there is even slightest doubt about thoroughness of the debridement or in severely contaminated wound it is better to keep wound open for daily dressing. Second look after 24 hrs with repeat debridement is performed.

Fracture Care

The fracture should be immobilized at the earliest as movement at fracture site will not allow control of infection. Following methods can be used for fracture management.

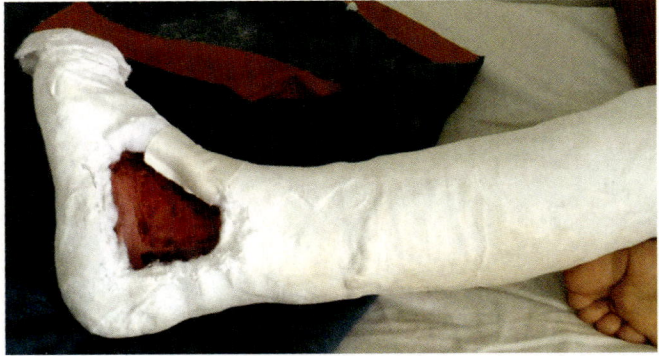

Fig. 5.2: Cast with window

1. Immobilization in plaster cast with window for wound care if acceptable stable reduction is achieved (Fig. 5.2).
2. Internal fixation—if patient presents with minimal contamination within 6 hrs of injury, then debridement of wound along with open reduction and internal fixation can be performed safely.
3. External fixation

External Fixator

It is a device by which a fracture can be stabilized in a frame outside the limb. The pins are passed percutaneously to hold the bone, and are connected to the rods by means of clamps. This method is useful when internal fixation is not possible due to risk of infection at the implant site in cases of open fractures. External fixator can be used temporarily until wound healing or can be used as a definitive method of fracture fixation.

Indication of External Fixator

1. *Wound consideration:* Large wound, severe internal degloving, gross contamination
2. *Fracture consideration:* Severe comminution, multiple fractures (as external fixator application takes less time).

Types of External Fixator

1. *Tubular external fixator:* Most commonly used device. It basically consists of multiple Schanz pins which are passed percutaneously into the bone. These Schanz pins are connected to tubular rods outside the bone with the help of clamps (Fig. 5.3).
2. *Ring external fixator:* This device consists of multiple pre-tensioned metal wires passed percutaneously, which are connected to externally placed metal or carbon rings forming a frame. This method is more versatile than tubular external fixator thus can be

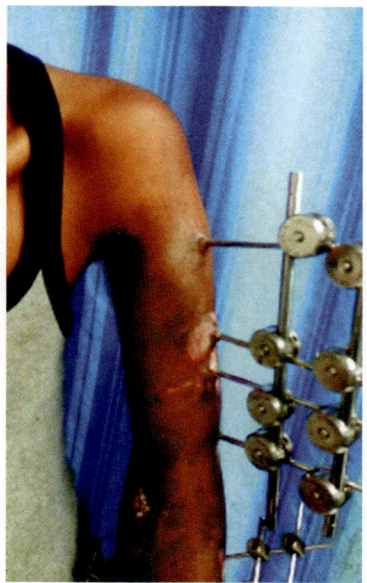

Fig. 5.3: Tubular external fixator

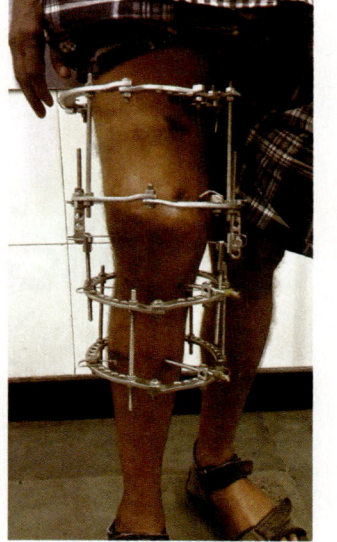
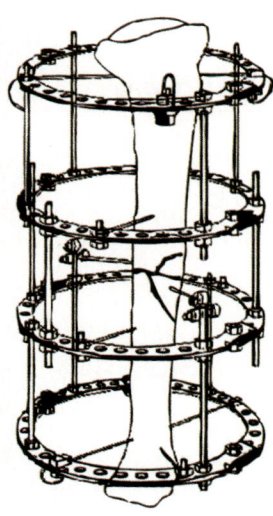

Fig. 5.4: Ilizarov ring fixator

used even for deformity corrections apart from open fracture fixation (Fig. 5.4).

3. *Hybrid external fixator:* It combines use of pre-tensioned wires and Schanz pins as per requirement and anatomy.

Advantages of External Fixator

1. Allows wound care.
2. Can be applied even in gross contamination with soft tissue loss.
3. Can be used as definitive way of fracture management.

Disadvantages of External Fixator

1. It is cumbersome for the patient.
2. May not allow reciprocating movements of the contralateral limb.
3. Continuous pin tract care is required to prevent pin tract infection.

Complications of External Fixator

1. Pin tract infection
2. Loosening of the pins
3. Loss of reduction
4. Osteomyelitis
5. Injury to adjacent nerve and vessels while passing pins or wires
6. Adjacent joint stiffness

Complications of Open Fractures

Open fractures are more prone for certain complications as compared to closed fractures.

1. Infection
2. *Delayed union/nonunion:* This is because of multiple reasons such as loss of haematoma, stripping of soft tissue compromising blood supply, infection, etc.
3. Stiffness
4. Shortening due to bone loss.

Complications of Fractures

The complications of fractures are classified as in Table 6.1.

Table 6.1: Classification of fracture complications

Immediate (at the time of sustaining fracture)	Early (within few days of fracture)	Late (weeks to months of fracture)
Hypovolemic shock	Compartment syndrome	Delayed union, Nonunion
Injury to vessels and nerves	DVT and Pulmonary embolism	Malunion
Injury to muscle and tendons	ARDS	Cross union
	Fat embolism	Stiffness of adjacent joints
	Crush syndrome	Avascular necrosis
	Osteomyelitis	Reflex sympathetic dystrophy
		Heterotopic ossification

IMMEDIATE COMPLICATIONS: HYPOVOLEMIC SHOCK

This complication is commonly seen in major bone fractures like femur or pelvis. Polytrauma patients are also likely to develop shock.

If there is open fracture, the blood loss is evident. However, in closed fractures also there is significant internal bleeding which usually is neglected, e.g. fracture pelvis may lead to internal blood loss up to 2 litres, fracture shaft femur up to 1.5 litres.

Classification and Diagnosis of Hypovolemic Shock (Table 6.2)

Table 6.2: Classification of hypovolemic shock

	Class I	Class II	Class III	Class IV
Blood loss (cc)	<750	750–1500	1500–2000	>2000
Percentage of blood volume loss	<15%	15–30%	30–40%	>40%
Pulse rate (beats/min)	<100	>100	>120	>140
Urine output	>30	20–30	3–15	Negligible

Management

1. As soon as patient with fracture arrives, resuscitation is started with crystalloid solutions (Ringer's Lactate is preferred) through large-bore intravenous lines and is monitored by urine output with a goal of 0.5 ml/kg/hr in adults. Central venous catheters and pulmonary catheters are used in severe trauma, chest trauma, and care of elderly patients. With more severe degrees of shock, venous constriction occurs, and it becomes necessary to use intravenous cut down of the saphenous or cubital veins.

2. Patients that have required large volumes of fluid for resuscitation will frequently develop hypothermia that leads to dysfunctions in coagulation. The warming of these patients is a critical part of their resuscitation and is achieved with the use of warm fluids, warming blankets, and warm inspired air.

3. Associated sites of bleeding like chest or abdominal cavity should be screened in case patient doesn't respond.

4. The fractures should be splinted immediately so as to decrease movements and further blood loss.

5. In case of fracture pelvis, emergency external fixator application is sometimes needed to stop bleeding from major vessels.

INJURY TO MAJOR BLOOD VESSELS

Vascular injuries are common orthopaedic emergencies. The neurovascular bundle of the limb lies in proximity of the bone, hence is likely to be injured along with bone (Table 6.3). The vessels are damaged either due to object causing fracture like cut injury or they are damaged due to displaced sharp spikes of the fractured bones (Fig. 6.1). Contusion and spasm of arteries is more common than anatomical severance of the blood vessels.

Table 6.3: Common fractures with vascular insults

Supracondylar humerus fracture	Brachial artery
Supracondylar femur fracture	Femoral artery
Dislocation of knee	Popliteal artery
Clavicle fracture	Subclavian artery

Diagnosis

1. In all the patients with fracture, distal arterial pulsations must be palpated. If there is vascular injury, the distal pulses won't be palpable, and the capillary circulation will be absent.
2. The patients presenting late may complain of excessive cramp like pain, paraesthesia and inability to move the limb. If left untreated for more than a few hours, gangrene may be established in the involved extremity
3. If distal pulsations are absent, immediate arterial Doppler of the limb should be performed.

Treatment

All the patients with vascular injuries should be treated as emergency.

1. Any tight splint or bandage should be removed immediately.

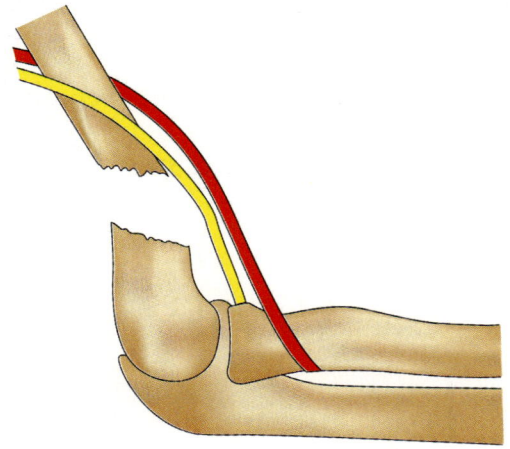

Fig. 6.1: Supracondylar humerus fracture may cause injury to brachial artery

2. If there is dislocation, it should be reduced. In cases of displaced fractures the fracture is reduced and held in grossly reduced position temporarily.
   If there is arterial spasm, pulse returns within an hour with these manoeuvres. Simultaneously preparation for exploration is done in case pulse does not return.
3. Before exploration of vessels, fracture needs to be fixed either internally or externally.

INJURY TO NERVES

As with arteries, nerves are also likely to be damaged with fractures and dislocations (Table 6.4). The degree of injury can be neuropraxia, axonotmesis or neurotmesis depending on the cause of nerve damage. Causes of nerve injury can be:

1. Insult causing fracture, e.g. sharp object
2. Damage due to sharp spike of fractured bone
3. Traction injury due to dislocation, e.g. sciatic nerve in case of posterior hip dislocation
4. Traction during reduction manoeuvre, e.g. radial nerve injury after reduction of fracture shaft humerus
5. Entrapment of the nerve in fracture
6. Entrapement of the nerve in the callus

Table 6.4: Common fractures causing nerve injuries

Supracondylar humerus fracture	Median nerve
Anterior shoulder dislocation	Axillary nerve
Posterior hip dislocation	Sciatic nerve
Shaft humerus fracture	Radial nerve (Holstein-Lewis lesion)

Diagnosis

All distal nerves must be assessed in all the cases of fractures and dislocations. It should be repeated after reduction and immobilization of the fracture. The diagnosis of nerve injury is clinical. Documentation of nerve damage can be done by electromyography and nerve conduction velocity study (EMG-NCV).

Treatment

If the nerve is more likely to be damaged due to insult causing fracture, e.g. cut injury then immediate exploration of the nerve is indicated. The fracture is fixed internally at the same time.

In cases of closed fractures usual pathology is neuropraxia, which generally recovers within 4 to 6 weeks. In such patients joints are immobilized in functional position to prevent deformities. Fracture is managed in conventional way in these cases.

INJURY TO MUSCLES AND TENDONS

Some injury to adjacent muscles and tendons is inevitable with fractures, e.g. EPL tendon rupture in

Colles' fracture. What is important is to rule out major tendon injury like patellar or quadriceps tendon cut injury, as they need urgent repair.

EARLY COMPLICATIONS: COMPARTMENT SYNDROME

Compartment syndrome is a painful, limb-threatening condition due to prolonged interruption of blood flow to a limb.

Definition

It is a condition in which the pressure within a closed osseo-fascial compartment increases progressively thus jeopardizing the blood supply of muscle and nerves of that compartment.

Pathogenesis

The limb contains muscles within compartment enclosed by bone, fascia and interosseous membrane (Fig. 6.2). If there is increase in the compartment pressure, it compresses the arteries as well as hampers the venous drainage of the extremity. This leads to inflammatory swelling of the muscles causing further increase in the compartment pressure, thus setting a vicious cycle.

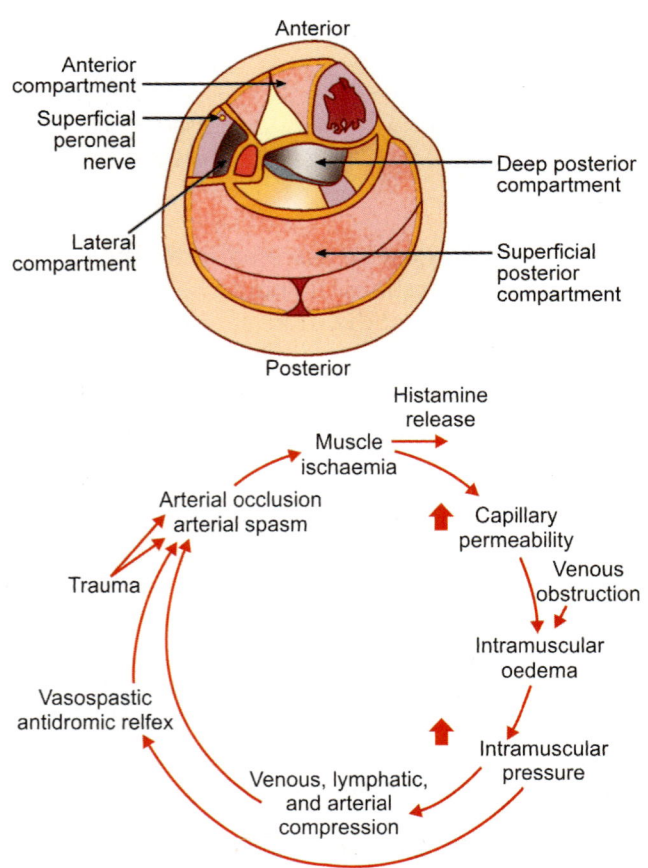

Fig. 6.2: Osseo-fascial compartment of the leg and pathogenesis of compartment syndrome

Clinical Features

Compartment syndrome is predominantly a clinical diagnosis. There is intense, disproportionate pain in the limb, worsened by passive stretching of the involved muscles. The classical sign of acute compartment syndrome is stretch pain—pain occurring in an extremity after an injury, especially when the muscle is stretched. Clinically characterized by the:

Five Ps
1. **P**ain (especially stretch pain)
2. **P**araesthesia
3. **P**allor
4. **P**ulselessness
5. **P**aralysis

Diagnosis

1. High degree of suspicion
2. Intra-compartmental pressure monitoring by wick catheter technique (Fig. 6.3).
   A handheld measuring instrument such as the slit catheter is used. Under local anesthesia, the catheter is inserted into the appropriate compartment, and the pressure is recorded. If there is difference of less than 30 mm Hg between the diastolic and tissue pressures, decompression of the affected compartments should be carried out.
3. Muscle oxyhaemoglobin level measured by using near-infrared wavelength reflection spectroscopy.

Treatment

This is an orthopaedic emergency and complete fasciotomy should be carried out.

Principles of Fasciotomy (Fig. 6.4)

1. *Long incisions:* Fasciotomy should not be undertaken subcutaneously through small skin incisions, as the intact skin may act as a constriction, further raising the pressure.
2. All compartments should be decompressed thoroughly.
3. Individual muscle sheets should also be opened to decompress the muscles

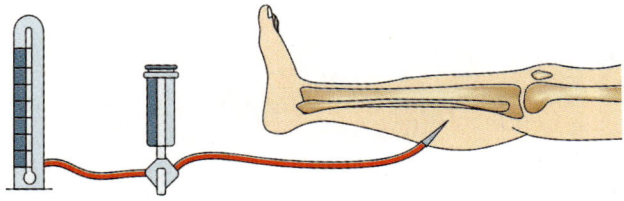

Fig. 6.3: Measurement of compartment pressure

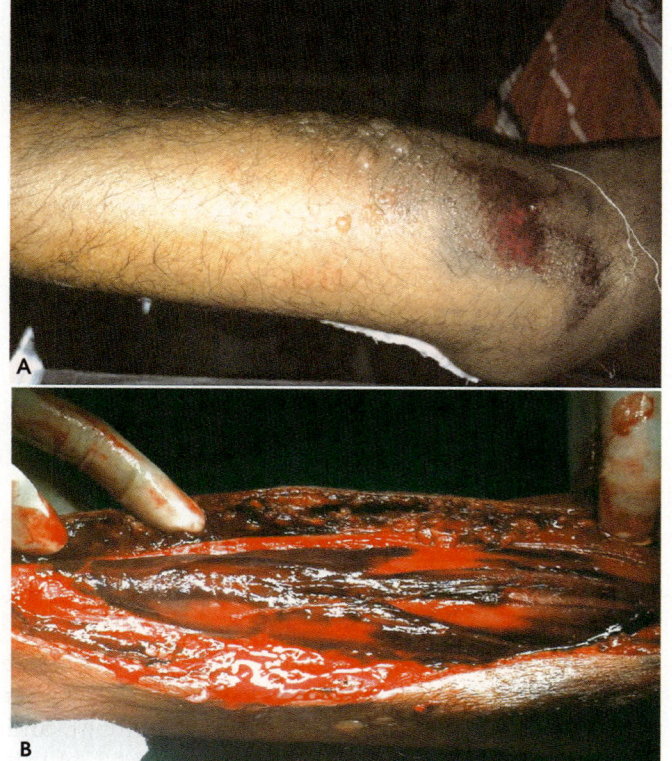

Fig. 6.4A and B: Fasciotomy of forearm

4. The wound should not be closed. It should be kept open for daily dressing followed by secondary closure or split thickness skin grafting.

VOLKMANN'S ISCHAEMIC CONTRACTURE

Volkmann's ischaemic contracture was described in 1881 by Richard van Volkmann as the end result of an ischemic injury to the muscles and nerves of a limb secondary to untreated or inadequately treated compartment syndrome.

A severe ischaemic insult has three possible outcomes.
1. Complete recovery may occur if there is good collateral circulation.
2. If no collateral circulation is present, limb necrosis leading to gangrene will be the end result. Gangrene involves all the tissues, especially the most distal (fingers and toes), and typically demarcates to a level determined by the location of the arterial insult.
3. A "middle course" may ensue and result in ischemic muscle contractures. A contracture is the result of selective ischaemia of the muscles and nerves of the distal segment of the limb (the arm below the elbow, or leg below the knee). Most distal tissues, such as the hand and foot, do not become ischemic, however, they are not immune to injury due to more proximal nerve damage.

Pathology

When the muscle becomes necrotic, they are eventually replaced by fibrous tissue that leads to muscle contracture. This is commonly seen in deep flexor compartment of the forearm, which are most likely to sustain this injury because of its tight fascial sheath. Other compartments that may be affected include the anterior tibial, peroneal, and deep posterior compartments of the leg.

Diagnosis

Volkmann's sign: This is based on principle of fixed length phenomenon. If the deep compartment of forearm is involved, the long flexors of fingers are contracted and shortened. This will cause flexion deformity at wrist and fingers. In this case if the wrist is flexed palmarly, then extension of fingers is possible. If the wrist is dorsiflexed, fingers will automatically be flexed and cannot be extended (Fig. 6.5).

Treatment

1. *Mild cases:* Stretching exercises, serial corrective casts, splints, etc. work.
2. *Moderate cases:* Need soft tissue release and excision of contracted muscles along with neurolysis (Max Page's procedure)
3. *Severe cases:* Need bony procedures like shortening of forearm or excision of carpals.

DEEP VENOUS THROMBOSIS AND PULMONARY EMBOLISM

Venous thromboembolism is multifactorial. The pathophysiology was originally described by Virchow as damage to the vessel wall, venous stasis, and hypercoagulability. All three of these factors are likely to be present in multiple injured patients. Venous stasis is due to immobilization associated with bedrest, damage to the vessel wall can occur at the time of the injury, and hypercoagulability is often present several days after injury.

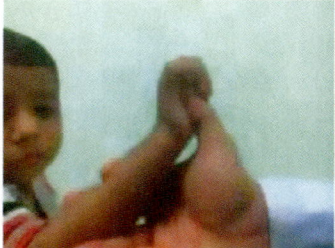
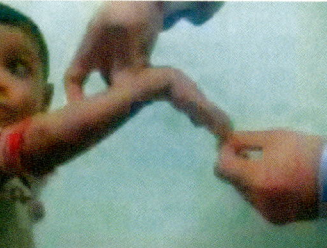

Fig. 6.5: Volkmann's sign/fixed length phenomenon

Diagnosis

Clinically DVT presents with pain and swelling in the calf. Calf tenderness and pain on passive dorsiflexion of foot (Homan's sign) are important signs. However, incidence of subclinical DVT is very high.

Best diagnostic modality is venous Doppler of the limb as it is noninvasive and very sensitive.

The clinical symptoms of pulmonary embolism (PE) include transient dyspnoea, chest pain, haemoptysis and, with larger occlusive emboli, symptoms of right-sided heart failure with syncope and hypotension. These symptoms are nonspecific, so pulmonary embolism is often missed clinically.

Ventilation perfusion scan and pulmonary angiography are investigations of choice for pulmonary embolism.

Treatment

DVT is treated with compression dressing, limb elevation and low molecular weight heparin. Pulmonary embolism requires ventilatory support along with heparin therapy.

FAT EMBOLISM

Fat embolism occurs in almost all patients who sustain a pelvic or long bone fracture. While the majority of patients remain asymptomatic, fat embolism syndrome (FES) develops in 0.5 to 3% of patients. Mortality rates of FES are as high as 20% in severe cases. The incidence increases in young adults with multiple injuries and rarely occurs in children or patients with upper extremity fractures.

Aetiology

1. *Mechanical obstruction theory:* Following a fracture, intramedullary fat is released into the venous circulation. These fat globules subsequently embolize to the end organs such as the lungs, brain and skin. Mechanical obstruction of the end-organ capillary beds has been proposed as a potential source of injury in FES.
2. *Inflammatory theory:* In this theory, fat emboli are metabolized to free fatty acids that, when present in high concentrations, induce an inflammatory reaction that damages end organs.

Clinical Presentation

All the cases have a latent period that ranges from 6 hours to several days after the injury. About 25% of patients develop symptoms in the first 12 hours and 75% have symptoms by 36 hours.

Table 6.5: Diagnostic features of fat embolism syndrome (FES)

Major criteria
Respiratory insufficiency
Altered mental status
Petechial rash

Minor criteria
Fever
Tachycardia
Retinal changes
Jaundice
Renal insufficiency
Anaemia
Thrombocytopenia
Elevated erythrocyte sedimentation rate

To make the diagnosis of FES, one major plus three minor criteria or two major and two minor criteria must be present (Table 6.5).

Pulmonary involvement is the earliest feature and is present in 75% of patients. It manifests as tachypnoea and dyspnoea that may be confused with pulmonary embolism. Hypoxia is present and the PO_2 is often <50 mm Hg. Moist rales may be noted over the lung fields on examination. The chest radiograph is normal in mild to moderate cases, but after an initial delay, bilateral diffuse pulmonary oedema develops in severe cases. The findings of high-resolution CT in mild cases of FES demonstrate ground-glass opacities. Mechanical ventilation will be necessary in 10% of patients. Pulmonary function recovers completely within 1 week.

Neurological symptoms range from restlessness to confusion or convulsions. Prolonged coma due to cerebral fat embolism has been reported, but in the majority of cases, symptoms resolve spontaneously. Recovery of higher cortical functions may be delayed. CT scan of the brain will be negative, but MRI may help in diagnosing cerebral fat embolism by revealing high-intensity signal abnormalities in watershed areas.

Petechiae are observed in 50% of patients with FES. The low specific gravity of fat globules is thought to predispose to embolization in nondependent areas of the skin. Therefore, petechiae are initially observed over the anterior axillary folds and the anterior surface of the neck and chest. They are also found in the buccal mucosa and conjunctiva. The distribution and intensity of the rash varies and resolution is usually noted within 1 week.

Treatment

The cornerstone of treatment is prevention and early detection. Open reduction with internal fixation within 24 to 48 hours of injury will prevent embolism. When a prolonged stay is necessary in the emergency department, the respiratory rate and pulse oximetry should be monitored continuously and treatment with supplemental oxygen should be administered at the first sign of any compromise.

Of patients that do develop FES, one-third of cases are mild and require only supportive treatment. The management of respiratory failure secondary to fat embolism is similar to the management of the adult respiratory distress syndrome. Respiratory support with oxygen is employed to keep the pO$_2$ above 70 mm Hg. There is insufficient controlled data to confirm the value of parenteral steroids in the treatment of this inflammatory condition, although some authors recommend intravenous methylprednisolone at a dose of 30 mg/kg. Controversy remains over the value of heparin, which is recommended by some as a lipolytic agent. The mainstay of treatment, however, is respiratory support, which must be started early.

CRUSH SYNDROME

Whenever there is massive crushing of the muscles there is release of myohaemoglobin in the circulation which gets precipitated in the renal tubules thus leading to acute renal failure. There is also release of potassium from crushed muscles leading to life threatening hyperkalemia and acidosis.

Diagnosis

By demonstrating myohaemoglobin in urine along with hyperkalemia and acidosis.

Treatment

Mild cases respond to forced alkaline diuresis. Severe cases need dialysis.

LATE COMPLICATIONS: DELAYED UNION AND NONUNION

Definition

When the fracture is taking more than usual time for union for that particular fracture, it is called delayed union.

When the process of bone healing comes to standstill and further healing is not expected unless intervened, it is called nonunion.

Causes of Delayed Union and Nonunion

Patient Related Factors

1. Old age, poor nutrition
2. Associated systemic comorbidities, e.g. malignancy, renal failure, diabetes mellitus, hypothyroidism, etc.

3. High alcohol intake, smoking
4. Radiation therapy, steroid therapy

Fracture Related Factors

1. *Open fractures:* These are more prone for nonunion for several reasons like loss of haematoma necessary for forming callus, more chance of infection, bone loss through wound, poor soft tissue cover and poor vascularity.
2. *Distraction at fracture site:* Distraction by muscles, e.g. fracture patella (Fig. 6.6). Distraction by gravity, e.g. fracture humerus
3. *Intra-articular fractures:* These are more prone for nonunion as haematoma is washed away by synovial fluid.
4. *Precarious blood supply:* Some regions of a few bones are known to have precarious blood supply and are more prone for nonunion, e.g. scaphoid fracture, distal third of tibia, lateral condyle humerus in children, etc.
5. Soft tissue interposition
6. *Infection* as the entire inflammatory process is diverted to control infection rather than forming bone.
7. Pathological fractures.

Treatment Related Factors

1. Inappropriate reduction.
2. Inadequate immobilization.
3. Excessive soft tissue dissection during surgery making fragments avascular.

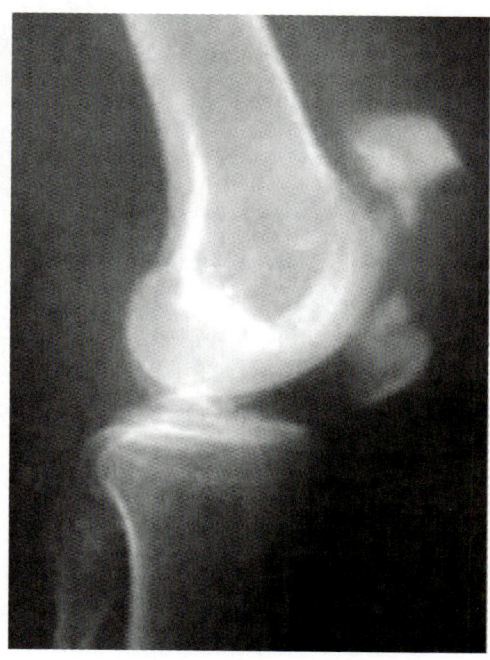

Fig. 6.6: Nonunion patella

Judet and Judet, Müller, Weber and Cech Classification of Nonunion

1. *Hypervascular nonunion* which is capable of biological reaction
2. *Avascular nonunion* which is not capable of biological reaction

Hypervascular nonunions are subdivided as follows (Fig. 6.7):

A. *"Elephant foot" nonunion.* These are hypertrophic and rich in callus. They result from insecure fixation, inadequate immobilization, or premature weight bearing in a reduced fracture with viable fragments.

B. *"Horse hoof" nonunion.* These are mildly hypertrophic and poor in callus. They typically occur after a moderately unstable fixation with plate and screws. The ends of the fragments show some callus, insufficient for union, and possibly a little sclerosis.

C. *Oligotrophic nonunion.* These are not hypertrophic, but are vascular, and callus is absent. They typically occur after major displacement of a fracture, distraction of the fragments, or internal fixation without accurate apposition of the fragments.

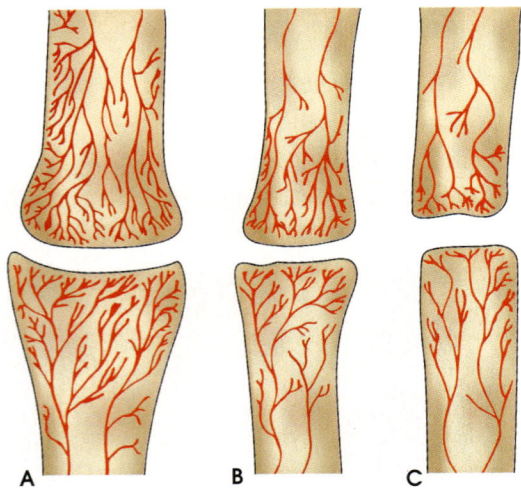

Fig. 6.7A to C: Hypervascular nonunion

Avascular nonunions are subdivided as follows (Fig. 6.8):

A. *Torsion wedge nonunion.* These are characterized by the presence of an intermediate fragment in which the blood supply is decreased or absent. The intermediate fragment has healed to one main fragment, but not to the other. These typically are seen in tibial fractures treated by plate and screws.

B. *Comminuted nonunion.* These are characterized by the presence of one or more intermediate fragments that are necrotic. The radiographs show absence of any sign of callus formation. Typically, these

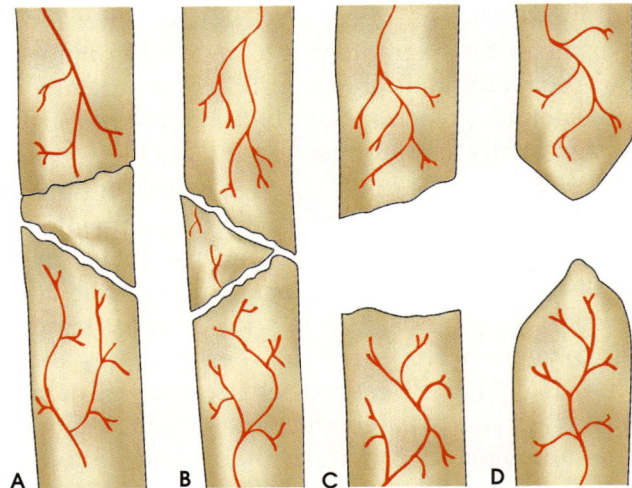

Fig. 6.8A to D: Avascular nonunion

nonunions result from the breakage of any plate used in stabilizing the acute fracture.

C. *Defect nonunion.* These are characterized by the loss of a fragment of the diaphysis of a bone. The ends of the fragments are viable, but union across the defect is impossible. As time passes, the ends of the fragments become atrophic. These nonunions occur after open fractures, sequestrectomy in osteomyelitis, and resection of tumours.

D. *Atrophic nonunion.* These usually are the final result when intermediate fragments are missing, and scar tissue that lacks osteogenic potential is left in their place. The ends of the fragments have become osteoporotic and atrophic.

Diagnosis of Nonunion

Clinical Diagnosis

1. Painless abnormal mobility is present
2. Fracture line is palpable
3. Loss of transmitted movements
4. Sufficient time lapsed since occurrence of fracture

Radiological Diagnosis (Fig. 6.9)

1. Persistent fracture line
2. Absence of bridging callus
3. Rounding of the fracture ends
4. Obliteration of medullary canal
5. Pseudoarthrosis formation

Management of Delayed Union

Most of the times continuing conservative management works for delayed union. However, if there is no progression, then bone grafting may be done.

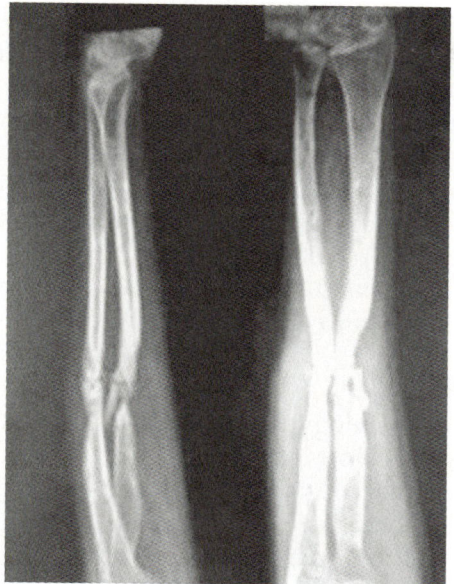

Fig. 6.9: Nonunion radius and ulna

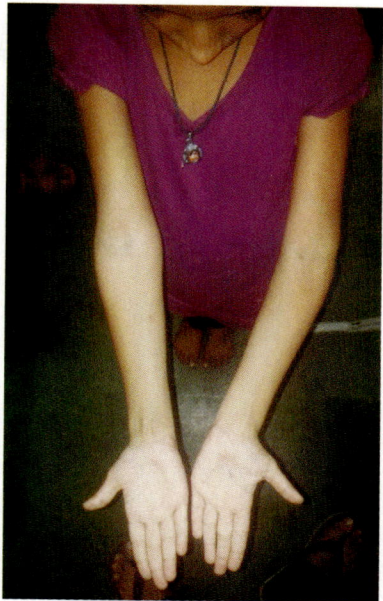

Fig. 6.10: Malunited supracondylar humerus fracture: Gun stock deformity

Management of Nonunion

Excision of the nonunion site, freshening the edges, opening up of the medullary canal, bone grafting and stable fixation is the treatment of nonunion in general.

At a few places the distal end of the bone can be excised, e.g. distal third of ulna.

Prosthetic replacement with bipolar hemi-arthroplasty is recommended for nonunion of transcervical femur fracture in elderly.

MALUNION

When the fracture does not unite in proper position, it is said to be malunited (Table 6.6).

A slight malunion is very common and is acceptable. In general varus malunion is not accepted anywhere in the body.

The malunion can lead to cosmetic deformity, shortening, loss of movements. At times it may not lead to any functional impairment.

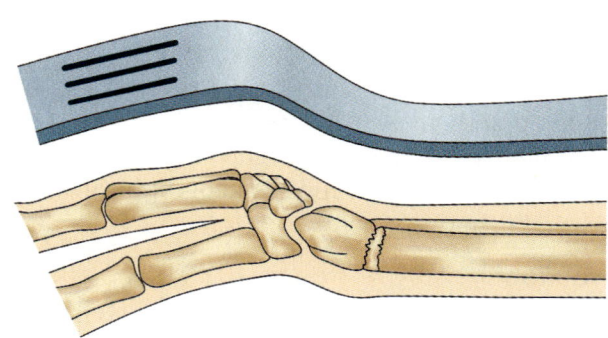

Fig. 6.11: Dinner-Fork deformity of malunited Colles' fracture

Table 6.6: Common sites of malunion (Figs 6.10 and 6.11)

Supracondylar humerus	Gun stock deformity
Colles' fracture	Dinner fork deformity

Treatment

It has to be individualized. Slight malunion causing no functional impairment can be accepted. Malunion causing shortening or restriction of motion should be treated. Various options available are:

1. Osteoclasis, i.e. refracturing the bone under anaesthesia. Used for maluniting fractures in children especially forearm fractures
2. Redoing the fracture surgically—original fracture lines are created, malunion corrected and fracture is fixed
3. Corrective osteotomy away from original fracture line, e.g. French osteotomy for malunited supracondylar humerus fracture.

AVASCULAR NECROSIS

Blood supply of some bones is precarious. Following fracture, blood supply to one of the fragments stops thus leading to avascular necrosis (Table 6.7). This leads to osteoarthritis of the adjacent joints (Fig. 6.12).

Diagnosis

1. *Radiographs:* It may take a few months to appear on X-rays (Fig. 6.12).

Table 6.7: Common sites of avascular necrosis

Head of femur	Transcervical femur fracture
Proximal part of scaphoid	Scaphoid waist fracture
Proximal part of talus	Talar neck fracture

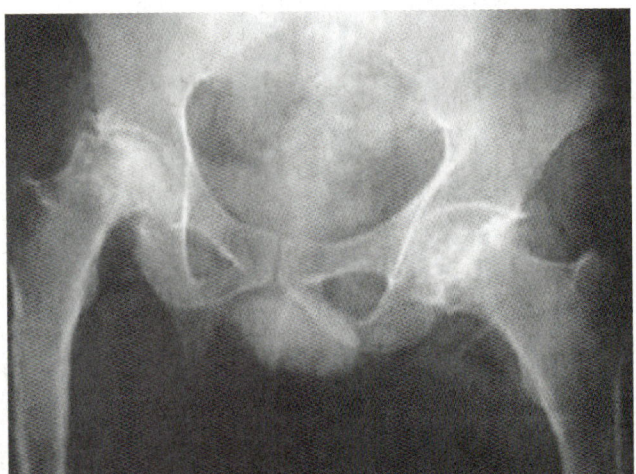

Fig. 6.12: Bilateral AVN hip

a. Affected part appears more sclerosed as compared to other areas
b. Collapse of the affected part
c. Osteoarthritis of the adjacent joint
2. Bone scan can pick up avascular necrosis much earlier than X-rays.
3. *MRI:* It is the investigation of choice as it detects AVN earlier than X-rays. It reveals geographical areas of avascularity prominently.

Prevention

Avascular necrosis can be prevented by earliest reduction and fixation of the fracture. During surgery, one must know vascular supply of that bone so as to preserve it.

Treatment

1. Delay weight bearing on necrotic bone so as to prevent collapse
2. Vascularised grafts, e.g. Meyer's procedure for AVN hip
3. Bisphosphonates have definite role in slowing down progression of AVN
4. Excision of necrosed part, e.g. scaphoid
5. Excision of necrosed part followed by prosthetic replacement, e.g. total hip arthroplasty
6. Arthrodesis.

COMPLEX REGIONAL PAIN SYNDROME (REFLEX SYMPATHETIC DYSTROPHY)

Previously known as reflex sympathetic dystrophy, the term complex regional pain syndrome (CRPS) was created to better describe this syndrome, which is not always associated with extremity dystrophy or involvement of the sympathetic nervous system. Other terms that have been used synonymously include post-traumatic reflex dystrophy, Sudeck's atrophy, reflex dystrophy, shoulder-hand syndrome, and causalgia.

CRPS is a painful condition of an extremity that follows trauma, infection, or surgery. It is most common in young adults and occurs in women more frequently than men by a ratio of 3:1.

Pathology

The pathophysiology of CRPS is not fully understood. Normally, following an extremity injury, the sympathetic nervous system is activated. Vasoconstriction in the limb leads to decreased blood flow. If sympathetic tone persists inappropriately, oedema, capillary collapse, and ischaemia result. These symptoms result in further pain, which re-excites the sympathetic nerves and creates a positive feedback circuit. This pathologic reflex of the sympathetic nervous system results in blood flow abnormalities, pain, and ultimately, atrophy (Fig. 6.13).

Stages of CRPS

1. *Acute stage:* The patient complains of a constant burning or aching pain in the extremity. A key feature to the early diagnosis of this syndrome is that the pain increases with external stimuli or motion and is out of proportion to the severity of the preceding injury. Over the ensuing months, the skin becomes cold and glossy with limited range of motion.
2. *Dystrophic stage* is characterized by the presence of chronic pain with neuropathic descriptors (burning, allodynia, dysesthesia, hyperalgesia to cold) in an extremity.

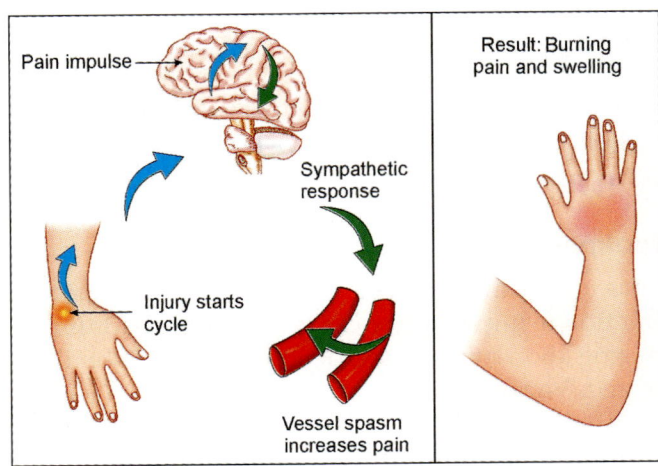

Fig. 6.13: Pathophysiology of CRPS

3. *Atrophic stage* is characterized by thinning and dryness of the skin and severely limited muscle and joint motion. The progression of these stages is variable in actual clinical practice.

Diagnosis

The diagnosis of CRPS is based primarily on history and physical examination. A history of recent or remote trauma is followed by pain that is abnormally prolonged or out of proportion to the inciting event. The syndrome is more common in the upper extremity, but the lower extremities may also be affected.

Physical Examination

1. Skin changes include shiny, stretched skin with mottling, discolouration, and sudomotor changes (abnormal dryness or perspiration).
2. Muscle weakness.
3. Stiffness in adjacent joints.
4. Allodynia, or pain due to an innocuous tactile stimulus, may be present.
5. Dystrophic changes may be seen in later stages, and includes abnormal nail and hair growth, glossy skin, or hyperkeratosis.

Radiology

The X-rays reveal generalised osteopenia in the involved region, which is most marked in periarticular areas (Fig. 6.14).

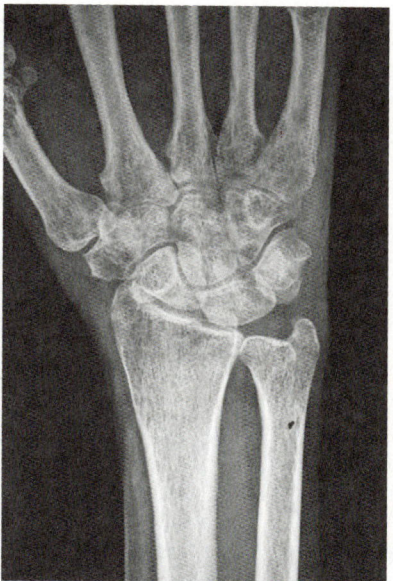

Fig. 6.14: X-ray picture in CRPS

Treatment

In patients with a mild form of CRPS, recovery may be spontaneous. Physical therapy is considered as first-line treatment and is probably more important than drug therapies. NSAIDs also help in most of the cases.

Severe cases may need intravenous blockade of the sympathetic nervous system, alpha-adrenergic blocking agents, beta-blockers, calcium channel blockers, antidepressants, and anticonvulsants.

Peripheral Nerve Injuries

ESSENTIAL ANATOMY

A typical peripheral nerve consists of numerous axons, each in a surrounding fibrous sheath called endoneurium. Axons are grouped together in small bundle, which is ensheathed by a structure called perineurium. Many such bundles are in turn surrounded by epineurium (Fig. 7.1).

NEURONAL DEGENERATION AND REGENERATION (Fig. 7.2)

- Any part of a neuron detached from its nucleus degenerates and is destroyed by phagocytosis.
- This process of degeneration distal to a point of injury is called secondary or Wallerian degeneration
- The reaction proximal to the point of detachment is called primary, traumatic or retrograde degeneration.
- During the first 3 days after injury, definite morphological changes become apparent in the axon. After 2 or 3 days, the distal segment becomes fragmented, and with subsequent fluid loss, the fragments begin to shrink and to assume a more oval

or globular appearance due to fragmentation and shrinkage of the myelin sheath.

- By day 7, macrophages have reached the area in greater numbers, and clearing of the axonal debris virtually is complete after 15 to 30 days. Schwann cell division by mitosis is evident by day 7, the cells increasing in number to fill the area previously filled by the axon and myelin sheath.
- The primary retrograde degeneration proceeds for at least an internode or more, depending on the degree of proximal insult, and it is histologically identical to wallerian degeneration.
- Chromatolysis with swelling of the cytoplasm and eccentric placement of the nucleus is commonly evident in the cell body. This reaction within the cell body is evident by day 7, and death or evidence of beginning recovery is apparent after 4 to 6 weeks. With recovery, the oedema begins to subside, the nucleus migrates toward the center of the cell, and Nissl substance begins to reaccumulate.
- Distal to the point of injury or to the proximal extent of retrograde degeneration, there is an endoneurial tube filled with Schwann cells to accept regenerating sprouts from the axonal stump.
- Axonal sprouting may occur within the first 24 hours after injury. If the endoneurial tube with its contained Schwann cells has been uninterrupted by the injury, the sprouts may pass readily along their former courses, and after regeneration the surviving cells innervate their previous end organs.
- If the injury has been severe enough to interrupt the endoneurial tube with its contained Schwann cells, sprouts that may number 100 from any one axonal stump may migrate aimlessly throughout the damaged area into the epineurial, perineurial, or adjacent regions to form a stump neuroma or neuroma in continuity.

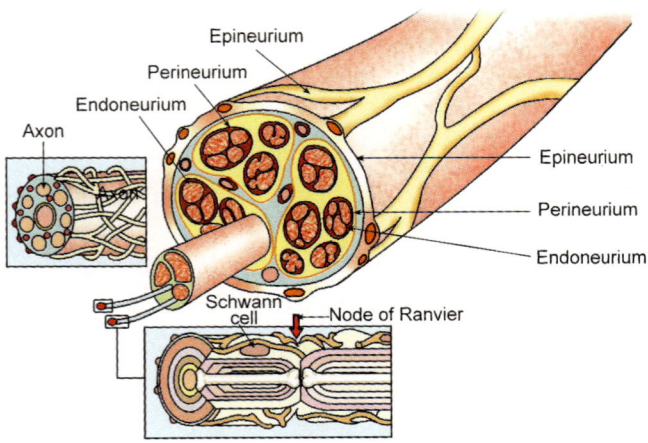

Fig. 7.1: Structure of peripheral nerve

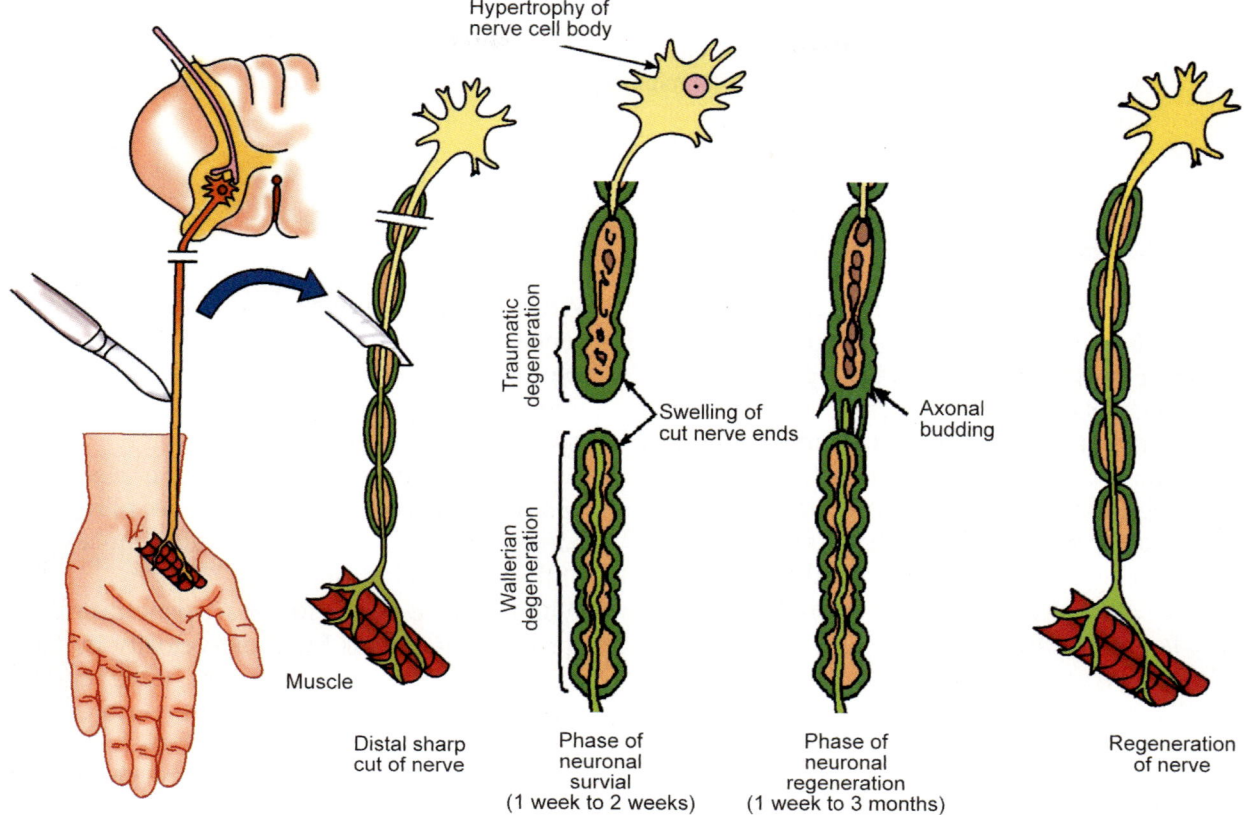

Fig. 7.2: Nerve degeneration and regeneration

- Lesser injuries without disruption of the endoneurial and Schwann cell sheaths are associated with excellent or acceptable anatomical regeneration. Conversely, more extensive injuries with complete disruption of the entire nerve, with wide separation of the ends of the nerve, and with the regenerating fibres obstructed by extensive scar tissue result in little or no return of function.

CLASSIFICATION OF PERIPHERAL NERVE INJURIES

The classification of nerve injuries proposed by Seddon in 1943 was generally accepted, but rarely used. He divided nerve injuries into three groups as follows:

1. *Neuropraxia*, designating minor contusion or compression of a peripheral nerve with preservation of the axis-cylinder, but with possibly minor oedema or breakdown of a localized segment of myelin sheath. Transmission of impulses is physiologically interrupted for some time, but recovery is complete in a few days or weeks.
2. *Axonotmesis*, designating more significant injury with breakdown of the axon and distal wallerian degeneration but with preservation of the Schwann cell and endoneurial tubes. Spontaneous regeneration with good functional recovery can be expected.

3. *Neurotmesis*, designating a more severe injury with complete anatomical severance of the nerve or extensive avulsing or crushing injury. The axon and the Schwann cell and endoneurial tubes are completely disrupted. The perineurium and epineurium also are disrupted to varying degrees. Segments of the latter two may bridge the gap if complete severance is not apparent. In this group, significant spontaneous recovery cannot be expected.

A more useful classification was described by Sunderland in 1951. This classification is more readily applicable clinically, each degree of injury suggesting a greater anatomical disruption with its correspondingly altered prognosis. In this classification, peripheral nerve injuries are arranged in ascending order of severity from the first to the fifth degree. Anatomically, the various degrees represent injury to (1) myelin, (2) axon, (3) the endoneurial tube and its contents, (4) perineurium, and (5) the entire nerve trunk (Table 7.1).

GENERAL CONSIDERATIONS OF TREATMENT

1. As in any other injury, initial management of a patient with peripheral nerve damage should begin with careful assessment of the vital functions. When

Table 7.1: Classification of peripheral nerve injuries

Degree of injury Sunderland	Seddon	Histopathological changes Myelin	Axon	Endoneurium	Perineurium	Epineurium	Tinel sign Present	Progresses
I	Neuropraxia	±					–	–
II	Axonotmesis	+	+				+	+
III		+	+	+			+	+
IV		+	+	+	+		+	–
V	Neurotmesis	+	+	+	+	+	+	–

indicated, appropriate actions to prevent cardiopulmonary failure and shock should be taken, and systemic antibiotics and tetanus prophylaxis should be provided.

2. An open wound in which a peripheral nerve has been injured should be cleaned and debrided thoroughly of any foreign material and necrotic tissue, using local, regional, or general anaesthesia. If the wound is clean and sharply incised, if the condition of the patient is satisfactory, immediate primary repair of the nerve is preferred.

3. When open wounds are caused by blasting, abrading, or crushing agents, and when contamination with foreign material is severe, the wound is cleansed and debrided thoroughly, and a sterile dressing is applied. If the ends of the nerve can be identified, they are marked with sutures, such as those of stainless steel, which can be easily identified later. Soft-tissue coverage of the wound consistent with the management of the injured part is carried out, and the nerve is repaired after 3 to 6 weeks when the soft tissues have healed adequately.

Several important factors that seem to influence nerve regeneration are:

1. *Age of the patient:* Younger patients do better than elderly.
2. *Gap between the nerve ends:* Regeneration occurs roughly at the rate of 1 mm per day.
3. *Delay* between the time of injury and repair.
4. *Level of injury:* Distal injuries recover better than proximal.
5. Condition of the nerve ends, e.g. severe crushing adversely affects regeneration.
6. Type of nerve injured, e.g. pure motor nerve recovers better than mixed nerve.

GENERAL CONSIDERATIONS FOR SURGERY

Indications

1. When a sharp injury has obviously divided a nerve, early exploration is indicated for diagnostic, therapeutic, and prognostic purposes. Neurorrhaphy can be done at the time of exploration or can be delayed.

2. When abrading, avulsing, or blasting wounds have rendered the condition of the nerve unknown, exploration is required for identification of the nerve injury and for marking the ends of the nerve with sutures for later repair.

3. When a nerve deficit follows blunt or closed trauma, and no clinical or electrical evidence of regeneration has occurred after an appropriate time, exploration of the nerve is indicated.

4. When a nerve deficit follows a penetrating wound, such as that caused by a low-velocity gunshot, the part is observed for evidence of nerve regeneration for an appropriate time. If there is no evidence of regeneration, exploration is indicated.

Conversely, delay in exploration of a nerve injury is indicated if progressive regeneration is evidenced by improvement in sensation, motor power, and electro-diagnostic tests and by progression of the Tinel sign.

EVALUATION OF NERVE INJURY

1. Attitude

Most of the peripheral nerve injuries present with peculiar attitude of the limb helping us in clinical diagnosis (Table 7.2).

Table 7.2: Specific attitude in various nerve injuries

Attitude	Nerve involved	Muscle involved
Flattening of Shoulder	Axillary nerve	Deltoid paralysis
Winging of Scapula	Long thoracic Nerve	Serratus Anterior palsy
Ape thumb	Median nerve	Opponens palsy
Pointing index	Median nerve	FDS, FDP palsy
Clawhand	Ulnar nerve	Interossei palsy
Wristdrop	Radial nerve	ECRL, ECRB palsy
Footdrop	Sciatic nerve, Common Peroneal nerve	Tibialis Anterior palsy

2. Wasting

Sometime after the nerve injury, the muscles supplied by the nerves start wasting due to disuse of that specific muscle (Table 7.3).

Table 7.3: Wasting of muscles in various nerve injuries

Area involved	Associated nerve injury
Flattening of the shoulder	Axillary nerve
Thenar eminence	Median nerve
Hypothenar eminence	Ulnar nerve
Arms/Biceps	Musculocutaneous nerve
Thigh/Quadriceps	Femoral nerve

3. Motor Examination for Grading of Power (as compared to normal side)

0–Total paralysis
1–Muscle flicker
2–Muscle contraction
3–Muscle contraction against gravity
4–Muscle contraction against gravity and minimal resistance, and
5–Normal muscle contraction.

4. Sensory Examination

a. Pain
b. Temperature
c. Touch
d. Position
e. Vibration

5. Other Tests

a. *Sweat test:* This is the test to detect sympathetic function of the nerve. Sympathetic fibres are most resistant to injury. The presence of sweating detected by starch or ninhydrin is the evidence that the nerve is not completely interrupted.

b. *Richter's dermometer and skin resistance test:* Both these tests determine the resistance offered by the skin surface to the dermometer. Normal skin gives less resistance because of sweat as compared to denervated skin which is dry offering more resistance.

c. *Tinel sign:* On gentle tapping with finger along the anatomical course of the nerve from distal to proximal, if patient gets sensation of paresthesia in the anatomical distribution of a sensory nerve Tinel's sign is positive, e.g., in a patient with median nerve injury, if patient has paresthesia on tapping at wrist, then it signifies that the regeneration has occurred up to wrist. A progressively advancing Tinel sign is positive indicator of nerve regeneration.

d. *Two-point discrimination test:* It is measured with a bent paper clip and compared with the opposite normal side. It gives an indication of how completely the nerve has recovered. Normally two-point discrimination is about 6 mm in upper extremity.

Electrodiagnostic Studies

1. Electromyography (EMG)
2. Nerve conduction velocity testing (NCV)
3. Somatosensory evoked potential (SSEP)

Electromyography

It is graphical recording of electrical activity of the muscle.

Normal EMG

At rest, normal muscle shows no electrical activity. With contractions, there are potentials which increase progressively with increasing strength of muscle contraction thus leading to interference pattern.

Denervated Muscle

At rest shows potential known as denervation potential. It takes 3 weeks for these activities to appear. Hence, EMG should be done only after 3 weeks of nerve injury.

Recovering Nerve Injury

The muscles supplied by recovering nerve will show peculiar pattern of positive sharp waves.

Uses of EMG

1. Documentation of injury, has medicolegal importance.
2. To confirm whether weakness is due to nerve injury or due to other reason such as myopathy.
3. To decide level of the injury by testing muscles in order of nerve supply.
4. To see whether injury is complete or incomplete.
5. To look for recovery.

Nerve Conduction Velocity Study (NCV)

It measures conduction velocity of the nerve which is around 70 metres/second for motor nerve. If the nerve is cut completely, there will be no conduction across that damaged segment. In partially injured nerve, the conduction velocity will decrease. Use of nerve conduction study in nerve injury:

1. Whether injury is present or not.
2. Whether it is partial or complete injury.
3. Whether it is recovering or not.

INDIVIDUAL NERVE INJURIES: RADIAL NERVE INJURY (C5–T1)

Anatomy

This nerve is continuation of the posterior cord of brachial plexus. In the axilla, it gives a branch to long head of triceps and enters the arm.

In the arm, it gives off posterior cutaneous nerve of the arm and branch to medial head of triceps. Then it travels along the radial groove along the posterior aspect of the humerus. Here it gives branches to the lateral head of triceps and anconeus.

At the junction and middle and lower thirds of the arm, it pierces the lateral intermuscular septum and enters the anterior compartment. Here, it supplies brachioradialis and ECRL muscles.

Before it crosses the elbow, it divides into two branches, just in front of lateral condyle. The superficial branch is sensory and supplies the posterior aspect of the wrist and the hand. The deep branch called the posterior interosseous nerve supplies ECRB, supinator and all the muscles of the posterior compartment of the forearm namely EPL, APL, EPB, EIP, EDC, EDQ and ECU (Fig. 7.3).

Muscles Paralysed (Fig. 7.4)

High radial nerve palsy: Brachioradialis, ECRL, ECRB, Supinator, EPL, APL, EPB, EIP, EDC, EDQ and ECU

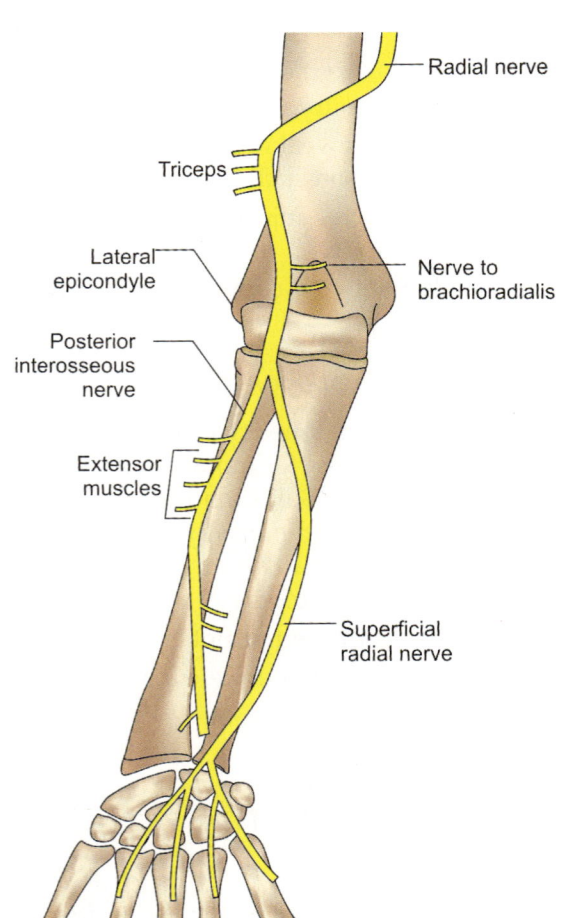

Fig. 7.3: Anatomy of radial nerve

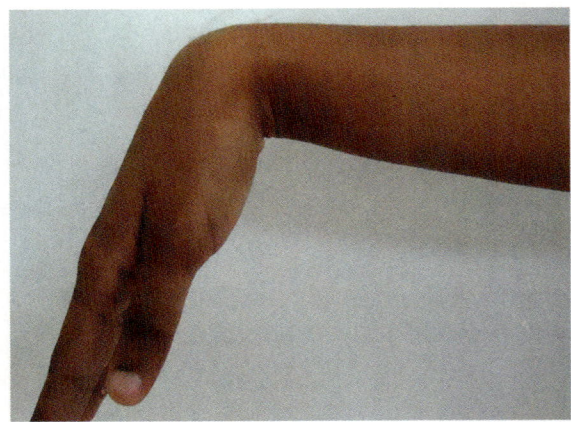

Fig. 7.4: Wrist drop due to radial nerve palsy

Low radial nerve palsy: Brachioradialis and ECRL are spared. ECRB, supinator, EPL, APL, EPB, EIP, EDC, EDQ and ECU are paralysed.

Triceps and anconeus may be affected in very high radial nerve palsy.

Movements Lost

Extension of elbow (very high radial nerve palsy), Extension of wrist joint, extension of MCP joints and thumb extension.

Muscle Testing

1. Elbow extension (very high radial nerve palsy).
2. Flexion of elbow in midprone (for brachioradialis – high radial nerve palsy).
3. Extension of wrist joint.
   Extension of MCP joints (high and low radial nerve palsy)
   Extension of thumb.

Sensory Areas Involved

Posterior aspect of arm and forearm, radial 3½ fingers on dorsal aspect upto DIP joint.

Autonomous area of radial nerve: 1st web space–dorsal aspect.

MUSCULOCUTANEOUS NERVE INJURY (C5–6)

Movements lost: Elbow flexion, weakness of supination of forearm

Sensory areas involved: Lateral aspect of forearm

MEDIAN NERVE INJURY (C5–T1)

Anatomy

It is formed from branches of both the medial and lateral cords of brachial plexus. In the arm, it travels along the course of brachial artery.

It enters the forearm between two heads of pronator teres and travels in the plane between flexor digitorum superficialis and flexor digitorum profundus. In the anterior compartment, it gives off anterior interosseous nerve just after exiting from the pronator teres, which supplies the muscles of the anterior compartment of the forearm.

In the hand, it passes below the flexor retinaculum. Here it supplies all the muscles of the thenar eminence except the adductor pollicis (Fig. 7.5).

Classification

High median nerve palsy: Injury proximal to the elbow.

Low median nerve palsy: Injury below the elbow.

Muscles paralysed:

High palsy: Pronator teres, FCR, PL, FDS, FPL, FDP, PQ, opponens pollicis APB, FPB, lateral two lumbricals.

Low palsy: Only hand muscles are affected, i.e. opponens pollicis, APB, FPB and lateral two lumbricals

Movements Lost

- Pronation of the forearm.
- Flexion of the wrist.
- Flexion of the index and long fingers at interphalangeal joints.
- Flexion of the thumb.
- Opposition of the thumb.

Muscle Testing

- *Pronator teres and pronator quadratus:* Pronation of forearm
- *FCR:* Flexion of wrist causes ulnar deviation of wrist in FCR palsy
- *FDS and lateral FDP:* Test flexion at PIP and DIP joints of individual fingers
- *FPL:* Flexion of thumb
- *Opponens pollicis:* Opposition of thumb
- *APB:* Pen test for thumb abduction (Fig. 7.6): Ask the patient to touch the pen which is kept at a slight higher level than the palm of the hand, with the thumb.

Sensory Areas Involved

Anterior aspect of forearm, radial 3½ digits on volar aspect and extending up to nail bed.

Autonomous area of median nerve: Tip of index finger–volar aspect.

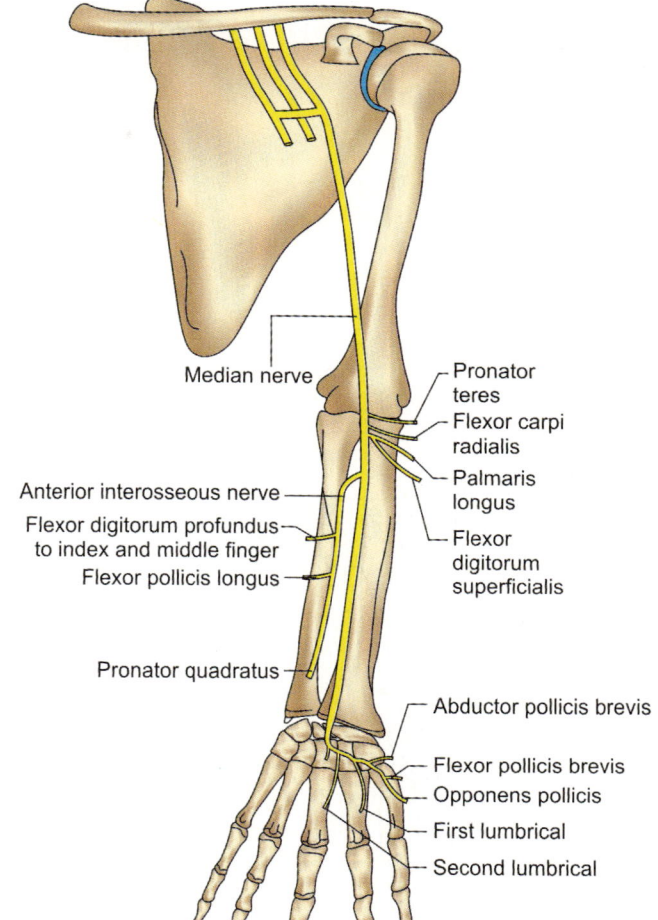

Median nerve — Pronator teres
— Flexor carpi radialis
— Palmaris longus
Anterior interosseous nerve —
Flexor digitorum profundus — to index and middle finger
Flexor pollicis longus —
— Flexor digitorum superficialis
Pronator quadratus —
— Abductor pollicis brevis
— Flexor pollicis brevis
— Opponens pollicis
— First lumbrical
— Second lumbrical

Fig. 7.5: Anatomy of median nerve

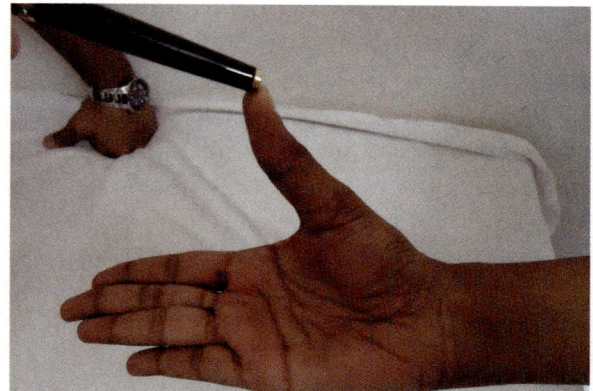

Fig. 7.6: Pen test for abductor pollicis brevis

ULNAR NERVE INJURY (C7–T1)

Anatomy

It arises from the medial cord of the brachial plexus. It passes medial to the brachial artery in the arm. In lower thirds of the arm, it pierces the medial intermuscular septum and enters the posterior compartment. It lies

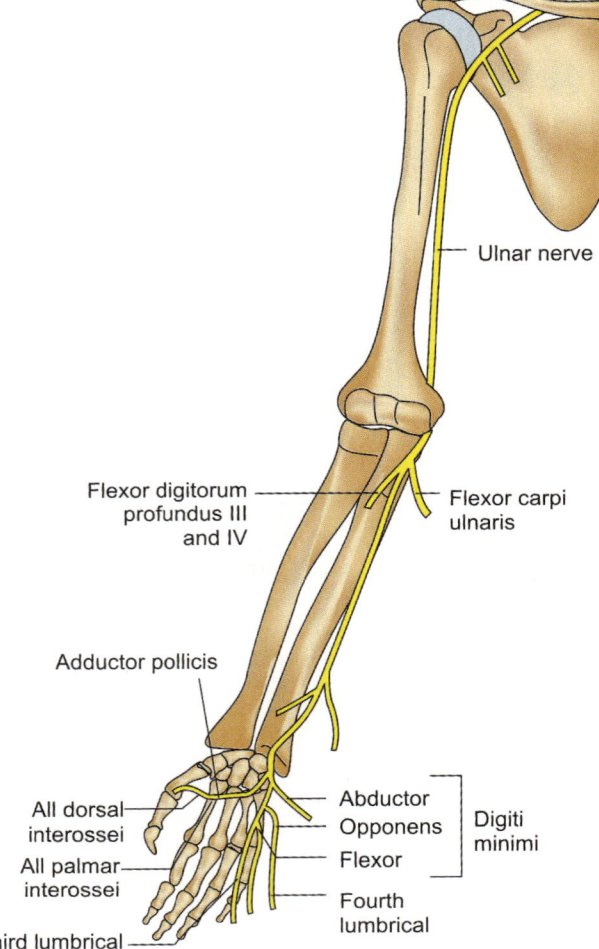

Fig. 7.7: Anatomy of ulnar nerve

posterior to the medial epicondyle, where it can be palpated over the posterior surface of the epicondyle.

In the forearm, it pierces the two heads of flexor carpi ulnaris muscle and then descends along the medial border of FDP muscles, along with the ulnar vessels.

In the hand, it passes superficial to flexor retinaculum and divides into a superficial sensory and a deep motor branch supplying the hypothenar muscles, medial lumbricals and dorsal as well as the palmar interossei muscles (Fig. 7.7).

Classification

- *High ulnar nerve plasy:* Injury proximal to elbow.
- *Low ulnar nerve plasy:* Injury distal to elbow.

Muscles Paralysed

High Ulnar Nerve Plasy

FCU, medial half of flexor digitorum profundus, adductor pollicis, hypothenar muscles, all dorsal and palmar interossei muscles and medial two lumbricals.

Low Ulnar Nerve Palsy

Forearm muscles are spared and only hand muscles are involved, i.e. adductor pollicis, hypothenar muscles, all dorsal and palmar interossei muscles and medial two lumbricals.

Movements Lost

- Adduction of thumb.
- Weakness of wrist flexion.
- Flexion of MCP joints (stabilization of MCP).
- Weakness of extension of fingers.
- Abduction of little finger.
- Adduction and abduction of the digits.
- This particular loss leads to deformity known as clawhand (Fig. 7.8). This clawing is more prominent in low ulnar nerve palsy than in high ulnar nerve palsy as medial half of flexor digitorum profundus is intact and add on to flexion at interphalangeal joints in low palsy. This is known as ulnar paradox.

Muscle Testing

Book Test for Adduction of Thumb (Fig. 7.9)

Ask the patient to grasp a book between the extended thumb and other fingers. In ulnar nerve palsy, the patient will hold the book by flexing thumb with the help of FPL called 'Fromet's sign'.

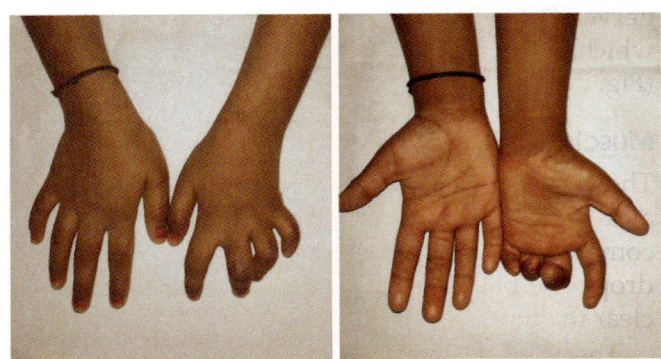

Fig. 7.8: Clawhand

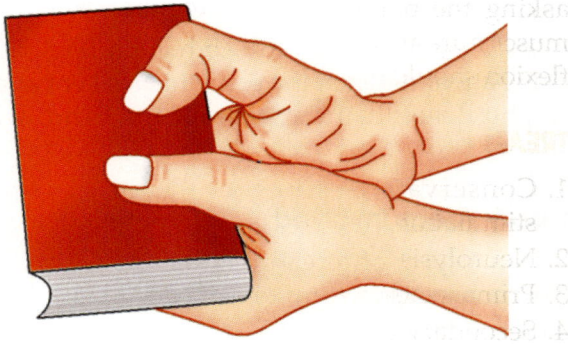

Fig. 7.9: Book test

Card Test for Adduction of Fingers (Fig. 7.10)

A card is inserted between the two fingers, same kept extended. The patient is asked to hold the card adducting these fingers as tightly as possible. Then try to pull the card out of the fingers for palmar interossei testing.

- Also check abduction of little finger.
- Wrist flexion causes lateral deviation of the hand.

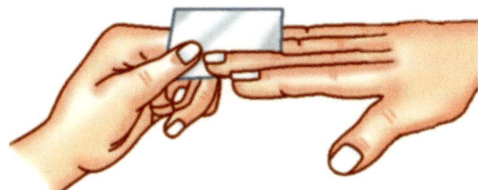

Fig. 7.10: Card test

Sensory Areas Involved

- Ulnar 1½ digits and ulnar one-third area of hand.
- *Autonomous zone:* Tip of little finger—volar aspect.

SCIATIC NERVE

Anatomy

It is formed by lumbar plexus (L2–S1). It has two distinct components, the common peroneal nerve and the tibial nerve. The common peroneal component is the one which gets injured in most of the sciatic nerve injuries (Fig. 7.11).

Muscle Testing

The common peroneal nerve supplies the dorsiflexors and evertors of the foot, and thus paralysis of this component leads to typical deformity known as foot-drop. The patient walks with a high steppage gait to clear the foot of the ground in such cases (Fig. 7.12).

The tibial component supplies the plantar flexors of the foot and ankle. This can be tested by asking the patient to plantar flex the foot against resistance or asking the patient to walk on toes. The hamstring muscles are also supplied by sciatic nerve and thus knee flexion should always be tested in sciatic nerve injury.

TREATMENT OF NERVE INJURIES

1. Conservative—dynamic splinting and nerve stimulation.
2. Neurolysis
3. Primary nerve repair—neurorrhaphy
4. Secondary nerve repair—nerve transfers
5. Tendon transfers

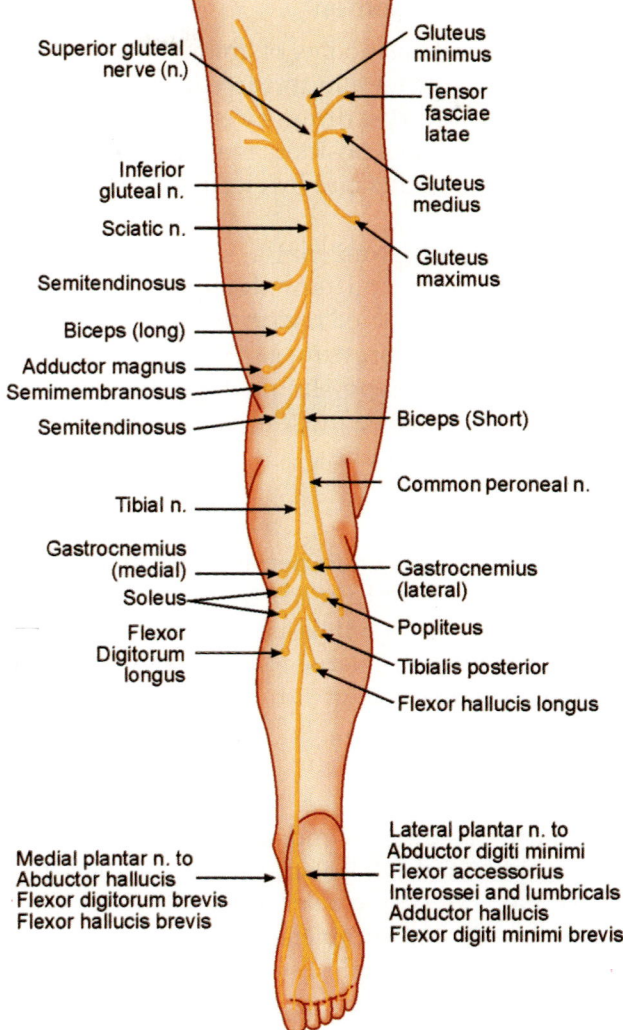

Fig. 7.11: Anatomy of sciatic nerve

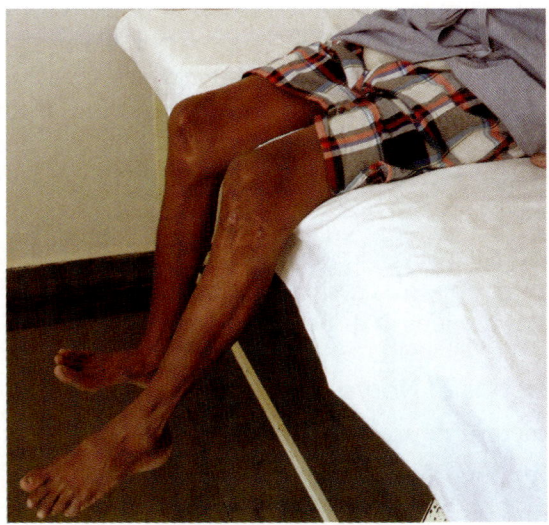

Fig. 7.12: Foot drop

Conservative Management

Maintaining neutral positioning of limbs and to prevent contractures is the main aim in early management of nerve injuries. This is done by splinting of the extremities in functional position, maintaining passive range of motion of joints and by electrical stimulation of nerves.

Care of the skin and nails should be done meticulously, as the patient does not have any sensations over the involved region and thus it is prone for trauma, burns and pressure sores.

Regular physiotherapy should be carried out to preserve tone of paralysed muscles and to prevent any contractures and deformities.

Neurolysis

This is done in cases when nerve is not transected completely, but is injured due to external factors which might be bony or due to soft tissue contractures as well as nerve impingements. Nerve is completely explored at the site of constriction and checked for any discontinuity.

Neurorrhaphy

Neurorrhaphy is end to end approximation of a transected nerve and in situ suturing of the nerve. It may be partial or a complete neurorrhaphy depending on partial transection, complete transection of nerve, or formation of a neuroma.

Primary nerve repair: This can be done when the nerve is cut with a sharp object and when wound is clean without any contamination. In such cases, nerve is immediately explored and the continuity is restored by means of neurorrhaphy.

Delayed primary nerve repair: It is done with nerve injuries with sharp objects and when there is some contamination, or if the patient reports late. In such cases, the wound is thoroughly debrided, and the nerve ends are tagged at first stage. Nerve repair is done at second stage at 2 weeks after the injury after healing of wound.

Secondary nerve repair: It is done in cases with gross contamination, blast injuries and in cases where there is loss of the length of nerve.

Techniques of Nerve Suturing

- Epineural neurorrhaphy.
- Epiperineural neurorrhaphy.
- Perineural neurorrhaphy.
- Fascicular neurorrhaphy.

Methods of Closing Gaps in Nerve Suturing

1. Mobilization of nerves on both sides of the gap.
2. Relaxation of the nerve by temporary positioning of the joints in attitude of flexion.
3. Alteration of the nerve through a short course, e.g anterior transposition of ulnar nerve.
4. Bone resection and shortening of the involved extremity.
5. Nerve grafting by nerve transfer from a donor site.

Nerve Transfers

This involves transfer of a nerve graft from a donor site to the injured nerve. This is required when primary approximation of the nerve cannot be done. Types of nerve grafts are:

   i. Trunk graft
   ii. Cable graft
   ii. Pedicle graft
   iv. Interfascicular grafting
   v. Pre-vascularised nerve grafting.

Tendon Transfers: Reconstructive Surgery

This is the final modality of treatment for nerve injuries when the regeneration potential of the nerve as well as the innervated muscle is lost. Usually we have to wait for a period of 1 year till we proceed with tendon transfer techniques.

OBSTETRICS BRACHIAL PLEXUS PALSY

Newborn babies can develop brachial plexus injury due to distraction of neck during passage through birth canal in a difficult or assisted delivery. This is called OBPP (Obstetric Brachial Plexus Palsy).

Rish factors:
- Breech presentation
- Diabetic mother
- Birth weight >4 kg
- Assisted delivery (forceps or vaccum)

Classification

1. **Upper plexus injury (Erb's palsy):** This involves C5 and C6 nerve root injury. Classical presentation in the newborn is shoulder adduction, elbow extension and wrist flexion. This is the commonest type of OBPP.
2. **Lower plexus injury (Klumpke palsy):** This involves C8 and T1 root injury. This type involves only handgrip weakness. This is a rare injury.
3. **Total plexus injury:** This involves C5 to T1 nerve roots and is the most devastating injury as the infant is left with clawhand along with flail and insensate

upper limb. This injury is common with assisted delivery.

Diagnosis

Diagnosis is mainly clinical. MRI or CT myelography are helpful for documenting the injury and to locate the exact site of injury. EMG—nerve conduction study is not very reliable in infants.

Management

Conservative: Early recognition of this condition is impoartant so that physiotherapy can be started at the earliest. Most of the patients recover gradually, large muscles such as deltoid and biceps recover faster than small hand muscles.

Surgical

Surgical intervention is indicated when there is no improvement in deltoid and biceps up to 3 months.

Types of Surgeries

  i. Exploration, evaluation and repair of the nerve

 ii. Tendon transfer in late presentation

Shoulder Injuries

SCAPULAR FRACTURES

These are relatively uncommon injuries that generally occur in patients between 40 and 60 years of age.

Essential Anatomy (Fig. 8.1)

Classification of Scapular Fractures

Scapular fractures are classified anatomically into fractures of the body or spine, acromion, neck, glenoid, and coracoid process.

Body or Spine Fractures

Mechanism of Injury

The mechanism involved is usually a direct blow over the involved area. Typically, there is little displacement due to the support of the investing muscles and the periosteum.

Examination

The patient presents with pain, swelling, and ecchymosis over the involved area. The involved extremity is held in adduction, and the patient resists abduction. Abduction past the first 90° is largely the result of scapular motion and, thus, will exacerbate the pain.

Imaging

Routine AP and transscapular lateral views (Y view) are generally adequate in defining these fractures (Fig. 8.2). A specialized view called Stryker notch view (45 degree cephalad) can be taken for coracoid process.

Associated Injuries

Scapular fractures involving the body or the spine are usually the result of large blunt forces and may be associated with several life-threatening injuries. Associated injuries to consider include:
1. Pneumothorax or pulmonary contusion.
2. Injuries to thoracic aorta.

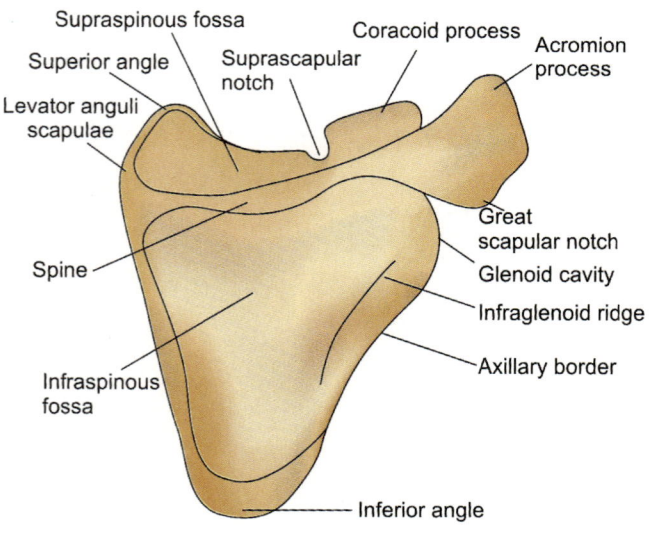

Supraspinous fossa
Coracoid process
Superior angle
Suprascapular notch
Acromion process
Levator anguli scapulae
Spine
Great scapular notch
Glenoid cavity
Infraglenoid ridge
Axillary border
Infraspinous fossa
Inferior angle

Fig. 8.1: Anatomy of scapula

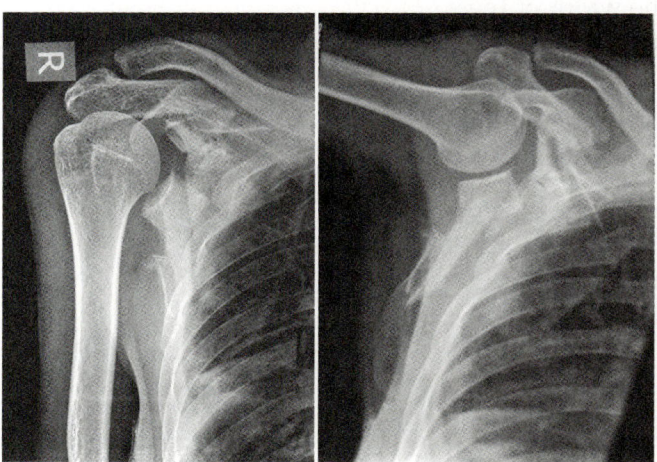

Fig. 8.2: Scapula fracture

3. Rib or vertebral compression fractures.
4. Both upper and lower extremity fractures.
5. Injuries to the axillary artery, nerve or the brachial plexus are rare.

Treatment

Nonoperative treatment is usually sufficient for scapula fracture as most of these fractures are undisplaced and scapula has good muscle coverage. The emergency management of these fractures includes sling, or sling and swathe immobilization with ice and analgesics. Early limited exercise is strongly recommended. After about 2 weeks, limited activity as tolerated is advised.

Operative treatment may be necessary for glenoid fractures depending on location, displacement and stability.

CLAVICLE FRACTURES

Clavicle fractures are one of the most common childhood fractures. These fractures are often encountered in newborn infants secondary to birth trauma. Clavicle fractures are distributed as follows:

Middle third	80%
Distal third	15%
Medial third	5%

Essential Anatomy

The clavicle is an oblong bone, the middle portion of which is tubular and the distal portion, flattened. It is anchored to the scapula by the acromioclavicular and the coracoclavicular ligaments. The sternoclavicular and the costoclavicular ligaments anchor the clavicle medially. The clavicle serves as points of attachment for both the sternocleidomastoid and the subclavius muscles (Fig. 8.3). The ligaments and the muscles act in conjunction to anchor the clavicle and, thus, maintain the width of the shoulder and serve as the attachment point of the shoulder to the axial skeleton. Both the subclavian vessels and the brachial plexus lie in close proximity to the clavicle. Displaced clavicle fractures can be associated with injuries to these vital structures.

Mechanism of Injury

Two mechanisms are commonly responsible for clavicle fracture.

1. *Direct blow:* A posteriorly directed force may result in a single fracture. If the force is directed inferiorly, the resulting fracture is often comminuted, with likelihood of neurovascular damage.

2. *Indirect injury:* Due to fall on the lateral shoulder or outstretched hand. The force gets transmitted via the

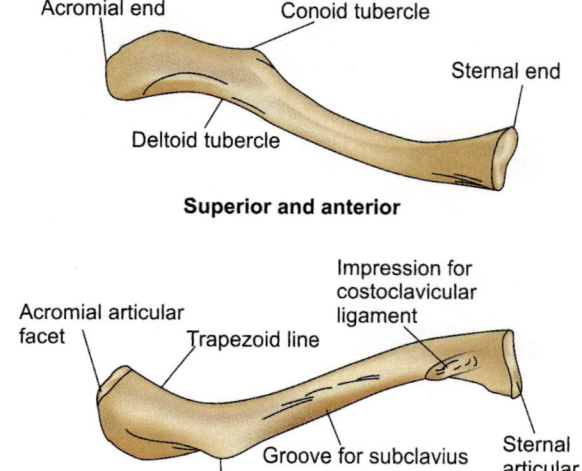

Fig. 8.3: Anatomy of clavicle

acromion to the middle third of clavicle due to its 'S' shape resulting in the middle one third fracture.

Examination

The clavicle is subcutaneous over nearly its entire extent and, therefore, fractures can be easily diagnosed on the basis of examination. Middle-third clavicle fractures usually result in a downward and inward slump of the involved shoulder due to loss of support. The proximal fragment is displaced superiorly due to the pull of the sternocleidomastoid.

Patients usually carry their arm adducted against the chest wall and resist motion of the extremity.

All clavicle fractures require examination and documentation of the neurovascular function distal to the injury.

Imaging

Routine AP views are usually adequate in demonstrating the fracture and any displacement if present (Fig. 8.4).

Apical lordotic view: An AP view with the tube directed 45° cephalad better defines the displacement.

Treatment

Most of these fractures can be managed conservatively using figure of 8 clavicle straps (Fig. 8.5). Commercial figure of eight splints is available. It is important to apply this splint while patient is pulling both the shoulders backwards (military position). The splints have to be retightened daily.

Operative management: Using K-wire or a reconstruction plate on the superior surface (Fig. 8.6).

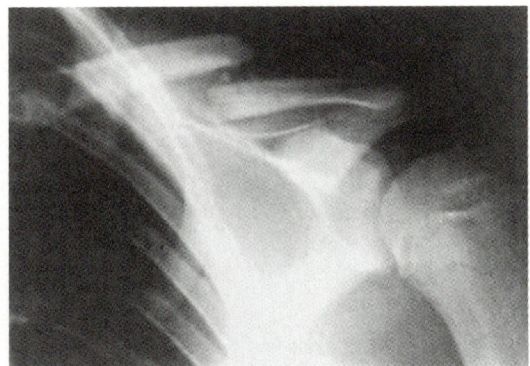

Fig. 8.4: Clavicle fracture

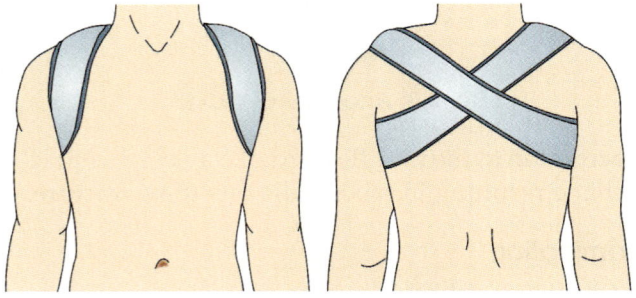

Fig. 8.5: Figure of 8 strapping

Indications

1. Shortening of the clavicle by >2 cm due to overlap.
2. Open fracture.
3. Vascular compromise, or neurologic injury.
4. Relative indications include <2 cm of displacement and intolerance to immobilization.

All displaced lateral-third clavicular fractures are associated with coracoclavicular ligament rupture and should be treated similar to an acromioclavicular joint dislocation discussed later.

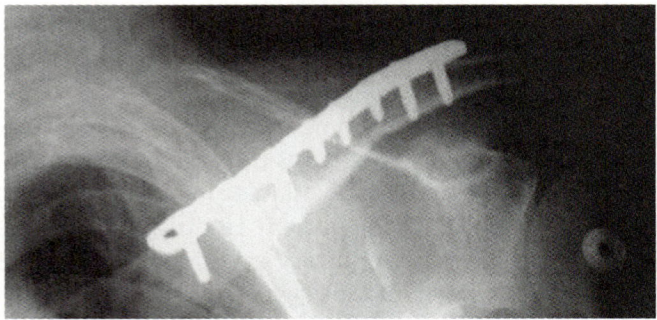

Fig. 8.6: Fracture clavicle treated with ORIF using reconstruction plate

Complications

1. Malunion is primarily a complication of adult fractures. In children, malunion is uncommon due to extensive remodelling of these fractures.
2. Excessive callus formation may occur resulting in a cosmetic defect
3. Nonunion is a rare complication. It is treated with open reduction and internal fixation along with bone grafting.

ACROMIOCLAVICULAR JOINT INJURIES

The acromioclavicular (AC) joint functions to elevate the arm and abduct it. Two ligaments provide stability at this joint—the acromioclavicular and the coracoclavicular ligaments. The coracoclavicular ligament is divided into the conoid and the trapezoid ligaments, which function together to anchor the distal clavicle to the coracoid process (Fig. 8.7).

Mechanism of Injury

1. *Direct:* Fall onto the point of shoulder with arm adducted to the side (common).
2. *Indirect:* Fall on the outstretched hand.

Examination

The deformity appears in the form of a prominence of the distal clavicle, indicating a tear of the AC and possibly the coracoclavicular (CC) ligaments. The upward displacement of the clavicle is due to downward pull of the shoulder caused by the weight of the arm and loss of the suspending coracoclavicular ligament.

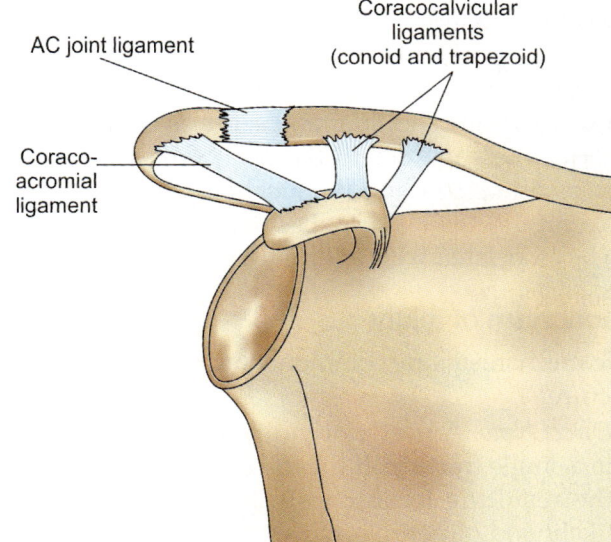

Fig. 8.7: Anatomy of acromioclavicular joint

Imaging

Simultaneous imaging of both shoulders on one large cassette is recommended in order to compare the injured with the normal side. Tilting the beam 10° to 15° toward the head will avoid superimposing the scapular spine and allow for more subtle detection of injuries (Fig. 8.8).

Classification and Treatment

Classification and treatment of acromioclavicular joint injuries are shown in Table 8.1 and Fig. 8.9.

GLENOHUMERAL JOINT INJURIES

Shoulder Dislocation

Shoulder is most commonly dislocated joint in human beings.
1. *Anterior dislocation:* 95% of cases.
2. *Posterior dislocation:* Remaining 5%.
3. Inferior dislocation (luxatio erecta): Extremely rare.

Anterior Shoulder Dislocation

There are four types of anterior dislocation (Fig. 8.10): (A) Subcoracoid (90%), (B) subglenoid, (C) subclavicular, (D) intrathoracic.

Mechanism of Injury

1. *Common:* Abduction accompanied by external rotation of the arm, which disrupts the anterior capsule and the glenohumeral ligaments.
2. Direct blow to the posterior aspect of the proximal humerus, displacing it anteriorly.
3. Atraumatic (4%), occurring while raising an arm or moving during sleep.

Examination

The patient presents with the arm held to the side and the clinical diagnosis can be made with following characteristics:
1. The acromion is prominent and there is loss of the normal rounded contour of the shoulder.

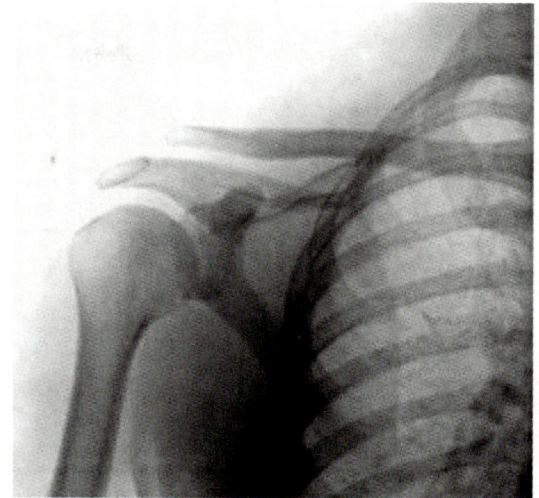

Fig. 8.8: AC Joint Injury

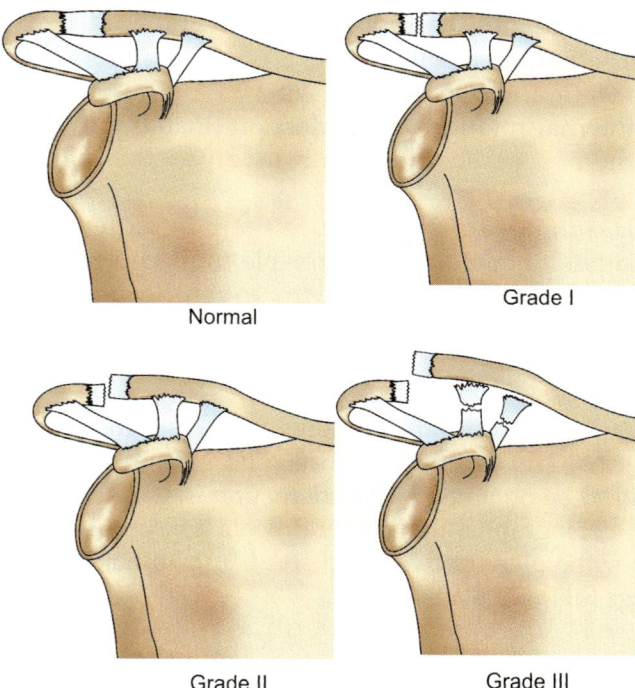

Normal

Grade I

Grade II

Grade III

Fig. 8.9: Grades of AC Joint Injury

Table 8.1: Classification of acromioclavicular joint injury		
Grade I injury	Incomplete tear of acromioclavicular ligament	Treated conservatively using rest, ice application and anti-inflammatory drugs
Grade II injury	Complete disruption of acromioclavicular ligament with subluxation of acromioclavicular joint	Treated conservatively similar to grade 1 injury. However, immobilization is necessary for 2–3 weeks
	Coracoclavicular ligament is intact.	
Grade III injury	Both acromioclavicular and coracoclavicular ligaments are disrupted. Clavicle migrates superiorly.	Can be treated conservatively; open reduction and coracoclavicular ligament reconstruction is required in athletes or if coracoclavicular separation is > 2 cm on X-ray

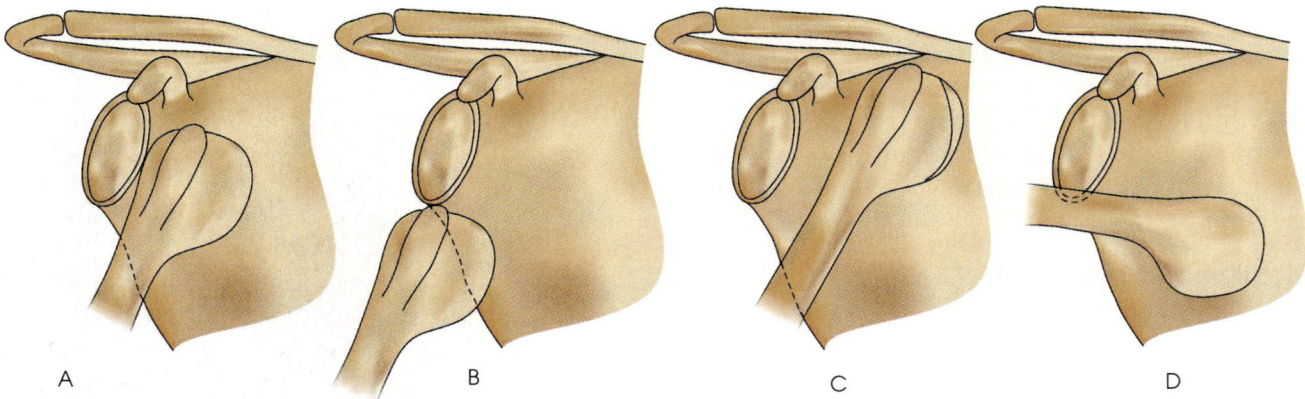

Fig. 8.10A to D: Types of anterior shoulder dislocation

2. There is absence of the humeral head in its usual location while palpating inferior to the acromion.

3. Fullness in the anterior shoulder may be palpated, indicating the presence of the humeral head.

4. The patient permits some abduction and external rotation of the arm, but resists any attempts at internal rotation and adduction (inability to reach the normal shoulder with involved side hand is known as Duga's sign.)

5. *Hamilton's ruler test:* Since there is flattening of shoulder contour, it is possible to place a ruler on the lateral aspect of arm touching acromion superiorly and lateral condyle of humerus inferiorly.

Imaging

Standard radiographic views of the shoulder (AP, internal and external rotation, and scapular Y view) should be obtained before reduction is attempted. On AP radiographs, the humeral head will be displaced from the glenoid fossa and fixed in external rotation (Figs 8.11 and 8.12).

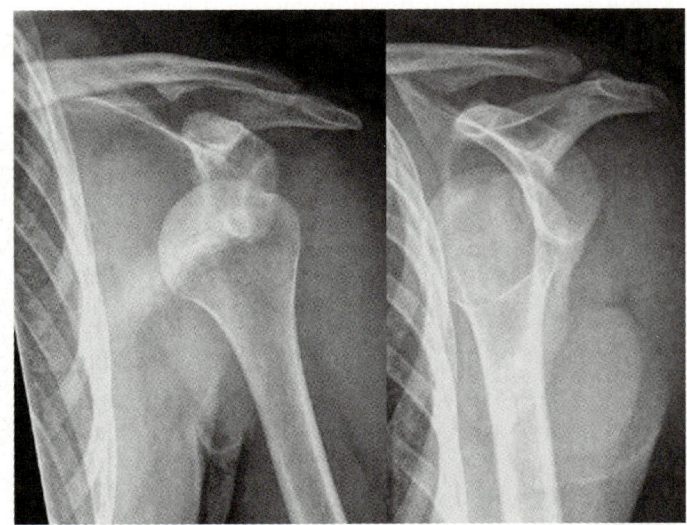

Fig. 8.12: Anterior dislocation of shoulder

Associated Injuries

1. *Hill-Sachs lesion (Fig. 8.13):* A defect in the posterior lateral portion of the humeral head. This defect, known as Hill-Sachs lesion is present in up to 50% of cases of anterior shoulder dislocation and is very common in recurrent shoulder dislocation (Figs 8.14 and 8.15). It occurs as a result of impaction of the soft base of the humeral head against the anterior glenoid (Fig. 8.13).

   The longer the humeral head is out of the glenoid fossa, the larger is the defect. If one suspects a Hill-Sachs lesion an internal rotation view can be obtained after the shoulder has been reduced for better delineation of the defect.

2. *Bankart's lesion:* Anteriorly dislocating humerus head causes stripping of the capsule, labrum and periosteum from the anteroinferior portion of the glenoid. This is known as Bankart's lesion and is the main culprit of recurrent dislocation (Fig. 8.16).

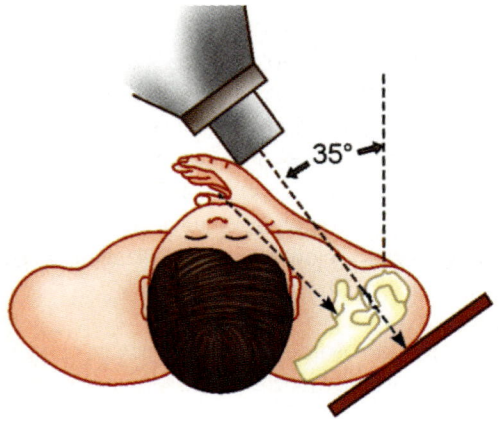

Fig. 8.11: True AP view of shoulder

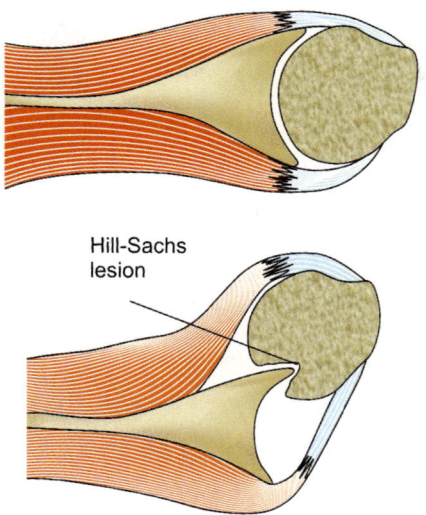

Fig. 8.13: Mechanism of Hill-Sachs lesion

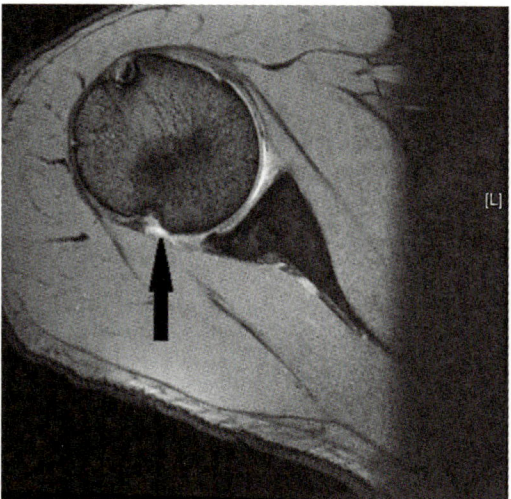

Fig. 8.15: MRI shoulder showing Hill-Sachs lesion

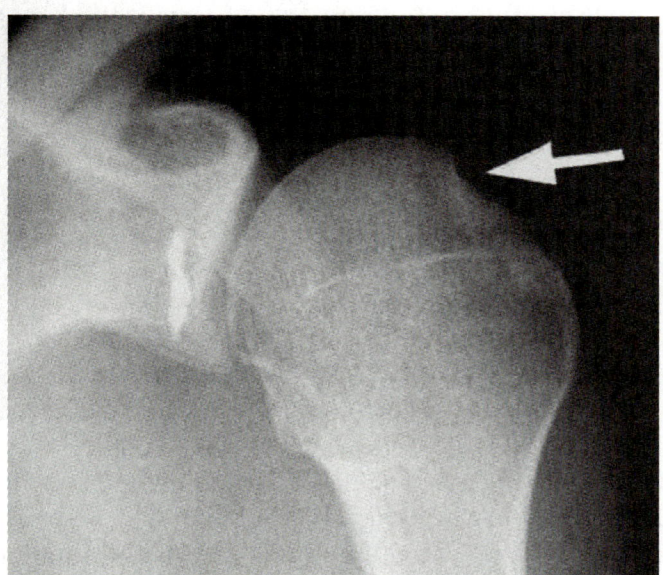

Fig. 8.14: Hill-Sachs lesion

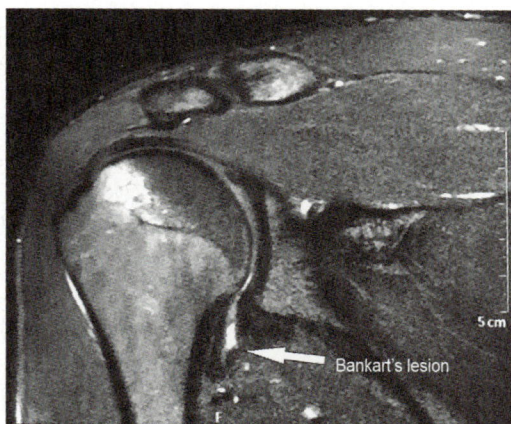

Fig. 8.16: T2W MRI of shoulder showing Bankart's lesion

3. *Eburnation of Glenoid rim:* This means that the anterior portion of glenoid becomes smooth due to bone loss.
4. Fractures of the greater tuberosity occur in 15% of patients with anterior shoulder dislocations especially in patients >45 years of age.
5. Glenoid rim fractures occur in approximately 5% of patients.
6. Rotator cuff tears occur in 50% of patients <40 years old and in 80% of patients >60 years old. Inability to abduct the arm following reduction of an anterior shoulder dislocation is a sensitive indicator of a rotator cuff tear. This test is not specific, however, because it may occur in patients with an axillary nerve injury.

7. Axillary nerve injury is the most common associated neurologic injury in anterior shoulder dislocations occurring in approximately 12% of cases. Injury to the axillary nerve can be assessed by testing motor strength of deltoid and pinprick sensation over the lateral aspect of the arm and comparing it with the other side. Careful testing will reveal a small area of numbness over the deltoid (the sergeant's patch)

Treatment

Once diagnosis of anterior shoulder dislocation is established, shoulder joint has to be reduced immediately under general anaesthesia. Without adequate analgesia and muscle relaxation, anterior shoulder dislocation reduction can be difficult. Several methods have been described for reducing anterior shoulder dislocations, some of which will be discussed.

1. *Traction and counter-traction:* In this method, an assistant applies counter-traction with a folded sheet

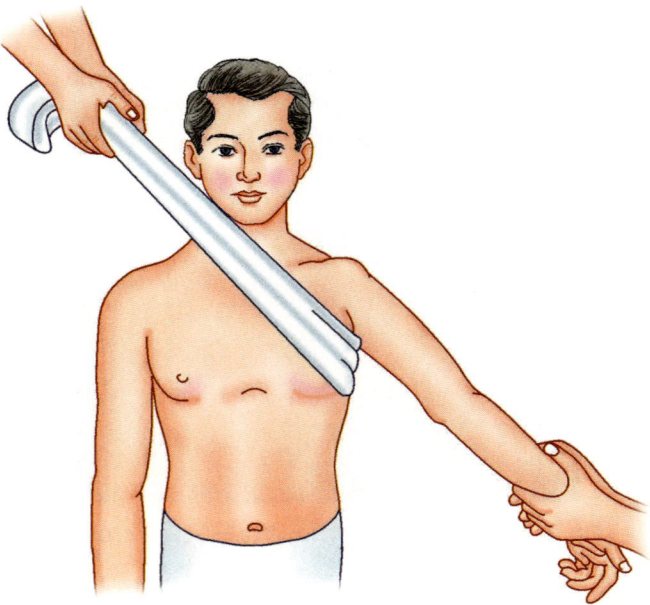

Fig. 8.17: Traction counter-traction method

wrapped around the upper chest, and the examiner applies traction to the arm in an inferolateral direction (Fig. 8.17).

2. *Traction and counter-traction with lateral traction:* In addition to traction and counter-traction as indicated above, a perpendicular force to the longitudinal axis of the humerus is applied to the proximal humerus in the axilla by a second assistant (Fig. 8.18A).

3. *Stimson technique:* The patient is placed in the prone position with the arms dependent over a pillow or folded sheets. A strap is added to the wrist or distal forearm and 10 to 15 lbs of weights are applied for a period of 20 to 30 minutes. If unsuccessful, the examiner may rotate the humerus gently, externally and then internally with mild force, which usually reduces the dislocation (Fig. 8.18B).

Other techniques like Kocher's manoeuvre, Hippocrate's manoeuvre or external rotation manoeuvre are no longer recommended due to high rate of complications.

Post-reduction Rehabilitation Protocol

Following reduction, the shoulder should remain adducted and internally rotated in a shoulder immobilizer.

In patients <30 years of age: 3 weeks of immobilization is advocated. After this, gentle active range of motion exercises can be instituted; however, external rotation and abduction should be prohibited for an additional 3 weeks after immobilization has been discontinued.

In patients >30 years of age: Immobilization for 7 to 10 days with circumduction (Codman) exercises, to

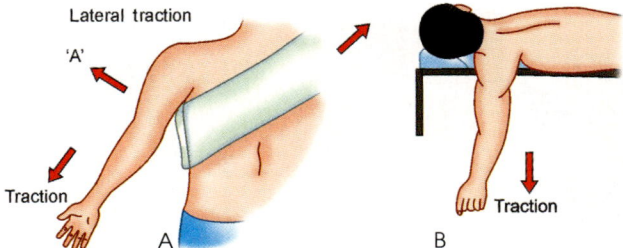

Fig. 8.18A and B: Traction and counter-traction with lateral traction and Stimson method

begin within 4 to 5 days of injury. The patient should avoid abduction and external rotation of the shoulder.

Complications

1. Axillary nerve palsy
2. *Recurrent dislocation:* This is the most common complication of anterior dislocation, which is seen in 60% of patients <30 years of age and approximately 10% in patients >40 years of age. The most important reason for recurrence after acute dislocation is inadequate immobilization or unnoticed Bankart's lesion.

RECURRENT ANTERIOR SHOULDER DISLOCATION

Patho-anatomy

Shoulder dislocation is highly prone for recurrence due to following reasons:

1. *Primary deficiency:* Shoulder is an inherently unstable joint as glenoid is much smaller, shallower as compared to humeral head. This articulation area is partly increased by glenoid labrum. Any injury to labrum thus renders shoulder unstable.

2. *Secondary deficiencies* which occur at the time of dislocation of shoulder making it more prone for subsequent dislocations. These are as follows:

   a. *Bankart's lesion:* In anterior dislocation the humeral head is forced anteriorly out of the glenoid cavity and tears not only the fibrocartilaginous labrum from almost the entire anterior half of the rim of the glenoid cavity, but also the capsule and periosteum from the anterior surface of the neck of the scapula. This traumatic detachment of the glenoid labrum has been called the Bankart's lesion. This renders shoulder highly prone for recurrent dislocations.

   b. *Eburnation of glenoid margin:* As humerus head dislocates it erodes the anterior margin of glenoid, making it further shallower (Fig. 8.19).

   c. *Hill-Sachs lesion:* It is basically a defect in posterolateral part of humerus head; if large in size makes shoulder prone for further dislocation.

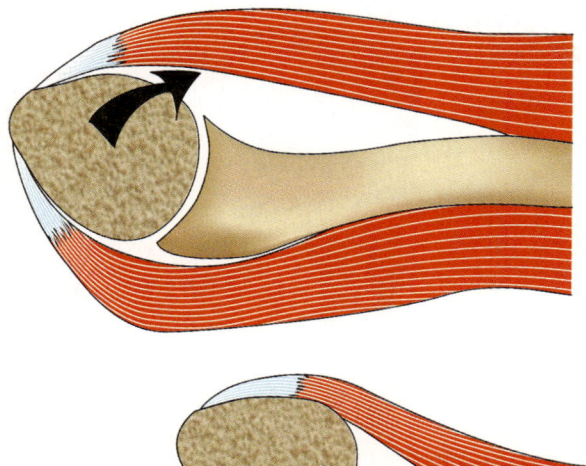

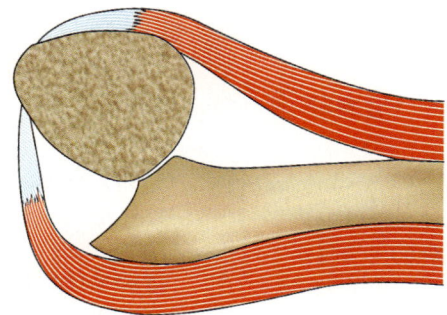

Fig. 8.19: Eburnation of glenoid

d. *Glenoid labrum tears:* Obviously affects shoulder stability.
e. Capsular stretching and laxity following dislocation may add on to recurrence.

Diagnosis

Clinical diagnosis: History of recurrent dislocations is quite obvious.

1. *Apprehension test:* With patient sitting or supine, examiner keeps patient's shoulder to 90 degrees of abduction and external rotation force applied to the extremity as anterior stress is applied to the humerus. This generally produces an apprehension reaction in a patient who has anterior instability .
2. *Anterior drawer test:* With patient sitting on couch, examiner compares anterior laxity with the opposite shoulder.

Radiological diagnosis

1. X-ray may reveal Hill-Sachs lesion.
2. MRI is more useful as it reveals Bankart's lesion and other associated lesions already described.

Treatment

Bankart's Repair

Principles

1. Maximizing the healing potential by abrading the scapular neck.
2. Restoring glenoid concavity.

3. Securing anatomical capsular fixation at the edge of the glenoid articular surface.
4. Recreating physiological capsular tension by superior and inferior capsular advancement and imbrication
5. Performing supervised goal-oriented rehabilitation.

Many other procedures like Bristow procedure (shifting tip of coracoid process to neck of scapula), Putti-Platt operation (lateral advancement of subscapularis) etc. are also described.

Posterior Shoulder Dislocation

Posterior dislocations are far less common than anterior dislocations, but are the most commonly missed major dislocations of the body. Posterior dislocations are missed partially because they are less common, but also because they present with less pain than anterior dislocations and the radiographic findings are subtle.

Mechanism of Injury

A violent internal rotational force such as would occur during a fall on the forward flexed internally rotated arm, e.g. seizure or an electric shock.

Examination

1. The cardinal sign of a posterior dislocation of the shoulder is that the arm is held in adduction and internal rotation.
2. Abduction is severely limited and external rotation of the shoulder is blocked.
3. On palpation of the shoulder girdle, the examiner will note a prominence in the posterior aspect of the shoulder accompanied by flattening of the normal shoulder contour.

Imaging

Plain X-ray shows internal rotation of the humeral head resulting in rotation of the greater tuberosity so that it is no longer in its normal lateral position. This is referred to as the "light bulb" or "ice cream cone" sign because the humeral head appears rounded, as though it sits on top of a cone—the humeral shaft (Fig. 8.20).

If there remains a question about dislocation, a scapular Y or axillary view can be obtained. A CT scan will also be diagnostic, but is not routinely performed.

Treatment

Closed reduction using flexion and adduction with axial traction on the arm is usually successful and can be performed in acute dislocations (<3 weeks) when there is a <25% articular surface defect. Direct anterior pressure on the posterior displaced humeral head may

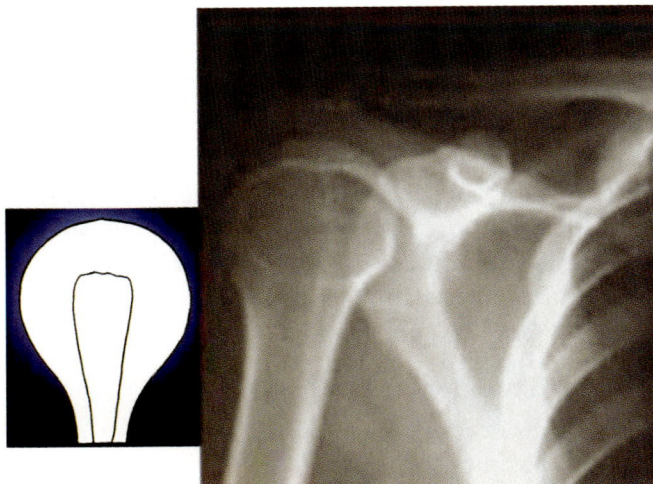

Fig. 8.20: Light bulb sign

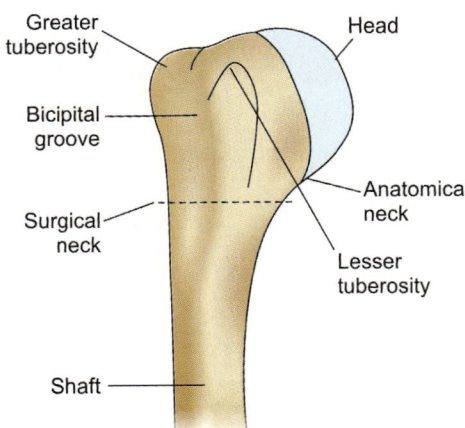

Fig. 8.21: Anatomy of proximal humerus

facilitate the reduction. Indications for surgical intervention include significant displacement of the greater tuberosity that is irreducible on reduction of the dislocation, an articular defect >25%, or a chronic dislocation (>3 weeks).

PROXIMAL HUMERUS FRACTURES

Essential Anatomy

Anatomically, proximal humerus fractures include all humerus fractures proximal to the surgical neck.

The humeral head articulates with the glenoid, forming the glenohumeral joint.

The articular surface ends at the anatomic neck; therefore, fractures located proximal to the anatomic neck are considered articular surface fractures. The surgical neck is the narrowed portion of the proximal humerus distal to the anatomic neck. The greater and lesser tuberosities are bony prominences located just distal to the anatomic neck (Fig. 8.21).

Mechanism of Injury

1. A direct blow on the lateral aspect of the arm such as during a fall may result in a fracture.
2. The indirect mechanism is more common and is usually secondary to a fall on the outstretched arm.

Imaging

Radiographs of the shoulder should include an AP and lateral view (Table 8.2).

Classification and Treatment

The treatment for proximal humerus fractures varies depending on the age of the patient and his or her lifestyle. Successful treatment of proximal humerus

Table 8.2: Special views of shoulder	
AP with the humerus in external rotation	Fractures of the greater tuberosity are best visualized
AP with the humerus in internal rotation	Fractures of lesser tuberosity are best visualized
Scapular Y view	Glenohumeral dislocations and scapular fractures are best visualized

fractures is dependent on early mobility. A compromise in anatomic reduction may be accepted so that prolonged immobilization can be avoided.

Non-displaced fractures, which comprise 80% of all proximal humerus fractures, may be treated with a sling and swathe or a sling alone. Early passive exercises are generally recommended. Active exercises are recommended during the later stages of healing. More complex, displaced, or angulated fractures often require operative management and are treated according to the classification system given by Neer et al.

According to Neer's classification system, the proximal humerus is divided into four segments (Fig. 8.22).
1. Surgical neck
2. Anatomic neck
3. Greater tuberosity
4. Lesser tuberosity

1. If all of the proximal humeral fragments are non-displaced and without angulation, the injury would be classified as a one-part fracture.
2. If a fragment has >1 cm of displacement or angulation >45° from the remaining intact proximal humerus, the fracture is classified as a two-part fracture.
3. If two fragments are individually displaced from the remaining proximal humerus, the fracture is classified as a three-part fracture.

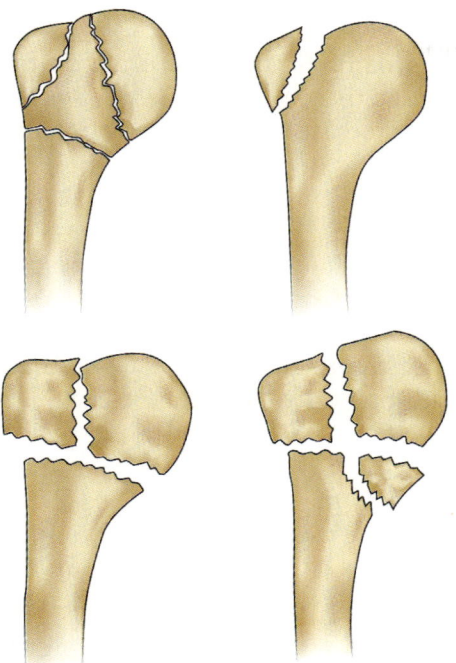

Fig. 8.22: Classification of proximal humerus fracture

4. If all four fragments are individually displaced, the fracture is a four-part fracture.

The three- and four-part fractures are often associated with dislocation.

Surgical Neck Fractures

Surgical neck fractures can be divided into three classes—nondisplaced fractures, displaced fractures, or comminuted fractures.

Examination

The patient will present with tenderness and swelling over the upper arm and shoulder. If, on presentation, the arm is held in adduction, the incidence of brachial plexus and axillary arterial injury is low. If the patient presents with the arm abducted, the incidence of neurovascular injury is much more significant.

Associated Injuries

Non-displaced surgical neck fractures may be associated with a contusion or tear of the axillary nerve. Axillary neurovascular injury and brachial plexus injuries are more common after displaced or comminuted fractures of the surgical neck.

Treatment

The normal neck shaft angle of humerus is 135 degrees. Angulation up to 45 degree from this is well tolerated especially by elderly. More severe angulations require reduction either closed or open.

Similarly displacement up to 1cm is well tolerated. More displacement requires open reduction and fixation using plate or multiple K wires.

Anatomic Neck Fractures

Anatomic neck fractures are through the area of the physis and can be divided into adult or childhood injuries. Adult injuries are rare and may be classified as non-displaced or displaced (>1 cm). Childhood injuries are generally limited to 8 to 14-year-old.

Treatment

Undisplaced fractures can be treated with immobilization in a sling and swathe, ice and analgesics, followed by early mobilization in adults. Fractures displaced >1 cm requires reduction and fixation using multiple K wires or specially designed locking plates. Childhood anatomic neck fractures are referred to as proximal humeral epiphyseal injuries and require immediate reduction.

GREATER TUBEROSITY FRACTURES

Anatomy

The supraspinatus, infraspinatus, and teres minor insert on the greater tuberosity and, when fractured, cause upward displacement of the fragment, causing mechanical block to abduction of the shoulder.

There are two types of greater tuberosity fractures—nondisplaced and displaced. A fracture of the greater tuberosity with displacement of >1 cm is often associated with a tear of the rotator cuff.

Imaging

AP radiographs are able to assess superior displacement. However, axillary lateral radiographs can be used to assess the amount of posterior retraction. A CT scan will accurately diagnose the degree of displacement.

Treatment

Nondisplaced (Fig. 8.23)

The management consists of ice, analgesics, sling immobilization.

Displaced

If associated with an anterior shoulder dislocation, reduction of the dislocation often corrects the displacement of the greater tuberosity and the fracture can then be managed as a nondisplaced fracture.

If displacement remains (Fig. 8.24) or a displaced fracture is present without a shoulder dislocation, the management of these injuries is dependent on the age

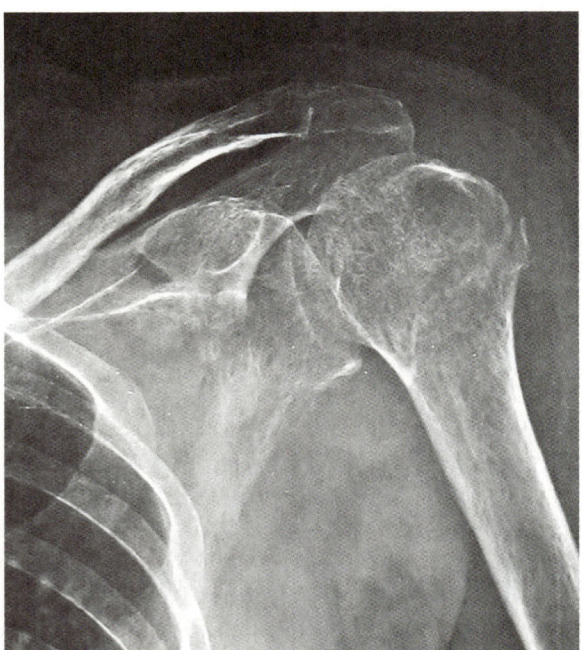

Fig. 8.23: Nondisplaced greater tuberosity fracture

and activity of the patient. Young patients require internal fixation of the fragment with repair of the torn rotator cuff. Good bone stock must be present for fixation with screws, but is frequently lacking in elderly patients. Older patients are usually not candidates for surgical repair and require ice, immobilization with a sling, analgesics. Early mobilization in the elderly patient is essential.

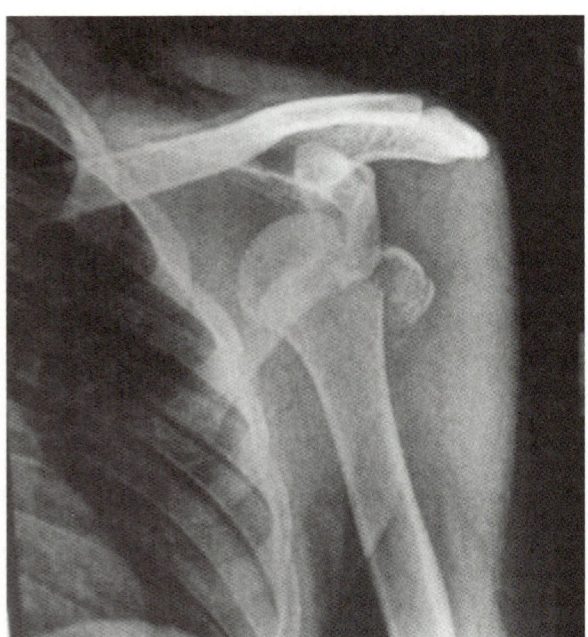

Fig. 8.24: Displaced greater tuberosity fracture with anterior dislocation of shoulder

Lesser Tuberosity Fractures

Lesser tuberosity fractures are uncommon. They commonly occur in conjunction with posterior shoulder dislocations. Fracture fragments may be small or large (>1 cm).

Mechanism of Injury

Lesser tuberosity fractures are usually associated with an indirect mechanism of injury such as a seizure or a fall on the adducted arm. Both of these situations result in an intense contraction of the subscapularis muscle and an avulsion of the lesser tuberosity.

Treatment

The emergency management of lesser tuberosity fractures includes ice, analgesics, sling immobilization. Most fractures can be treated with sling immobilization for 3 to 5 days followed by gradually increasing range of motion exercises.

PAINFUL SHOULDER CONDITIONS

The frequency of painful shoulder conditions has been ascertained from several reports. The incidence of common syndromes is as follows (Fig. 8.25).

Subacromial bursitis/supraspinatus tendinitis	60%
Rotator cuff tears	10%
Bicipital tendinitis	4%
Adhesive capsulitis	12%
Acromioclavicular joint osteoarthritis	7%
Other conditions	7%

Impingement of muscles and tendons under the acromion and rigid coracoacromial arch is a common underlying pathology that exists in a number of these conditions. Supraspinatus tendinitis, bicipital tendinitis, and eventual degeneration and tearing of the rotator cuff tendons may all be secondary to impingement.

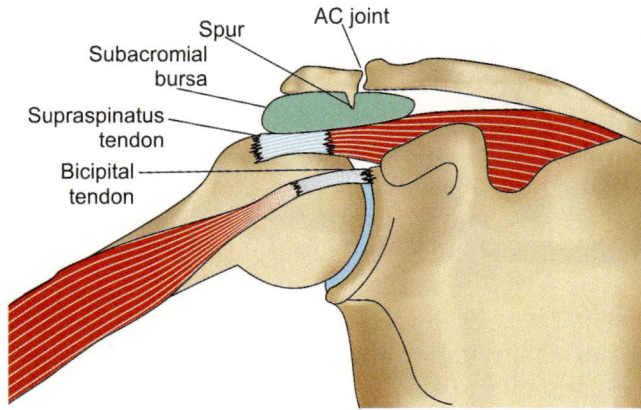

Fig. 8.25: Common causes of painful shoulder

Supraspinatus Tendinitis and Subacromial Bursitis

Introduction

Supraspinatus tendinitis is the most common cause of shoulder pain and is usually caused by degenerative changes in that tendon with advancing age and impingement.

Aetiology

- Impingement (75%)
- Chronic overuse (10%)
- Acute strains (5%)

The pathogenesis of supraspinatus tendinitis is along a continuum that will ultimately lead to subacromial bursitis. As the supraspinatus tendon traverses under the acromion and the coracoacromial arch, small tears occur. The repair process is associated with inflammatory cells that lead to tendonitis. The patient seen at this stage usually complains of a deep ache in the shoulder with increasing pain on abduction and internal rotation. The inflammatory cells cause significant swelling, and eventually calcium deposits within the tendon. The swelling of the tendon causes worsening impingement on the subacromial bursa that forms the roof of the supraspinatus tendon (Fig. 8.26). At this stage the tendon becomes an obstacle to pain-free abduction and the patient complains of increasing pain in the shoulder. Attempts to abduct the arm to 70° cause severe pain.

As the process continues, a severe inflammatory reaction occurs within the bursa, leading to bursitis. As the subacromial bursa swells, partial abduction and adduction is restricted. The arm is held at approximately 30° of abduction. Further adduction or abduction causes increasing pain, and the patient resists any attempt to elevate the arm beyond this point. If the process is allowed to continue, the patient may experience a chronic bursitis leading eventually to adhesive pericapsulitis.

Clinical Presentation

- *Age:* 35–50 years.
- F > M
- A deep ache in the shoulder referred to the deltoid region and the pain may radiate to the entire limb. There is usually point tenderness between the coracoid process and acromion, at the site of the supraspinatus tendon.
- Pain is increased on abduction and internal rotation of the arm.
- Onset is usually gradual, but may be acute after overuse of the shoulder, especially in an overhead position. Within 2 to 3 days the pain becomes increasingly intense at the point of the shoulder.

Treatment

Most patients improve with conservative therapy. Treatment consists of avoidance of the inciting activity, non-steroidal anti-inflammatory medications, ice, and exercises that prevent muscle atrophy. The patient should be encouraged to initiate range of motion, starting with pendulum exercises. A very important part of therapy is never to place the shoulder in immobilization for any prolonged period, as this will induce adhesive capsulitis.

Bicipital Tendinitis

Introduction

The long head of the biceps traverses between the greater and lesser tuberosities within the bicipital groove ensheathed by the capsule of the glenohumeral joint and inserts on the glenoid rim. This position makes the tendon subject to constant trauma and irritation from motions of the shoulder and impingement as described previously. Inflammation around the tendon increases until it moves reluctantly.

Clinical Presentation

- Pain in the biceps region and anterior aspect of the shoulder that radiates down toward the forearm.
- Abduction and external rotation are the most painful motions and snap extension of the elbow increases the pain markedly.

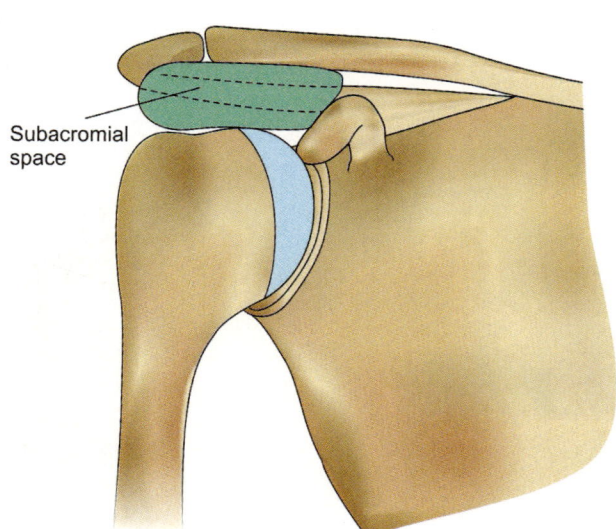

Subacromial space

Fig. 8.26: Subacromial space

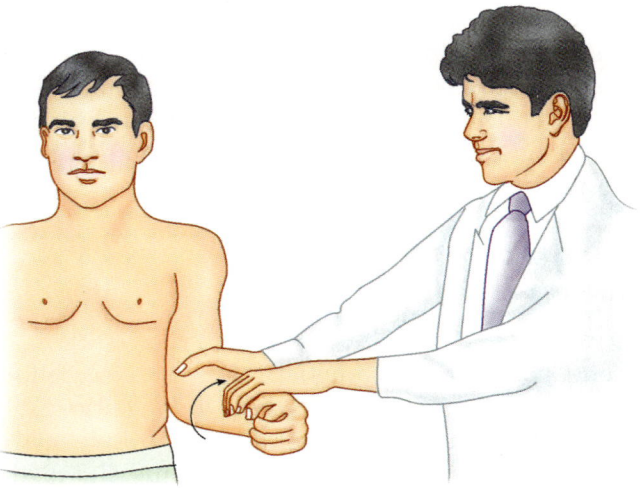

Fig. 8.27: Yergason's test

- Tenderness to palpation in the bicipital groove.
- Yergason test (Fig. 8.27), the patient's elbow is held at 90° of flexion. The patient is asked to supinate the forearm as the examiner resists this attempt. This causes pain along the intertubercular groove and is a reliable test to distinguish tenosynovitis of the long head of the biceps from subacromial bursitis.

Treatment

The treatment includes immobilization in a sling and injection of the bicipital canal with an anesthetic and steroid solution. One must be careful not to inject the tendon itself. The injection is usually carried out at several points along the route of the tendon within the bicipital groove. Analgesics and anti-inflammatory agents may be administered as well.

Humeral Shaft Fractures

Anatomy

The humeral shaft extends from the insertion of the pectoralis major to the supracondylar ridges. The extensive musculature surrounding the humeral shaft may result in distraction and displacement of the bony fragments after a fracture.

A fracture proximal to the pectoralis major insertion may be accompanied by abduction and external rotation of the humeral head because of the action of the supraspinatus. A fracture between the insertion of the pectoralis major and the deltoid will usually result in adduction of the proximal fragment secondary to the pull of the pectoralis major. Fractures distal to the deltoid insertion usually result in abduction of the proximal fragment secondary to the pull of the deltoid muscle (Fig. 9.1).

The neurovascular bundle, which supplies the forearm and the hand, extends along the medial border

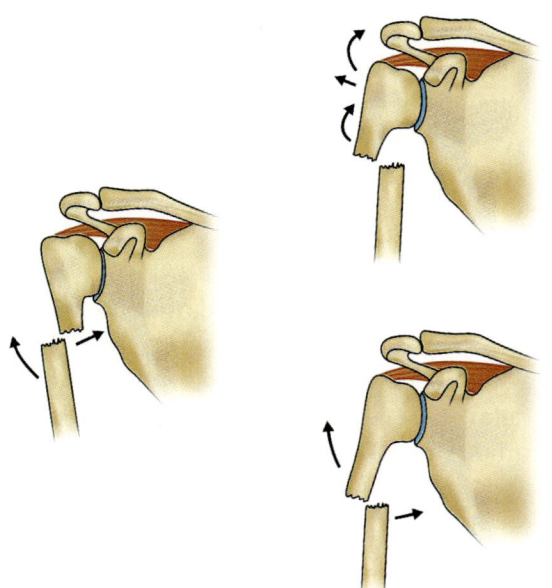

Fig. 9.1: Deforming forces of humerus fracture

of the humeral shaft. The radial nerve lies in close proximity to the humeral shaft at the junction of its middle and distal thirds. Fractures in this area are often accompanied by radial nerve impairment.

Examination

Symptoms

Pain and swelling over the area of the humeral shaft.

Signs

1. Shortening
2. Obvious deformity
3. Abnormal mobility with crepitation.

It is imperative that a thorough neurovascular examination accompanies the initial assessment of all humeral shaft fractures.

The examiner should give particular emphasis to the radial nerve function and document the time at which radial nerve injury is first detected. This information is important because:

1. Damage at the time of injury is most often a neurapraxia.
2. Damage detected after manipulation or immobilization may lead to axonotmesis if the pressure is not relieved.
3. Damage detected during healing is typically due to a slowly progressive axonotmesis.

Treatment

Treatment is often nonsurgical. Closed management of humeral shaft fractures is initially with sugar tong cast followed by a Sarmiento-type brace (Fig. 9.2).

These methods provide dependency traction with the goal that they will correct angulation and displacement. Rigid immobilization and perfect alignment are not essential for adequate healing. Indications for continued closed treatment include less than 20 degrees of anterior

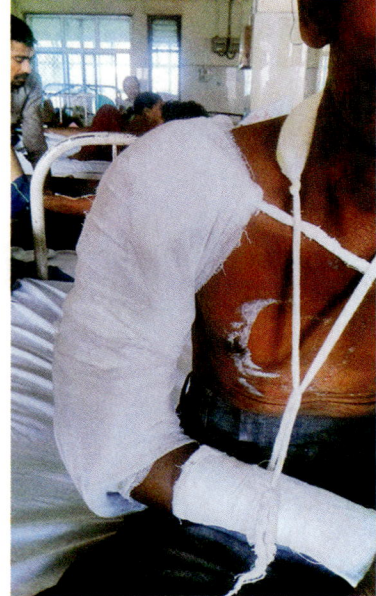

Fig. 9.2: Sugar tong cast

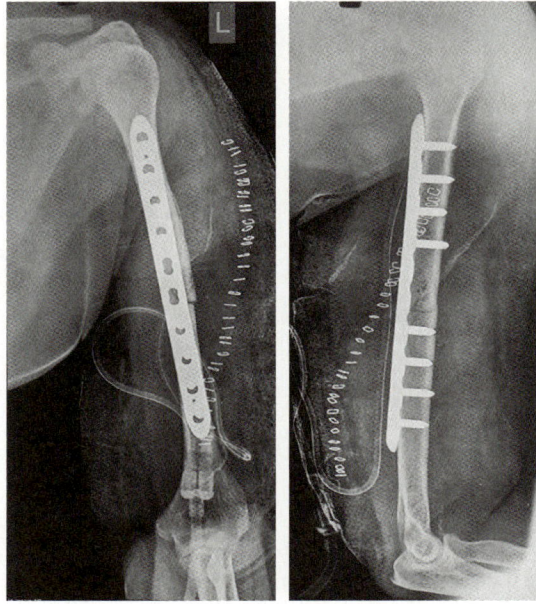

Fig. 9.3: Humerus fracture treated with ORIF using DCP

or posterior angulation, less than 30 degrees of varus, and less than 3 cm of shortening. Closed management of these injuries has resulted in a 98% union rate with good functional restoration and minimal deformity; however, success depends on a compliant patient.

Operative Treatment

Indications

1. Failed closed treatment
2. Open fractures
3. Vascular or neurologic injury
4. Segmental fractures
5. Floating elbow
6. Bilateral humeral shaft fractures
7. Pathological fractures
8. Ipsilateral brachial plexus injuries
9. Polytrauma patients
10. Parkinson disease.

Techniques for humeral shaft fracture fixation include plate osteosynthesis, intramedullary interlocking nail fixation and external fixation. External fixation is indicated for severe open fractures with soft tissue injury, burns or infected nonunions, and humeral shaft fracture with neurovascular injury. Plate fixation provides the best functional results (Fig. 9.3).

Radial nerve injury is present in 6 to 15% of humeral shaft fractures. These injuries are commonly associated with spiral fractures of the distal third, but may also be seen in middle-third fractures or after fracture patterns other than spiral (i.e. transverse). The injury may be partial or complete and may involve motor or sensory fibres. Complete motor dysfunction is present in over one-half of cases. The majority of cases of radial nerve dysfunction occur at the time of injury, but up to 20% will develop during treatment.

Radial nerve palsies after humeral shaft fractures were historically an indication for operative exploration, but this treatment has fallen out of favour because

1. Transection is present in only 12% of cases
2. Spontaneous nerve regeneration is common
3. Delayed operative intervention does not adversely affect outcome.

Complications

1. The development of shoulder adhesive capsulitis may be prevented by early circumduction exercises
2. Myositis ossificans of the elbow may develop. This can be avoided by using active routine exercises.
3. The delayed development of radial nerve palsy.
4. Nonunion or delayed union.

Elbow Injuries

Essential Anatomy

The elbow is a hinge joint composed of three articulations: humero-ulnar, radio-humeral, and radio-ulnar. These articulations provide a high degree of inherent stability (Fig. 10.1).

The distal humerus consists of two columns of bone whose terminal ends make up the condyles. The coronoid fossa is the area of very thin, sometimes transparent bone that connects the two condyles of the distal humerus. The articular surface of the medial condyle is called the trochlea, whereas the lateral articular surface is the capitellum. The nonarticular portions of the condyles are called epicondyles, and serve as points of attachment for the muscles of the forearm. Those muscles concerned with forearm flexion insert on the medial epicondyle, whereas those of extension insert on the lateral epicondyle. The bone distal to and including the supracondylar ridges is anatomically defined as the distal humerus.

Three bursae around the elbow are of clinical significance: one between the olecranon and the triceps, another between the radius and the insertion of the biceps tendon, and finally the olecranon bursa, which lies between the skin and the olecranon process. Bursitis about the elbow most commonly involves the olecranon bursa.

The functional ROM of the elbow is 30 to 130 degrees of extension and flexion and 50 degrees of pronation supination, each.

T–Y ELBOW FRACTURES

Intercondylar fractures generally occur in patients over the age of 50. This is actually a supracondylar fracture with a vertical intra-articular component. The terms T and Y indicate the direction of the fracture line. T fractures have a single transverse line, whereas Y fractures present with two oblique fracture lines through the supracondylar humeral column (Fig. 10.2). Classification is based on the amount of separation

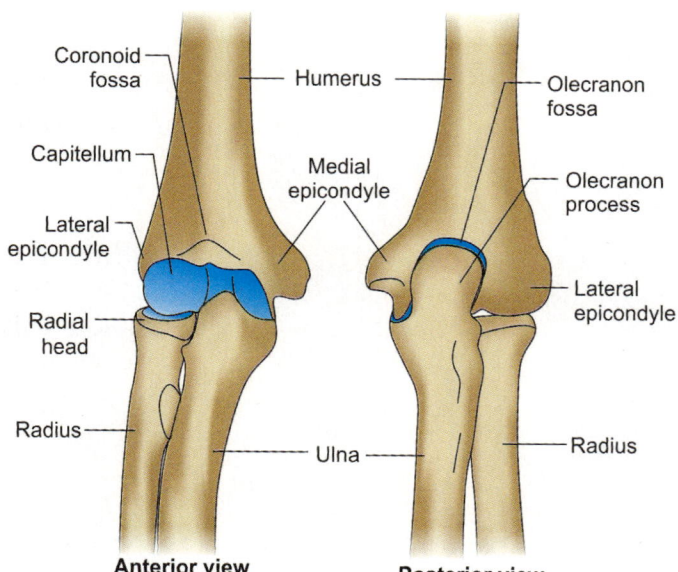

Fig. 10.1: Anatomy of elbow

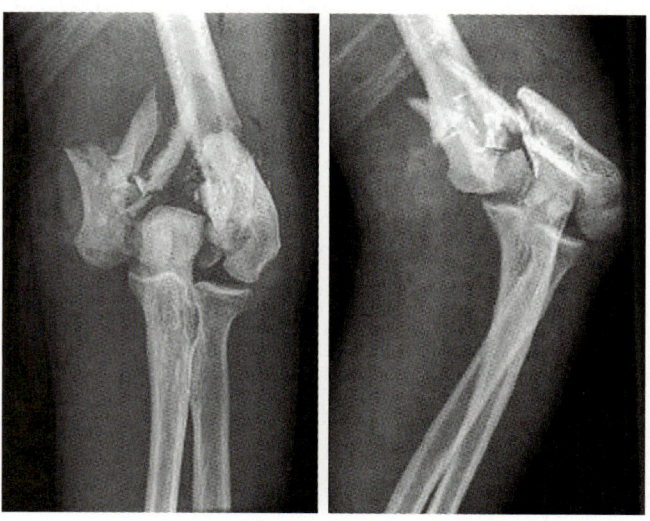

Fig. 10.2: T–Y fracture

between the fracture fragments and is broadly divided into (1) nondisplaced fractures and (2) displaced, rotated, or comminuted fractures.

Mechanism of Injury

Usually a direct blow driving the olecranon into the distal humerus at the trochlea.

Imaging

AP and lateral views may demonstrate comminution, and overlapping bony edges may make interpretation difficult. X-ray views taken with traction or computed tomography (CT) is often helpful to the surgeon in planning operative treatment.

Nondisplaced

This is a stable fracture and can be treated with a long-arm posterior splint with the forearm in neutral position. Active motion exercises can be started within 2 to 3 weeks.

Displaced, Rotated, or Comminuted

These fractures are difficult to treat. Operative treatment in the form of plating, is the treatment of choice (Fig. 10.3). In patients with contraindications to surgery, other means of treatment such as olecranon pinning with traction may be used.

Complications

1. Loss of elbow range of motion
2. Post-traumatic arthritis
3. Neurovascular complications (rare)

4. Malunion and nonunion
5. Wound dehiscence

Capitellum Fracture

Capitellum fractures constitute only 0.5 to 1% of all elbow injuries.

Mechanism of Injury

The fracture mechanism is usually the result of a blow inflicted on the outstretched hand. The force is transmitted up the radius to the capitellum. The capitellum has no muscular attachments and consequently, the fragment may be nondisplaced. In some circumstances, secondary displacement occurs from elbow motion (Fig. 10.4).

Associated Injuries

1. Radial head fractures common.
2. Rupture of the ulnar collateral ligament in 70%.

Treatment

An accurate reduction is imperative to ensure normal motion of the radio-humeral joint. Large fracture fragments are treated with fixation using specialized screws known as Herbert screws (Fig. 10.5). Small comminuted fragments should be excised.

Complications

1. Post-traumatic arthritis
2. Avascular necrosis of the fracture fragment
3. Restricted range of motion

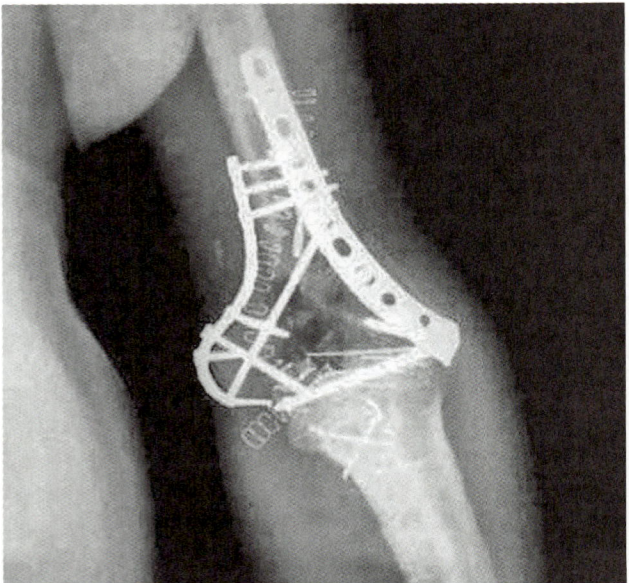

Fig. 10.3: T–Y fracture treated with bipillar plating

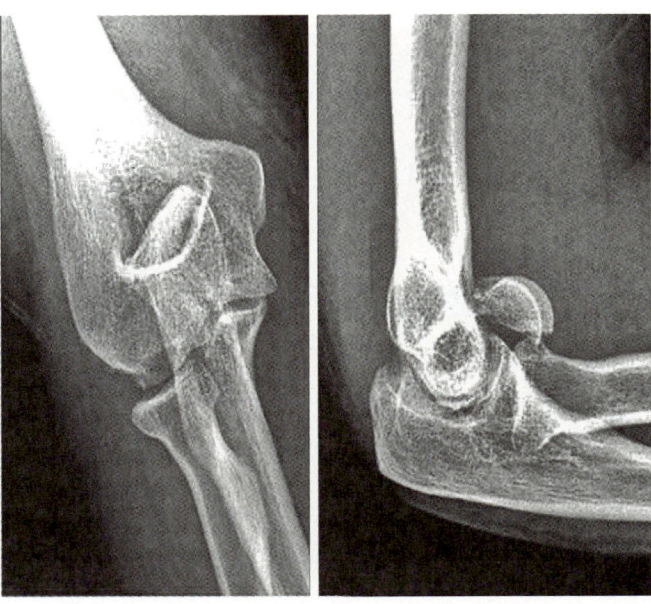

Fig. 10.4: Capitellum fracture

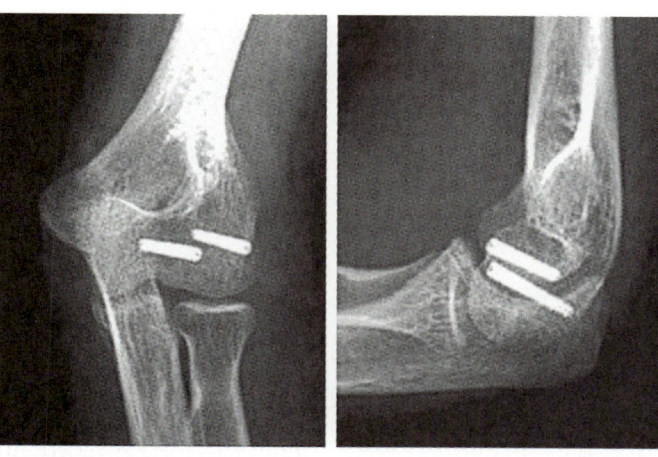

Fig. 10.5: Capitellum fracture treated with ORIF using Herbert screws

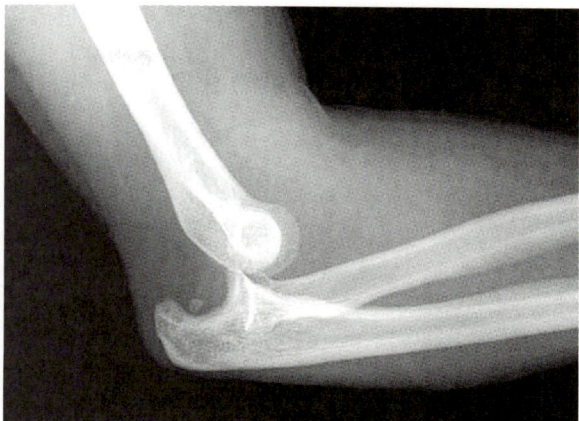

Fig 10.6: Posterior dislocation of elbow

ELBOW DISLOCATION

Elbow dislocations are among the most commonly seen dislocations in the body, second in frequency only to dislocations of the shoulder and the fingers. 90% are posterior dislocations.

Posterior Dislocation

Mechanism of Injury:
Fall on the extended and abducted arm.

Examination

1. Pain with the upper limb held in flexion
2. The olecranon is prominent posteriorly
3. The triceps tendon appears taut like a cord (*cord sign*)
4. Swelling and deformity at the joint
5. It is important to differentiate between dislocation and supracondylar fracture on examination. If one palpates the two epicondyles and the tip of the olecranon in patients with a supracondylar fracture they will be in the same plane, whereas with dislocations, the olecranon will be displaced from the plane of the epicondyles on palpation.

Imaging

Plain radiographs are diagnostic, and reveal an empty olecranon fossa posterior to the distal humerus (Fig. 10.6). Associated fractures include the coronoid process, radial head, and occasionally the humeral epicondyles or capitellum. Small fractures of the coronoid are common and should not impact management. When both the coronoid and radial head are fractured in a posterior elbow dislocation, the injury is referred to as the *"terrible triad"*.

Associated Injuries

1. Ulnar nerve injury occurs in 8 to 21% of patients, hence function should be checked before and after reduction.
2. Injury to the brachial artery (rare).

Treatment

Early reduction under anaesthesia is advocated, as delay may damage the articular cartilage or result in excessive swelling or circulatory compromise. One must be careful to avoid forceful manipulation during reduction, as this can result in myositis ossificans.

After reduction of the elbow, the ligaments are stress tested and the elbow is immobilized at 90° in a long-arm posterior splint for 3 weeks.

Complications

1. *Neurovascular injuries:* The most common are ulnar nerve injuries that usually resolve with conservative management.
2. *Post-traumatic joint stiffness:* Loss of the terminal 15° of elbow extension after dislocation is common.
3. *Heterotopic ossification:* This is common after posterior elbow dislocation (>75% of patients), but limits motion in <5%.
4. Lateral elbow instability.

Anterior Dislocations

Anterior dislocations are far less common, occurring from a blow to the flexed elbow that drives the olecranon forward.

On examination, the arm appears shortened and the forearm is elongated and held in supination. The elbow is usually held in full extension. The olecranon fossa is often palpable anteriorly.

All of these patients should be splinted, and the vascular and neurologic status assessed. Many of these dislocations are open, and vascular damage is quite common. Complete avulsion of the triceps mechanism is another commonly associated soft-tissue injury.

OLECRANON FRACTURES

All fractures of the olecranon should be considered intra-articular and to have disrupted the integrity of the joint (Fig. 10.7).

Classification

1. Transverse
2. Oblique
3. Comminuted

Mechanism of Injury

1. Direct blow: Results in a comminuted fracture.
2. Indirectly, a fall on the outstretched hand: results in a transverse or oblique fracture (Fig. 10.7).

Associated Injuries

1. Ulnar nerve injury
2. Elbow dislocation
3. Concomitant fractures of the radial head, radial shaft, and distal humerus.

Treatment

Nondisplaced

Nondisplaced fractures are those fractures with <2 mm of separation or articular incongruity. These are treated with immobilization in a long-arm splint with the elbow in extension and the forearm in supination.

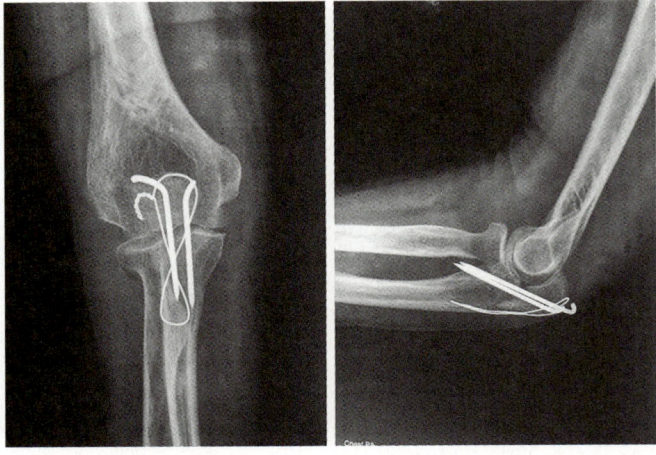

Fig. 10.8: Olecranon fracture treated with ORIF using K wires and TBW

Displaced Fractures

They require open reduction and internal fixation using K wires and tension band wire (TBW) (Fig. 10.8) or specialized hook plates.

RADIAL HEAD AND NECK FRACTURES

Mechanism of Injury

The most common mechanism is a fall on the outstretched hand (indirect). With the elbow in extension the force drives the radius against the capitellum, resulting in a marginal or radial neck fracture. As the force increases, comminution, dislocation, or displacement may occur . The fracture pattern in adults and children is variable, due to differences in the strength of the proximal radius. In adults, marginal or comminuted fractures of the radial head or neck with articular involvement are common (Fig. 10.9). In children, displacement of the radial

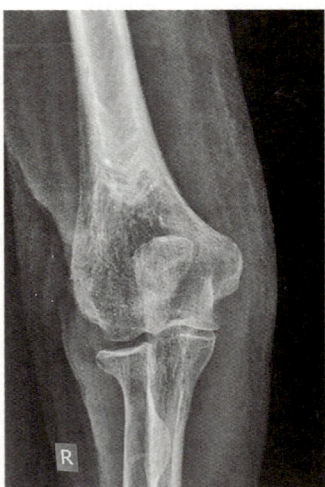
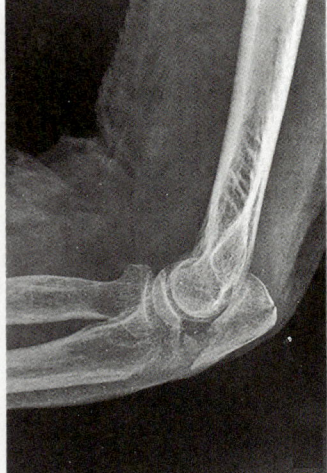

Fig. 10.7: Olecranon fracture

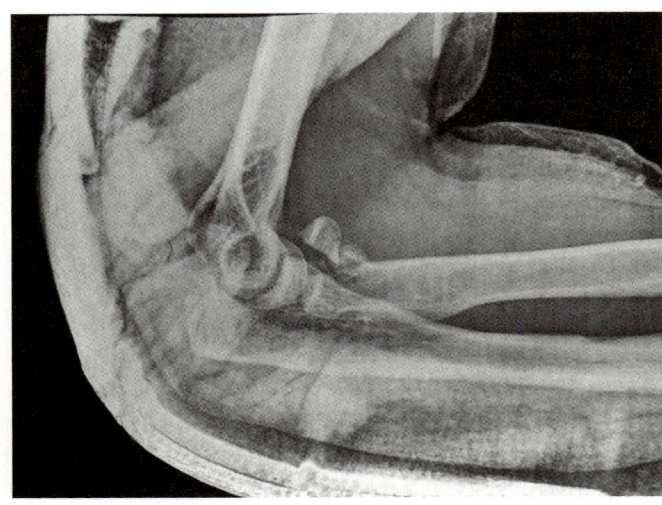

Fig. 10.9: Radial head fracture

epiphysis is common, whereas articular involvement is rare.

Examination

Tenderness is present over the radial head with swelling secondary to haemarthrosis. Pain is exacerbated by supination and associated with reduced mobility. Children with epiphyseal injuries may have very little swelling, but pain will be elicited with palpation or motion. If the patient has associated wrist pain, disruption of the distal radioulnar joint should be suspected (*Essex Lopresti lesion*).

Mason Classification for
Radial Head Fractures (Table 10.1)

Table 10.1: Classification of radial head fractures (Fig. 10.10)		
Type	Displacement	Description
I	Nondisplaced, less than 2 mm of articular step-off	No block to movement
II	Displaced more than 2 mm	Internal fixation possible
III	Displaced, severely comminuted	Usually irreparable; often requires excision to allow elbow movement

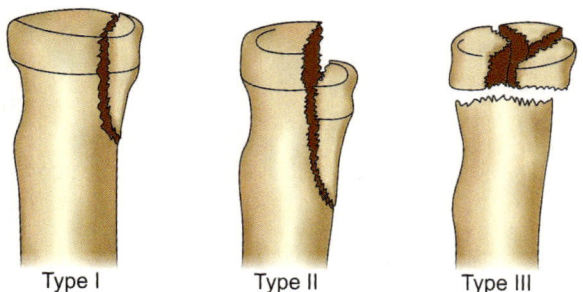

Type I   Type II   Type III

Fig. 10.10: Mason classification

Treatment

Marginal (Intra-articular)

Nondisplaced: Marginal radial head fractures with displacement of <2 mm (marginal fractures or minimal depression fractures) are treated with a sling or a long-arm posterior splint for 3 to 4 days. Early motion exercises are recommended if pain can be tolerated.

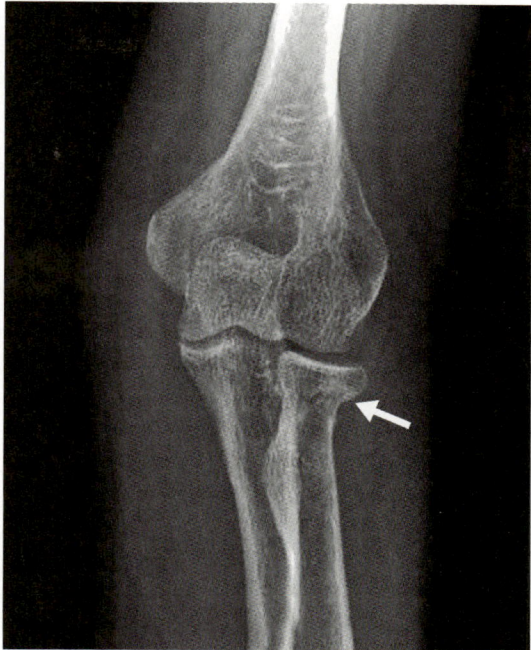

Fig. 10.11: Radial neck fracture

Displaced: When there is displacement or depression of >2 mm with over one-third of the articular surface involved, operative treatment is required. Displaced fractures with less than one-third of the articular surface involved are reduced and fixed with Herbert screws and followed by early motion.

Neck

Non-displaced: Neck fractures without displacement and angulation of <30° are treated with immobilization in a sling or a long-arm posterior splint (Fig. 10.11).

Displaced: With angulation >30° or significant displacement, operative fixation using specially designed T shaped plate is recommended.

Comminuted

Non-displaced: Non-displaced comminuted fractures of the head and neck can be treated conservatively with a long-arm posterior splint. Early motion exercises are recommended.

Displaced: With severe comminution of the head, excision of fragments or a prosthetic head replacement are the recommended therapies.

Paediatric Elbow Injuries

The elbow is a common site for fractures in children. The typical history is a fall on the outstretched hand with hyperextension at the elbow and resultant injury to the distal humerus.

Radiologic evaluation of a child's elbow is made more complicated because of the six ossification centres around the elbow, which appear at different ages (Table 11.1). So, comparison with opposite side X-ray is often helpful to differentiate between fracture fragment and ossification centre.

Table 11.1: "CRITOE" age of appearance of ossification centres around elbow (Fig. 11.1)	
Capitellum	1 to 8 months
Radial head	3 to 5 years
Internal (medial) epicondyle	5 to 7 years
Trochlea	7 to 9 years
Olecranon	8 to 11 years
External (lateral) epicondyle	11 to 14 years

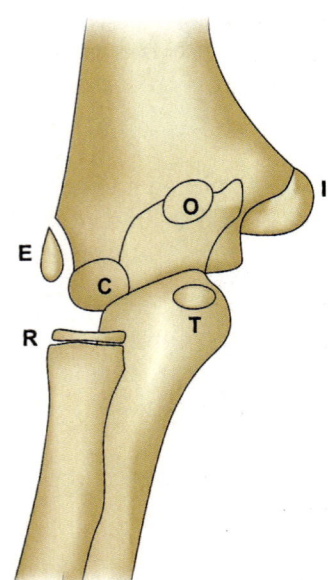

Fig. 11.1: Ossification centres around elbow

SUPRACONDYLAR HUMERUS FRACTURE

Supracondylar fractures are extra-articular, account for 50 to 70% of all elbow fractures, and are most commonly seen in children between the ages of 3 and 11 years.

Mechanism of Injury

1. Indirect Injury

After fall on outstretched hand, elbow goes into hyperextension due to ligament laxity and the force is transmitted through olecranon process onto olecranon fossa leading to supracondylar fracture (*extension type*) (Fig. 11.2).

2. Direct Injury

Fall on a flexed elbow can also lead to supracondylar fracture (*flexion type*).

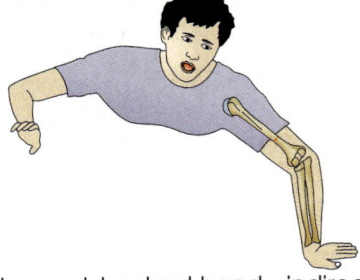

Fig. 11.2: Fall on outstreched hand—indirect injury

Classification

Extension type: Around 98%
Flexion type: Around 2% (Fig. 11.5)
Each type is further classified by *Gartland* (Fig. 11.3).

Type I: Non-displaced or minimally displaced.
Type II: Only one cortex fractured and angulation of the distal fragment.
Type III: Fractures of both cortices and are completely displaced (Fig. 11.4).
Type IV: Like type III but extremely unstable in flexion and extension.

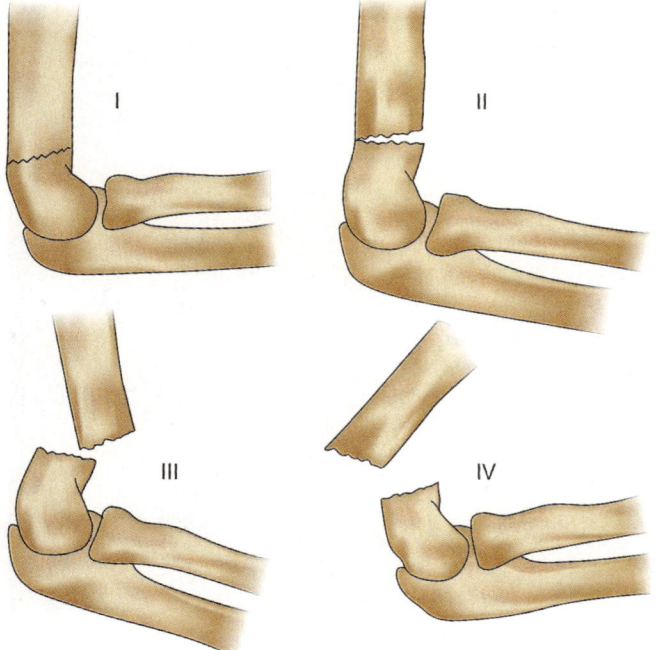

Fig. 11.3: Gartland classification

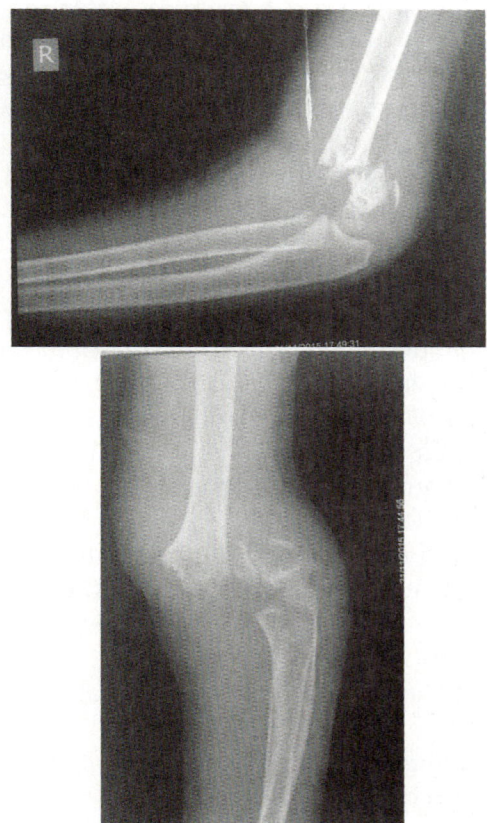

Fig. 11.4: Type III supracondylar humerus fracture

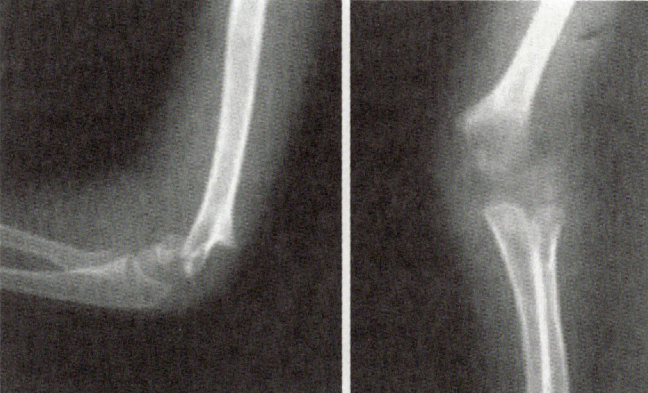

Fig. 11.5: Flexion type supracondylar humerus fracture

2. In early presentation, the displaced distal humeral fragment can often be palpated posteriorly and superiorly because of the pull of the triceps muscle. As swelling increases, this injury can easily be confused with a posterior dislocation of the elbow resulting from the prominence of the olecranon and the presence of a posterior concavity. In supracondylar humerus fracture 3 point bony relationship is maintained, while in posterior elbow dislocation it is disturbed.

3. The involved forearm may appear shorter when compared with the uninvolved side.

4. Detailed examination of radial and ulnar artery pulses, capillary circulation of hand and examination of all the three nerves of upper limb is must in supracondylar humerus fracture. These fractures are frequently associated with neurovascular complications, even in the absence of displacement. The most commonly injured structures are the anterior interosseous component of median nerve and the brachial artery. These structures are injured either due to sharp spike from proximal fragment or due to compartment syndrome secondary to fracture (Fig. 11.6).

Imaging

Routine views must include AP and lateral projections with comparison to the uninvolved extremity in children.

Subtle changes, such as the presence of an abnormal fat pad sign, may be the only radiographic clue to the presence of a fracture especially type 1 (Fig. 11.7).

Elevation of the fat pad in the coronoid fossa (anterior fat pad sign) and olecranon fossa (posterior fat pad sign more reliable than anterior) occur due to an effusion from trauma.

Examination

1. General signs of fracture like swelling, tenderness, crepitus are present. The typical deformity in extension type is 'S'shaped deformity.

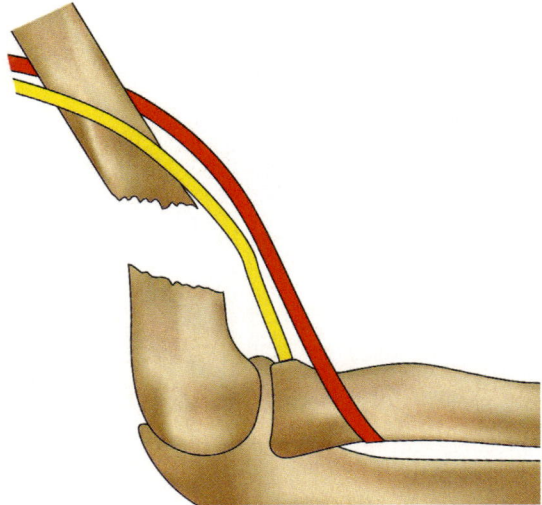

Fig. 11.6: Sharp spike of proximal fragment impinging neurovascular structures

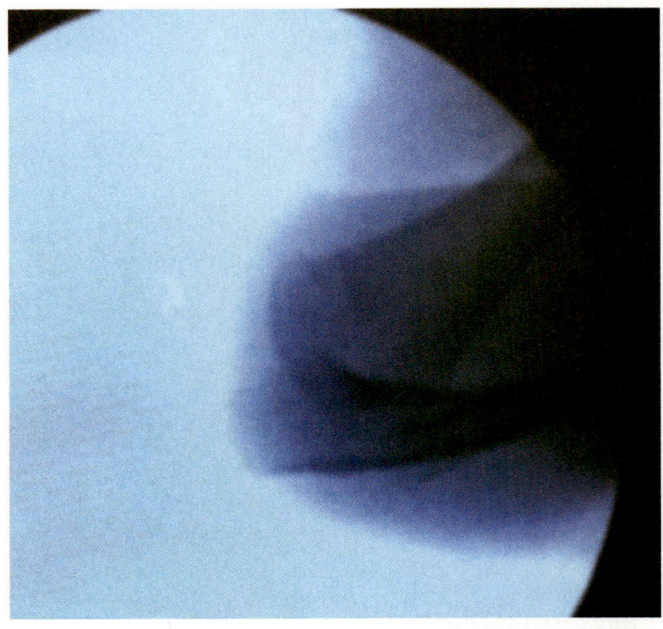

Fig. 11.8: Jones view

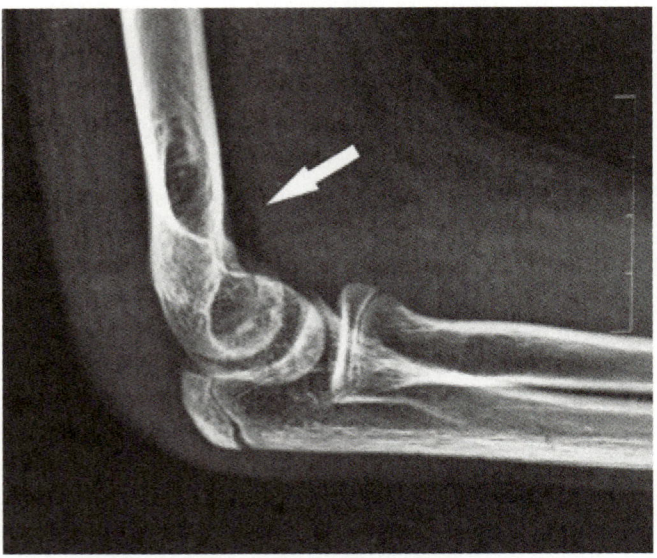

Fig. 11.7: Fat pad sign

Specialized view known as *Jones view* is AP view taken with elbow in hyperflexion. It is useful intra-operatively to judge the reduction (Fig. 11.8).

Treatment

Non-displaced (type I) fractures are treated with immobilization for 3 weeks in a posterior long-arm splint with the elbow in over 90° of flexion. The distal pulses should be checked and, if absent, the elbow is to be extended 5° to 15° or until the pulses return.

Type 2 fracture should be close reduced under anaesthesia and immobilized in above elbow cast. Extension type fracture should be immobilized in flexion and flexion types fractures should be immobilized in extension of elbow. Distal pulses should be checked as in type 1 fractures after reduction. Repeated X-rays are taken to check for loss of reduction. If primary reduction is unstable or it is lost subsequently then re-reduction and percutaneous pinning should be done.

Type 3 fractures should be close reduced under anaesthesia and fixed using either cross K wires (Fig. 11.9) or lateral divergent K wires.

Reduction technique for extension type supracondylar humerus fracture (Fig. 11.10).

A. Patient under general anaesthesia in supine position. Reduction is done under C arm imaging.
B. *Dis-impaction:* With assistant giving countertraction by holding patient's proximal arm, surgeon holds the hand and gives traction in extension of elbow to disimpact fragments.
C. *Reduction:* Surgeon now gives pressure on olecranon process to correct the extension. With this pressure maintained, he flexes the elbow more than 90 degrees.
D. *Locking:* The reduction is held by final pronation of the forearm.

It is mandatory to check distal pulses after reduction, before proceeding for pinning.

Open Reduction with Internal Fixation

Indications

1. Inability to achieve a satisfactory closed reduction
2. Complicating fractures of the forearm
3. Vascular compromise

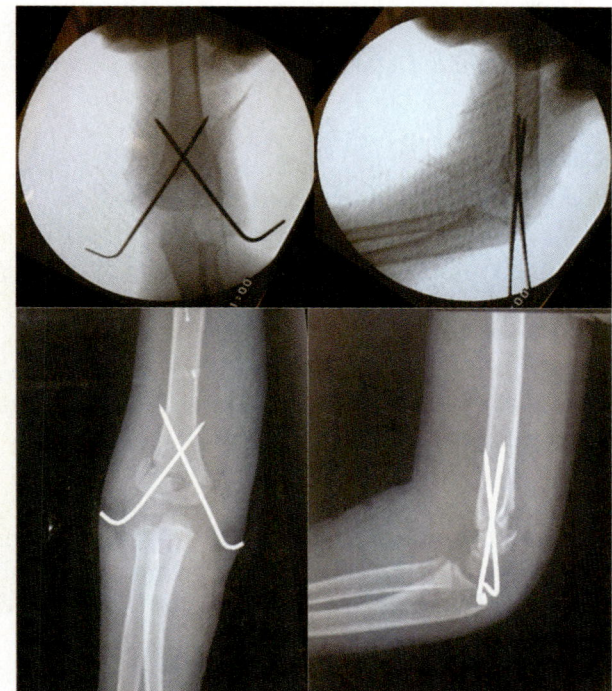

Fig. 11.9: Supracondylar fracture treated with closed reduction and cross K wires

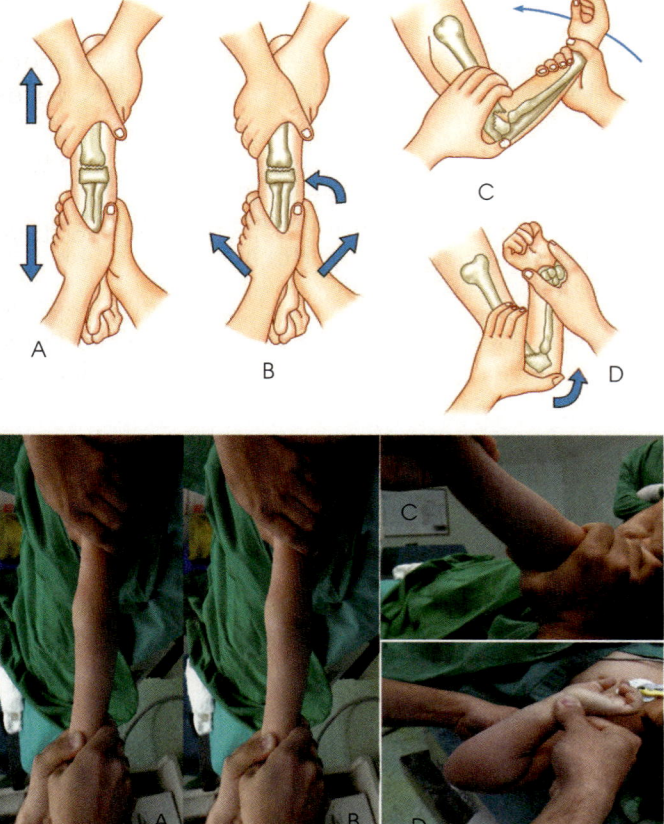

Fig. 11.10A to D: Reduction technique for extension type fracture

Complications

This fracture is also known as fracture of complications.

Early Complications

1. *Neurological injuries* (7 to 10%): Anterior interosseous component of median nerve is commonest nerve involved followed by radial nerve. Ulnar nerve injuries are seen in flexion type of fractures. Most of the injuries are neuropraxia and recover spontaneously.

   The causes of nerve injuries can be injury due to prominent bone spikes, traction or entrapment in fracture during reduction, ischaemia due to compartment syndrome or entrapment in the callus.

2. *Vascular injury* (0.5%): This may be direct injury or secondary to swelling in antecubital fossa. After reduction of fracture even if pulses are absent but hand is well perfused, only observation is recommended. If perfusion is also compromised, then it demands urgent open reduction and repair of artery.

3. *Compartment syndrome:* This is rare complication occurring most commonly due to immobilisation in hyperflexion.

Late Complications

1. *Malunion:*

   Cubitus varus or gun stock deformity: This is a common complication of improperly treated supracondylar fracture. Normally the long axis of forearm forms a valgus of 10 to 15 degrees with long axis of arm. This is known as *carrying angle* and this is necessary for clearing pelvis while walking.

   Usually in supracondylar humerus fracture, there is comminution on posteromedial aspect.So non-anatomical reduction, improper fixation or inadequate immobilisation can lead to malunion with varus, extension and internal rotation of distal fragment. If amount of varus is less then there is just loss of carrying angle. If varus is significant then there is gun stock deformity. This deformity is non-progressive (Fig. 11.11).

   Treatment: Extension deformity usually remodels well, so can be observed. Gun stock deformity however; doesn't remodel and requires corrective lateral close wedge osteotomy(French osteotomy), step-cut osteotomy or dome osteotomy (Fig. 11.12).

2. *Myositis ossificans:* occurs due to repeated attempts of close reduction or massaging. It restricts range of motion.

3. *Stiffness:* It is not common as fracture is extra-articular.

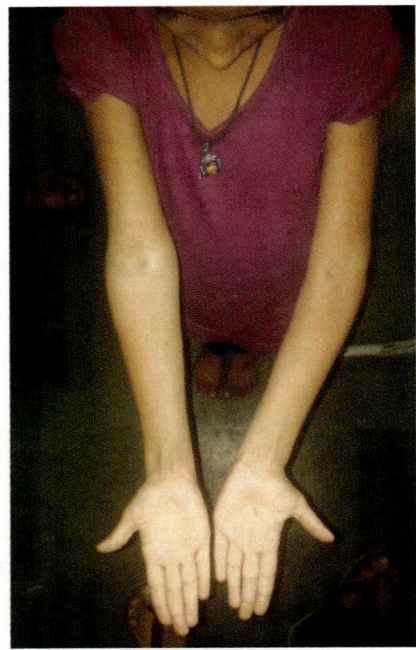

Fig. 11.11: Cubitus varus or gun stock deformity

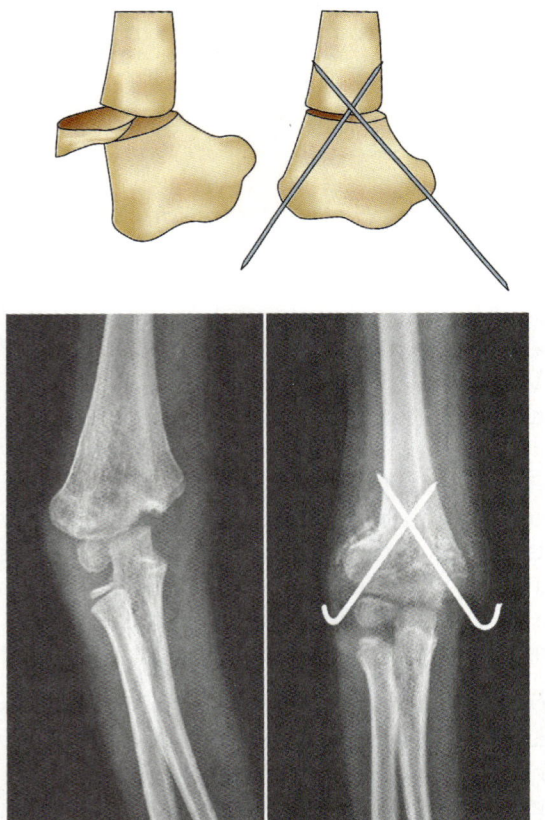

Fig. 11.12: Corrective lateral close wedge osteotomy for cubitus varus

4. *Avascular necrosis of trochlea:* Extremely rare complication leading to progressive cubitus varus and fish tail deformity of trochlea.

LATERAL CONDYLE FRACTURE

It is intra-articular distal humerus fracture, also known as *fracture of necessity.*

Mechanism

Pull theory: Due to pull of extensors attached to it.
Push theory: Fall on outstreched hand; load being transmitted from radial head to lateral condyle.

Examination

Symptoms and signs at times can be very subtle due to deeper location. But the 3 point relationship is disturbed in this fracture.

Imaging

Apart from routine AP and lateral X-rays, internal oblique view, varus stress view and arthrogram can be useful to differentiate between normal ossification centre and fracture of lateral condyle.

Classification

Milch Classification (Fig. 11.13)

Type 1: Salter Harris type 4 injury. Fracture line courses lateral to trochlea. It is a stable fracture as trochlea is intact.

Type 2: Salter Harris type 2 injury. Fracture line extends into apex of trochlea. It is an unstable fracture.

Treatment

Nonoperative: Undisplaced or minimally displaced (<2 mm) can be treated in above elbow cast with elbow in 90 degree flexion and forearm in neutral for 4 weeks followed by mobilization.

Operative: Displaced fractures need open reduction and internal fixation using K wires or cancellous screw to maintain articular congruity.

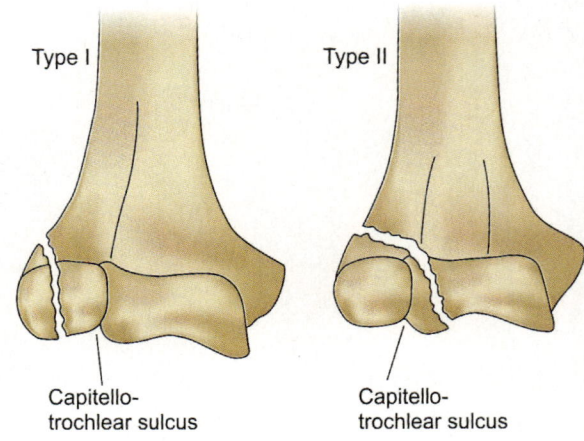

Fig. 11.13: Milch classification

Complications

1. *Delayed union and nonunion:* Common complication as fracture is intra-articular being bathed by synovial fluid and there is continuous pull of extensors (Fig. 11.14). Also the blood supply to lateral condyle is precarious.
2. *Malunion:* Leading to cubitus valgus deformity. Since ulnar nerve passes behind medial epicondyle, valgus deformity causes gradual stretching of ulnar nerve *(Tardy ulnar nerve palsy).* This may lead to sensory symptoms in ulnar nerve distribution. Motor deficits are rare.

   This can be treated by transposition of the ulnar nerve anterior to medial epicondyle.
3. *Cubitus pseudo-varus* occurs due to ossification of the raised lateral periosteal flap leading to lateral condyle prominence.
4. *Osteonecrosis of trochlea and fishtail deformity:* Usually iatrogenic complication due to excessive dissection.

NURSEMAID'S/PULLED ELBOW

Nursemaid's elbow (radial head subluxation) is a common orthopaedic injury occurring in early childhood. The peak incidence is in the toddler years; however, the condition does occur in the first year of life and has been described as late as 6 years of age. The annular ligament provides support for the radial head, maintaining the head in its normal relationship with the humerus and the ulna. In children, there is little structural support between the radius and the humerus. With sudden traction of the hand or the forearm usually occurring when a parent pulls a child up by the arm to prevent a fall, the annular ligament is pulled over the radial head and is interposed between the radius and the capitellum (Fig. 11.15).

Children with nursemaid's elbow present because of disuse of the affected arm and will be noted to hold the arm at their side with the forearm in a pronated position. It is important to note that patients with nursemaid's elbow do not have swelling, warmth, or ecchymosis about the elbow.

Treatment

Two different methods are commonly used for reducing a nursemaid's elbow.

Hyperpronation Technique

The hyperpronation method involves the examiner cradling the child's elbow with one hand (with thumb or forefingers overlying the radial head) while the other hand is used to hyperpronate the child's forearm by holding and turning the child's hand into a hyperpronated position. With successful reduction, a "click" will be felt about the child's elbow by the examiner.

Supination/Flexion Technique

The supination/flexion technique involves the examiner cradling the child's elbow with one hand (again with thumb or forefingers over the radial head) and supinating the patient's hand completely. The examiner then fully flexes the child's elbow by bringing the supinated hand up toward the shoulder. With successful reduction, a "click" will be felt near the elbow.

Regardless of which reduction technique is used, the child will typically begin to use the arm normally within 15 minutes.

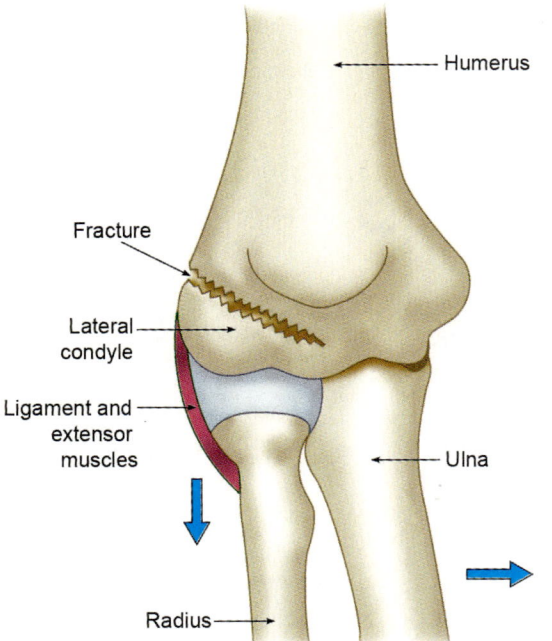

Fig. 11.14: Deforming forces on lateral condyle fracture

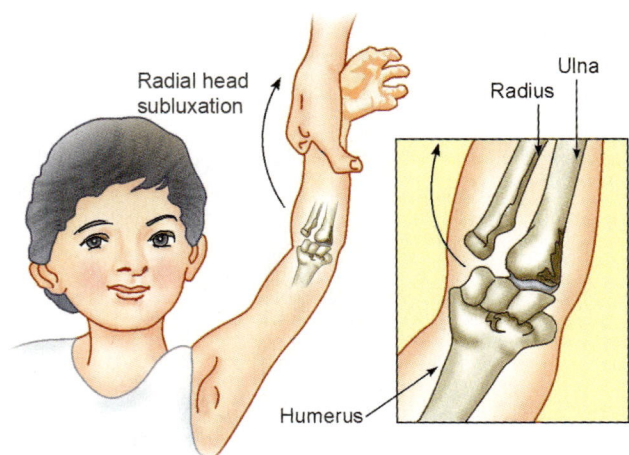

Fig. 11.15: Pulled elbow

Forearm Fractures

Essential Anatomy

Forearm is formed by 2 bones, radius and ulna.

These bones are bound together by joint capsules at the elbow and the wrist. Additionally, they are attached at their proximal ends by the anterior and posterior radioulnar ligaments. Distally, the radioulnar ligaments form a joint that contains a fibrocartilaginous articular disc. Throughout the mid shaft of both bones is a strong interconnecting fibrous interosseous membrane (Fig. 12.1).

The forearm is like a ring; a fracture that shortens either the radius or ulna results either in fracture or dislocation of fellow bone either at proximal or distal radioulnar joint.

When considering treatment of these fractures, careful attention must be paid to the maintenance of length and alignment. The ulna is a fixed straight bone around which the radius rotates. The radius, to the contrary, has a lateral bow that must be preserved to allow full pronation and supination after healing.

The shafts of the radius and the ulna are surrounded by four primary muscle groups whose pull frequently results in fracture displacement or nullification of an adequate reduction (Fig. 12.2).

RADIAL SHAFT FRACTURES

Radial shaft fractures can be divided into three groups on the basis of muscular attachments and consequent fragment displacement after a fracture.

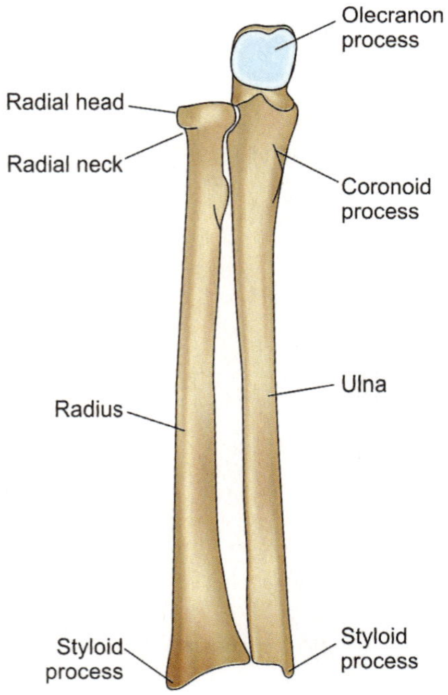

Fig. 12.1: Anatomy of forearm

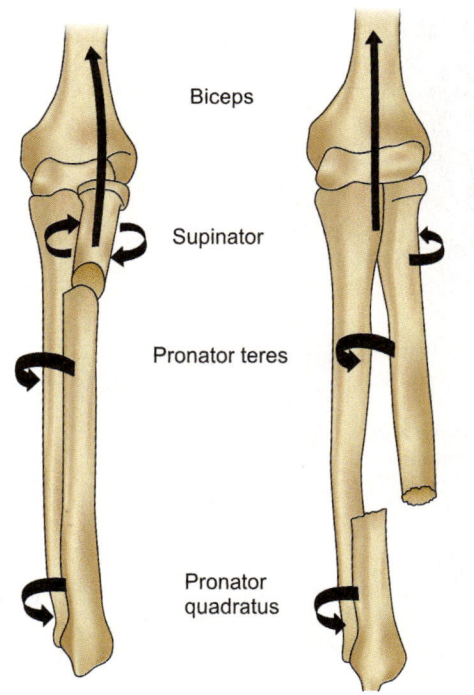

Fig. 12.2: Deforming forces of forearm fracture

- *Proximal one-third* just distal to the insertion of the supinator and the biceps brachii where both of these muscles exert a supinating force
- *Middle one-third* where the pronator teres exerts a pronating force.
- *Distal one-third* where the pronator quadratus exerts a pronating force on the fracture fragment.

Mechanism of Injury

Usually a fall from standing height, a direct blow or a road traffic accident.

Examination

Tenderness is present along the fracture site and can be elicited with direct palpation or longitudinal compression. Tenderness over the distal radioulnar joint may be secondary to subluxation or dislocation and should alert the emergency physician to the possibility of a *Galeazzi fracture* (fracture of radius with dislocation of distal radioulnar joint).

Imaging

Routine anteroposterior (AP) and lateral views including elbow and wrist are usually adequate (Fig. 12.3).

There are four reliable radiographic signs of injury to the distal radioulnar joint:
1. Fracture of the base of the ulnar styloid.
2. AP view: Widening of the distal radioulnar joint space.

3. Lateral view: Dislocation of the distal radius relative to the ulna.
4. Shortening of the radius by >5 mm.

Treatment

Nonoperative

Undisplaced fracture in adults can be treated with well moulded above elbow cast. Proximal third fractures are immobilized in supination, middle third in neutral and distal third in pronation to neutralize the deforming muscular forces.

In children most of the fractures are treated conservatively.

Operative

Displaced fractures in adult demand open reduction and internal fixation using dynamic compression plate.

In children if acceptable closed reduction is not possible or if it is unstable then it can be treated using specially designed intramedullary nails.

Galeazzi fracture dislocation requires urgent reduction of fracture as well as distal radioulnar joint either by closed or open method.

ULNA FRACTURE

This can be either isolated fracture or associated with dislocation of proximal radioulnar joint i.e. Monteggia fracture dislocation (Fig.12.4).

Mechanism of Injury

1. A direct blow is the most common mechanism, and the resulting fracture is often referred to as a *"nightstick fracture,"* because it appears as if an individual was holding up the arm to protect the face from being struck by a nightstick. This mechanism is common in automobile accidents or fights.
2. Excessive pronation or supination can also result in ulnar shaft fractures.

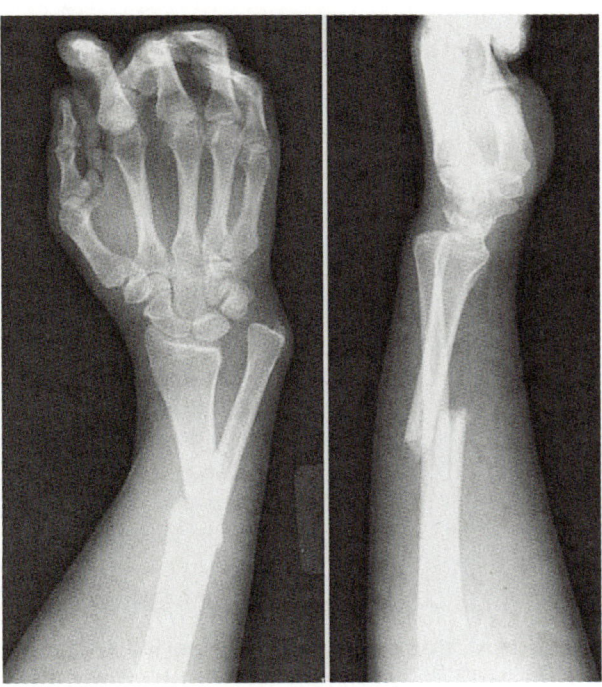

Fig. 12.3: Galeazzi fracture dislocation

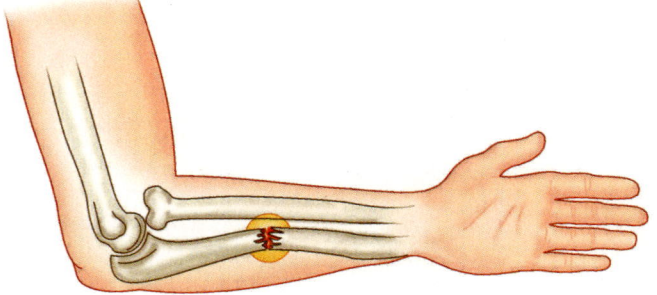

Fig. 12.4: Monteggia fracture dislocation

Monteggia fractures are due to forces that fracture the ulna and dislocate the radial head. These injuries do not require high-energy forces, and can occur after low-energy mechanisms such as falls.

Examination

Swelling and tenderness to palpation are evident over the fracture site. Pronation and supination will be painful.

Monteggia fractures often will reveal shortening of the forearm due to angulation. The radial head may be palpable in the antecubital fossa following anterior dislocations.

Imaging

AP and lateral views will generally demonstrate the fracture. In any fracture of the ulna, especially proximal fractures, it is important to evaluate the *radiocapitellar line* on the lateral radiograph. A line drawn down the centre of the shaft and head of the radius should intersect the middle of the capitellum, irrespective of the position of elbow in flexion-extention. If this intersection does not occur, the proximal radioulnar joint is disrupted (Fig. 12.5).

Treatment of Ulna Fracture

Nonoperative

Closed reduction and immobilization in above elbow cast gives excellent union in undisplaced and minimally displaced (<5 mm) fractures.

Operative

Open reduction internal fixation using dynamic compression plate is recommended for displaced fractures in adults (Fig. 12.6).

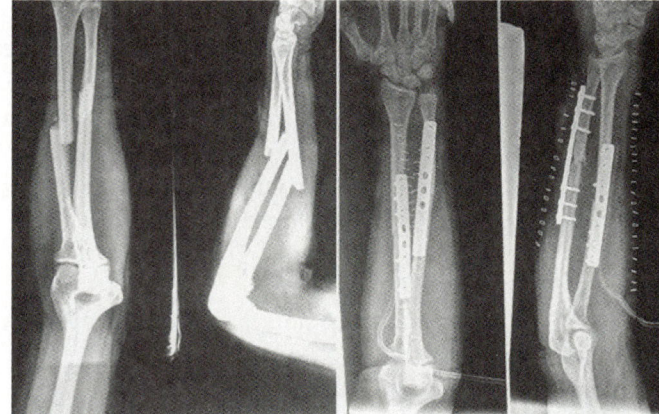

Fig. 12.6: Fracture of radius ulna treated with ORIF using DCP

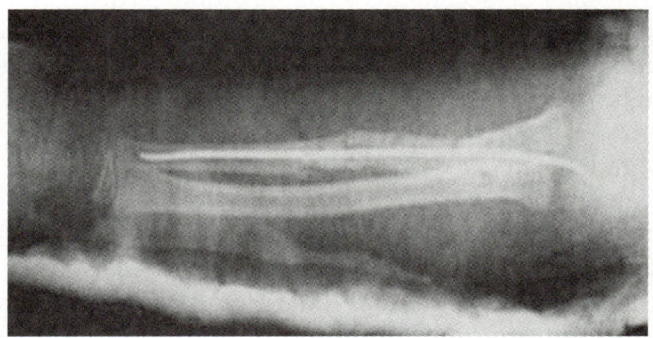

Fig. 12.7: Fracture ulna treated with CRIF using intra-medullary nail

In children if closed reduction is not possible or is unstable, then intramedullary nails can be inserted (Fig. 12.7).

MONTEGGIA FRACTURE DISLOCATION

Bado's Classification (Fig. 12.8 and Table 12.1)

Table 12.1: Classification of Monteggia fracture dislocation		
Type	Rate of occurrence	Description
I	60%	Anterior radial head dislocation, anterior angulation of ulna
II	15%	Posterior radial head dislocation, posterior angulation of ulna
III	20%	Lateral dislocation of the radial head, lateral angulation of ulna
IV	5%	Anterior radial head dislocation, both bones forearm fracture

In children, this requires urgent closed reduction of fracture as well as dislocation along with immobilization in above elbow cast.

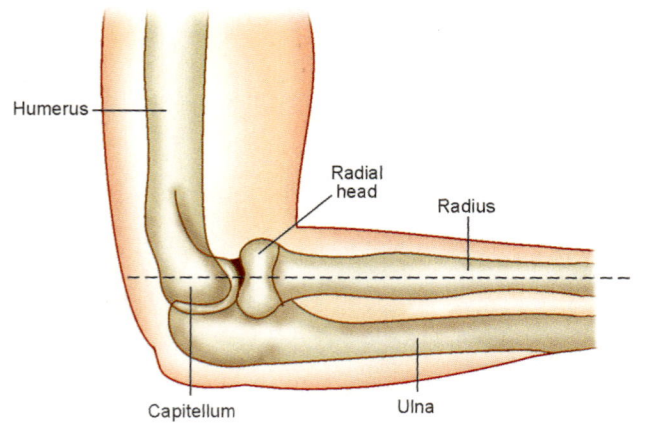

Fig. 12.5: Radio-capitellar line

Humerus

Radial head

Radius

Capitellum   Ulna

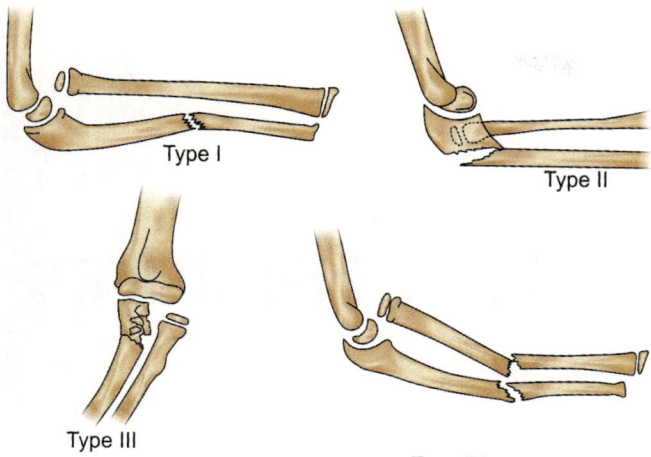

Type I

Type II

Type III

Type IV

Fig. 12.8: Bado's classification for Monteggia fracture dislocation

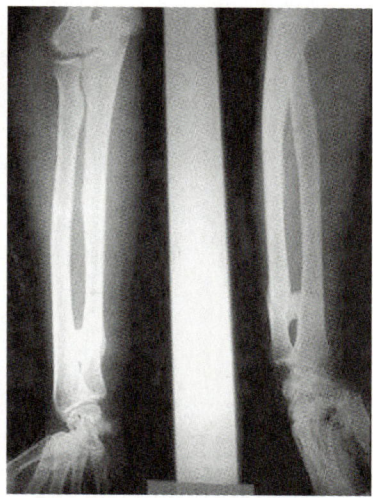

Fig. 12.9: Radio-ulnar synostosis following ulna fracture

Adults require open reduction internal fixation of ulna using dynamic compression plate. Anatomical reduction of fracture is mandatory; radial head usually reduces automatically with this. Rarely open reduction of radial head is required.

Complications

1. Infection is commonly seen with open fractures.
2. Nerve damage is uncommon in closed injuries, but is frequently seen with open fractures. There is an equal frequency of involvement between the radial, ulnar, and median nerves.

3. Vascular compromise is an uncommon complication because of the presence of arterial collaterals.
4. Non-union or malunion may be secondary to inadequate reduction or inadequate immobilization.
5. Compartment syndromes can occur following combined shaft fractures. It is important to recognize that distal pulses may remain intact despite elevated compartment pressures and compromised capillary flow. The treatment is emergent referral for fasciotomy.
6. Pronation and supination may be impaired if fractures are malunited or there is cross-union (Fig. 12.9).

Wrist Fractures

Essential Anatomy (Fig. 13.1)

1. Articulation between distal end of radius with scaphoid and lunate
2. Ulnar styloid process provides attachment to triangular fibrocartilage complex (TFCC). This TFCC in turn supports triquetrum.
3. Distal end of ulna articulates with sigmoid notch of radius.
4. 80% load is transmitted by radius and 20% by ulna.

DISTAL END RADIUS FRACTURES

These are among the most common fractures of upper limb. Though this can be seen even in toddler, incidence increases sharply in 6th decade due to osteoporosis especially in females.

Important Radiological Parameters (Fig. 13.2)

1. *Radial length/Ulnar variance*

   This is the most important parameter and correlates best clinically. This measurement is drawn

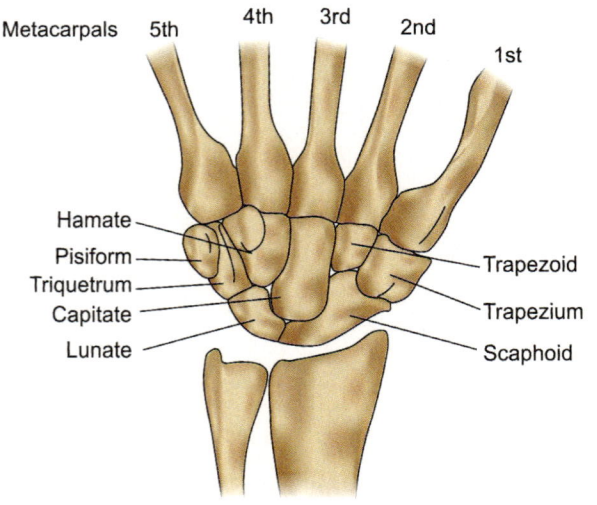

Fig. 13.1: Anatomy of wrist

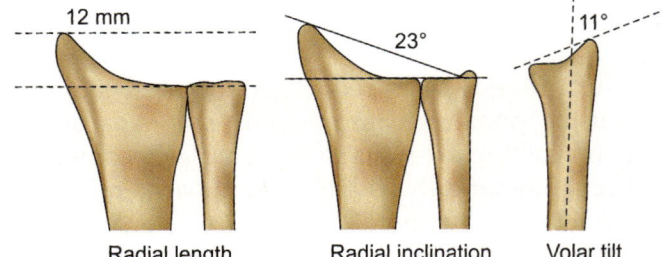

Fig. 13.2: Radiological parameters of distal radius–ulna

perpendicular to the radial shaft and is the distance from the tip of the radial styloid to the distal articular surface of the ulna. Normal radial length is 12 mm.

2. *Radial inclination*

   Usually distal radial angulation of the radioulnar joint, seen on the PA view of the wrist, is around 23°. The evaluation of this angle is essential when treating fractures of the distal forearm because failure or incomplete reduction with loss of this angle will result in an inhibition of ulnar deviation.

3. *Volar tilt*

   The normal radiocarpal joint angle on the lateral view is around 11° in a palmar direction.

Classification

Many classification systems are described for fractures of the distal radius. *Fernandez* classification is based on mechanism of injury and has added benefit of offering guidelines for treatment (Fig. 13.3). This system is as follows:

Type I   Extra-articular metaphyseal bending fractures—Colles (dorsal angulation) and Smith (volar angulation)

Type II   Intra-articular shearing fractures Barton (dorsal and volar)

Type III Intra-articular compression fractures Complex articular and radial pilon fractures

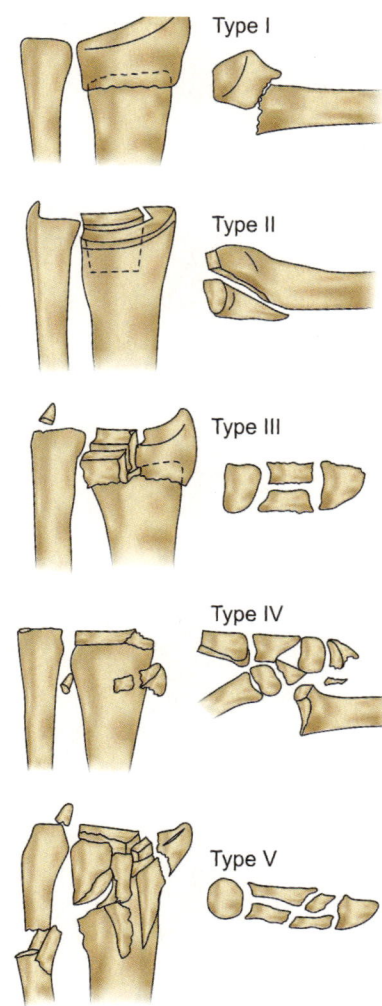

Fig. 13.3: Fernandez classification

Type IV	Avulsion fractures
	Radiocarpal fracture—dislocations
Type V	High-velocity mechanism with extensive injury

Frykman classification based on individual involvement of the radiocarpal and radioulnar joint.

Type I	Extra-articular fractures
Type II	Extra-articular fractures with ulnar styloid fracture
Type III	Radiocarpal articular involvement
Type IV	Radiocarpal articular involvement with ulnar styloid fracture
Type V	Radioulnar involvement
Type VI	Radioulnar involvement with ulnar styloid fracture
Type VII	Radiocarpal and radioulnar involvement
Type VIII	Radiocarpal and radioulnar involvement with ulnar styloid fracture

COLLES' FRACTURE

Classical Colles' fracture is extra-articular distal end radius fracture occurring at cortico-cancellous junction and is associated with classical displacements like dorsal tilt, dorsal shift, radial tilt, radial shift, impaction and supination (Fig. 13.4).

Mechanism of Injury

Most distal forearm fractures are the result of a fall on the outstretched hand (indirect mechanism). The amount of comminution and location of the fracture line is dependent on the force of the fall and the brittleness (age) of the bone.

Examination

Examination reveals pain, swelling, and tenderness of the distal forearm. The displaced angulated fracture typically resembles a *'dinner fork'* (Fig. 13.5). Documentation of the neurologic status with special emphasis on median nerve function should be stressed.

Imaging

PA and lateral views are usually sufficient for demonstrating the fracture fragments and one should always look for classical displacements described.

Associated Injuries

1. 60% are accompanied by ulnar styloid fractures.
2. Fractures of the ulnar neck.

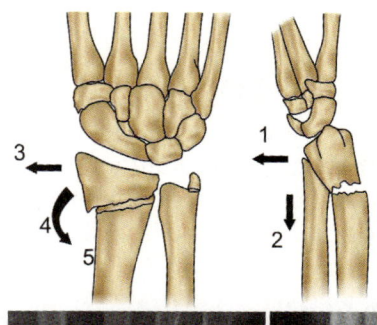

1. Dorsal tilt
2. Dorsal displacemet
3. Radial displacement
4. Radial tilt
5. Shortening

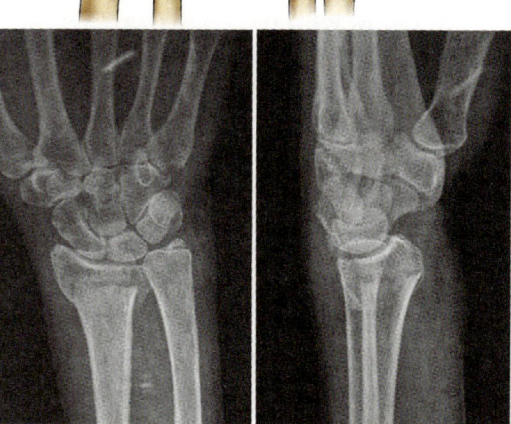

Fig. 13.4: Displacements in Colles' fracture

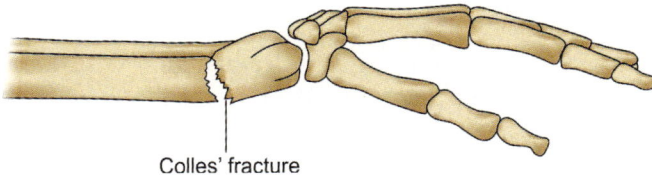

Colles' fracture

Fig. 13.5: Dinner fork deformity

3. Carpal fractures.
4. Distal radioulnar subluxation.
5. Flexor tendon injuries.
6. Median and ulnar nerve injury must be excluded. If the median nerve function is abnormal, carpal canal pressures should be documented to distinguish an acute carpal tunnel syndrome from a median nerve contusion.

Treatment

In reducing distal metaphyseal forearm fractures, three principles must be remembered:
1. Radial length is most important and easiest parameter to achieve.
2. The normal volar tilt is around 11°. Dorsal angulation is not acceptable.
3. The normal radial tilt is around 23°. The angle is easily achieved with reduction but difficult to maintain during the healing phase unless positioned properly. If the reduction cannot be maintained, internal fixation may be required.

Most of these fractures can be treated conservatively by closed reduction and immobilization in below elbow cast for 6 weeks.

Reduction Technique (Fig. 13.6)

1. Adequate anaesthesia should be provided with a haematoma block or procedural sedation.
2. Disimpaction. With assistant giving countertraction at arm, surgeon holds patient's hand in 'Shake hand' manner and gives traction to disimpact fragments. This achieves radial length.
3. While maintaining traction, pressure is applied over the distal fragment in a volar direction with the thumbs, and dorsally directed pressure over the proximal segment with the fingers.
4. The forearm is immobilized in a position of pronation or neutral position with the wrist in 15° of volar flexion and 15° of ulnar deviation.
5. The forearm is immobilized in well fitting and well moulded below elbow cast.
6. Post-reduction radiographs must be obtained to ensure proper positioning (Fig. 13.7A and B). In addition, after reduction the function of the median nerve must be documented.

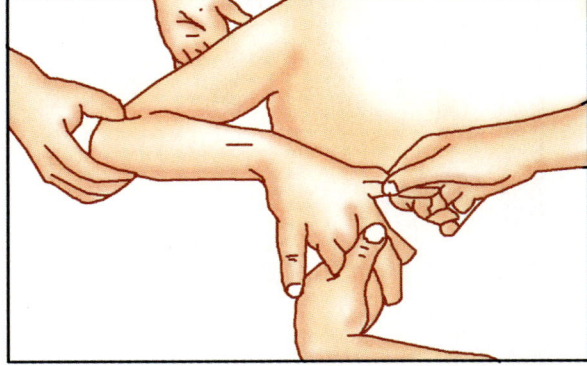

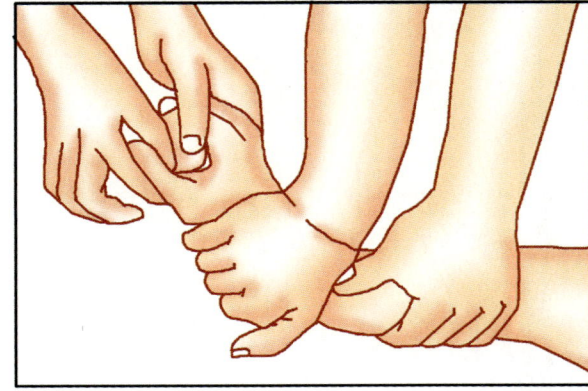

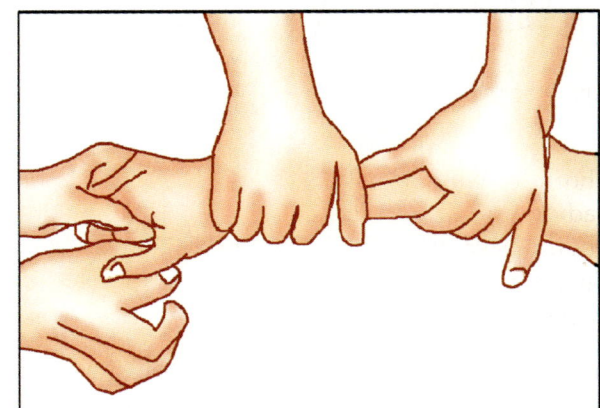

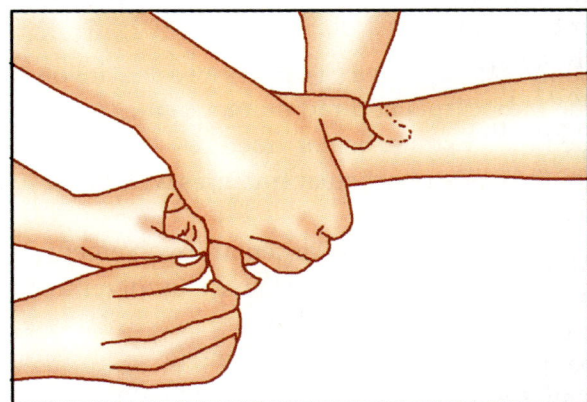

Fig. 13.6: Reduction technique for Colles' fracture

7. After reduction, the arm should remain elevated for 72 hours to keep swelling at a minimum. Finger and

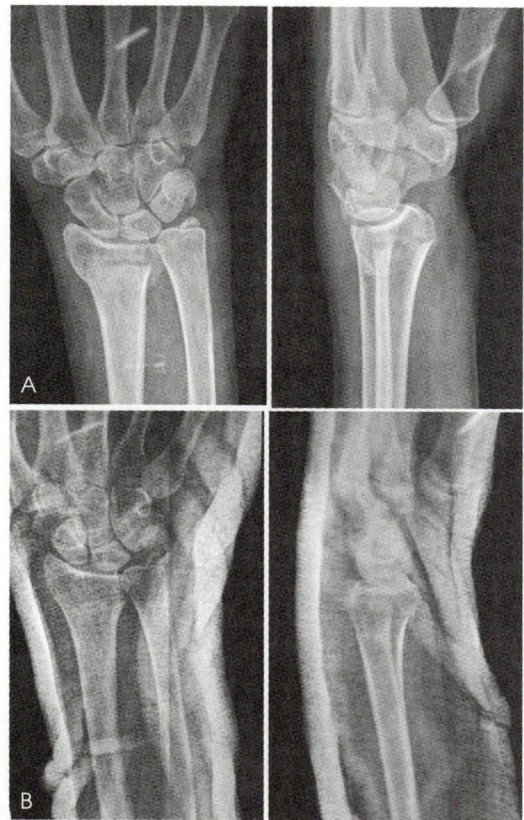

Fig. 13.7A and B: Colles' fracture treated using closed reduction and cast

shoulder exercises should begin immediately and radiographs for documentation of proper positioning should be obtained at 3 days and 2 weeks post-injury.
8. Severely comminuted fractures require additional percutaneous pinning (Fig. 13.8).

Complications

These are very common. Limitation of wrist function after these fractures has been reported as high as 90%. Early adequate reduction of the fracture is the most important means of avoiding complications. Complications of these fractures are described as early and late.

Early Complications

1. *Median nerve compression:* The patient will complain of pain and paresthesias over the distribution of the median nerve. If casted, the cast and padding should be split and the arm elevated for 48 to 72 hours. If the symptoms persist, a carpal tunnel syndrome should be suspected, and surgical release is then indicated.
2. Tendon damage secondary to trauma
3. Ulnar nerve contusion or compression must be diagnosed early.

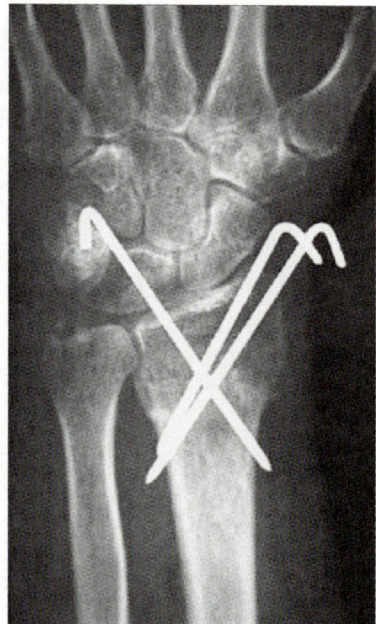

Fig. 13.8: Closed reduction and percutaneous K wires fixation

4. Post-reduction swelling with secondary compartment syndromes.
5. Fragment displacement after reduction and immobilization

Late Complications

1. Stiffness of the fingers, shoulder, or radiocarpal joint: *shoulder hand syndrome.*
2. Reflex sympathetic dystrophy.
3. Rupture of the extensor pollicis longus: *Drummer's palsy.*
4. *Malunion:* Secondary to inadequate immobilization or incomplete reduction.
5. Flexor tendon adhesions secondary to trauma and immobilization can be a debilitating complication.

SMITH'S FRACTURE

This fracture has often been described as a reverse Colles' fracture. It is an uncommon fracture, compared to Colles' fractures.

Mechanism of Injury

1. Fall on the supinated forearm with the hand in dorsiflexion, a punch with the fist clenched and the wrist slightly flexed (Fig. 13.9).
2. A direct blow to the dorsum of the wrist or distal radius with the hand flexed and the forearm in pronation.

Examination

Pain and swelling will be apparent over the volar aspect of the wrist. The clinical appearance of this fracture is

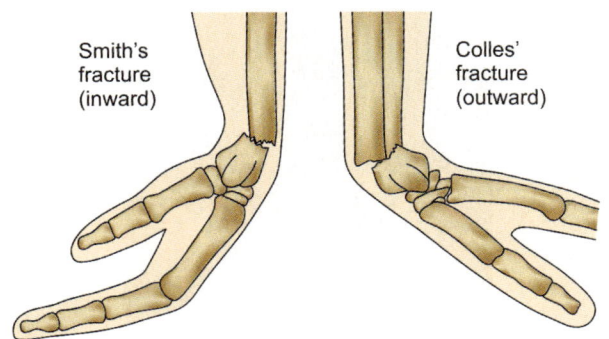

Fig. 13.9: Mechanism of injury: Colles' and Smith's fracture

Smith's fracture (inward)

Colles' fracture (outward)

described as a *'garden spade'* deformity. The presence and function of the radial artery and median nerve should be examined and documented (Fig. 13.10).

Imaging

Routine PA and lateral views are adequate for demonstrating this fracture (Fig. 13.11).

Treatment

Closed reduction under anaesthesia and immobilization in above elbow cast is recommended. Results are usually good.

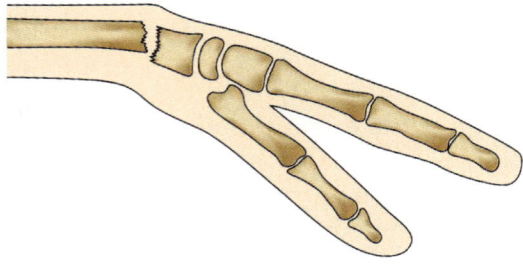

Fig. 13.10: Garden spade deformity

DORSAL AND VOLAR RIM FRACTURE (BARTON)

These fractures are intra-articular and involve the dorsal or volar rim of the radius (Figs 13.12 and 13.13)

Mechanism of Injury

Extreme dorsiflexion of the wrist accompanied by a pronating force may result in a dorsal rim fracture.

Examination

The distal dorsal radius is tender and swollen. Occasionally radial nerve sensory branch may be compromised and present as paresthesias in the area of distribution.

Imaging

Lateral radiographs adequately demonstrate the fracture fragment and the degree of displacement.

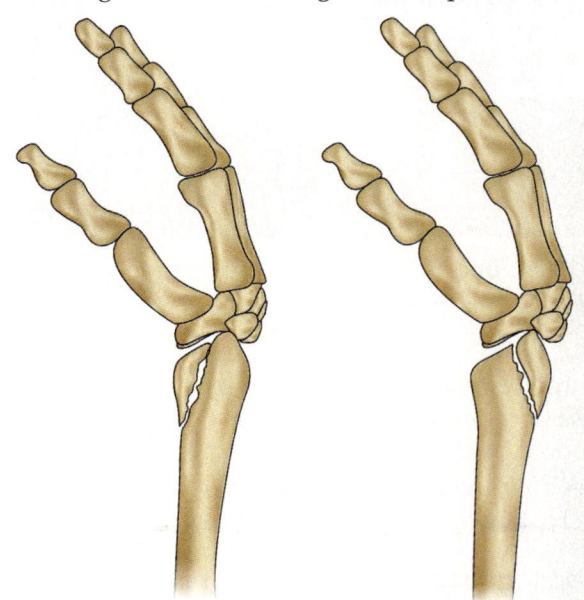

Fig. 13.12: Volar and dorsal Barton fracture

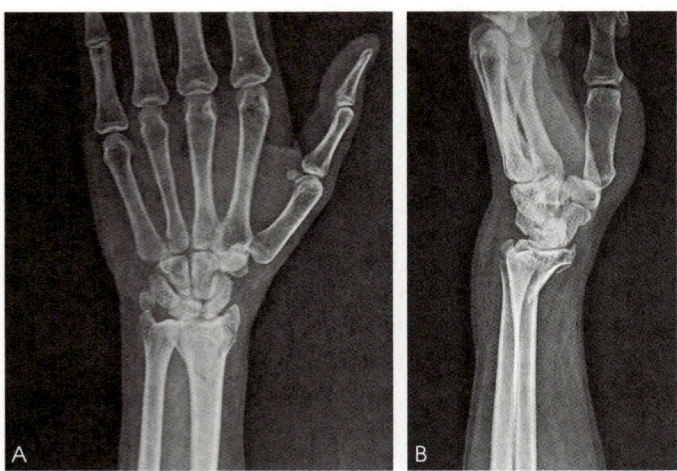

Fig. 13.11A and B: Smith's fracture

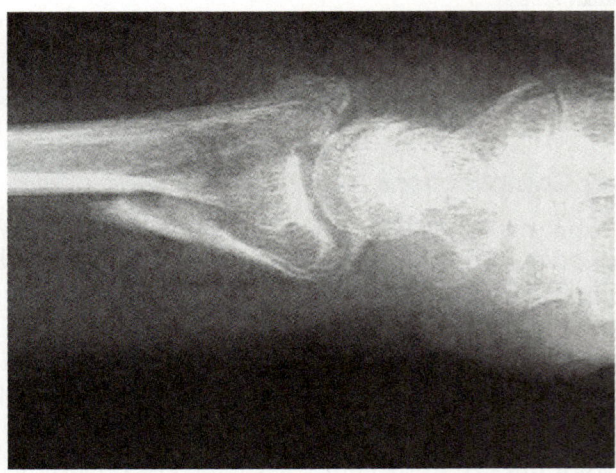

Fig. 13.13: Volar Barton fracture

Treatment

These are highly unstable fractures and often require open reduction and internal fixation.

Volar Barton is fixed using buttress plate (Fig. 13.14) while dorsal Barton is fixed using multiple K wires.

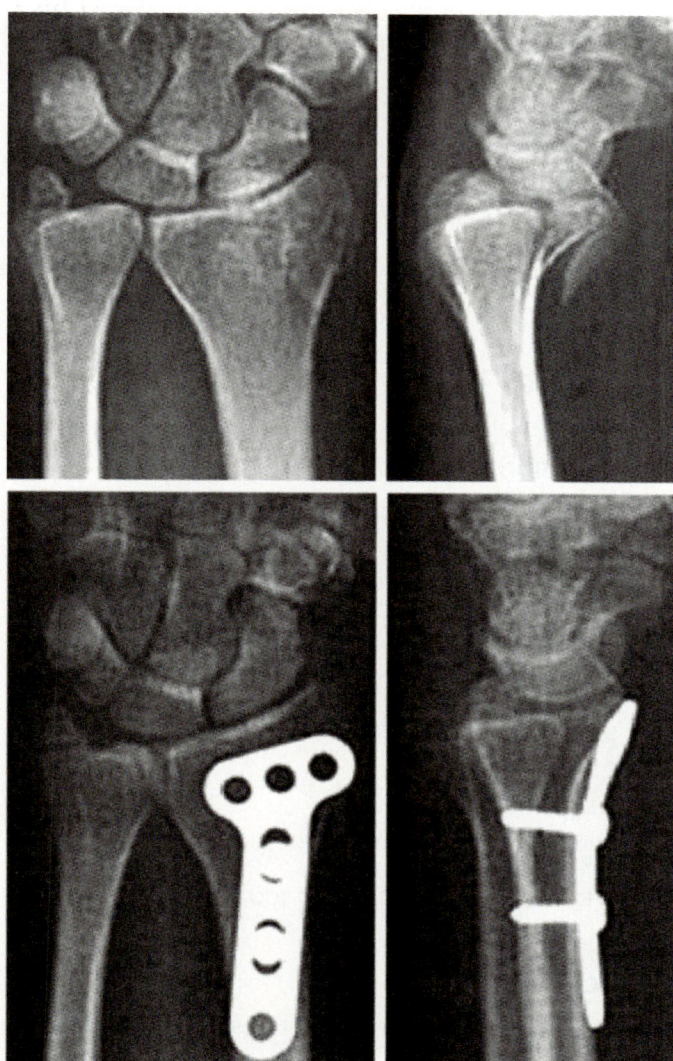

Fig. 13.14: Volar Barton fracture treated with volar buttress plate

CARPAL FRACTURES

The carpals are a complex set of bones that form multiple articulations. Because radiographs often reveal significant bony overlap, a careful history and a meticulous clinical examination are necessary to accurately diagnose these fractures. The scaphoid, triquetrum and lunate are the most frequently fractured bones of wrist in the decreasing order of frequency.

Essential Anatomy (Fig. 13.15)

Of the forearm bones only the radius articulates with the carpal bones. The ulna has a nonosseous

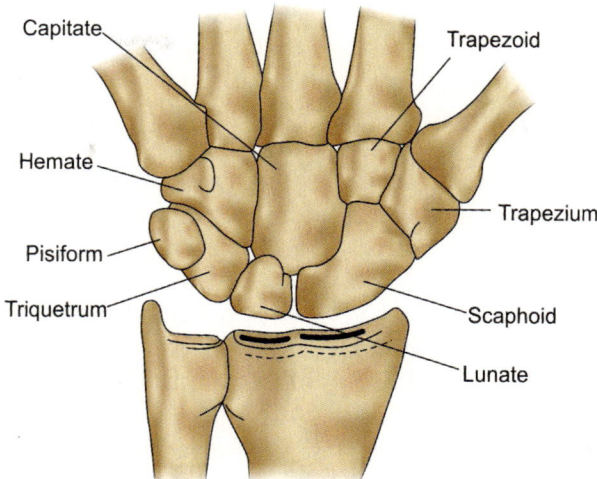

Fig. 13.15: Anatomy of carpal bones

fibrocartilaginous union with the triquetrum and the radius, known as the triangular fibrocartilage complex (TFCC). The ulna articulates with the radius at the distal radioulnar joint (DRUJ)

The ligaments of the wrist are considered extrinsic if they join the carpal bones to the radius, ulna, or metacarpals and intrinsic when they link the carpal bones to one another. The ligaments of the wrist are also classified as dorsal, volar, or interosseus. The volar ligaments are stronger than their dorsal counterparts and provide the greatest stability (Fig. 13.16).

Many important neurovascular structures pass through the palmar canal formed by the pisiform and the hook of the hamate. A fracture to either the hamate or the capitate may result in neurovascular bundle damage and subsequent impairment of normal

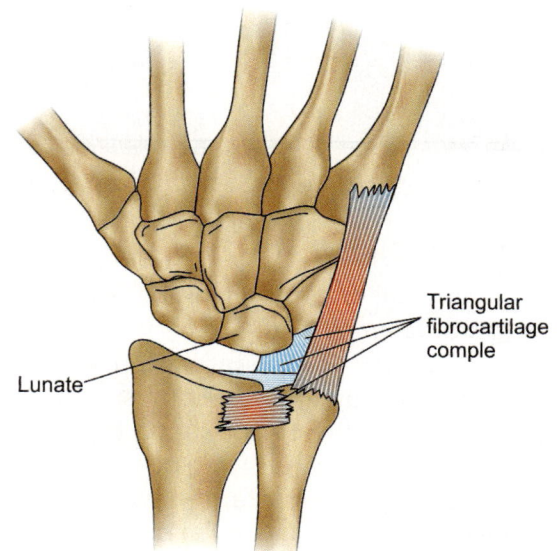

Fig. 13.16: Anatomy of DRUJ

function. The median nerve lies in close proximity to the volar surfaces of the lunate and the capitate and may be injured following a fracture.

Imaging

The minimum number of radiographic views includes a posteroanterior (PA), lateral, and oblique with the wrist in a neutral position. The carpal bones are visualized best in the PA view. Additional views may be obtained to better visualize suspected fractures. A PA with maximum ulnar deviation *(scaphoid view)* will allow better visualization of the scaphoid (Fig. 13.17).

The *carpal tunnel view* is used to detect fractures of the hook of the hamate and pisiform. This radiograph is obtained with the wrist hyperextended and the beam directed across the volar aspect of the wrist. An additional oblique film with the hand supinated 45° will better demonstrate the pisiform and the palmar aspects of the triquetrum and hamate.

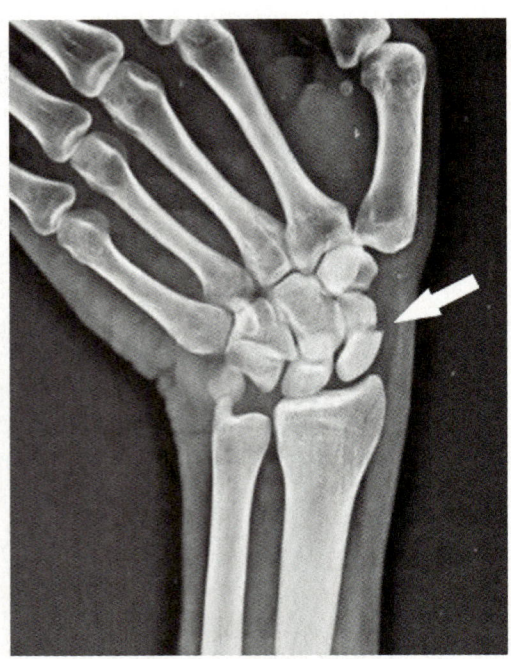

Fig. 13.17: Scaphoid view of wrist showing fracture

SCAPHOID FRACTURES

The scaphoid is the most commonly fractured carpal bone, accounting for 60 to 70% of carpal injuries.

The blood supply to the scaphoid penetrates the cortex on the dorsal surface near the tubercle waist area. Therefore, there is no direct blood supply to the proximal portion of the bone (Fig. 13.18). Because of this tenuous blood supply, scaphoid fractures have a tendency to develop delayed union or avascular necrosis. The more proximal the scaphoid fracture, the greater the likelihood the bone will develop avascular necrosis.

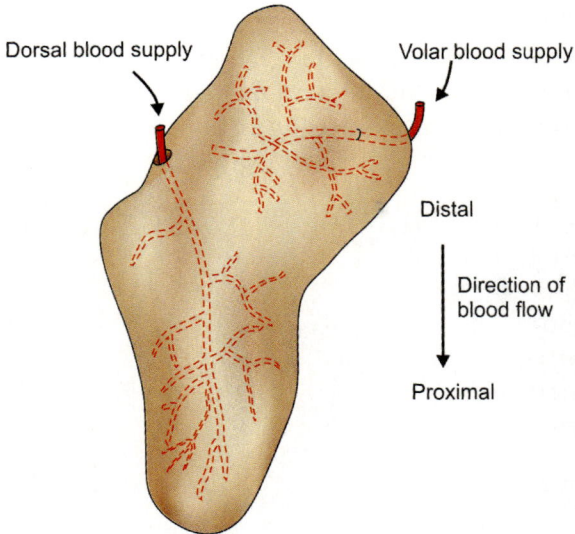

Fig. 13.18: Blood supply of scaphoid

Classification (Fig. 13.19)

- Distal 1/3rd fracture: Rare in adults, common in children
- Middle 1/3rd fracture (waist): 70 to 80%
- Proximal 1/3rd fracture: 10 to 20%

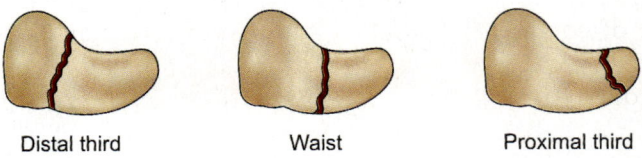

Fig. 13.19: Classification of scaphoid fracture

Mechanism of Injury

Scaphoid fractures commonly result from forceful hyperextension of the wrist.

Examination

1. There is maximum tenderness over the floor of the anatomic snuffbox (most sensitive).
2. Palpation of the scaphoid tubercle for tenderness. This test is performed by radially deviating the wrist and palpating over the palmar aspect of the scaphoid.
3. Axial compression of the thumb in line with the first metacarpal and supination against resistance may also elicit pain from a scaphoid fracture.
4. Ulnar deviation of the pronated wrist has been shown to produce pain in the anatomic snuffbox in patients with a scaphoid fracture.

Imaging

Routine radiographs including PA, lateral, and scaphoid views may demonstrate the fracture. If a fracture is suspected clinically, an ulnar-deviated scaphoid view should be obtained (Fig. 13.20).

Despite this additional film, a fracture may not be demonstrated radiographically for up to 6 weeks post injury. Up to 30% of scaphoid fractures are not demonstrated on any view in the acute setting. Therefore, after 7 to 10 days, a repeat physical and radiographic examination should be performed. Alternative methods for the early detection of occult fracture include bone scan, CT and MRI.

Treatment

Nonoperative

Indication

1. Undisplaced fractures
2. Tuberosity fractures

These are best treated by a long-arm thumb spica cast. The spica should extend from the interphalangeal joint of the thumb to an area proximal to the elbow with the elbow in 90° of flexion (glass holding position) after 6 weeks, a short-arm thumb spica cast is applied for the remaining duration of immobilization (Fig. 13.21), totalling 8 to 12 weeks. Due to their higher rate of complications, proximal third fractures are immobilized for a greater duration (12 to 16 weeks) than middle or distal third fractures (8 to 12 weeks).

Operative

Indications

1. Displacement >1 mm

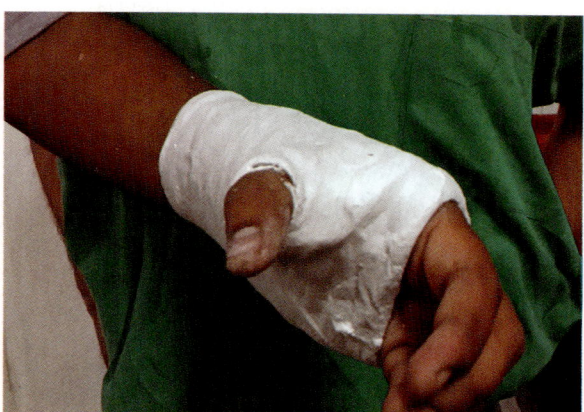

Fig. 13.21: Scaphoid cast

2. Angulation >15 degrees
3. Nonunion

Principle of operative management is to reduce fragments and achieve interfragmentory compression with the help of headless Herbert screw (Fig. 13.22). This can be done by percutaneous or open technique.

For nonunion and comminuted fractures, open reduction and bone grafting is recommended.

Complications

1. Avascular necrosis is associated with proximal third fractures, displaced fractures that are inadequately reduced, and comminuted fractures or fractures that are inadequately immobilized.
2. Delayed union, malunion, or non-union may be encountered despite optimal management. The most important factor in cases of non-union is early discontinuation of immobilization.
3. Radiocarpal arthritis with subsequent wrist pain and/or stiffness.

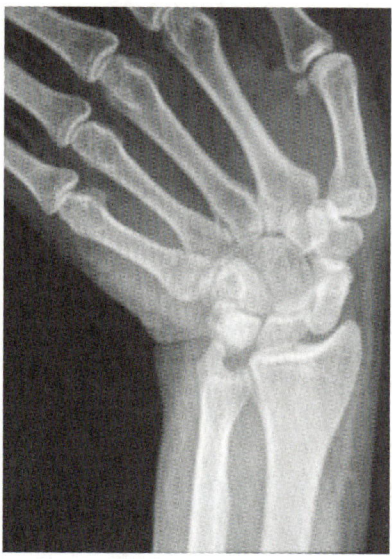

Fig. 13.20: PA view with ulnar deviation

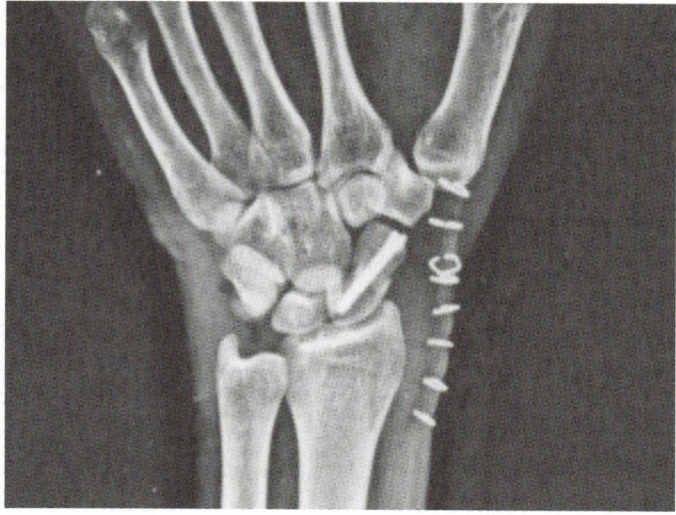

Fig. 13.22: Scaphoid fracture treated with Herbert screw fixation

Hand Injuries

Essential Anatomy

Anatomically, the hand is a group of highly mobile gliding bones connected by tendons and ligaments to a "fixed centre." This fixed centre consists of the second and third metacarpal bones. The remainder of the hand is suspended from these two relatively immobile bones. All of the intrinsic movements of the hand are relative to and dependent on the stability and immobility of these two bones (Fig. 14.1).

Mobility is a critical consideration in the management of fractures. Those bones with a high degree of mobility can withstand a greater degree of angulation with the retention of normal function. Those bones with less mobility (second and third metacarpals) require a much more precise reduction in angulation to ensure a return to full function.

Imaging

A minimum of three views should be obtained when a hand fracture is suspected (anteroposterior—AP, lateral, and oblique). Metacarpal injuries may require special views for adequate radiographic visualization, e.g. fractures of the fourth and fifth metacarpals are frequently undetected until a lateral view with 10° of supination is obtained. Second and third metacarpal injuries are often detected on a lateral view with 10° of pronation. Finger injuries require a true lateral view without superimposition of the other digits.

Protected or Functional Position of Hand

Hand joints are highly prone for stiffness even with immobilization as short as 1 week. So it is mandatory to immobilize hand in a position in which all the ligaments of the hand are optimally stretched. This is known as *functional position* of hand and is as follows:

The wrist in 15° of extension, the metacarpophalangeal (MCP) joints in 50° to 90° of flexion, and the interphalangeal (IP) joints in extension (Fig. 14.2). The thumb is typically immobilized, slightly abducted, and neither flexed nor extended.

SPECIFIC FRACTURES

Metacarpals

Metacarpal Head

Most of these require anatomical reduction to minimize arthritis.

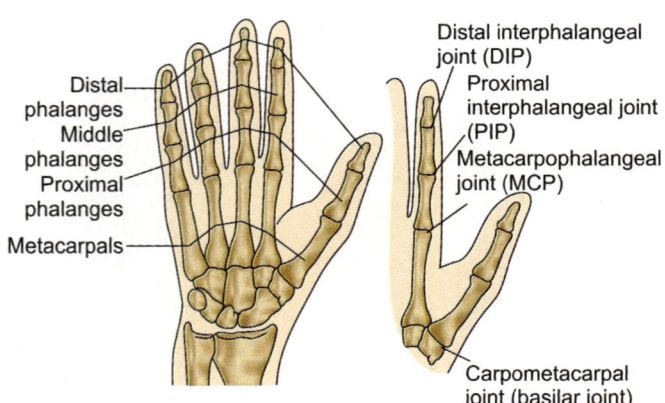

Fig. 14.1: Anatomy of hand

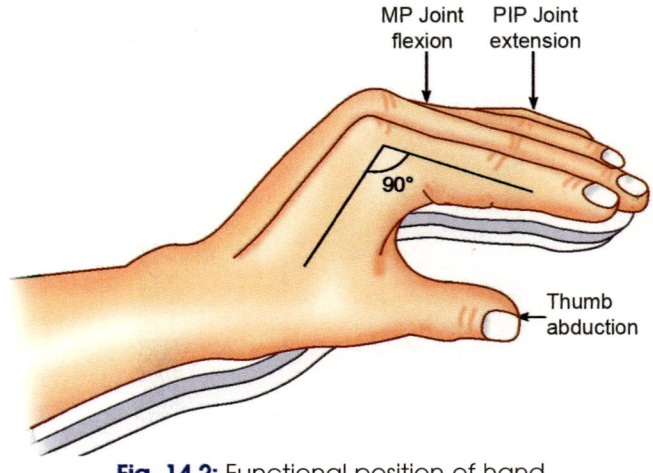

Fig. 14.2: Functional position of hand

1. Stable fractures can be splinted in functional position of hand with MP joint flexion >70 degree.
2. Unstable fractures can be fixed with percutaneous K wires.
3. Comminuted fractures require distraction by external fixator.

Metacarpal Neck

Usually result from direct trauma leading to dorsal angulation. Most of these can be managed by closed reduction using technique demonstrated in Fig. 14.3.

Angulation up to 10 degree is acceptable for 2nd and 3rd metacarpal and up to 30 degree for 4th and 5th metacarpals.

Unstable fractures may require fixation.

Metacarpal Shaft

Undisplaced or minimally dispalced fractures can be immobilized in functional position. Indications for surgery (Fig. 14.4)
1. Rotational deformity >10 degree.
2. Dorsal angulation >10 degree for 2nd and 3rd metacarpal >40 degree for 4th and 5th metacarpal.

Metacarpal Base

Base of 2nd, 3rd and 4th metacarpals can be treated by splinting in functional position.

Base of 5th metacarpal fracture or *reverse Bennett's* fracture usually requires open reduction internal fixation due to continuous pull of extensor carpi ulnaris.

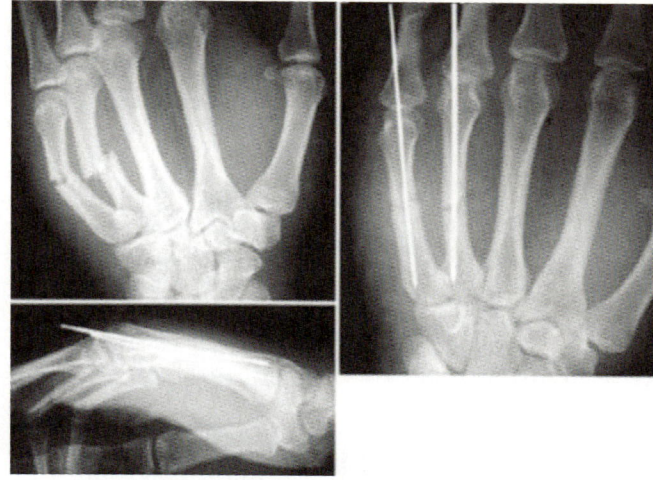

Fig. 14.4: Metacarpal shaft fractures treated with CRIF using K wires

THUMB FRACTURES

Extra-articular Fractures

These can be transverse or oblique and most can be managed by closed reduction and casting. Unstable fractures may require closed reduction and percutaneous pinning.

Intra-articular Fractures

Type 1: *Bennett's fracture* (partial articular): Fracture line seperates major part of metacarpal from volar lip fragment, producing a disruption of first carpometacarpal joint; 1st metacarpal is pulled proximally by abductor pollicis longus (Fig. 14.5).

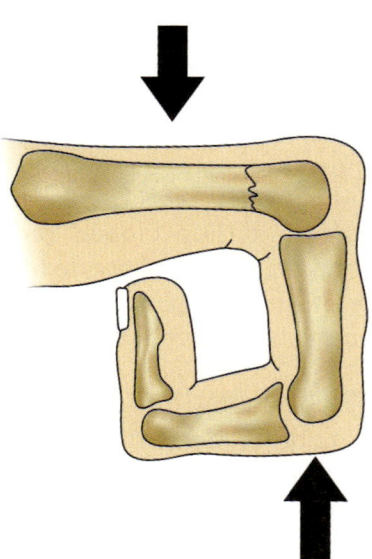

Fig. 14.3: Reduction technique for metacarpal neck fracture

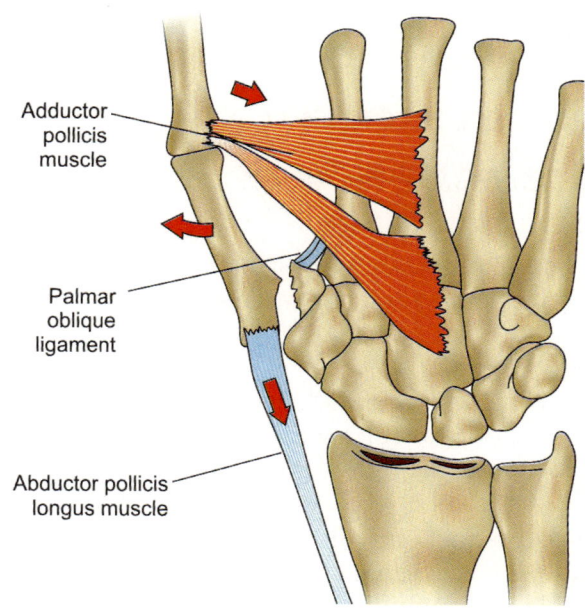

Fig. 14.5: Deforming forces of Bennett's fracture

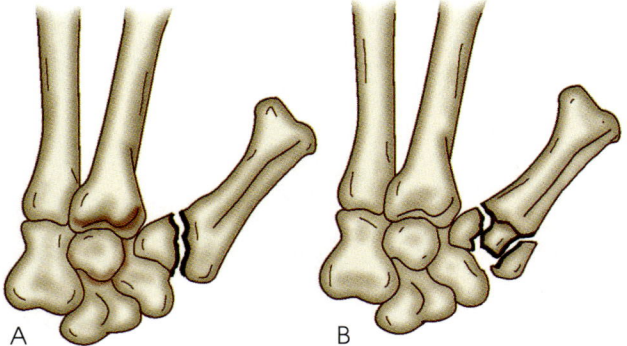

Fig. 14.6A and B: (A) Bennett fracture; (B) Rolando fracture

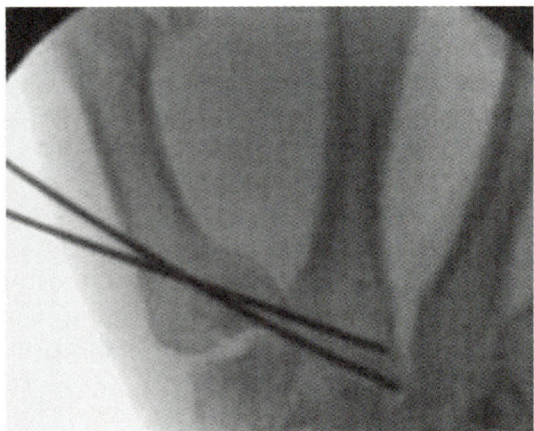

Fig. 14.7: Bennett's fracture treated with CRIF using K wires

Type 2: *Rolando fracture* (complete articular) is comminuted Bennett fracture; can have T/Y or dorsal and palmar fragments (Fig. 14.6).

Treatment

Both these fractures require closed reduction and percutaneous pinning (Fig. 14.7).

PHALANGEAL FRACTURES

Proximal and Middle Phalanx

Intra-articular Fractures

Anatomical reduction is must; open reduction internal fixation is necessary if displacement > 1mm.

Extra-articular Fractures

Fractures at the base of middle phalanx tend to angulate with the apex dorsal, whereas fractures at the neck angulate with the apex volarly owing to the pull of sublimis (Fig. 14.8).

Closed reduction with traction followed by buddy strapping is sufficient in most cases. If reduction is unstable, percutaneous pinning or open miniplate application can be done (Fig. 14.9).

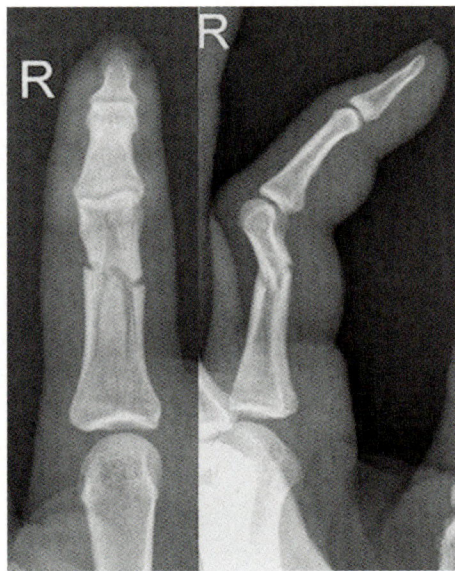

Fig. 14.8: Proximal phalanx fracture with volar angulation

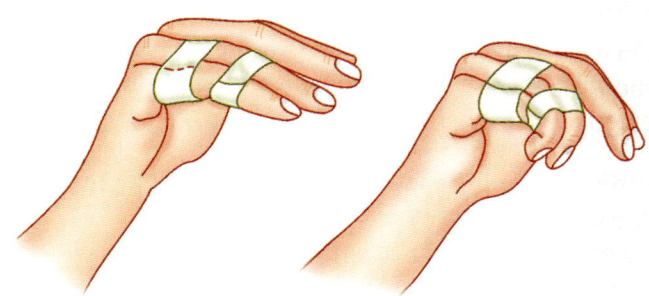

Fig. 14.9: Buddy strapping

Distal Phalanx

Intra-articular Fractures

Dorsal lip fracture results in *mallet finger*. Classical mallet finger otherwise is pure tendinous disruption of the extensor tendon.

Most of these are managed with splinting in extension for 6 to 8 weeks. If > 25 percent of articular surface is involved then closed reduction and percutaneous pinning is recommended.

Volar lip fractures leading to *Jersey finger* usually require open reduction internal fixation (Fig. 14.10).

Extra-articular Fractures

Most of these can be treated with closed reduction and splinting with commercially available splints.

MALLET FINGER

It results from forced flexion of the distal phalanx with the finger in taut extension. The fracture is commonly

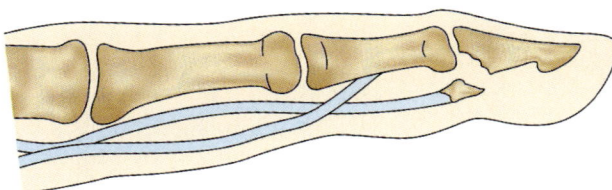

Fig. 14.10: Jersey finger

seen in basketball, baseball, and softball players when the ball accidentally hits the tip of the finger causing forced flexion. Three associated injuries are possible to the extensor tendon.

1. The tendon may stretch, resulting in a 15° to 20° loss of extension.
2. The tendon may rupture, resulting in up to a 45° loss of extension (soft-tissue mallet finger).
3. The tendon may avulse a bone fragment from the distal phalanx, resulting in up to a 45° loss of extension (bony mallet finger) (Figs 14.11 and 14.12).

Examination

On examination, there is swelling and tenderness over the dorsal aspect of the joint. There is loss of active extension at the distal interphalangeal (DIP) joint.

Imaging

A true lateral view is essential for avulsion fractures to determine if the fragment is displaced and involves >25% of the articular surface.

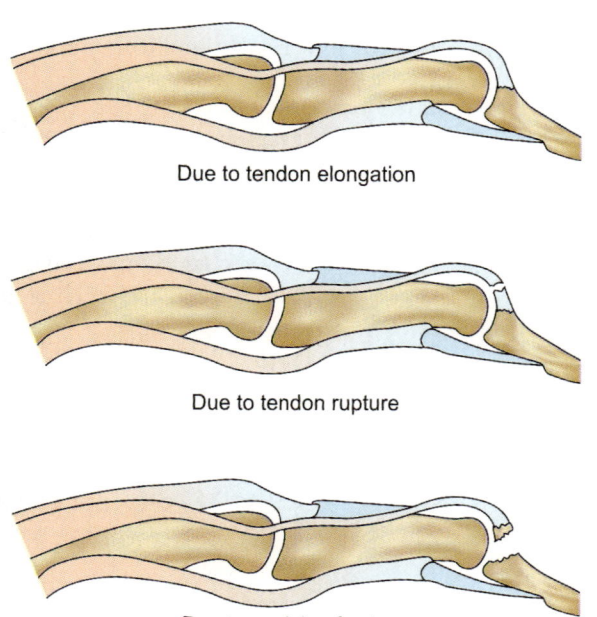

Due to tendon elongation

Due to tendon rupture

Due to avulsion fracture

Fig. 14.11: Mallet finger

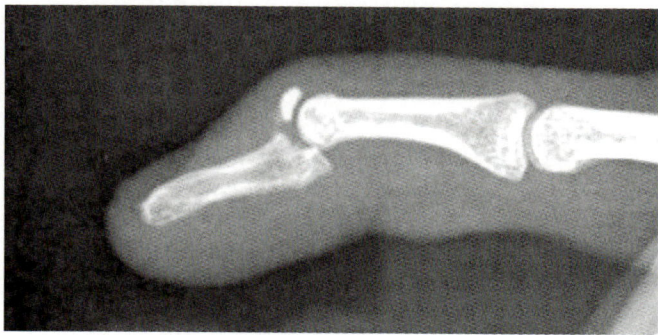

Fig. 14.12: Mallet finger

Treatment

Management is dependent on three variables: Patient reliability, the size of the avulsion fragment, and degree of displacement.

Undisplaced

In a reliable patient, the treatment is conservative, with either a volar or dorsal splint (Fig. 14.13). Dorsal splints provide better fixation, as there are fewer soft tissues between the splint and the fracture.

The DIP joint is extended with flexion permitted at the proximal phalangeal (PIP) joint. The finger must be maintained in this position for 6 to 8 weeks. Flexion of the DIP at any point during this period may result in a chronic flexion deformity. To stress this point, the patient is instructed to hold the tip of the finger in extension against the top of a table when changing the splint. After 6 to 8 weeks, the splint can be removed during the daytime with the patient cautioned against finger flexion for an additional 4 weeks.

If the patient is unreliable, the hand and finger is casted to ensure that the DIP joint is kept in extension. The cast remains in place for 6 weeks followed by 2 to 3 weeks of splinting of the digit.

Displaced and >25% of Articular Surface Involvement

This fracture is frequently associated with some degree of subluxation of the DIP joint. Closed reduction and internal fixation with Kirschner wires is usually necessary.

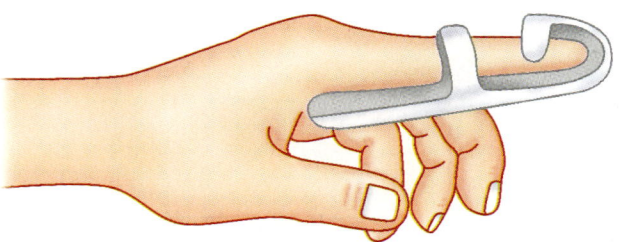

Fig. 14.13: Volar splint for mallet finger

Pelvic Injuries

Introduction

Pelvic fractures are life-threatening injuries. Patients who survive a pelvic fracture are at risk of significant complications such as chronic pain, leg length discrepancy, sexual dysfunction, or nerve palsy. Pubic rami fractures are the most common pelvic fractures with the superior ramus more frequently involved than the inferior ramus.

Anatomy

In 1615, Hook described pelvis as consisting of the two haunch bones, or innominate bones, joined with the holy bone, or sacrum, to form a bony dish that contains part of the gut, bladder, and womb (Fig. 15.1). This remarkable bony structure enables locomotion and protects the pelvic viscera. The pelvic bones support five joints as follows:

1. *Symphysis pubis* lies anteriorly and is the articulation between the two innominate bones.

2. *Sacroiliac joints* lie posteriorly and are the articulation between the sacrum and the innominate bones to its left and right.

3. *Acetabula* lie on the lateral surface of each innominate bone, and are formed at maturity from contributions by the ilium, ischium, and pubis.

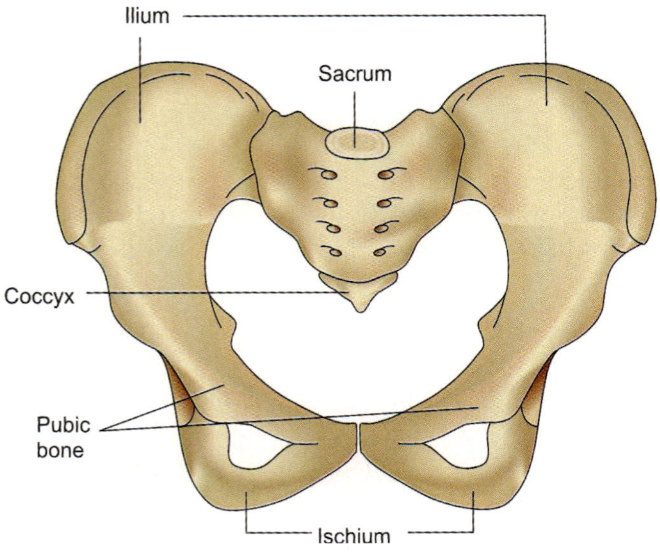

Mechanism of Injury

High-energy pelvic fractures result most commonly from motor vehicle accidents, falls, automobile-pedestrian encounters, and industrial crush injuries.

Classification

Tile classification system of pelvic ring injuries (Fig. 15.2).

Type A: Stable pelvic ring injury.

Type B: Rotationally unstable, vertically stable pelvic ring injury.

Type C: Rotationally and vertically unstable pelvic ring injury.

Fig. 15.1: Anatomy of pelvis

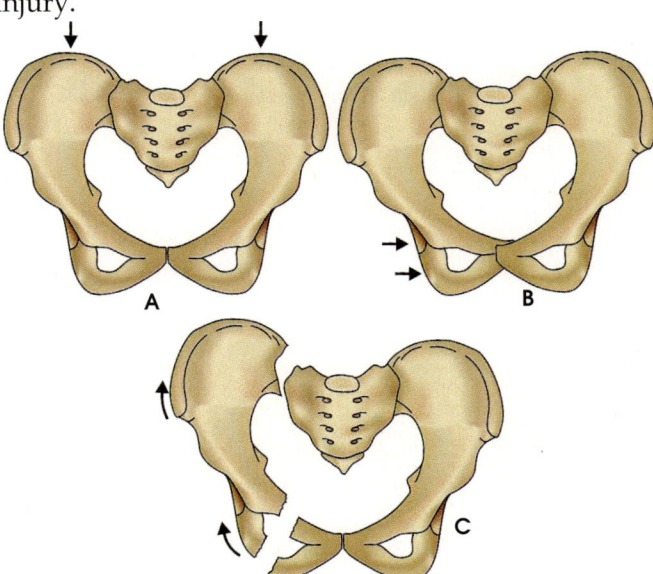

Fig. 15.2A to C: Pelvis fracture classification

Clinical Evaluation

Primary survey: It consists of ABCs (airway, breathing, and circulation), i.e. haemodynamic status. The goal of this primary survey is to identify and begin treatment of immediately life-threatening injuries.

Secondary survey: The pelvis is assessed by palpation at the anterior superior iliac spines. The examiner gently compresses the iliac wings together to expose instability in internal rotation, and then gently pulls the wings apart to expose instability in external rotation (Fig. 15.3). This examination should be performed only once, because fracture motion can disturb the pelvic haematoma and may lead to further bleeding.

Associated Injuries

Associated injuries include neurological damage, visceral injuries, and the Morel-Lavalle lesion. Neurological injury most commonly occurs at L5 and S1. Look for injuries to the bladder and urethra. Clinical signs include blood at the meatus or a high-riding prostate or eventual swelling of scrotum and labia.

Morel-Lavallè Lesion

A careful evaluation of the skin overlying the hip, pelvis, and thigh may show an area of subcutaneous degloving. This is recognized by a fluid wave on palpation or may be later identified by the presence of a fluctuant, circumscribed area of cutaneous anesthesia and ecchymosis. These injuries, even when closed, are associated with a significant incidence of positive bacterial culture. Initial debridement of the lesions and delayed acetabulum fracture fixation is recommended if the fracture surgery must be performed though such a lesion.

Management

Diagnosis

X-rays

1. Pelvis with both hips—anteroposterior view and lateral view should be taken.
2. Pelvis inlet view and outlet view help understand the fracture anatomy better (Fig. 15.4).

CT scan: Computed tomography (CT) is used to gather more information about fracture anatomy and to reveal the size and location of pelvic haematoma. It helps in the diagnosis of visceral injuries in patients sustaining pelvic fractures.

Additional investigations are needed in certain cases.

Pelvic angiography: To occlude a bleeding pelvic vessel.

Retrograde urethrogram: To assess status of urethral tear.

Retrograde cystogram: To assess integrity of urinary bladder.

Treatment

Treatment is based on instability. The sacrum is the keystone to the bony stability of the pelvis.

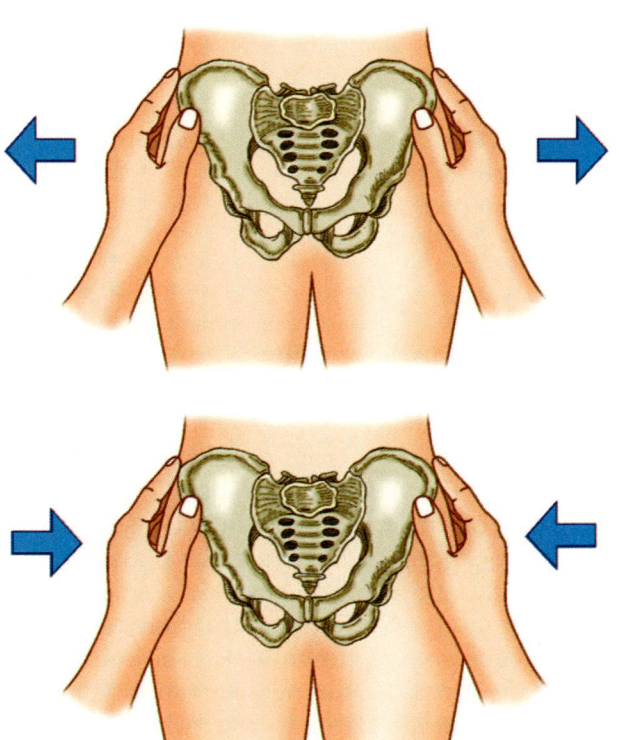

Fig. 15.3: Pelvic disrtraction and compression test

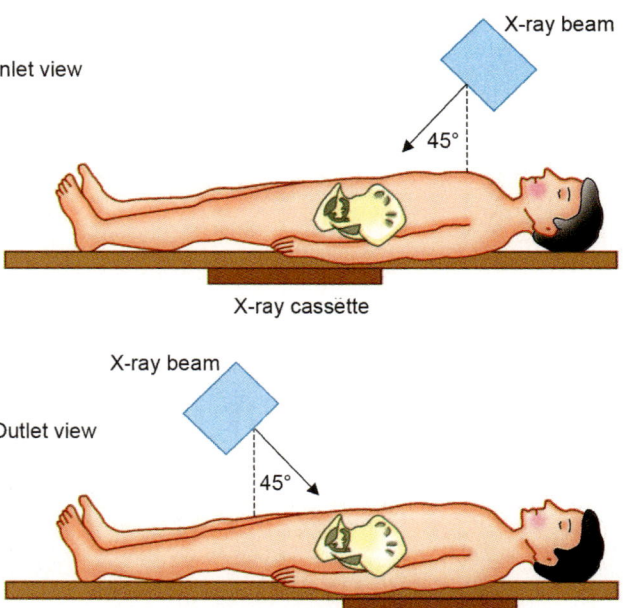

Fig. 15.4: Pelvis inlet and outlet views

Nonoperative Treatment

Indicated for fractures with less than 2.5 cm of anterior diastasis (opening of symphysis pubis). Patients are followed with serial radiographs to assure fracture stability and are allowed to weight-bear with support.

Operative Treatment

Fractures with greater than 2.5 cm anterior diastasis are treated with anterior plating of the pubic symphysis (Fig. 15.5). Sacroiliac joint instability requires stabilization posteriorly and may need additional treatment anteriorly.

Pelvic Damage Control

Closed reduction of the pelvis at admission
- External fixation (Fig. 15.6)
  - Wrapping pelvis with sheets with internal rotation and slight flexion of knees
  - External fixator
  - Pelvic C-clamp
  - Pneumatic antishock garment
- Control of haemorrhage
  - Pelvic packing
  - Angiography

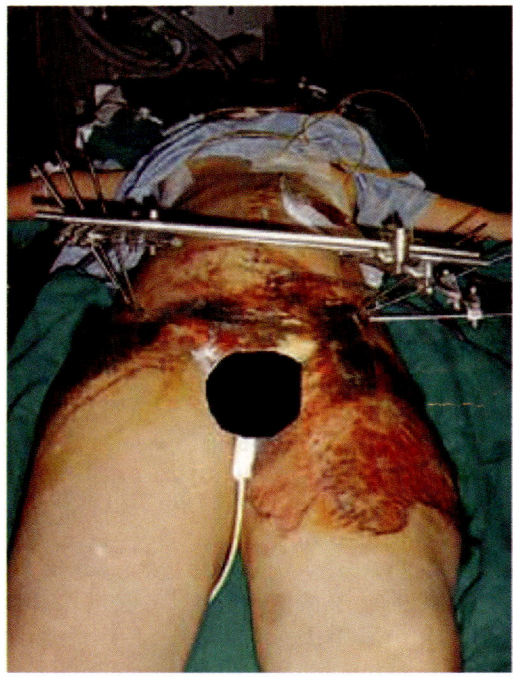

Fig. 15.6: Pelvic injury with severe ecchymosis treated with external fixator

- Control of contamination
  - Repair of genitourinary and rectal injuries
  - Debridement of necrotic tissue in the case of open injury

Complications

1. Post-traumatic arthritis is common.
2. Malunion or nonunion.
3. Pulmonary or fat emboli may develop during the early stages of healing.
4. A perforated viscera secondary to trauma may later become a source of sepsis.

JUMPER'S FRACTURE

Forceful axial loading of the spine and pelvis may lead to pelvic ring injury that is called the jumper's fracture, or suicidal jumper's fracture. The injury is often seen after a fall from height, as in a suicide attempt. The mechanism may be thought of as a dissociation of the central portion of the sacrum from the lateral portions. Simply put, the patient hits the ground with both feet. The legs, hips, and sacral ala stop immediately, while the sacral body and spinal column keep moving downward. The sacrum fails at its weakest points, the neural foramina. Careful neurologic examination is crucial, because the fracture can cause injury to the sacral nerve roots or cauda equina.

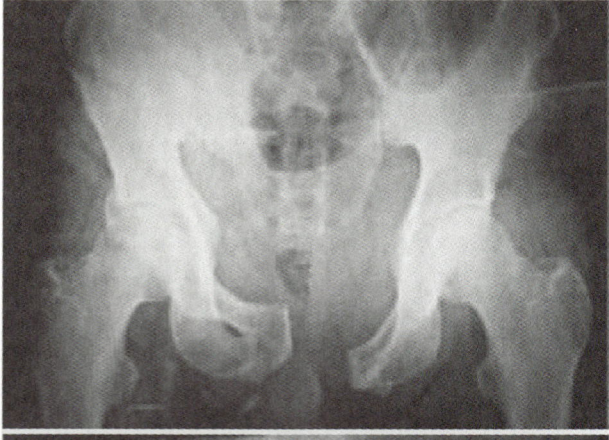

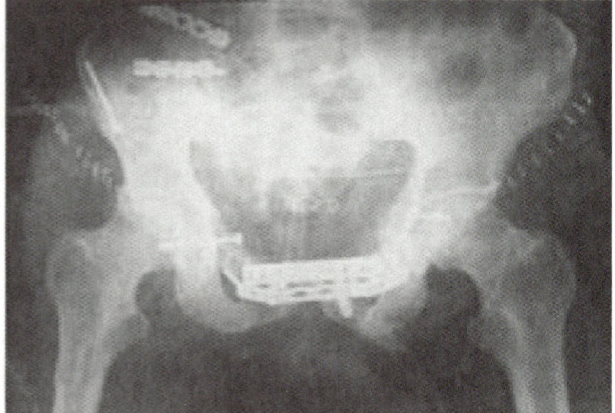

Fig. 15.5: Symphysis pubis disruption treated with plating

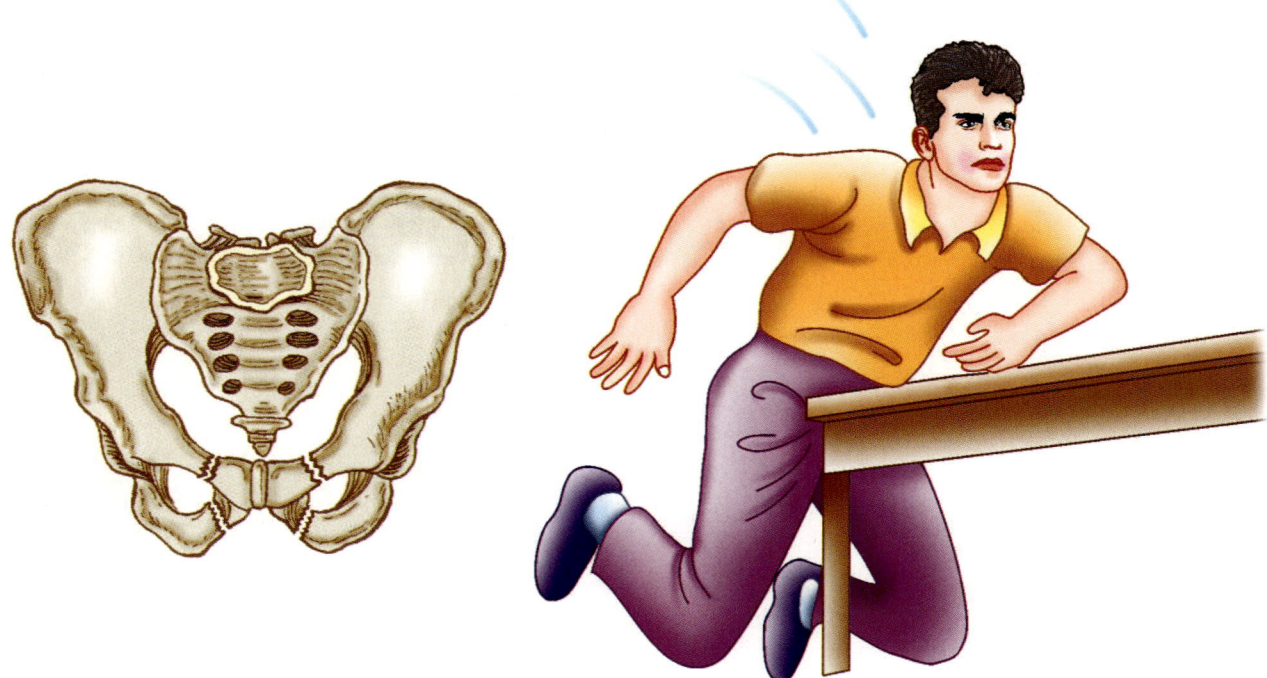

Fig. 15.7: Straddle injury

STRADDLE INJURY

Bilateral superior and inferior pubic rami fractures are known as straddle injury. This was originally described in horseback riders and is the result of direct trauma. Nearly one-third of these fractures have an associated lower urinary tract injury (Fig. 15.7).

Emergency management of these fractures includes immobilization and stabilization, including fluid therapy and the exclusion of serious associated injuries. The physician's priority must be directed at the identification and stabilization of life-threatening associated injuries. Operative fixation of the anterior pelvis is necessary after straddle injuries.

Acetabulum Injuries

Anatomy

The acetabulum follows an inverted Y, 2-column concept (Fig. 16.1).

1. *Anterior column:* Extends from the anterior iliac crest to the symphysis pubis and consists of an iliac segment, acetabular segment, and pubic segment.
2. *Posterior (ilioischial) column:* Extends from the greater sciatic notch to the inferior ischium.

Mechanism of Injury

Acetabulum fractures occur as force is transmitted from the femur to the pelvis via the femoral head. The fracture pattern, therefore, is dependent on the position

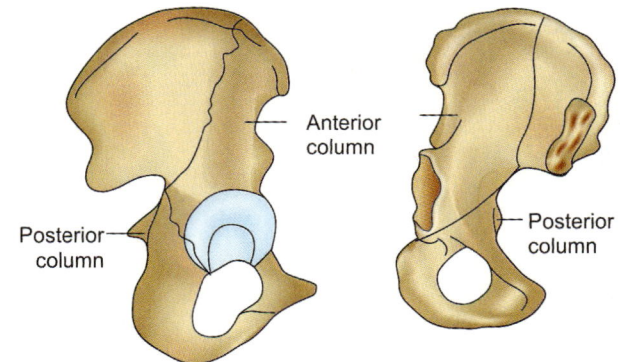

Fig. 16.1: Anatomy of acetabulum

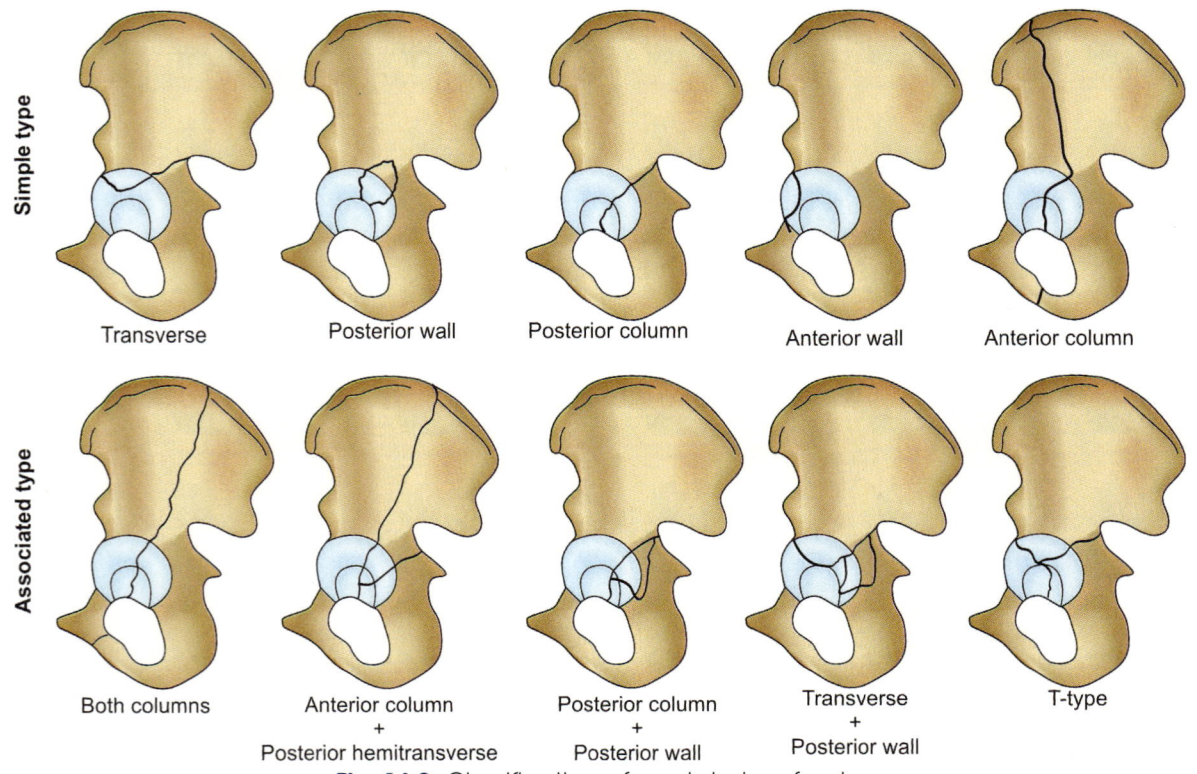

Simple type

| Transverse | Posterior wall | Posterior column | Anterior wall | Anterior column |

Associated type

| Both columns | Anterior column + Posterior hemitransverse | Posterior column + Posterior wall | Transverse + Posterior wall | T-type |

Fig. 16.2: Classification of acetabulum fractures

of the hip at the time of injury, as well as the direction and magnitude of the impact.

Classification

Fracture classification of Letournel and Judet (Fig. 16.2).

Elementary Fractures

- Posterior wall
- Posterior column
- Anterior wall
- Anterior column
- Transverse fractures

Associated Fractures

- Posterior column + wall
- Anterior + posterior hemitransverse
- Transverse + posterior wall
- T-shaped
- Associated both columns

Clinical Examination

General Clinical Evaluation

1. Rule out other life-threatening injuries.
2. Look for associated abdominal, urogenital, and neurological injuries.
3. Identify associated musculoskeletal injuries to the knee such as patellar fractures, chondral injuries, or ligamentous injuries.
4. Morel-Lavalle lesion as described in pelvic injury chapter.
5. Neurological injuries occur in up to 30% of cases especially with posterior dislocation of femoral head, and are usually partial injuries to the sciatic nerve. The peroneal division is more commonly injured than the tibial division.

Local Clinical Evaluation

1. The lower extremity may be externally rotated or in neutral position and only slight shortening is present.
2. If associated femoral head dislocation is present then flexion deformity of the hip with internal rotation of the lower limb will be present.

Management

A. Radiographic Evaluation

Following X-rays should be taken:
1. Pelvis with both hips anteroposterior view
2. Judet views: These are 45 degree oblique views called obturator oblique view and iliac oblique view obtained by rolling the patient 45 degrees in relation to the X-ray beam (Fig. 16.3).

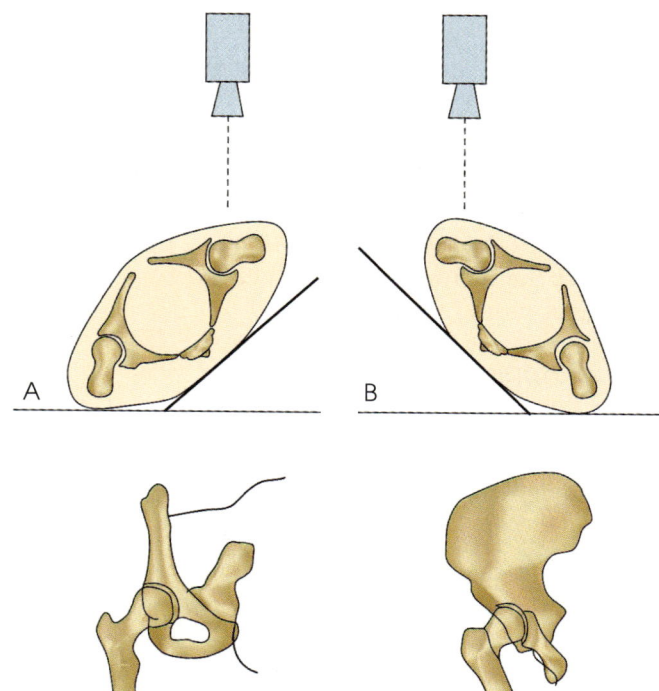

Fig. 16.3A and B: Judet views. (A) Obturator oblique view; (B) Iliac oblique view

B. Computed Tomography (CT) Scan of the Pelvis

Defines rotational displacements, intra-articular fragments, marginal articular impactions, and associated femoral head injuries, nowadays 3D CT scan shows better anatomy of the fractures.

Treatment

Nonoperative

Indications

1. Minimally displaced fractures with <2 mm displacement
2. Congruence of the femoral head to the intact acetabulum.

Method

Longitudinal skeletal traction through a distal femoral or proximal tibial pin pulling axially in neutral position. Postreduction radiographs are obtained. If the reduction is judged acceptable, traction is maintained for 6–8 weeks until bone healing is evident. Another 6–8 weeks is necessary before full weight bearing can be attempted during which period physiotherapy to strengthen muscles of the hip and knee can be carried out.

Operative

Goal: To achieve an anatomical and congruous reduction.

Indications
1. Loss of congruence between the femoral head and the acetabulum on any view (AP or Judet X-rays)
2. Displacement of greater that 2 mm within the superior articular surface (weight bearing dome)
3. Retained intra-articular fragments
4. Greater than 25% of the width of the posterior wall of acetabulum fracture on CT.

Surgical Approaches to Hip

1. *Kocher-Langenbeck:* A posterior approach to the acetabulum.
2. *Ilioinguinal:* An anterior approach to the acetabulum.

Implants used for acetabulum fixation are:
1. 6.5 mm cannulated or non-cannulated screws:
2. Reconstruction plates.

Complications

1. *Post-traumatic arthrosis:* Post-traumatic arthritis is a common complication especially, after poor articular reductions.
   Treatment: Total hip arthroplasty
2. *Avascular necrosis of femoral head:* Most commonly associated with posterior dislocation of the femoral head leading to the disruption of femoral head blood supply.
   Treatment: Total hip arthroplasty.

3. *Heterotopic ossification:* Heterotopic ossification is related to the degree of soft tissue disruption, from either the injury or the surgical approach.

Factors associated with the formation of heterotopic ossification:
a. Head injury
b. Prolonged mechanical ventilation
c. Male gender
d. Use of an extensile approach also contributes to the formation of heterotopic ossification caused by the amount of muscle dissection and elevation from the ilium. *Treatment:* Most patients who develop heterotopic ossification after acetabulam fractures do not have functional restrictions of their hip motion. Prophylactic treatments for heterotopic ossification include 6 weeks of indomethacin use (25 mg tid), single dose external beam radiotherapy (700 cGy), or a combination of both.

4. *Venous thromboembolism:* Deep venous thrombosis (DVT) and pulmonary embolism are common complications after pelvic or acetabulam fractures treated without prophylaxis.

5. *Neurological injury:* Sciatic nerve injury may occur in up to 30% of acetabulam fractures. Its chances also increase with posterior dislocation of the hip or associated posterior wall or column fractures. The sciatic nerve may be damaged during posterior surgical approach used to treat the acetabulum fractures.

Injuries around the Hip

FEMORAL NECK FRACTURES

Anatomy

The average neck-shaft angle is 130 ± 7 degrees, and the average anteversion is 10 ± 7 degrees. The **Calcar Femorale** is a dense vertical plate of bone extending from the posteromedial portion of the femoral shaft under the lesser trochanter and radiating lateral to the greater trochanter, reinforcing the femoral neck posteroinferiorly. The calcar femorale is thicker medially and gradually thins as it passes laterally (Fig. 17.1).

Blood Supply of Femoral Head

Medial and lateral circumflex femoral arteries, arising from the profunda femoris artery form the extracapsular vascular ring around the base of the neck, which sends intracapsular vessels (retinacular vessels). It is the most important ring in maintaining perfusion to the femoral head (Fig. 17.2).

1. Femoral circumflex and retinacular arteries

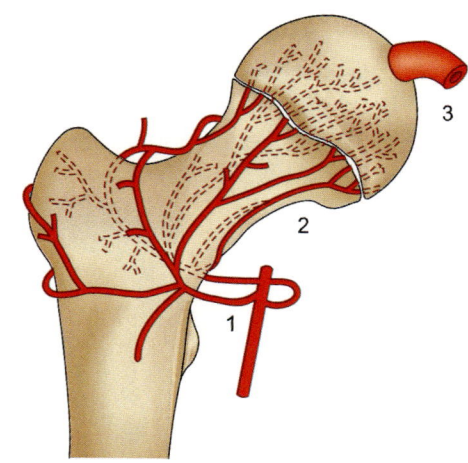

Fig. 17.2: Blood supply of femoral head (1 to 3: *see* text)

2. Medullary vascularture
3. Vessel of the ligamentum teres.

Clinical Significance of Femoral Neck Fractures

Following are the important four reasons why femoral neck fractures should be treated as a true orthopaedic emergency and treated promptly and why the incidence of non-union and avascular necrosis of femoral head is high after femoral neck fracture.

1. Femoral neck fractures are *intracapsular*, the synovial fluid bathing the fracture interferes with the healing process. Angiogenic-inhibiting factors in synovial fluid also can inhibit fracture repair.
2. Femoral neck has *no periosteal layer*, all healing is endosteal. Periosteum is required for fracture union.
3. The *blood supply* to the femoral head is very *precarious* and closely associated to the femoral neck, hence disruption of the blood supply in femoral neck fractures leads to high incidence of nonunion of femoral neck fractures.
4. The *tamponading effect* of the intracapsular haematoma leads to impairment of blood supply.

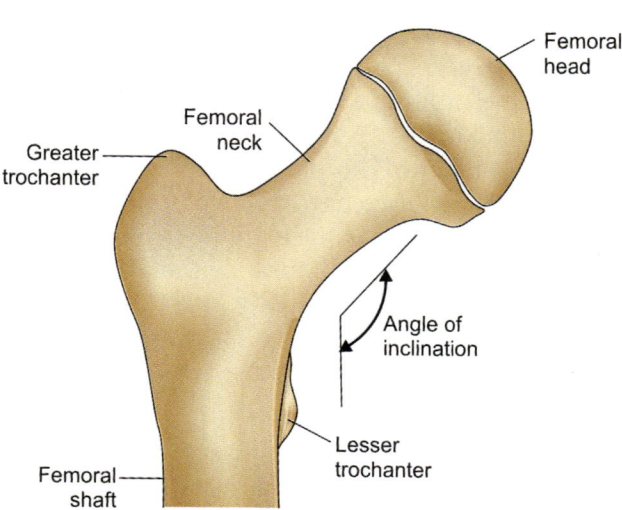

Fig. 17.1: Anatomy of proximal femur

Femoral head

Femoral neck

Greater trochanter

Angle of inclination

Lesser trochanter

Femoral shaft

Mechanism of Injury

Young individuals: Major trauma.

Old individuals: Low energy injuries.

The term *"insufficiency fractures"* is used to describe femoral neck fractures in elderly individuals with osteoporosis.

Classification

The three common systems:

a. Anatomical Classification (Fig. 17.3)

1. *Subcapital:* Occur immediately beneath the articular surface of the femoral head along the old epiphyseal plate. *Highest incidence of nonunion and avascular necrosis* among all types of fracture neck femur.
2. *Transcervical:* Pass across the femoral neck between the femoral head and the greater trochanter.
3. *Basicervical:* It is extracapsular and occurs at the base of the femoral neck.

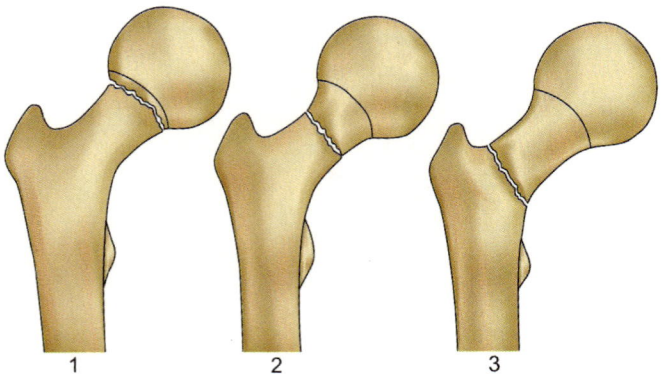

Fig. 17.3: Anatomical classification

b. Pauwel's Classification (Fig. 17.4)

Based on the direction of the fracture line across the femoral neck.

Type I: 30° from the horizontal

Type II: 50° from the horizontal

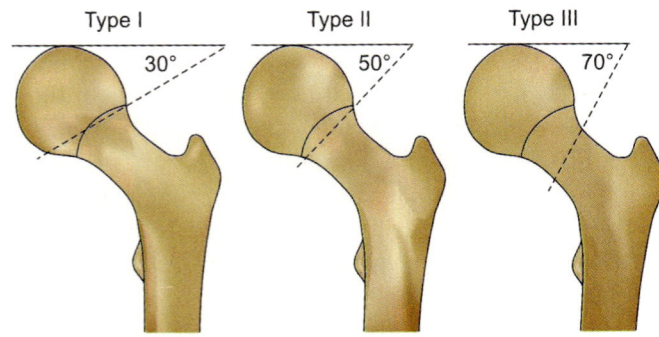

Fig. 17.4: Pauwel's classification

Type III: 70° from the horizontal. Pauwel attributed nonunion in type III to the increased shearing force of this vertical fracture.

c. Garden's Classification (Fig. 17.5)

Based on the fracture displacement

Type I Incomplete or impacted fracture

Type II Complete, but nondisplaced fracture

Type III Partially displaced or angulated fracture

Type IV Displaced fracture with no contact between the fragments.

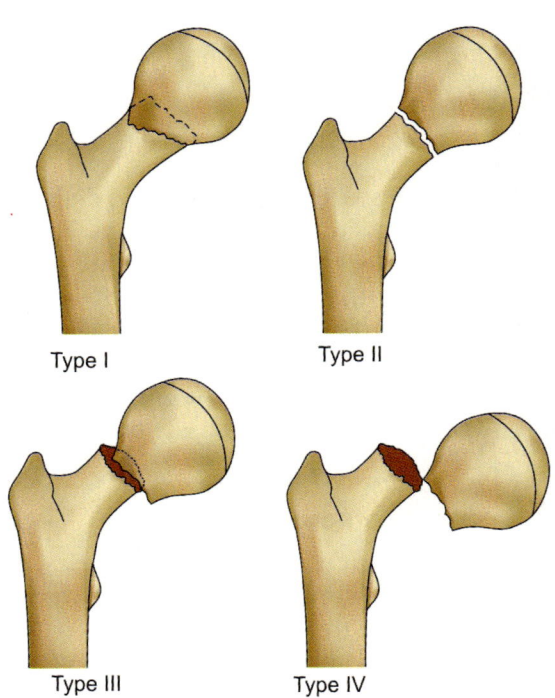

Fig. 17.5: Garden's classification

Clinical Evaluation

1. History of fall.
2. Pain in the groin or referred pain along the medial side of the knee.
3. Attitude of limb: The patients lie with the leg in *external rotation, abduction, and slight shortening.* These patients may not have the extreme deformity that is present in dislocations of the hip or intertrochanteric fractures because of a partially intact capsule.

Management

Diagnosis

1. **X-rays:** Pelvis with both hips X-ray, anteroposterior view with 15 degree internal rotation of both the lower limbs should be taken.15 degree internal rotation of lower limb is done as in this position, the

entire *length* of the femoral neck is visible and helps to identify the fracture line better.

2. **CT scan** is helpful in the diagnosis of occult fractures about the hip.

Treatment

The standard of care is operative for all femoral neck fractures. The decision regarding type of operative intervention is based on patient characteristics (young versus elderly) and fracture characteristics (stable versus unstable).

1. Closed Reduction and Internal Fixation

It should be preferred and done under visualization of C-arm machine by one of the following two techniques:

a. *Leadbetter technique*: Performed with hip in 90 degree flexion.

b. *Whitman technique*: Performed with the hip in extension.

After achieving closed reduction, internal fixation is done with cannulated cancellous screws, in age less than 65 years, preferably within 24 hours (Fig. 17.6).

2. Open Reduction and Internal Fixation

It is resorted to only when anatomical closed reduction is not attainable and the patient is not a good candidate for a hemiarthroplasty with a femoral head prosthesis.

3. Arthroplasty

This is the modality of treatment for elderly patients (age >65 yrs).

It involves replacing part of the hip joint.

a. *Hemiarthroplasty*—if only the femoral head is replaced (Fig. 17.7).

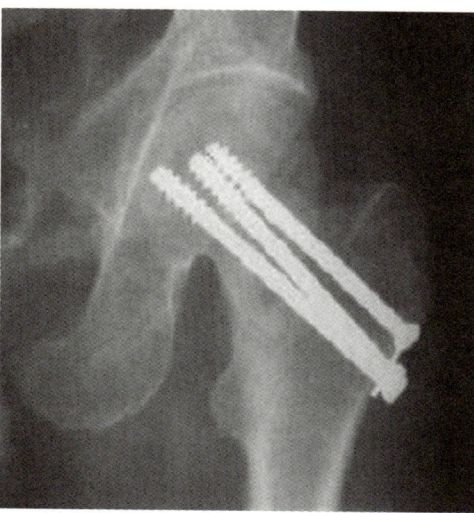

Fig. 17.6: Femur neck fracture treated with CRIF using 6.5 mm cannulated cancellous screw

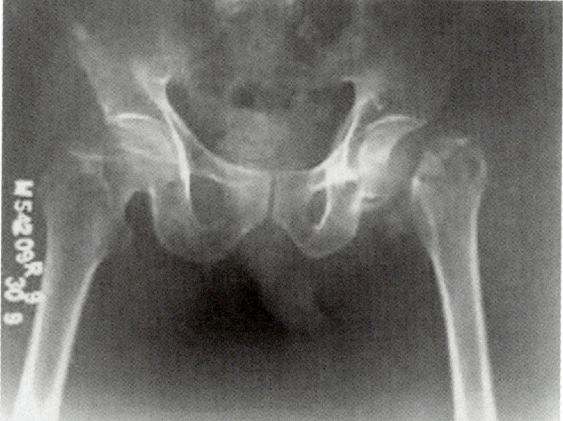

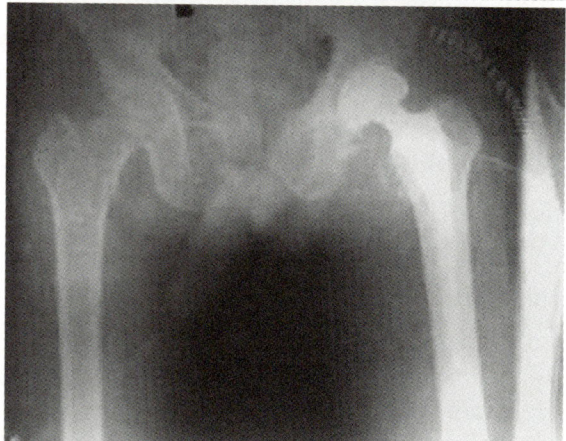

Fig. 17.7: Femur neck fracture in elderly treated with bipolar hemireplacement arthroplasty

Prostheses used—Austin-Moore and Thompson prosthesis (unipolar) or bipolar prosthesis (widely used now).

b. *Total hip arthroplasty*—both, the femoral head and the acetabulum are replaced.

Complications

1. Non-union

Risk factors for non-union are:

1. Posterior comminution
2. Initial displacement
3. Inadequate reduction
4. Noncompressive fixation

The treatment of nonunions in the elderly is arthroplasty. In *younger patients, a valgus-producing osteotomy* is an option in those with varus alignment or with limb shortening. In those with normal alignment, bone graft with repeat open reduction and internal fixation with cannulated screws is suggested.

2. Avascular Necrosis

The treatment of AVN includes total hip arthroplasty.

INTERTROCHANTERIC FRACTURES

Anatomy

The intertrochanteric region of the hip extends from the extracapsular portion of the femoral neck to the inferior border of the lesser trochanter. Majority of intertrochanteric fractures occur in patients older than 65 years. Osteoporosis is an important risk factor. Intertrochanteric fractures are extracapsular and involve the cancellous bone between the greater and lesser trochanters (Fig. 17.8). The vascular supply to this region is very good, owing to the large amount of surrounding musculature and the presence of cancellous bone. The internal rotators of the hip remain attached to the proximal fragment whereas the short external rotators remain attached to the distal segment.

Mechanism of Injury

Young: High energy injury
Old: Low energy injury, trivial trauma or fall.

Classification

Tronzo classification of intertrochanteric fractures (Fig. 17.9)

Type I: Incomplete fracture.

Type II: Non-comminuted fractures, with or without displacement; both trochanters fractured.

Type III: Comminuted fractures, large lesser trochanter fragment; posterior wall exploded; neck beak impacted in shaft. Variant: As above, plus greater trochanter fractured off and separated.

Type IV: Posterior wall exploded, neck spike displaced outside shaft.

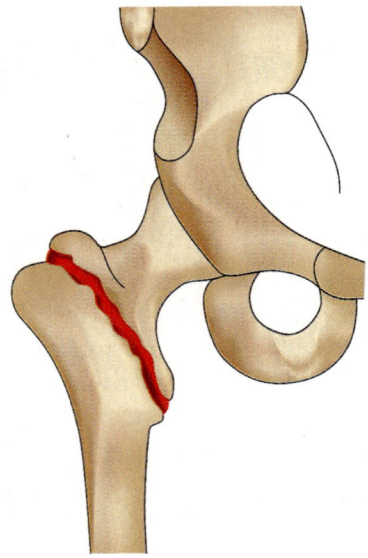

Fig. 17.8: Intertrochantric fracture

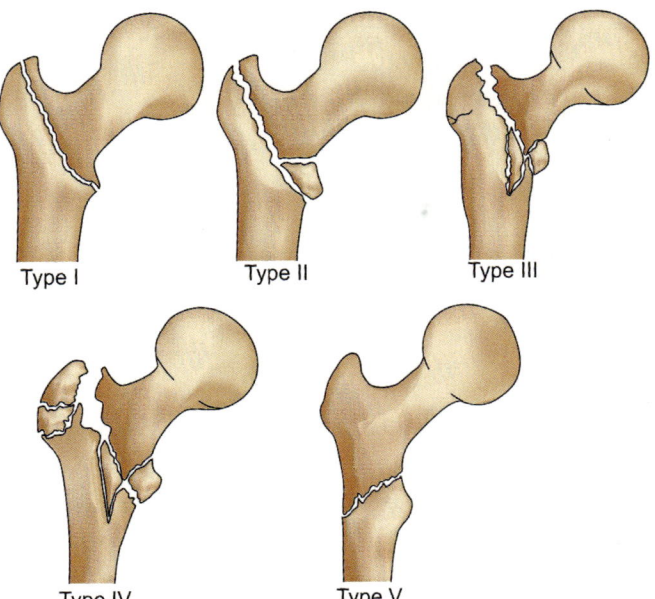

Fig. 17.9: Tronzo classification

Type V: Reverse oblique fracture, with or without greater trochanter separation.

Stable fracture patterns: The posteromedial cortex remains intact or has minimal comminution, making it possible to obtain a stable reduction.

Unstable fracture patterns: Characterized by greater comminution of the posteromedial cortex. The reverse obliquity pattern is inherently unstable because of the tendency for medial displacement of the femoral shaft.

Clinical Evaluation

The patient will present with tenderness, swelling and ecchymosis over the hip. There is usually *significant leg shortening with external rotation* (compared to patients with femoral neck fracture who have lesser degree of leg shortening and less external rotation deformity).

Diagnosis

X-ray of pelvis with both hips—anteroposterior view and lateral view of affected hip should be taken.

Treatment

Nonoperative Treatment

Indication: An elderly person whose medical condition carries an excessively high risk of mortality from anaesthesia and surgery. Non-operative treatment consists of prolonged bedrest in traction until fracture healing occurs (usually 10 to 12 weeks). In elderly patients, this approach is associated with high complication rates like decubitus ulcers, urinary tract infection, joint contractures, pneumonia, and thrombo-embolic complications, resulting in a high mortality rate.

In addition, fracture healing is generally accompanied by varus deformity and shortening because of the inability of traction to effectively counteract the deforming muscular forces.

Operative Treatment

Treatment of choice for the vast majority of inter-trochanteric fractures.

Goal of operative treatment: To obtain a stable reduction with internal fixation that permits immediate mobilization of the patient.

Options

1. Dynamic Compression Hip Screw (DHS)
(Fig. 17.10)

Advantages
- Can be used for majority of fractures
- It allows compression at fracture site

Indication for DHS
1. Stable fracture
2. Basicervical fracture

2. Proximal Femoral Nail (Intramedullary Nail)
(Fig. 17.11)

Advantages
- It has decreased implant bending strength.
- It can be used by percutaneous technique.

Indications
- Reverse oblique fracture
- Unstable fracture

3. Hemiarthroplasty (Fig. 17.12)

Indications: In elderly patients with
1. Pathological fracture
2. Severe osteopenia

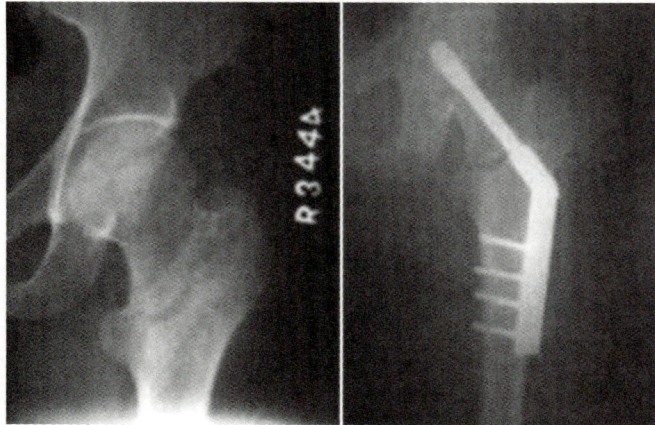

Fig. 17.10: Intertrochanteric fracture treated with CRIF using DHS

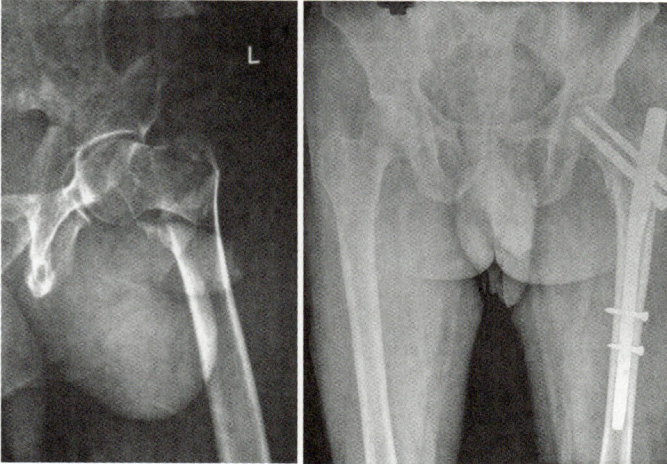

Fig. 17.11: Proximal femoral nail

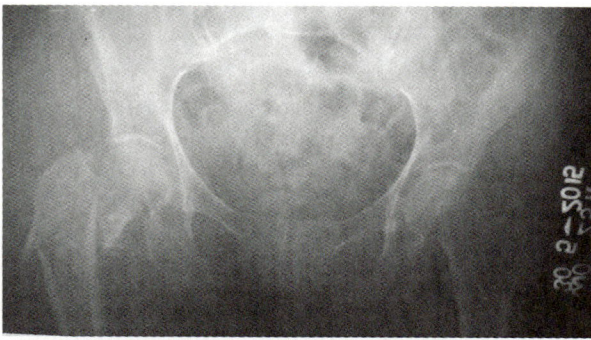
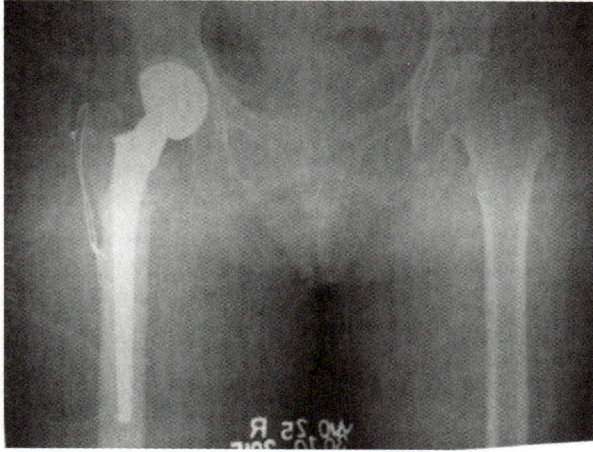

Fig. 17.12: Intertochanteric fracture treated using bipolar hemiarthroplasty and greater trochanteric reconstruction using wire

3. Severe comminution
4. Rheumatoid arthritis

Complications of Intertrochanteric Fractures

1. Malunion–due to nonoperative treatment–external roatation and varus deformity of hip with shortening of lower limb.

2. Implant failure—in cases of osteoporotic bones where dynamic hip screw is inserted and the bone quality is weak, the implant may cut out due to poor purchase in the bone. In such cases hemiarthroplasty should be preferred.

HIP DISLOCATIONS

The hip joint is inherently stable, requiring significant force to dislocate.

Mechanism of Injury

Hip dislocations are usually the result of high energy trauma.

Posterior dislocation is the most common type of hip dislocation. It occurs with an axial load applied to the femur while the hip is flexed. Most commonly, it is the result of a dashboard impact on the knee.

The blood supply is compromised due to dislocation, hence early intervention should be carried out to limit vascular insult to bone.

Clinical Evaluation

1. *Posterior hip dislocation:* **F**lexion, **AD**duction and **I**nternal **R**otation (FADIR) of affected extremity (Fig. 17.13).
2. *Anterior hip dislocation:* **F**lexion, **AB**duction and **E**xternal **R**otation (FABER) of affected extremity.

Associated injuries include distal femoral contusions or fractures, patella fractures, foot and ankle injuries (especially when the knee is extended), and sciatic nerve injury in up to 10% of patients.

Management

Diagnosis

1. **X-rays:** Pelvis with both hips—anteroposterior view and lateral view of affected hip.

It shows femoral head not centred in acetabulum. If the head appears *larger*, then the dislocation is *anterior*, but if it appears *smaller*, then the dislocation is *posterior* (Fig. 17.14).

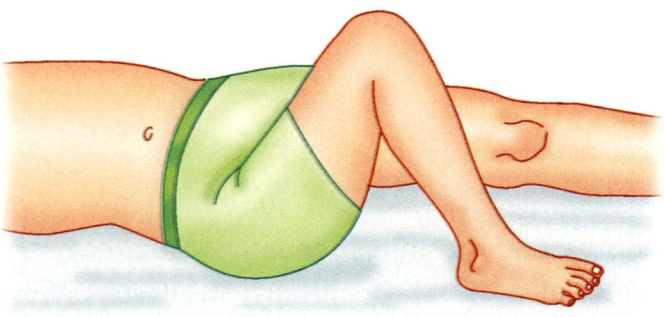

Fig. 17.13: Attitude of hip in posterior hip dislocation

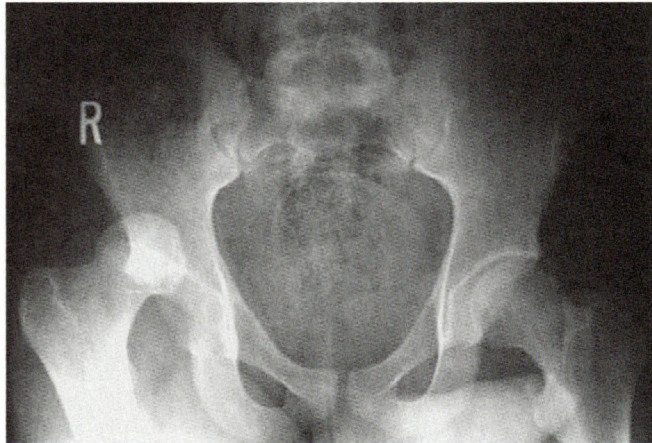

Fig. 17.14: X-ray pelvis with both hips showing posterior hip dislocation

2. **CT scan:** It is necessary to assess the postreduction status of the hip, identify nondisplaced fractures, determine the congruity of reduction, and visualize and determine the size intra-articular fragments.

Treatment

Posterior hip dislocations are best managed with immobilization and emergent reduction within 6 hours. Delay in reduction increases the rate of AVN of the femoral head and the risk of sciatic nerve injury.

Closed reduction is achieved with the following manoeuvres.

Allis manoeuvre is performed with the patient in supine position with the pelvis stabilized. The hip is flexed to 90 degrees, and increased traction is placed with the hip adducted and extremity internally rotated and the hip joint is reduced back in position (Fig. 17.15).

Stimson manoeuvre is performed with the patient prone as the hip is flexed and the leg is placed off the stretcher (Fig. 17.16).

Indications for Operative Treatment

1. Irreducible dislocation
2. Dislocation with femoral neck fracture
3. Intra-articular fragment
4. Incongruent reduction
5. Unstable hip after reduction

Post-reduction Management

X-rays should always be taken after any joint is reduced to check for adequate acceptable reduction. The patient is immobilized in a Thomas' splint for 6 weeks, then mobilized with crutches initially with touch-down weight bearing and resumption of full weight bearing after pain has subsided.

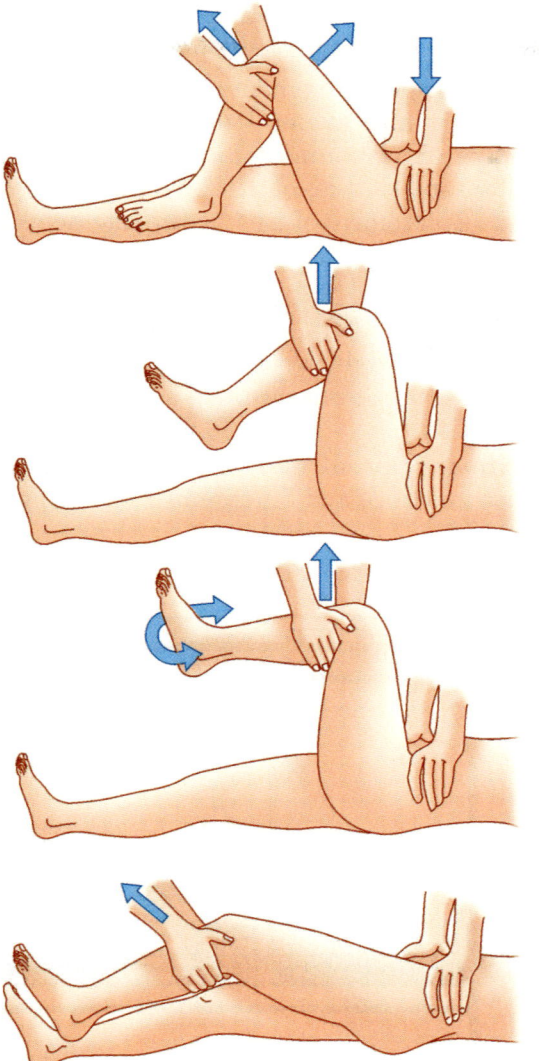

Fig. 17.15: Allis manoeuvre for reduction of posterior hip dislocation

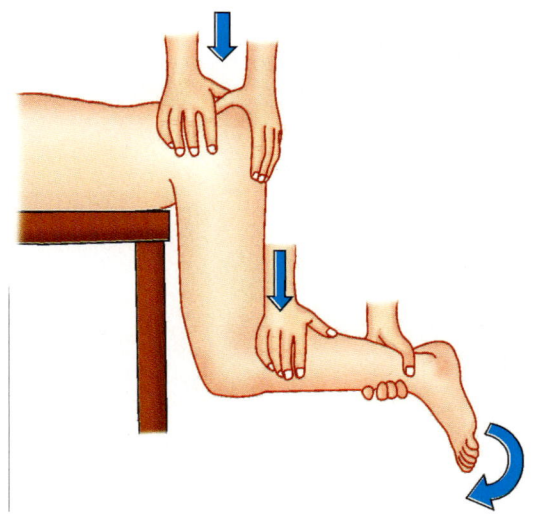

Fig. 17.16: Stimson's manoeuvre for reduction of posterior hip dislocation

Complications

1. *Avascular necrosis* (1 to 20%) is correlated with the duration of dislocation, but the best results are obtained if the hip is reduced within 6 hours.
2. *Post-traumatic osteoarthritis (OA)* has increased incidence with concomitant femoral head or acetabular fractures, and anatomic reduction is key to prevent abrasive wear of cartilage.
3. *Sciatic nerve injury:* A deficit of the sciatic nerve is present in 10 to 13% of posterior hip dislocations.

SUBTROCHANTERIC FRACTURES

Definition

Subtrochanteric fractures occur below the lesser trochanter to 5 cm distally in the shaft of the femur.

Anatomy

Muscle Attachment

The causes of fracture fragment displacement are due to the unbalanced muscle pull after a closed fracture (Fig. 17.17).

In the proximal fragment, the iliopsoas, with its insertion on the lesser trochanter, causes the proximal segment to become externally rotated and flexed.

The short abductors of the hip muscles on the greater trochanter also cause proximal segment abduction.

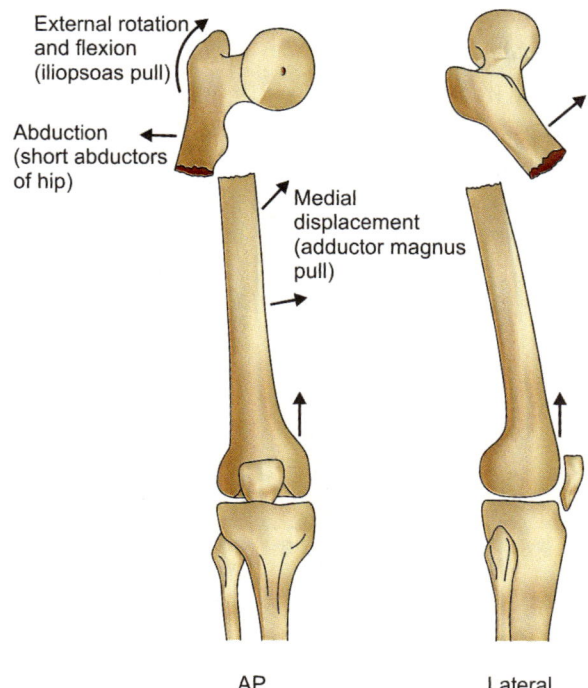

Fig. 17.17: Deforming muscle forces of subtrochanteric fracture

The distal segment, because of the unopposed pull from the adductor magnus, always displaces medially and further aggravates the deformities of the two fracture fragments.

Mechanism of Injury

Young: High energy injury
Elderly: Low energy.

Classification (Fig. 17.18)

Fielding's classification of subtrochanteric fractures (Fig. 17.18):

Type I: At the level of the lesser trochanter
Type II: 2.5 to 5 cm below the lesser trochanter
Type III: 5 to 7.5 cm below the lesser trochanter

Clinical Evaluation

- Swelling in upper thigh region
- External rotation deformity and shortening of lower limb (both are more than femoral neck and inter-trochanteric fracture).
- Look for other associated injury to pelvis and knee joint
- Look for signs and symptoms of hypovolemic shock.

Management

Diagnosis

X-rays of affected extremity anteroposterior and lateral views, including hip and knee.

Treatment

First priority is given to stabilization of the patient haemodynamically and other associated life threatening injuries, if present.

Non–operative Methods or Initial Treatment (Fig. 17.19)

Transosseous pin through lower end of femur or upper end of tibia and skeletal traction. Nonoperative methods are not favoured as long time to fracture union is required and chances of non-union are very high due to gross displacement of the fracture fragments present usually.

Operative Methods

1. **Dynamic condylar screw system:** Open reduction and fixation done under direct observation (Fig. 17.20).
2. **Proximal femoral nail:** Closed reduction under C-arm guidance and intramedullary nailing is done (Fig. 17.21).

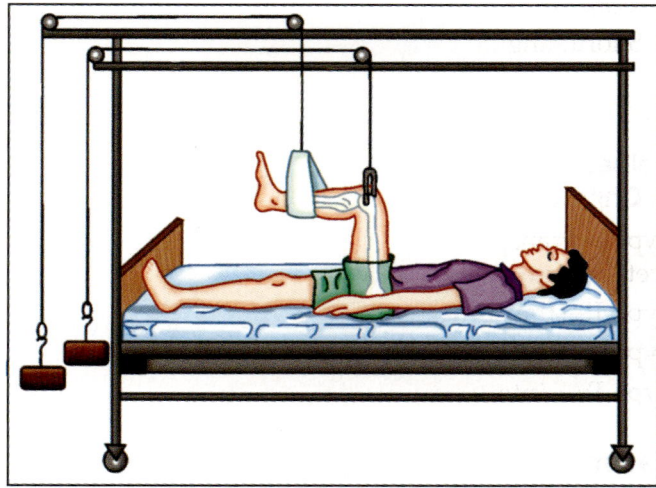

Fig. 17.19: Traction technique for subtrochanteric femur fracture

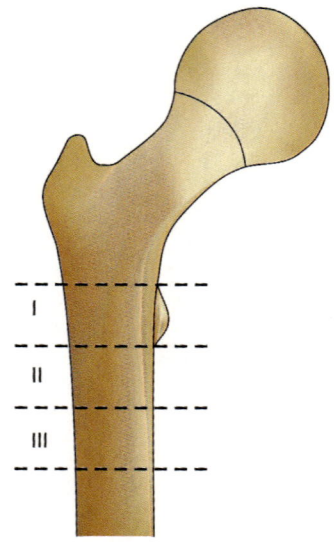

Fig. 17.18: Fielding's classification

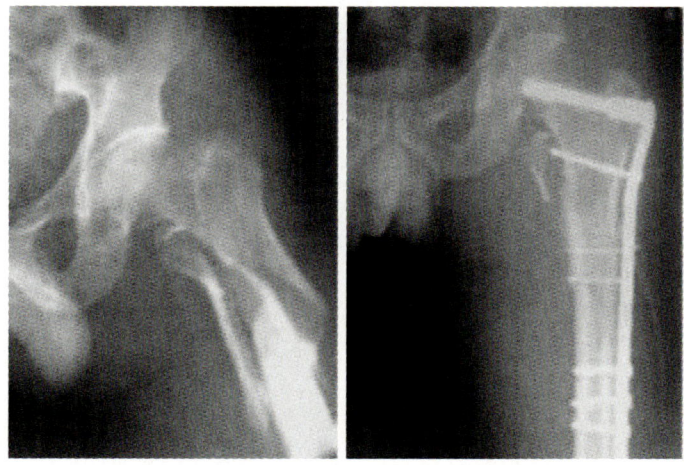

Fig. 17.20: Subtrochanteric fracture treated using dynamic condylar screw system

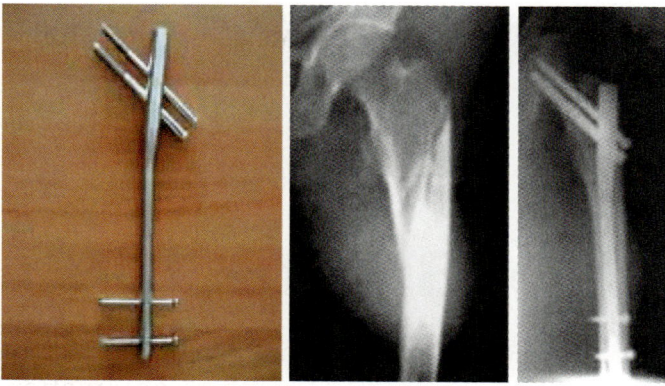

Fig. 17.21: Subtrochanteric fracture treated using proximal femoral nail

Complications of Subtochanteric Fractures

1. Non-union
2. *Malunion:* Coxa vara deformity
3. Shortening of lower limb

HIP FRACTURES IN CHILDREN

Delbet Classification of Hip Fractures in Children (Fig. 17.22)

Type I—transphyseal, with or without dislocation from acetabulum

Type II—transcervical

Type III—cervicotrochanteric (basicervical)

Type IV—intertrochanteric

Treatment

1. *Type I,* transphyseal: Gentle closed reduction and internal fixation; with dislocation–gentle closed reduction, if unsuccessful, immediate open reduction and fixation with pins or cannulated hip screws.
2. *Type II,* transcervical: Closed reduction and internal fixation regardless of the amount of displacement.
3. *Type III,* cervico-trochanteric fractures: If displaced–gentle closed reduction and internal fixation; if not displaced–abduction spica cast.

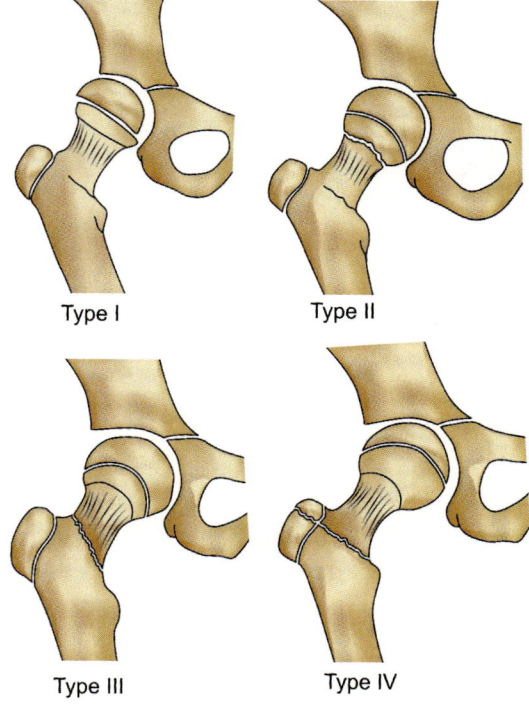

Type I   Type II

Type III   Type IV

Fig. 17.22: Delbet classification

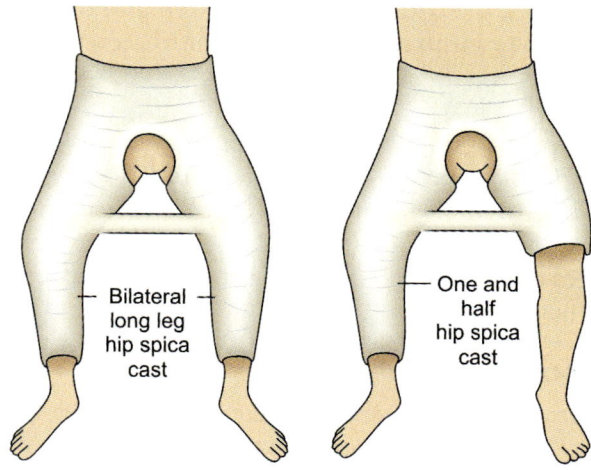

Bilateral long leg hip spica cast

One and half hip spica cast

Fig. 17.23: Hip spica cast

4. *Type IV,* intertrochanteric fractures: Skin or skeletal traction, abduction spica cast (Fig. 17.23).

Femoral Shaft Fracture

Introduction

Due to increase in the number of vehicular accidents, this is one of the most frequently encountered fractures in clinical practice. Fractures of the femoral shaft lead to massive internal blood loss, as they are high velocity injuries. Other severe associated injuries may be present which should be looked for, diagnosed promptly and emergent treatment carried out. The type and location of the fracture, the degree of comminution, the age of the patient, the patient's functional demands and other factors may influence the method of treatment.

Anatomy

Muscle forces across the femoral shaft (especially important in fracture alignment) include the iliopsoas, leading to flexion of the proximal fragment; the adductors, leading to shortening of the femur; and the gluteal muscles, which abduct and extend the proximal fragment.

Mechanism of Injury

Femoral shaft fractures are secondary to a *high-energy force*, such as a direct blow or an indirect force transmitted through the flexed knee. Automobile collisions are the most common cause. Fracture of the femur following a *low-energy mechanism is rare*, and the clinician should suspect a pathologic fracture if a patient presents with trivial trauma but a femoral shaft fracture.

Management

Diagnosis

X-rays of the affected extremity—anteroposterior and lateral views. Additional X-ray of the pelvis and the knee would help to treat the associated injuries.

Initial Management

Hypovolemia is likely due to major blood loss. It should be treated first, blood volume should be restored and maintained.

Treatment

Initial treatment in casualty would be splinting the affected lower limb in Thomas splint or by giving skeletal traction through a Steinmann pin inserted through lower femur or upper tibia transversely under local anaesthesia.

Techniques of Internal Fixation

a. Interlocking Intramedullary Nailing

Currently treatment of choice due to excellent rotational stability provided by it (Fig. 18.1).

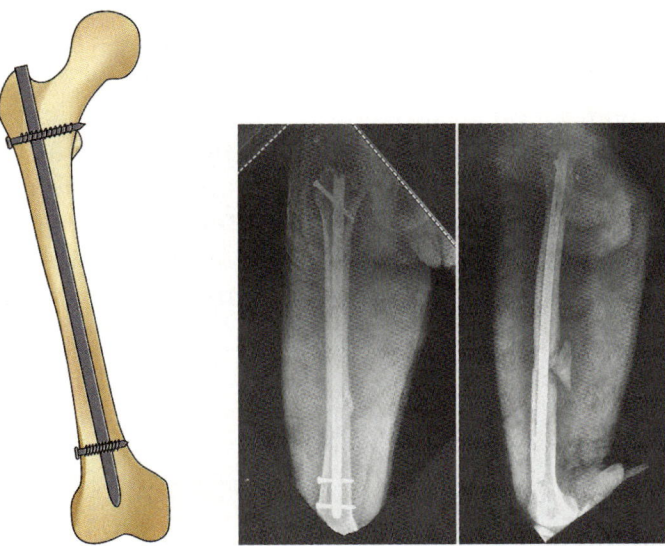

Fig. 18.1: Femur shaft fracture treated with interlocking nail

b. *Kuntscher Nail*

Known popularly as "K" nail. It is the first generation nail. It was used commonly for stabilisation of transverse femoral fractures in the region of isthmus.

c. *External Fixators*

External fixators are commonly used in compound fractures and help in early wound healing (Fig. 18.2).

d. *Plating for Femoral Fractures*

Commonly used for paediatric femoral fractures where nail insertion should not be carried out as, the *physes are open* and nail insertion might *damage the physes* situated at the end of diaphysis (Fig. 18.3).

e. *TENs (Titanium Elastic Nails)*

Used for paediatric femoral fractures (Fig. 18.4).

Complications of Femoral Fractures

1. Nonunion
2. Malunion which can be angular or rotational
3. Fat embolism
4. Compartment syndrome.

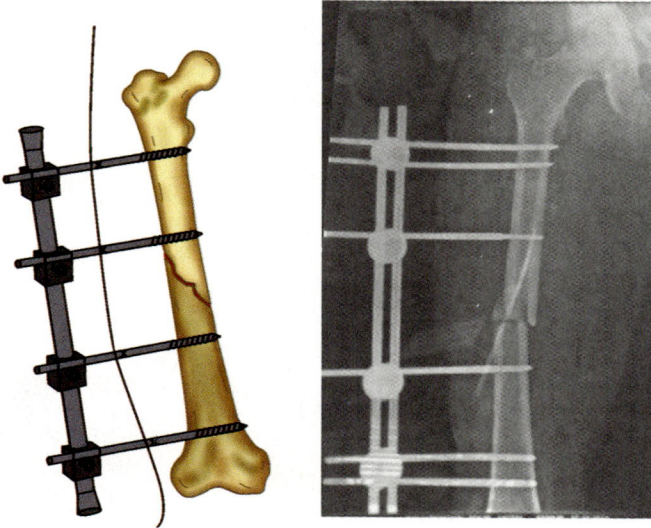

Fig. 18.2: Femur shaft fracture treated with external fixator

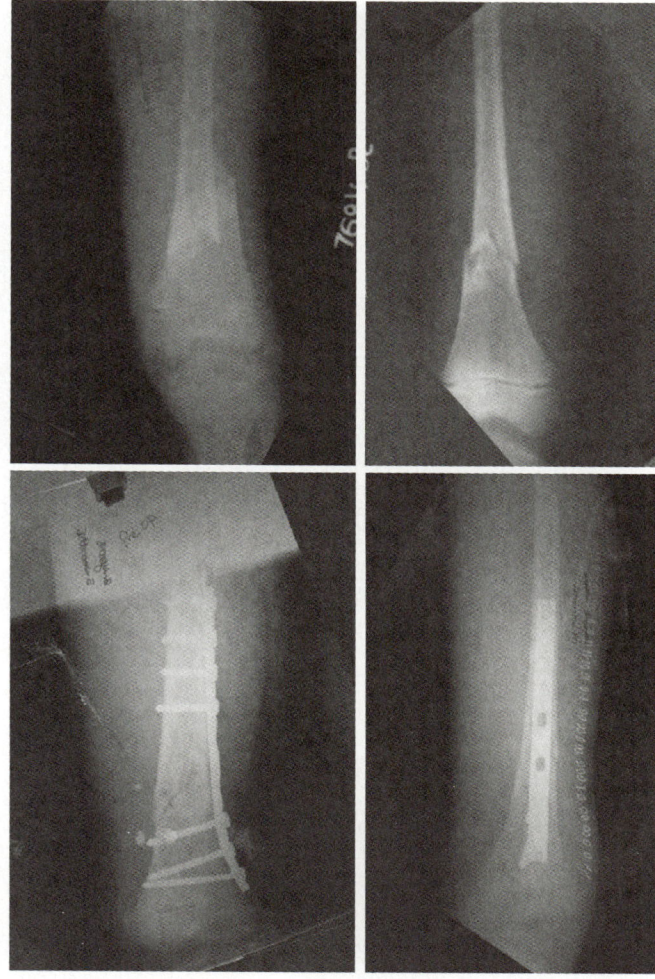

Fig. 18.3: Femur shaft fracture treated with DCP

FRACTURE SHAFT FEMUR IN CHILDREN

Gallow's Traction

Gallow's traction (Bryant's traction) is a sliding skin traction used to stabilize femoral shaft fracture in children under the age of 2 (Fig. 18.5).

		Table 18.1: General treatment guidelines in children with femoral shaft fractures		
Age	<1 yr	1–6 yrs	6–13 yrs	Adolescents
Preferred Treatment	Pavlik harness or Gallow's traction	Early spica casting	Elastic Intramedullary nail	Intramedullary Interlocking nail (trochanteric entry)

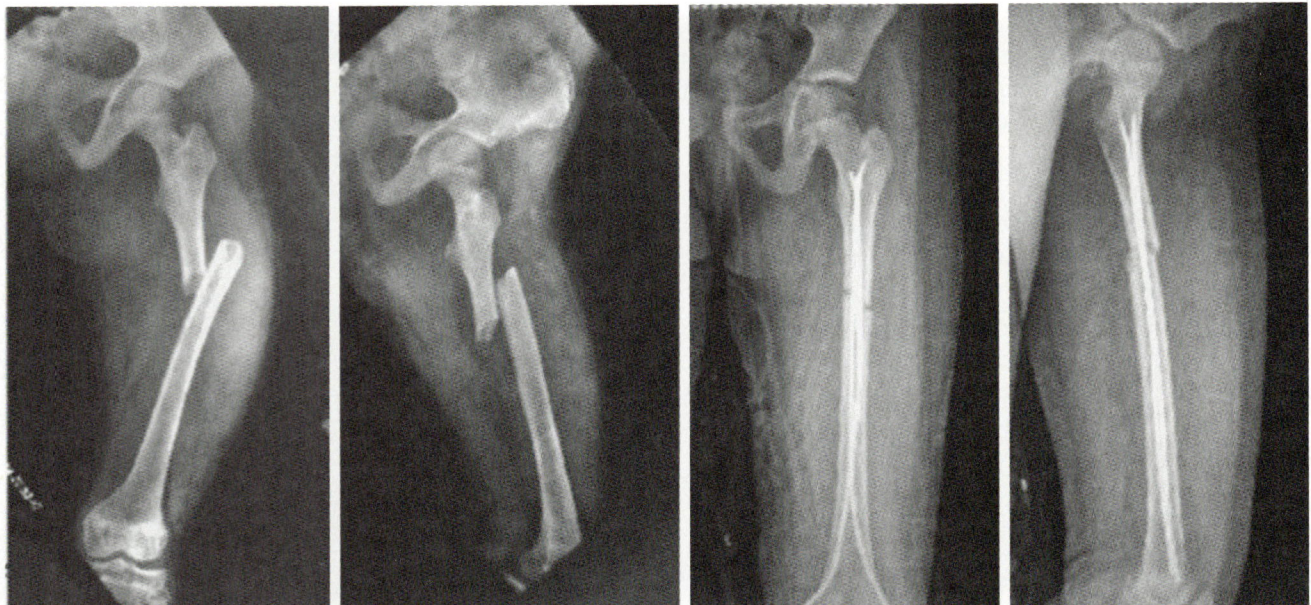

Fig. 18.4: Paediatric femur shaft fracture treated using TENS

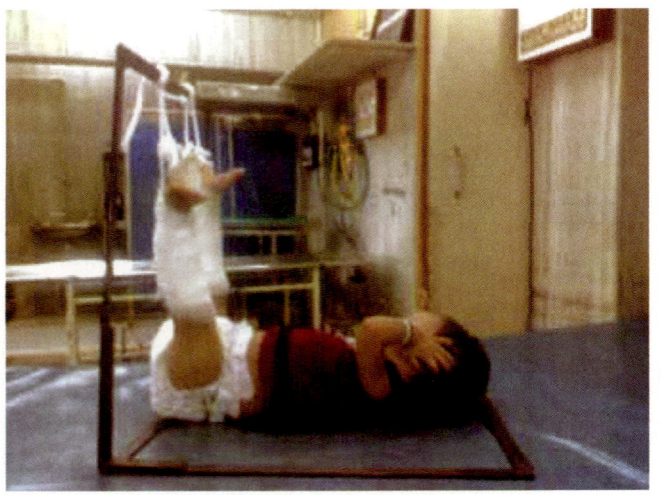

Fig. 18.5: Gallow's traction

Pavlik Harness

Pavlik harness is a dynamic flexion abduction orthosis used to treat developmental dysplasia of hip (DDH) in infants up to 6 months of age. But it can also be used for fracture shaft femur in infants (Fig. 18.6).

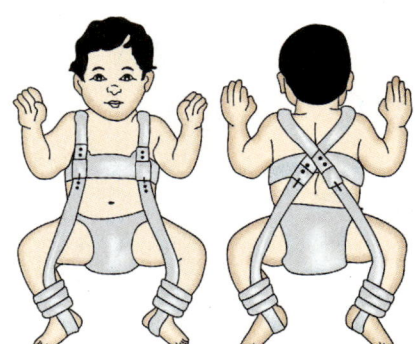

Fig. 18.6: Pavlik harness

Injuries around the Knee

SUPRACONDYLAR FEMUR FRACTURES

Definition

The supracondylar area of the femur is defined as the zone between the femoral condyles and the junction of the metaphysis with the femoral shaft. This area comprises the distal 9 to 15 cm of the femur (Fig. 19.1).

Mechanism of Injury

Supracondylar femur fractures occur as a result of severe axial load with varus, valgus, or rotation. In young patients, it occurs due to high-energy trauma such as motor vehicle collisions and fall from height. In elderly patients, the force from a minor slip and fall on a flexed knee causes such fractures.

Classification

The AO/OTA classification for supracondylar femur fractures divides the fractures into 3 groups (Fig. 19.2).
Type A: Supracondylar with no articular extension (extra-articular),
Type B: Unicondylar (intra-articular),
Type C: Supracondylar with intercondylar extension.

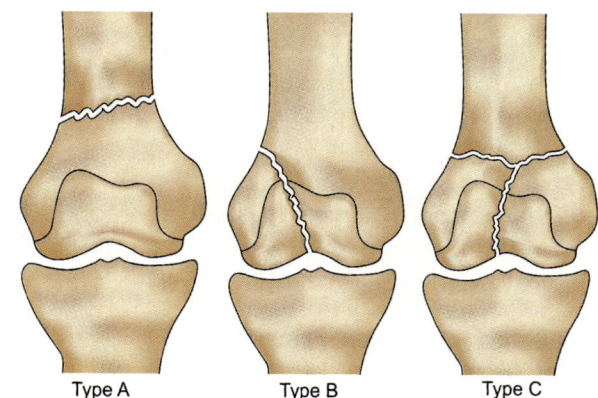

| Type A | Type B | Type C |

Fig. 19.2: AO classification of supracondylar femur fracture

Clinical Evaluation

Pain, swelling around the knee with deformity of the lower limb.

The typical fracture displacement in fractures of the supracondylar region of the distal femur is caused by the traction of the hamstrings and quadriceps muscles in one direction and the traction of the gastrocnemius muscle on the distal fragment, producing posterior angulation and displacement (Fig. 19.3).

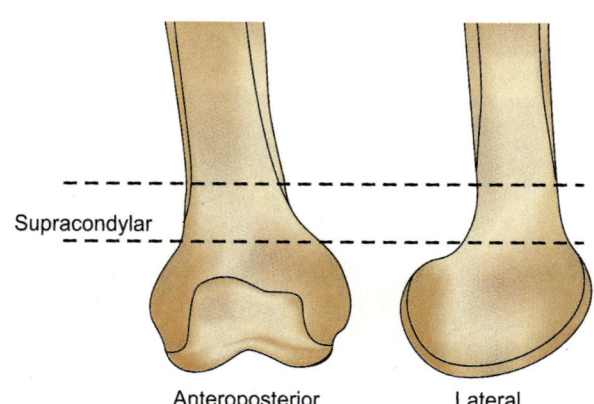

Supracondylar

Anteroposterior   Lateral

Fig. 19.1: Supracondylar region of femur

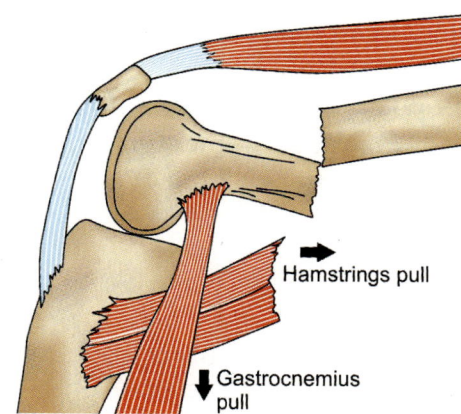

Hamstrings pull

Gastrocnemius pull

Fig. 19.3: Deforming forces of supracondylar femur fracture

Management

Diagnosis

1. X-rays of the affected part anteroposterior (AP) and lateral views.
2. *CT scan:* In cases of articular involvement or for planning the sequence of fracture fixation, 3D CT scans are helpful to understand the geometry of the fracture.

Treatment

Goals of treatment

1. Restore the articular anatomy.
2. Restore the mechanical axis.

1. Intramedullary Nailing (retrograde entry through knee joint) (Fig. 19.4)

For fractures in supracondylar femur region.

2. Plating

It can be performed via direct visualization of the joint during fixation, which also allows for restoration of the mechanical axis (with a fixed device) (Fig. 19.5).

Complications of Supracondylar Femoral Fractures

1. Non-union
2. Malunion
3. Knee stiffness due to intra-articular fracture.
4. Injury to popliteal vessels due to fracture displacement.

PATELLA FRACTURES

Anatomy

Salient features of patella

1. It is the largest sesamoid bone of the human body.
2. It helps to transmit forces across the knee joint
3. It is an important component of the knee extensor mechanism.
4. The distal pole is non-articular.
5. The patella translates approximately 7 cm from flexion to extension with 13 to 38% of the patellar surface in contact with the femur at any given time through the ROM.

Mechanism of Injury

1. Direct blow (e.g. dashboard injury) leads to comminution or articular damage.
2. Rapid knee flexion with quadriceps resistance can result in a simple, transverse fracture.

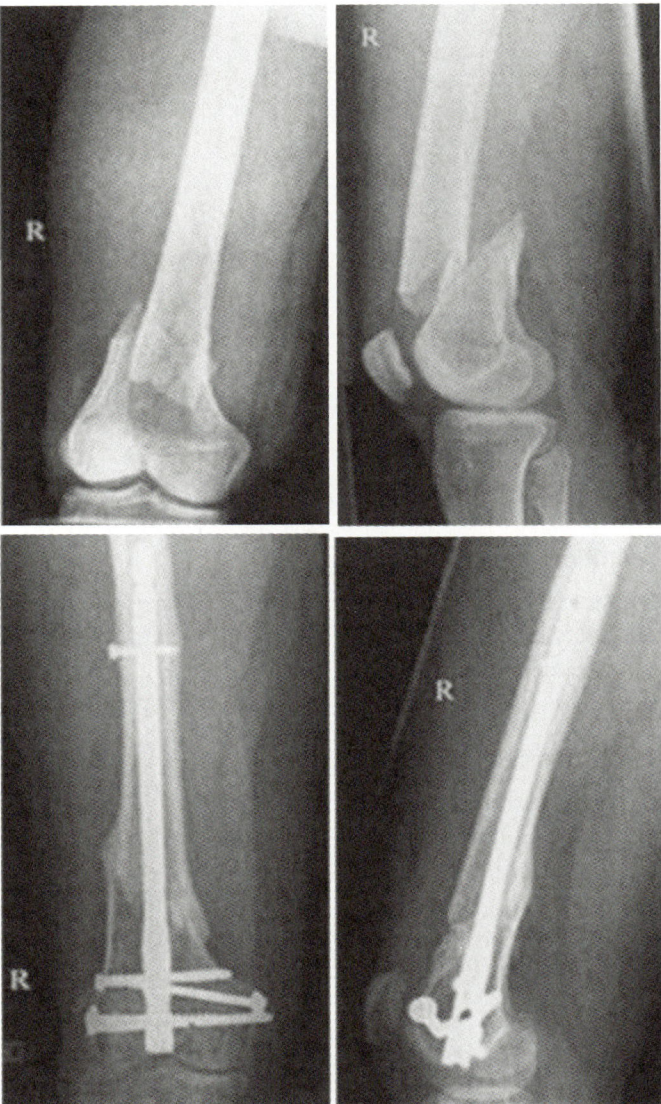

Fig. 19.4: Supracondylar femur fracture treated with retrograde intramedullary nail

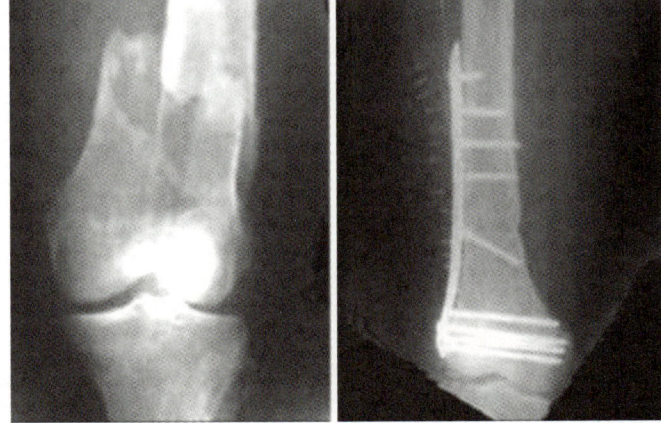

Fig. 19.5: Supracondylar femur fracture treated with locking plate

Classification (Fig. 19.6)

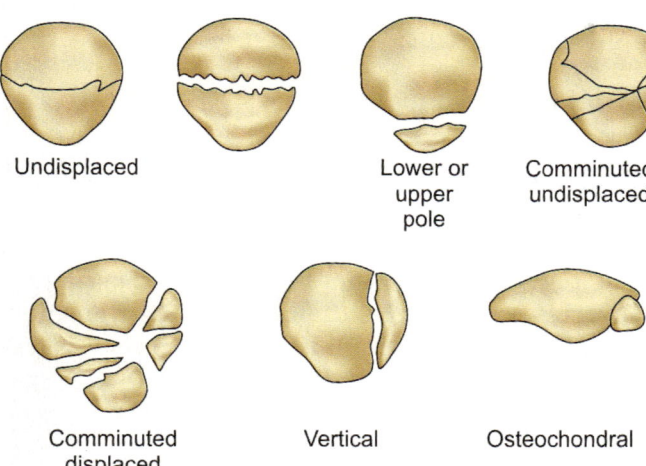

Undisplaced

Lower or upper pole

Comminuted undisplaced

Comminuted displaced

Vertical

Osteochondral

Fig. 19.6: Classification of patella fractures

Clinical Evaluation

Depending on the type and mechanism of injury, a palpable defect or a soft tissue component may exist. The extensor mechanism can be evaluated by having the patient extend the knee against gravity or maintain knee extension against gravity. Inability to extend the knee signifies disruption of extensor mechanism of the knee.

Management

Diagnosis

X-rays

1. Anteroposterior and lateral views of the knee joint.
2. Oblique X-rays of the knee joint should always be taken to rule out associated fractures of the femoral condyles and distal femoral articular surface.

   The examiner should be aware of the bipartite patella, which is a normal variant that involves the superolateral corner of the patella because of an accessory ossification centre. Radiographs of the other knee often reveal bilaterality.

Nonoperative Treatment

Indications

1. Nondisplaced fractures
2. Minimally displaced fractures in the elderly
3. Patients with multiple medical problems.

   Nonoperative treatment includes a long-leg cylinder cast for 4 to 6 weeks (consider knee immobilizer for the elderly) with immediate weight bearing as tolerated after cast application.

Operative Treatment

1. *Tension-band wiring:* For transverse, noncomminuted fractures.
2. Lag-screw fixation.
3. *Partial patellectomy:* It is indicated for fractures with extensive comminution not amenable to fixation.
4. *Complete patellectomy:* It is indicated for displaced, comminuted fractures not amenable to reconstruction, but it usually results in extensor lag and loss of strength.
5. *Fractures of inferior pole of patella:* Treated with suturing by strong material like Ethibond, or bone wire. If comminuted, it can be removed along with suturing the patellar tendon to the remaining portion of the patella.

Complications

1. Knee stiffness (most common complication)
2. Osteoarthritis of knee
3. Nonunion

TIBIAL PLATEAU FRACTURES

Anatomy

Tibial plateau consists of medial and lateral plateau (Fig. 19.7). *Salient features of the medial tibial plateau:*

1. It is larger and more distal than the lateral plateau
2. It is concave in shape with a 10-degree posterior slope
3. It has 3 mm of articular cartilage
4. The bone has greater density because it bears 75% of the weight.

Salient features of the lateral plateau: Slopes posteriorly 7 degrees with 4 mm of articular cartilage covering the surface.

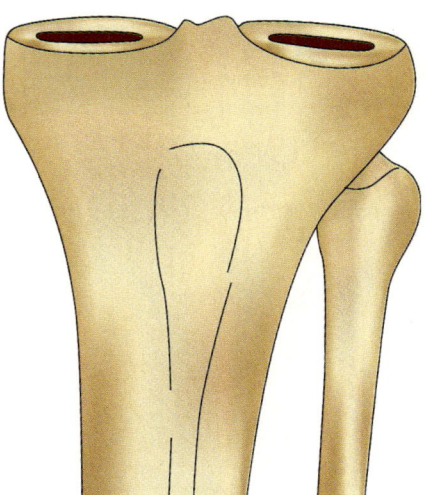

Fig. 19.7: Anatomy of tibial condyles

The lateral meniscus lies atop the lateral plateau. It is more circular in shape and covers more of the articular surface than the medial meniscus. The lateral meniscus bears more of the joint reactive force than the bone on the lateral side.

The medial meniscus is C-shaped, attached to the deep portion of the MCL, and biomechanically bears load equal to that of bone with respect to joint reactive forces.

Mechanism of Injury

Tibial plateau fractures occur in a bimodal distribution, with younger patients being injured secondary to high-energy injuries (e.g. MVA) and older patients due to low-energy injuries (e.g. fall from standing). The most common fracture pattern is split-depression of the lateral tibia.

Classification

Tibial plateau fractures can be classified according to Schatzker classification on the basis of the location and type of fracture pattern (Fig. 19.8).

Type I (split fracture): Pure split of lateral plateau.

Type II (split-depression): Split and depression of lateral plateau.

Type III: Pure central depression fracture of the lateral tibial plateau.

Type IV: Involves the medial tibial plateau.

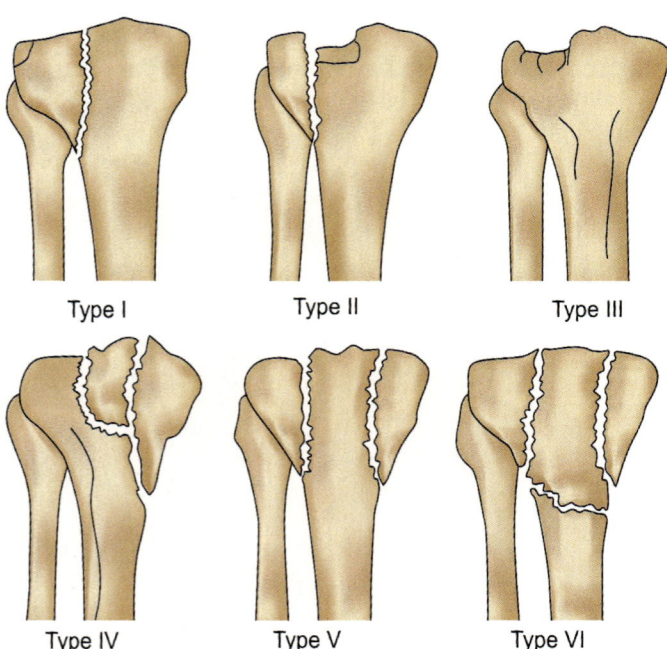

Fig. 19.8: Schatzker classification

Type V: Bicondylar fracture.

Type VI: Bicondylar fracture with extension into tibial diaphysis.

Clinical Evaluation

1. Evaluate the soft-tissues.
2. Evaluate the polpliteal artery by palpating and visualizing the pulsations of popliteal artery and distally of posterior tibial and dorsalis pedis arteries. The popliteal artery is at risk with medial plateau injuries or fracture/dislocations of the knee. Therefore, the examination should also assess compartment and knee stability.
3. Evaluation of the peroneal nerve should be done by asking the patient to dorsiflex the ankle and great toe.
4. *Compartment syndrome:* Always look out for compartment syndrome especially in cases of closed type V and type VI injuries as after fracture the blood through bone seeps into the surrounding soft tissues and since the leg consists of sleeve of fascia, it leads to increase in the intracompartmental pressure. This is an emergency which should be adequately treated by release of the compartments of leg. It carries priority over fracture treatment.

Management

Diagnosis

X-rays
a. Anteroposterior, lateral, and oblique views of the knee and the entire length of the tibia.
b. Traction radiographs provide valuable information regarding fracture patterns in complex plateau fractures.

CT scan
a. Helps understand the anatomy of the fracture better.
b. Helps in better preoperative planning.

A. Treatment: Nonoperative Treatment

Indications: Undisplaced fractures. Treated with above knee plaster in 30 degree knee flexion for 6 to 8 weeks.

B. Operative Treatment

Principles of fixation are:
1. Restoration of the varus and valgus alignment of the proximal tibia.
2. Maintaining the meniscus.
3. Reconstruction of incompetent ligamentous structures.
4. Restore the articular congruity.

Methods of Fixation

1. *Screws:* 6.5 mm cannulated or noncannulated screws for isolated, noncomminuted condylar fractures.
2. Implants of choice for tibial plateau fractures are T and L-shaped plates which can be simple plates used as buttressing plates (Fig. 19.9).

   New implants are locking plates used again as T or L plates, in this the threads of the screw head locks in thread of the plate hole–their advantage being more stability to the implant–fracture configuration.
3. *External fixators:* Indications for use include fractures with poor skin condition. External fixators that span the knee joint may include either half-pins or smooth wires. These constructs can be used temporarily to allow time for the soft tissue envelope to heal.

Complication of Tibial Plateau Fractures

Early Complications

1. *Skin dehiscence:* Preoperative attention to skin status is important. Adequate time should be given for abrasions or post-traumatic skin blisters to heal before surgery to prevent such complication occurring postoperatively.
2. Infection
3. Meniscal injuries
4. Injuries to anterior or posterior cruciate ligament-leading to instability of the knee and later osteoarthritis. These should be promptly suspected, diagnosed and treated by repair in acute setting or reconstruction at a later suitable time by open or arthroscopic techniques, which is widely popular nowadays for treatment of such injuries.

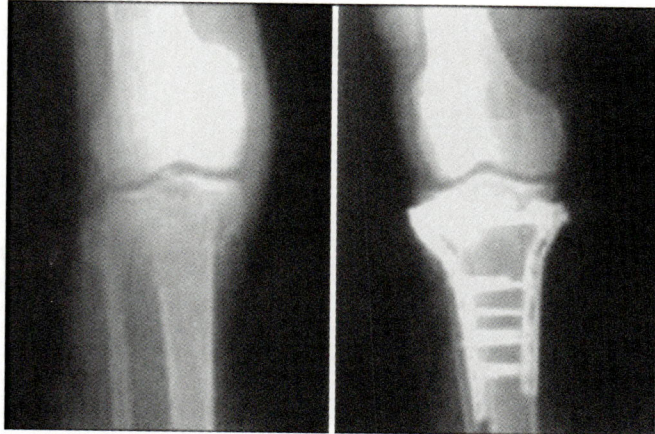

Fig. 19.9: Bicondylar (Type V) tibia plateau fracture treated with dual plates

Late Complications

1. *Non-union* in cases of untreated plateau fractures due to meniscal interposition or in those fractures with involvement of the tibial diaphysis.
2. *Malunion* either in untreated fractures or where adequate attention to restoration of the axial alignment in not given at the time of surgery.
3. *Osteoarthritis of the knee:* Potential complication in cases of intra-articular fractures of upper tibia, lower femur, and patella. Final solution in cases of patients with severe pain due to post-traumatic arthritis of knee would be total knee arthroplasty.
4. *Implant failure* in osteoporotic bones, hence nowadays better implants called locking plates are available.
5. *Painful hardware* that can be treated with implant removal to be done one year after initial surgery and after the fracture has healed.

Tibial Shaft Fractures

Tibia fractures are one of the most common long bone fractures and also the most common open fractures.

Anatomy

The anteromedial aspect of the tibia is almost *subcutaneous* being devoid of good muscle cover. This renders it very susceptible to severe bone and soft tissue injury and high incidence of open fractures. The blood supply to the tibial shaft arises from a single nutrient artery and periosteal arteries. The tibial canal expands, and the cortex thins proximally and distally at the metaphyseal diaphyseal junctions.

Mechanism of Injury

Direct trauma is a common cause of injury and usually results in associated soft-tissue injury. These fractures are frequently secondary to automobile collisions and typically result in transverse or comminuted fractures. Indirect trauma is associated with rotary and compressive forces, as from skiing or a fall, and usually result in a spiral or oblique fracture.

Classification

There is no special classification for shaft tibia fractures (Fig. 20.1).

Clinical Evaluation

Tibial shaft fractures usually present with pain, swelling, and deformity. Although neurovascular damage is not commonly seen after these injuries, documentation of distal pulses as well as peroneal nerve function should always be done. The dorsalis pedis pulse should be palpated and compared with the uninjured extremity. The patient should always be evaluated for "compartment syndrome". Tibia fractures are the most common cause of compartment syndrome.

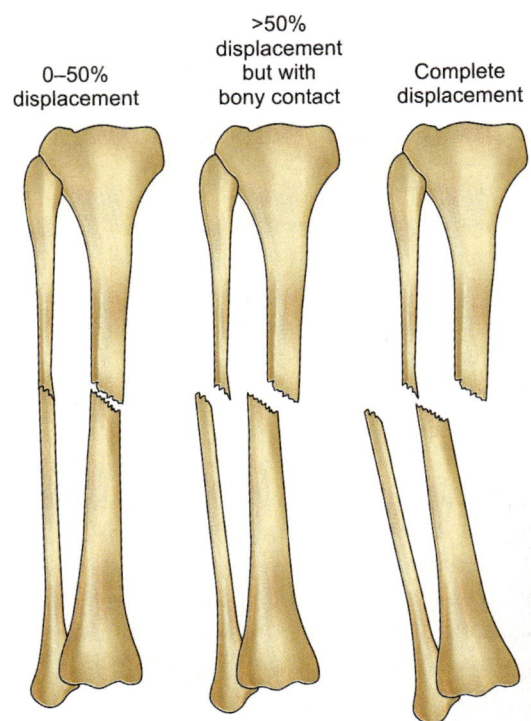

Fig. 20.1: Displacement of tibia fractures

Associated injuries: Associated injuries occur in up to 30% of patients; an ipsilateral fibula fracture is the most common additional injury. The ligamentous structures of the knee are at high risk in high-energy injuries.

Management

Diagnosis

X-rays-Anteroposterior and lateral views of the tibia along with X-ray of one joint above and below, i.e. knee and ankle X-ray should always be taken.

Treatment

Indications for nonoperative management

Fractures with:

1. Less than 50% displacement
2. Less than 10 degrees of anteroposterior angulation
3. Less than 5 degrees of varus and valgus angulation
4. Less than 2 cm of shortening

Techniques of Nonoperative Treatment

1. Long leg casts
2. Patellar tendon-bearing casts (allow knee movement)
3. Functional braces, which permit both knee and ankle movement.

Closed tibial fractures associated with intact fibulas are treated with cast immobilization.

Indications for Operative Treatment

Displacement of tibial shaft fractures with rotational or angular deformities.

Techniques

1. Intramedullary Nailing

Most preferred for majority of tibial shaft fractures. It is inserted inside the medullary canal through an entry point made in the proximal tibia. It is a load sharing device as it lies along the mechanical axis of the tibia and hence the lower limb (Fig. 20.2).

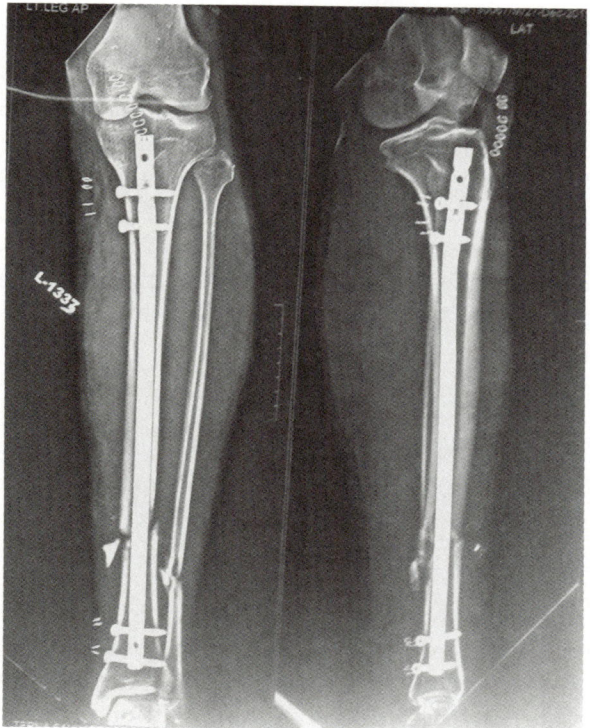

Fig. 20.2: Fracture tibia treated with intramedullary interlocking nail

2. Open Reduction and Internal Fixation(ORIF)

a. *Dynamic compression plates (DCP):* These plates cause compression at the fracture site as the screws inserted through the plate are tightened.
b. *Locking plates:* Latest new technology includes locking plates especially for osteoporotic fractures or technique of slide plating called *MIPPO (minimally invasive percutaneous plate osteosynthesis)* (Fig. 20.3).

Complications

a. *Nonunion:* Nonunion or delayed union is common especially when there is:
   • Severe displacement

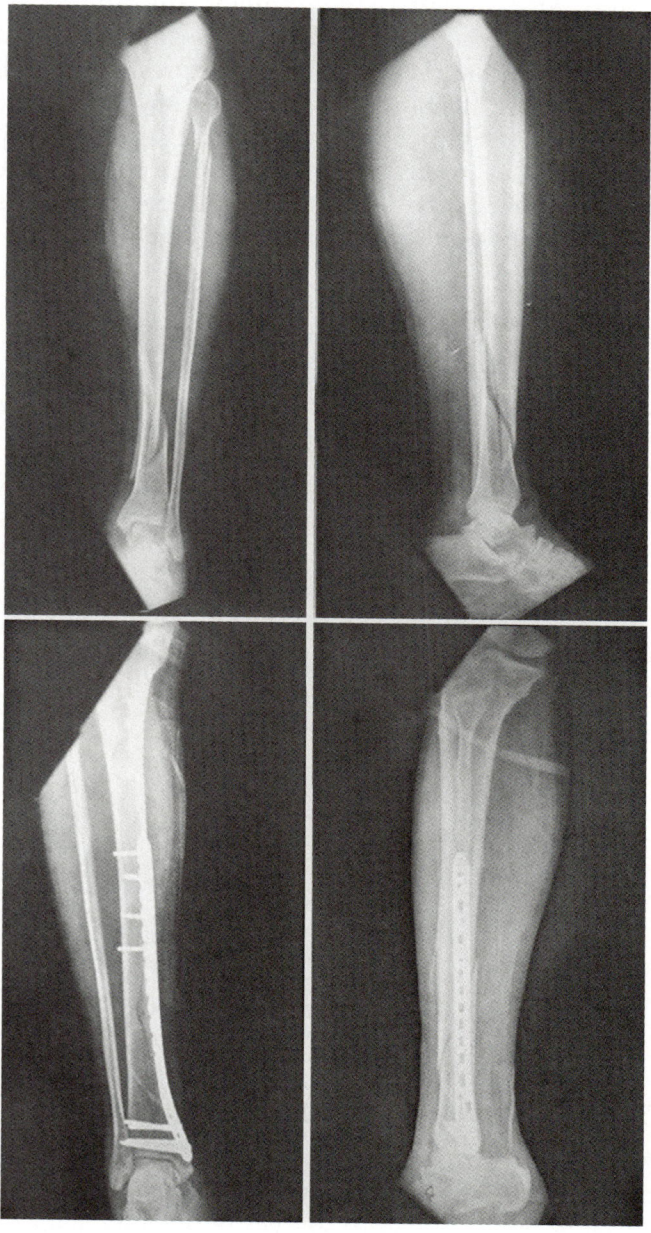

Fig. 20.3: Fracture tibia treated with locking plate

- Comminution
- Open fracture or severe soft-tissue damage
- Infection

b. Malunion
c. *Joint stiffness.* Most common complication after intra-medullary nailing of the closed fracture of shaft of the tibia is anterior knee pain. This is treated by removal of the implant after the fracture has united.
d. *Compartment syndrome:* It occurs in 5 to 15% of closed tibial shaft fractures, which are often associated with a history of high-energy or crush injury.

Treatment: This is an orthopaedic emergency and complete fasciotomy should be carried out. A two-incision approach is recommended with the anterior and lateral compartments being decompressed through the lateral incision and the superficial and deep posterior compartments decompressed through the medial incision. Fasciotomies should not be undertaken subcutaneously through small skin incisions, as the intact skin may act as a constriction, further raising the pressure. All four compartments should be decompressed thoroughly (Fig. 20.4).

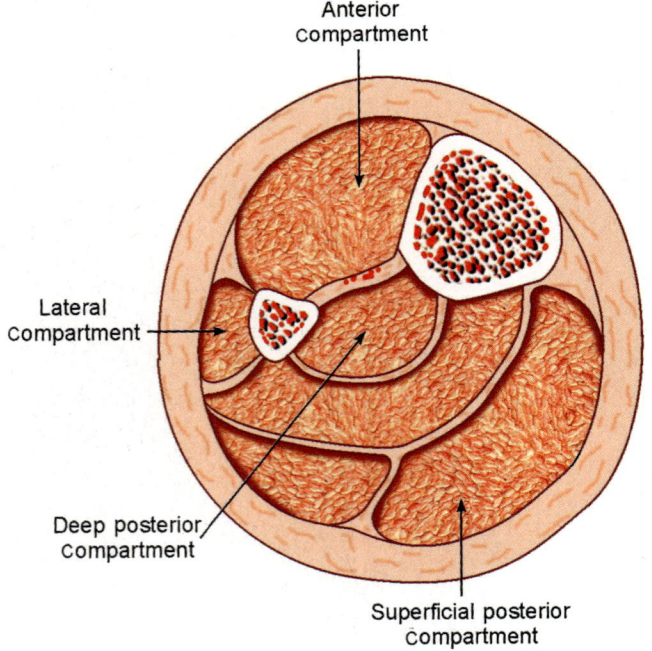

Fig. 20.4: Compartments of leg

OPEN TIBIAL SHAFT FRACTURES

As mentioned earlier in the anatomy of the tibia, the tibia is anteromedially devoid of good soft tissue envelope which renders it susceptible to open fractures due to its subcutaneous location.

Clinical Examination

Careful examination of the open wound, skin condition and fracture is important to determine the extent of debridement, need for plastic surgery and the procedure required for restoring the soft tissue envelope as well as the modality of fracture fixation technique required. The surgeon should digitally palpate the open wound, keeping in mind that any space that can be entered by a finger is potentially contaminated and must be opened.

Treatment

1. Thorough debridement
2. Skeletal stabilization by external fixation devices
3. Need for plastic surgery in the form of flaps or skin grafting.

Some surgeons recommend primary flap cover after debridement and stabilization of open fractures. A second look procedure is advocated 36 to 48 hours after the initial debridement, but delay beyond 72 hours should be avoided.

The goals of skeletal immobilization are as follows:
- Restore length and alignment of long bones.
- Reduce articular surfaces displaced by fracture.
- Allow access to the traumatic wound.
- Facilitate further reconstruction procedures.
- Allow early use of the limb.
- Facilitate fracture union and return of function.

Decision for Amputation

The necessity for amputation is directly related to the severity of the fracture. Primary amputation after tibial diaphyseal fractures should never be required in Gustilo type I or II fractures. In type IIIA fractures, the requirement for primary amputation is very rare. It should be stressed that primary amputation under these circumstances should only be performed if there is concern about the patient's survival if the leg is to be salvaged.

Absolute Indication for Amputation

1. Transection of the posterior tibial nerve and
2. Crush injuries with a warm ischaemia time of more than 6 hours.

Relative Indications

Serious associated polytrauma, severe ipsilateral foot trauma, and an anticipated protracted course to obtain soft tissue and tibial reconstruction. An attempt to assess and predict the need for amputation resulted in the development of the **mangled extremity severity score (MESS)** .

Mangled Extremity Severity Score (MESS)

This score is based on the

1. Type of skeletal and soft tissue injury
2. The degree of shock
3. Limb ischaemia
4. Patient's age

The MESS score is used as an aid to prediction of amputation. The decision to amputate should be made by two experienced orthopaedic surgeons.

MESS score of greater than or equal to 7 has a 100% predictable value for amputation.

PILON FRACTURE

Definition

The terms tibial plafond fracture, pilon fracture of amputation. The distal tibial explosion fracture all have been used to describe intra-articular fractures of the distal tibia.

Anatomy and Overview

The incidence of pilon fractures has increased with the advent of air bags. Most commonly, it occurs in age group of 15–30 years with males being involved predominantly. A tibial plafond fracture is typically secondary to a fall from height that drives the talus up into the tibia. The soft tissue component predominantly drives injury management (particularly anteromedially) because of the thin skin, lack of adipose tissue, and lack of deep veins over the distal tibia.

Classification

The *Ruedi-Allgower* classification system is used to describe these injuries (Fig. 20.5 and Table 20.1)

Table 20.1: Classification of pilon fractures

Type	Description
I	Articular fracture without significant displacement
II	Articular fracture, displaced with minimal comminution
III	Articular fracture with significant comminution and central depression

Clinical Evaluation

Pain, swelling, deformity. Bad skin condition with oedema, ecchymosis and blistering may be present. The extremity should be examined carefully for signs of vascular injury, and compartment syndrome.

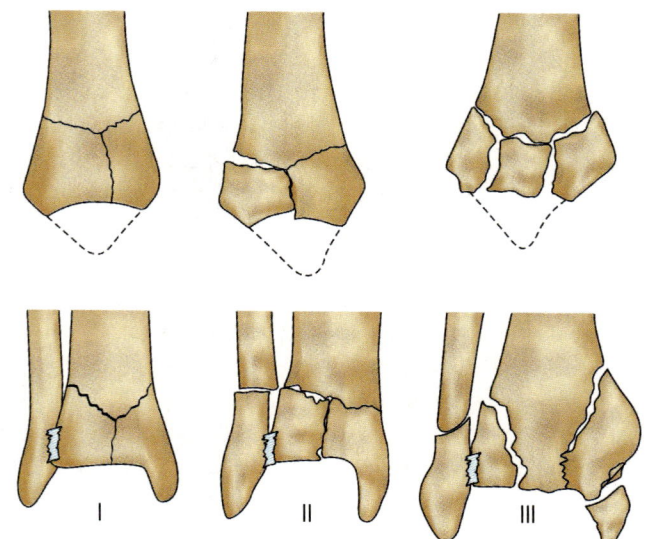

Fig. 20.5: lassification of tibial pilon fractures

Diagnosis

X-rays of the ankle anteroposterior and lateral views should be taken.

Management

Management of the soft tissue is the first priority in these injuries. Definitive surgical treatment should be delayed until the presence of a wrinkle sign (i.e. appearance of wrinkles when swelling subsides). Spanning external fixation should be applied until definitive treatment.

Goals of Treatment

• Anatomic reduction of intra-articular component
• Stable internal fixation
• Atraumatic technique with percutaneous or limited approaches
• Early pain-free mobilization

Fixation options include

• External fixation
• Plating-minimally invasive percutaneous plate osteosynthesis (MIPPO) is a good option done under C-arm guidance (Fig. 20.6).

Complications of Pilon Fractures

1. *Malunion at the fracture site:* This leads to secondary osteoarthritis of the ankle if proper attention to restoring the articular congruity and axial alignment is not maintained.
2. *Nonunion:* Mostly in cases of associated fibular fractures, this is due to poor soft tissue envelope of distal tibia.

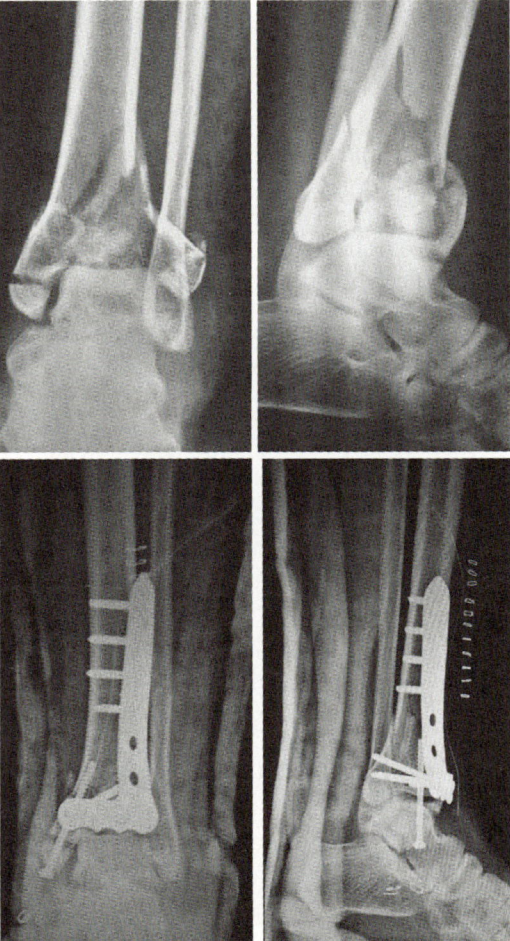

Fig. 20.6: Tibial pilon fracture fixed with distal tibia locking plate

Complication of Plating

1. Skin Breakdown

If due attention is not given to the preoperative status of the skin, there are high chances of skin breakdown in the lower tibial plafond region, which may be treated by plastic surgery in the form of flaps taken from calf region.

2. Infection

Due to poor soft tissue cover, chances of infection are high if meticulous surgical technique is not followed."

Ankle Fractures

Anatomy

Intrinsic stability of ankle is due to anatomy of the bones and muscles of the ankle joint. The ligaments and capsule of the ankle joint give extrinsic stability (Fig. 21.1). The talar dome and the tibial plafond are trapezoidal in shape (2.5 mm wider anteriorly). The ankle joint allows for triplane motion, tolerating 4 times body weight at stance. Normal range of motion is dorsiflexion 20 degrees (10 degrees is needed for normal gait) and plantar flexion 40 degrees.

Common Terms associated with Ankle Fractures

- **Pott's fracture:** Bimalleolar fracture (medial and lateral malleolus)

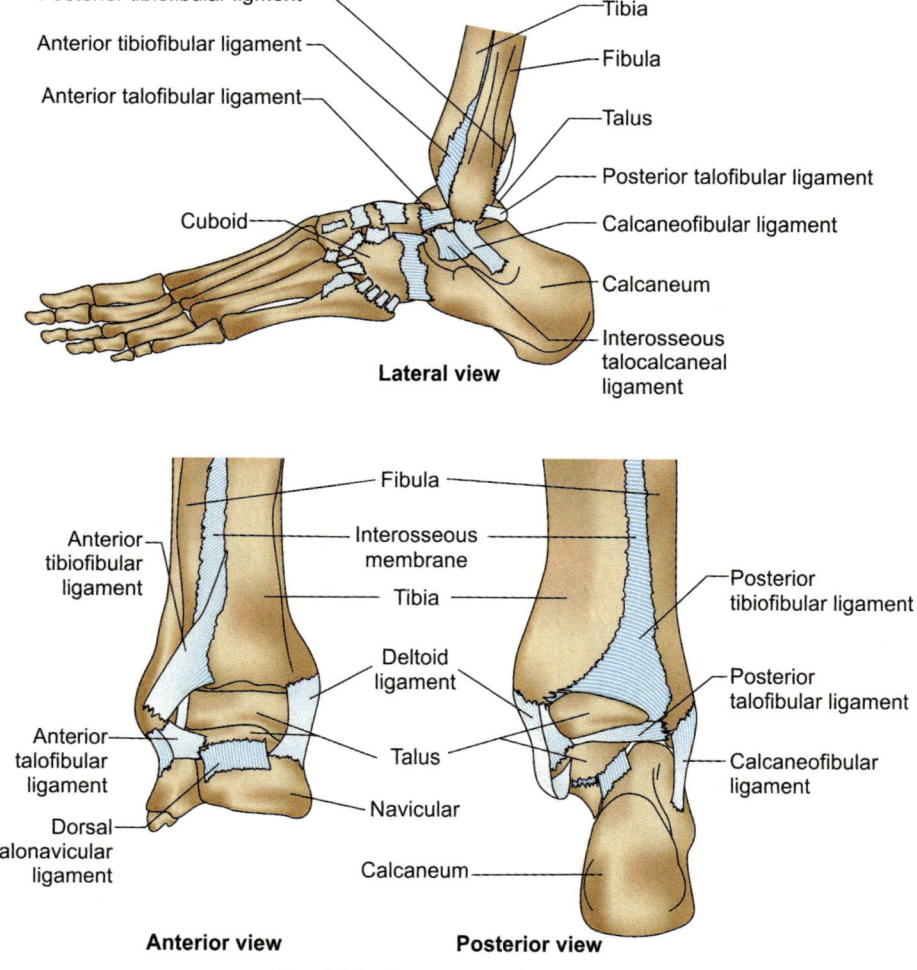

Fig. 21.1: Anatomy of ankle

- **Cotton's fracture:** Trimalleolar fracture (Pott's plus posterior malleolus)
- **Tillaux Chaput fracture:** Avulsion of tibial end of anterior tibiofibular ligament.
- **Lefort-Wagstaffe fracture:** Avulsion of fibular end of anterior tibiofibular ligament.

POTT'S FRACTURE

Mechanism of Injury

They occur commonly in elderly women. Incidence has increased nowadays due to use of high heels by females.

Classification

Weber Classification

Weber classification system is more simplified and is based on the location of fibula fracture with respect to the mortise .
A: Distal to the mortise (pronation abduction)
B: At the level of the mortise (supination external rotation)
C: Proximal to the mortise (pronation external rotation)

Lauge-Hansen Classification (Fig. 21.2)

1. Supination–adduction (SA)
2. Supination–eversion (external) rotation (SER)
3. Pronation–abduction (PA)
4. Pronation–eversion (external) rotation (PER)

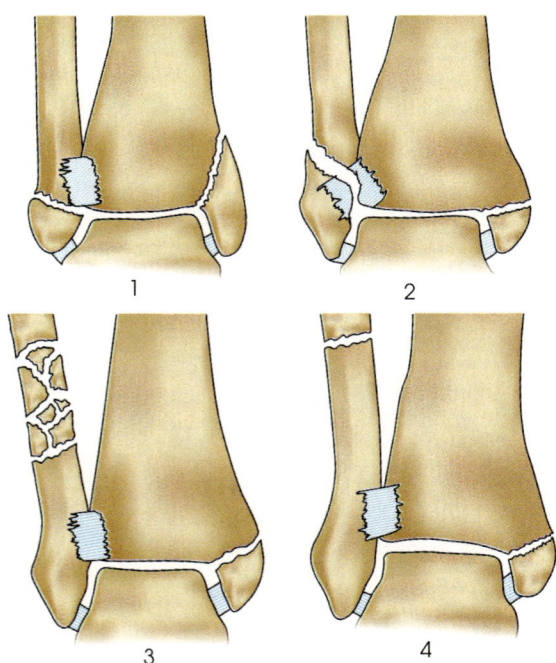

Fig. 21.2: Classification of ankle fractures

Lauge-Hansen classification is the commonest classification used for ankle fractures. There are four categories described by two words each. The first word describes the position of the foot at the time of injury, while the second word refers to the direction of the deforming force.

1. *Supination–adduction*
   - At the time of injury, if the foot is in supination, deltoid ligament is relaxed and lateral ligaments are tight.
   - When an adduction force is applied to supinated foot, talofibular ligament is injured first, followed by transverse low fibular fracture.
   - If adduction force continues further, deltoid ligament injury or vertical fracture of medial malleolus occurs.
2. *Supination–external rotation*
   - When external rotation force is applied to supinated foot, injury begins laterally at the anterior tibiofibular ligament and proceeds externally.
   - There is sequential involvement of lateral malleolous (oblique fracture above syndesmosis), posterior malleolus and finally medial structures (deltoid ligament or transverse medial malleolus fracture)
3. *Pronation–abduction*
   - At the time of injury, if foot is in pronation, medial structures are tight and hence subjected to avulsion. The lateral structures are injured due to bending force.
   - If abduction force is applied to a pronated foot, deltoid ligament is torn or medial malleolus undergoes avulsion fracture.
   - Lateral malleolus, due to bending force, develops comminuted fracture.
4. *Pronation–external rotation*
   - Pronated foot subjected to external rotation force leads to avulsion fracture of medial malleolus.
   - Further force sequentially injures anterior inferior tibiofibular ligament and finally lateral malleolus above syndesmosis.

Clinical Evaluation

- First inspect the soft tissues.
- Palpate the medial and lateral malleoli.
- Then assess the ligamentous stability.
- *Syndesmotic injury:* Pain during palpation of the entire course of the fibula or pain with side-to-side compression of the tibia and fibula at least 5 cm above the joint is indicative of a syndesmotic injury.
- *Associated injuries:* To fifth metatarsal or calcaneum.

Management

Imaging

1. X-rays anteroposterior, lateral, and mortise views.
   The mortise view is taken with the patient's leg internally rotated approximately 15 degrees, so the beam of the X-ray is perpendicular to the transmalleolar axis (Fig. 21.3).
2. Computed tomography (CT) scans help to delineate bony anatomy, especially in patients with plafond injuries.
3. Magnetic resonance imaging (MRI) may be used for assessing periankle occult cartilaginous, ligamentous, or tendinous injuries.

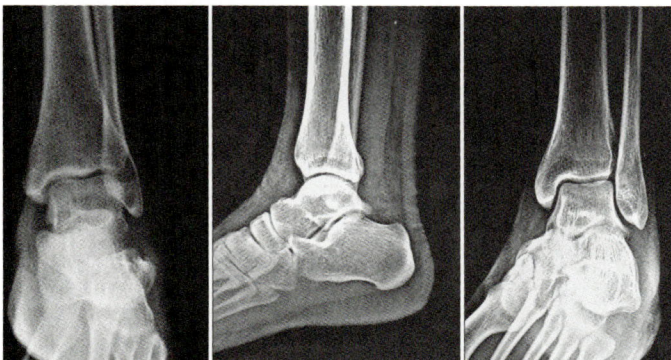

Fig. 21.3: AP, lateral and mortise view of ankle

Treatment

Nonoperative Treatment

Indications: Nondisplaced stable fractures with an intact syndesmosis or for medically unstable patients.

Treatment involves casting for 4 to 6 weeks with serial X-rays and subsequent conversion to a short-leg walking cast.

Operative Treatment

Indications
1. Talar subluxation
2. Joint incongruity

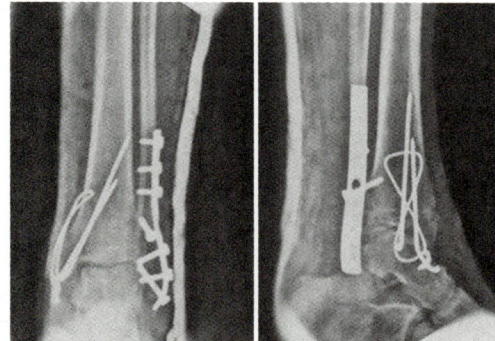

Fig. 21.4: Pott's fracture treated with K wires and tension band wiring

3. The posterior malleolus should be fixed if 25% of the joint surface is involved. This is associated with the pull of the posterior tibiofibular ligament (the fragment usually larger laterally than medially).
4. Syndesmotic injury

Implants for Fixation (Figs 21.4 and 21.5)

1. Malleolar screws: 4.5 mm screws and usually non-cannulated screws.
2. Tension band wiring.
3. *Plates:* Reconstruction plates.

Complications

Most common is malunion which leads to accelerated development of ankle arthritis.

Eventual treatment of ankle arthritis in a patient with severe pain would be ankle arthrodesis.

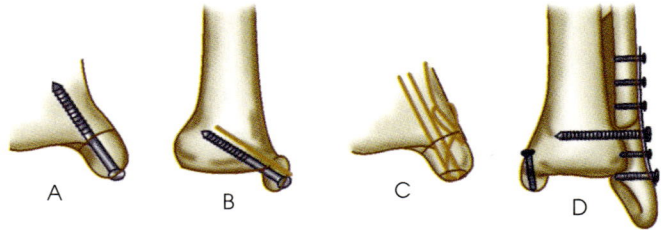

Fig. 21.5: Different modalities of fixation for ankle fractures. (A and B) Malleolar screw, (C) Tension band wire, (D) Plate

Complications of Surgery

1. Wound necrosis
2. Infection

BOSWORTH FRACTURE

The distal end of the proximal fragment of the fibula may be displaced posterior to the tibia and locked by the tibia's posterolateral ridge; the bone cannot be released by manipulation because of the pull of the intact interosseous membrane (Fig. 21.6).

Treatment is open reduction and internal fixation of the fibula fracture.

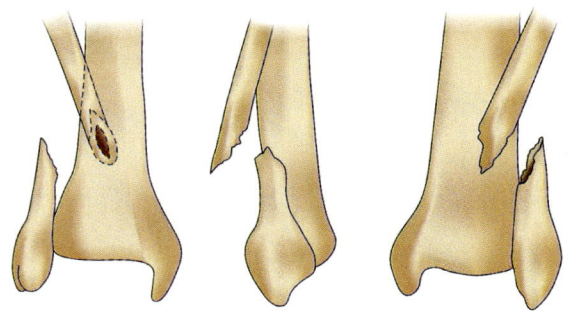

Fig. 21.6: Bosworth fracture

Injuries around Foot

TALUS FRACTURES

Anatomy

The talus is divided anatomically into three segments: head, neck, and body. It is held in place by ligaments and has no sites of muscle insertion. The vascular supply to the bone enters by way of the deltoid ligament, the talocalcaneal ligament, the anterior capsule, and the sinus tarsi. The blood supply is, tenuous and avascular necrosis is very common after displaced fractures. Proximal talar fractures are particularly predisposed to develop avascular necrosis of the proximal fragment (Fig. 22.2).

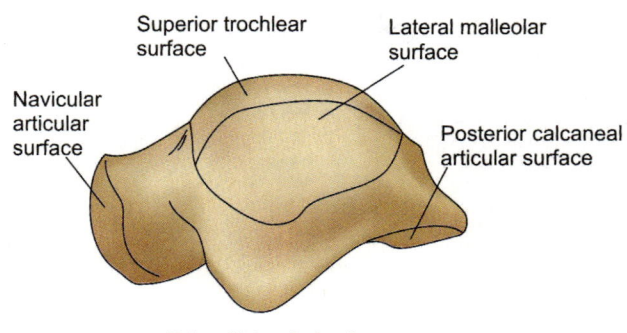

Talus (lateral view)

Fig. 22.2: Anatomy of talus

Mechanism of Injury

Most *serious* fractures of the talus are high-energy injuries. Fractures of the talar neck are commonly the result of a hyperdorsiflexion-type injury.

Classification

1. Minor talus fractures
   - Avulsion fractures
   - Posterior facet fractures
   - Osteochondral fractures
2. Major talus fractures
   - Talar head fractures
   - Talar neck fractures (Fig. 22.3)
   - Talar body fractures

Clinical Evaluation

Pain, swelling, ecchymosis, and tenderness.

Diagnosis

X-ray of ankle—lateral view is important. Oblique views of ankle help to identify the fracture better.

CT Scan: To evaluate the fracture anatomy.

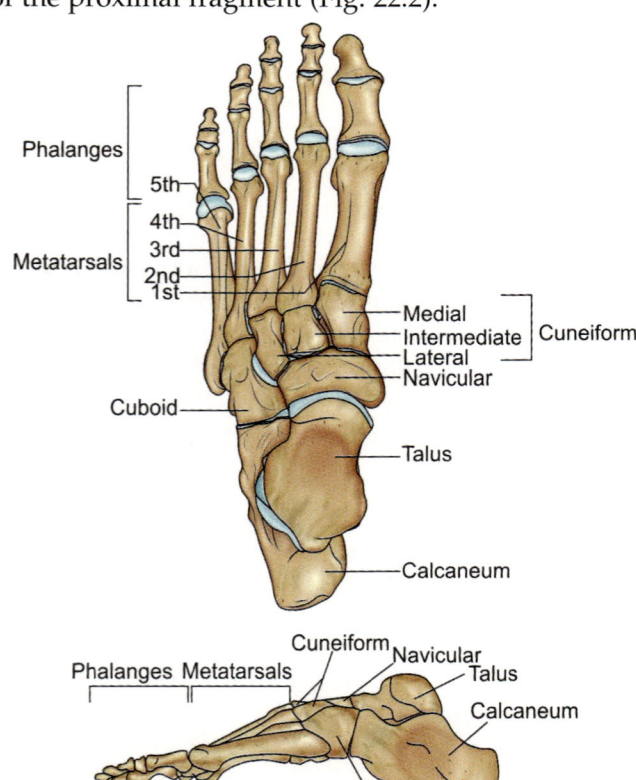

Fig. 22.1: Bones of foot

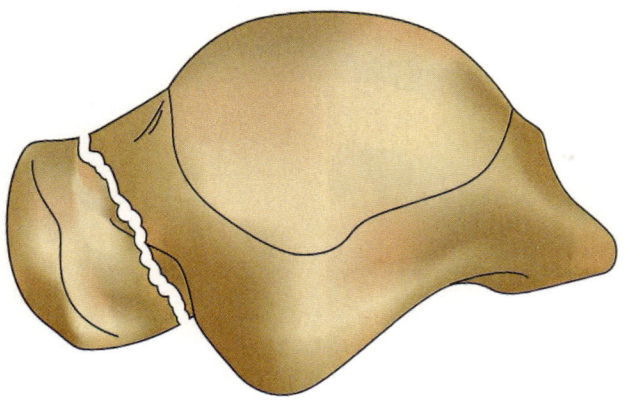

Fig. 22.3: Talar neck fracture

Treatment

Emergency management of this fracture should include ice, elevation, immobilization.

Nonoperative Treatment

Indicated for nondisplaced fractures. Nonweight bearing below knee cast for 6 to 8 weeks is the preferred mode of treatment.

Operative Treatment (Fig. 22.4)

Open reduction and internal fixation with cancellous screws is recommended if the fragment
1. causes instability of the talonavicular joint.
2. is displaced resulting in an articular step off.
3. is larger than 50% of the articular surface.

Complications

1. Avascular necrosis of talus.
2. Ankle and subtalar arthritis.

CALCANEUM FRACTURES

The calcaneum is the largest of the tarsal bones and serves as a springboard for locomotion and as an elastic support for the weight of the body. It is the most frequently fractured tarsal bone.

Anatomy

The anterior portion of the calcaneum is the body. The posterior portion of the calcaneum is the tuberosity. The Achilles tendon inserts on the posterior portion of the tuberosity. The principal articulation of the calcaneum is with the talus, forming the subtalar joint. Three articular surfaces exist as anterior, middle, and posterior articular facets. The sustentaculum talus is a medial extension of the calcaneum that supports the anterior and middle articular facets (Fig. 22.5).

Mechanism of Injury

Bilateral calcaneum fractures are usually observed along with spinal fractures in fall from height or high energy injuries in motor vehicular accidents.

Classification

1. Intra-articular
   • Body
2. Extra-articular
   • Anterior process
   • Sustentaculum tali
   • Lateral calcaneal process and peroneal tubercle
   • Medial calcaneal process
   • Tuberosity
   • Body

Clinical Evaluation

Pain, swelling, widening of heel, ecchymosis.

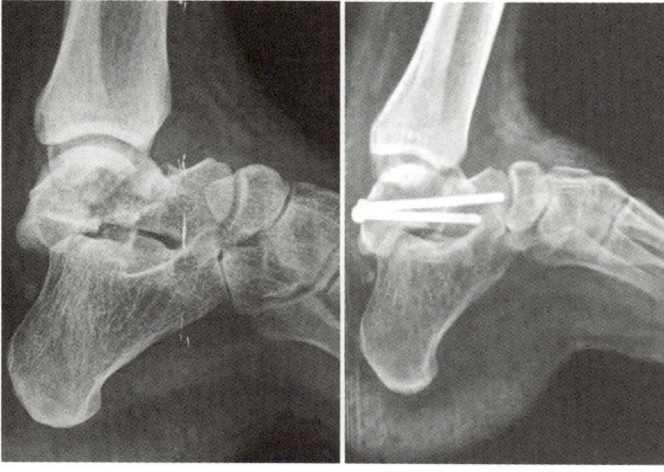

Fig. 22.4: Fracture talus treated with ORIF using screws

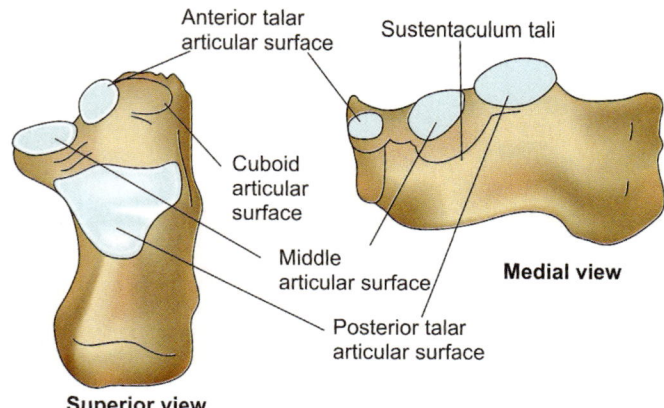

Fig. 22.5: Anatomy of calcaneum

Diagnosis

X-rays: AP, lateral and *Harris view* taken with the ankle dorsiflexed and the X-ray beam angled obliquely across the plantar aspect of the heel. It is helpful in defining the extent of intra-articular involvement and degree of depression of the fracture fragments.

Normal radiological measurements (Fig. 22.6)
a. *Gissane's angle:* Between 95 and 105°
b. *Bohler's angle:* Between 20 and 40°

Management

Emergency management of calcaneum fractures includes ice, elevation, and immobilization in a bulky compressive dressing with a posterior splint (to prevent soft-tissue injuries, such as fracture blisters and skin sloughing, which ultimately delay surgery).

Nonoperative treatment is for nonarticular and undisplaced fractures, with maintained Bohler's and Gissane's angle. It consists of nonweight bearing below knee cast for 6–8 weeks.

Operative treatment: It is indicated for displaced and intra-articular fractures. Goal of treatment is to restore the articular congruity and re-establish Bohler's and Gissane's angle as far as possible. It is achieved with screws or specially designed calcaneal plates (Fig. 22.7).

Complications

- Malunion
- Subtalar arthritis with stiffness and chronic pain

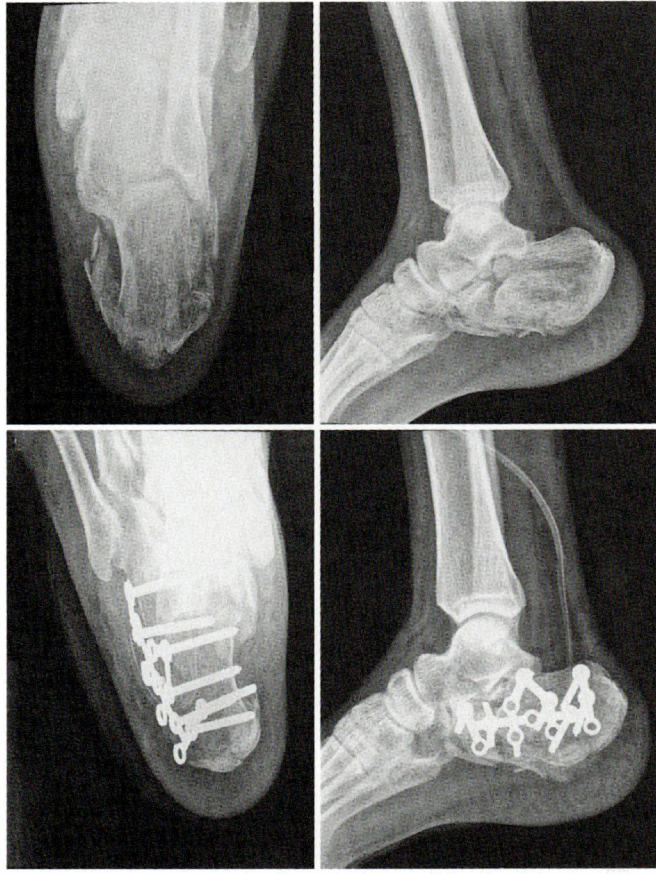

Fig. 22.7: Fracture calcaneum treated with ORIF using specially designed plate

FOOT INJURIES

Tarsometatarsal fracture-dislocations are also referred to as *Lisfranc fracture-dislocation*. These injuries are associated with a high incidence of chronic pain and

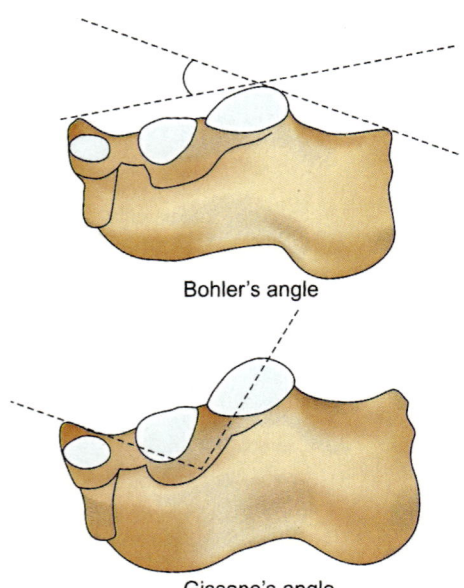

Bohler's angle

Gissane's angle

Fig. 22.6: Radiological parameters of calcaneum

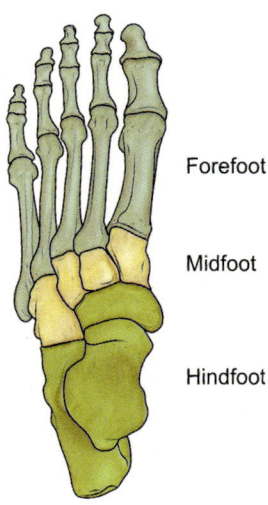

Forefoot

Midfoot

Hindfoot

Fig. 22.8: Different regions of foot

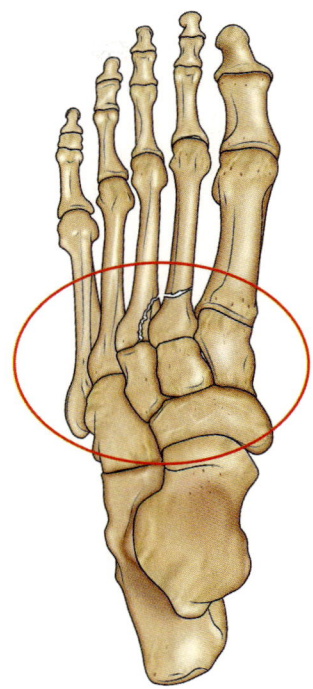

Fig. 22.9: Lisfranc fracture dislocation

functional disability. A fracture of the base of the second metatarsal indicates tarsometatarsal joint disruption until proven otherwise (Fig. 22.9).

These injuries generally occur after a high-energy trauma such as a fall from great height or motor vehicle collision.

Clinical Evaluation

The patient presents with severe pain, tenderness, and swelling over the involved area. Foot motion will exacerbate the pain. Dislocations present with a palpable deformity and severe pain.

Diagnosis

X-rays of the affected part—AP and lateral views. Oblique views help in some cases.

Management

Emergency management of these fractures includes ice, elevation, and a posterior splint.

Displaced fractures require open reduction and internal fixation with K wires (Kirschner wires) or screws to produce a stable, anatomical reduction in the active ambulatory patient.

Nonambulatory patients may be treated symptomatically with a compressive dressing.

Compound fractures require good debridement and dressing with external fixator as definitive treatment. Plastic surgery consultation may be required in cases of severe soft tissue injuries.

METATARSAL STRESS FRACTURE

Stress fractures of the metatarsals are called *March fractures*. The patient gives a history of an increase in physical activity with no clear history of preceding trauma.

On examination, there is tenderness at the middle of the shaft of the third metatarsal, which is the one most commonly involved. The pain is worse with ambulation and flexion or extension of the toes and subsides with rest. Initial radiographs are negative but within 2 weeks, callus is seen in the midshaft of the metatarsal.

When the fracture involves the first, third, fourth, and distal aspect of the second metatarsals, the treatment is symptomatic with relative rest. Stress fractures at the base of the second metatarsal should be treated with non-weight bearing for a period of 6 weeks. Diaphyseal fractures of the fifth metatarsal are prone to nonunion and these patients should be non-weight bearing for 6 to 10 weeks.

JONES FRACTURE

Tuberosity avulsion fractures, also called *pseudo-Jones' fracture*, are the most common and account for approximately 90% of fractures at the base of the fifth metatarsal.

An acute fracture at the junction of the diaphysis and metaphysis is termed the *Jones' fracture*, named after Sir Robert Jones, who described these fractures. These fractures involve the articular facet between the fourth and fifth metatarsal. Jones' fractures are unique and important to distinguish from the tuberosity fracture because they may disrupt the tenuous blood supply to the distal portion of the proximal fragment (Fig. 22.10).

Emergency management of these fractures includes ice, elevation, immobilization, and non-weight bearing. Definitive management consists of a short-leg, non-weight-bearing cast for 6 to 8 weeks. Displaced fractures are treated by operative fixation with a screw.

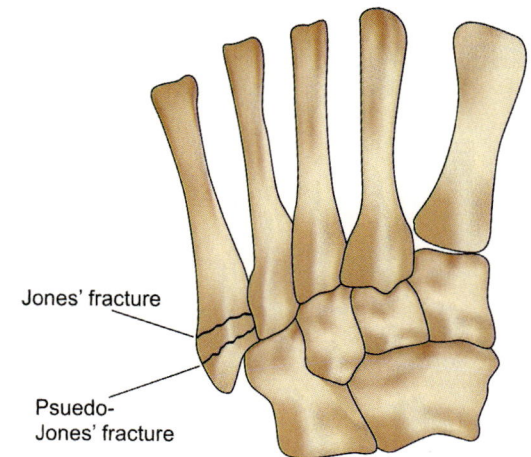

Jones' fracture

Psuedo-Jones' fracture

Fig. 22.10: Jones' and pseudo-Jones' fractures

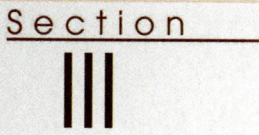

Infection of Bones and Joints

Osteomyelitis is defined as infection of bone as well as the bone marrow by micro-organisms.

Classification

1. *Depending on time duration*
   a. Acute osteomyelitis
   b. Subacute osteomyelitis
   c. Chronic osteomyelitis
2. *Depending on route of infection*
   a. Endogenous, i.e. haematogenous
   b. Exogenous, i.e. from open wound, postoperative.

ACUTE HAEMATOGENOUS OSTEOMYELITIS

Acute haematogenous osteomyelitis is the most common type of bone infection, especially seen in children. It usually involves metaphysis of the long bones, most commonly around the knee joint.

Relevant Anatomy

Metaphysis of the long bones is a highly vascular region. The medullary arteries traverse from diaphysis to growth plate, supply it, and form veins which drain again in diaphysis thus forming a hair pin loop. This leads to stagnation of blood supply, thus favouring seeding of bacteria (Fig. 23.1).

In most of the joints, the capsule is attached at the junction of epiphysis with metaphysis, i.e. the metaphysis is extra-articular. However, in some joints like hip, metaphysis is intra-articular. In such cases the infection can easily spread from metaphysis to joint causing septic arthritis (Fig. 23.2).

Causative Organisms

Staphylococcus aureus is the most common organism. Certain organisms have predilection for particular age group.

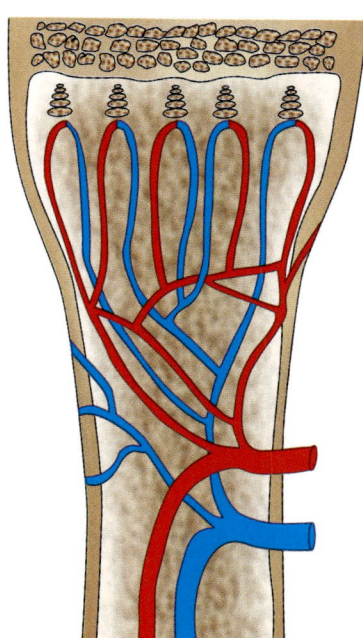

Fig. 23.1: Metaphysis of long bone

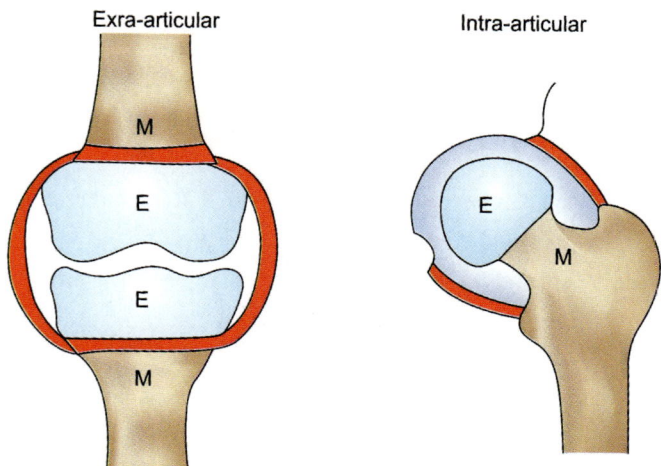

Fig. 23.2: Types of metaphysis affecting the location of infection (E: epiphysis, M: metaphysis)

1. Older children and adults—*Staphylococcus aureus* (most common infecting organism)
2. Infants—*Staphylococcus aureus* is most common, followed by group B Streptococcus and gram-negative coliforms.
3. 6 months to 2 years old child—*H. influenzae*
4. Vertebral body infections in adults—Gram-negative bacteria
5. Intravenous drug abusers—*Pseudomonas aeruginosa*
6. Chronically ill patients with long-term IV therapy or parenteral nutrition—fungal osteomyelitis
7. Haemoglobinopathies like sickle cell disease—*Salmonella osteomyelitis*.

Pathogenesis

The bacteria reach bones via haematogenous route. Due to various factors already discussed, the bacteria get lodged in the metaphysis of the long bones. Distal metaphysis of femur is most commonly affected site, other common sites being upper tibial, upper femoral and upper humeral metaphysis.

Once lodged, bacteria start proliferating in the metaphysis. This initiates inflammatory response thus forming pus. The pus thus formed in the metaphysis can spread in following directions (Fig. 23.3):

1. *Medullary cavity:* Pus travels rapidly along medullary cavity thus causing rapid spread of infection along with thrombosis of medullary vessels.
2. *Subperiosteal:* The pus can spread via Volkmann's canals to subperiosteal region thus stripping periosteum off the bone.
3. *Via growth plate:* In children younger than 2 years, some blood vessels cross the physis and may allow the spread of infection into the epiphysis. For this reason, infants are susceptible to limb shortening or angular deformity if the physis or epiphysis is damaged from the infection. Otherwise, the physis acts as a barrier that prevents the direct spread of a metaphyseal abscess into the epiphysis.
4. *Adjacent joints* like hip joint when the involved metaphysis is intra-articular.

The involved cortex of metaphysis undergoes rapid necrosis because its periosteal blood supply is hampered by subperiosteal abscess and endosteal blood supply is cut off due to thrombosis of medullary vessels. If the treatment is not started immediately, this part of bone becomes dead thus forming sequestrum, leading to chronic osteomyelitis.

Diagnosis

The diagnosis is mainly clinical.

History

- Pain around the involved limb.
- *Pseudoparalysis:* Child does not move involved limb due to severe pain.
- Localized swelling, redness.
- Fever with chills.

Clinical Features

- Tenderness of the involved region.
- Localized swelling.
- Increased local temperature.
- Decreased range of motion.
- Generalised symptoms and signs such as child being irritable or drowsy, not feeding well.

Laboratory Features

- Increased ESR, CRP.
- Raised leucocyte count.
- Blood culture.

Radiographic Features

Standard radiographs generally are negative initially, but may show soft-tissue swelling. Skeletal changes, such as periosteal reaction or bony destruction, are seen on plain films after around 10 to 12 days (Fig. 23.4).

Newer Diagnostic Modalities

Technetium-99 m bone scans can confirm the diagnosis 24 to 48 hours after onset in 90 to 95% of patients. Gallium scans and indium-111 labelled leukocyte scans are more specific for infections.

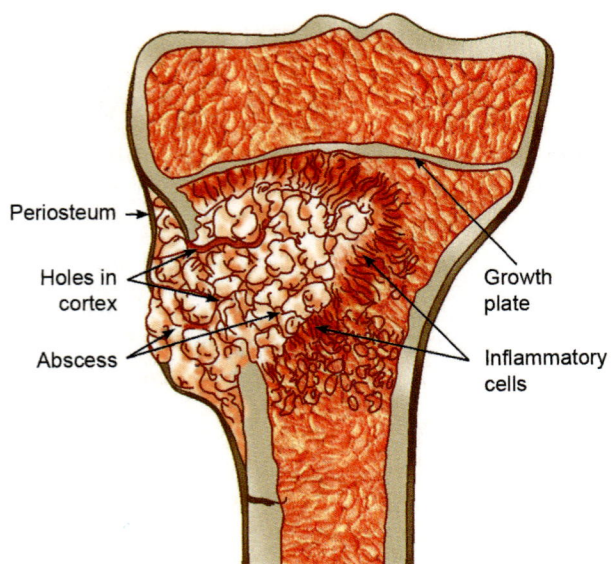

Periosteum

Holes in cortex

Abscess

Growth plate

Inflammatory cells

Fig. 23.3: Pathology of acute osteomyelitis

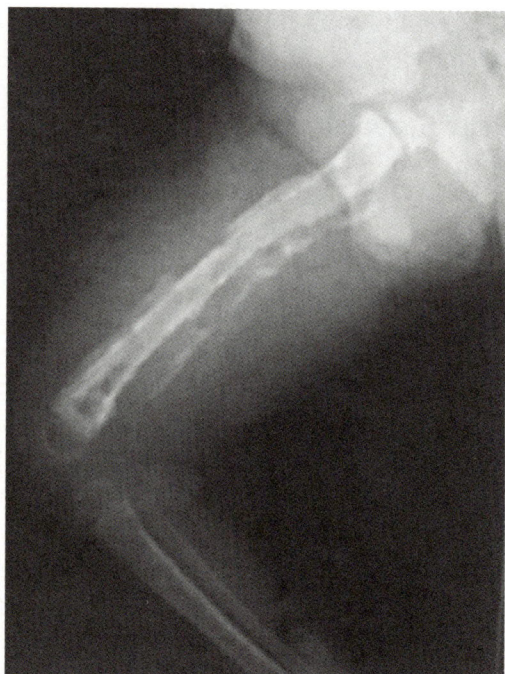

Fig. 23.4: X-ray picture of acute osteomyelitis

MRI can show early inflammatory changes in bone marrow and soft tissue. It may also locate the intra-osseous abscess, thus helping in drainage.

Role of aspiration: If a child presents with fever and localized redness, swelling and pain over a bone, then acute osteomyelitis should be suspected. In such cases, X-rays will not reveal anything. If higher radiological imaging is not available, under aseptic precautions the involved bone can be aspirated with large bore needle. If this aspiration reveals pus, then a proper incision and drainage is planned.

Treatment

Appropriate treatment shortly after onset of acute haematogenous osteomyelitis can significantly lower morbidity. Surgery and antibiotic treatment are complementary, and in some patients antibiotic treatment alone cures the disease.

It has been well established that sequestered abscesses demand surgical drainage, and areas of simple inflammation without abscess formation can be treated with antibiotics alone.

Thus if patient presents within 48 hours of symptoms, broad spectrum antibiotics should be started intravenously. Second generation cephalosporin like cefotaxime or cefazolin (100–150 mg/kg of body weight), plus aminoglycosides like amikacin (15 mg/kg of body weight) are effective in most cases. Later on antibiotics can be changed according to blood culture sensitivity report.

If patient presents 48 hours later without any treatment then it is assumed that pus has already formed and such patients usually need surgical drainage along with antibiotics for a period of 6 weeks.

Principles of Surgical Drainage

The objective of surgery is to drain any abscess cavity and remove all nonviable or necrotic tissue. When a subperiosteal abscess is found in an infant, several small holes should be drilled through the cortex into the medullary canal. If intramedullary pus is found, a small window of bone is removed. The skin is closed loosely over drains, and the limb is splinted. The limb is protected for several weeks to prevent pathological fracture. Intravenous followed by oral antibiotics should be continued postoperatively for a period of 6 weeks.

Complications of Acute Osteomyelitis

Immediate Complications

1. *Sepsis:* The infection may spread to other organs and can be fatal.
2. *Acute septic arthritis:* It occurs either because of spread through physis or if the metaphysis is intra-articular, e.g. hip joint. It is a serious complication requiring urgent arthrotomy and debridement. If untreated or treated late, it may lead to damage of cartilage and chronic arthritis.

Late Complications

1. Chronic Osteomyelitis

This is probably the commonest complication of acute osteomyelitis. It develops if the acute osteomyelitis is untreated or inadequately treated.

2. Growth Disturbance

In children less than 2 yrs of age, the physis is not effective barrier for spread of infection, so the infection spreads easily from metaphysis to growth plate thus damaging it and causing growth disturbances and deformities.

SUBACUTE HAEMATOGENOUS OSTEOMYELITIS

Compared to acute osteomyelitis, subacute hematogenous osteomyelitis has a more insidious onset and lacks the severity of symptoms. This makes the diagnosis of this disorder difficult and it is typically delayed for more than 2 weeks.

Aetiopathogenesis

The indolent course of subacute osteomyelitis is thought to be the result of increased host resistance, decreased bacterial virulence, or the administration of antibiotics before the onset of symptoms. It is speculated that the combination of an organism of low virulence with a strong host response may allow the inflammation to persist in bone without producing significant signs or symptoms.

Diagnosis

Systemic signs and symptoms are minimal. Temperature is only mildly elevated if at all. Mild-to-moderate pain is one of the only consistent signs suggesting the diagnosis. White blood cell counts generally are normal. The erythrocyte sedimentation rate is elevated in only 50% of patients, and blood cultures usually are negative.

Roberts and Drummonds Classification of Subacute Osteomyelitis (Fig. 23.5)

1. Central metaphyseal lesion
2. Eccentric metaphyseal lesion with cortical erosion
3. Diaphyseal cortical lesion
4. Diaphyseal lesion with periosteal new bone formation, but without definite bony lesion
5. Primary subacute epiphyseal osteomyelitis
6. Subacute osteomyelitis crossing physis to involve metaphysis and epiphysis.

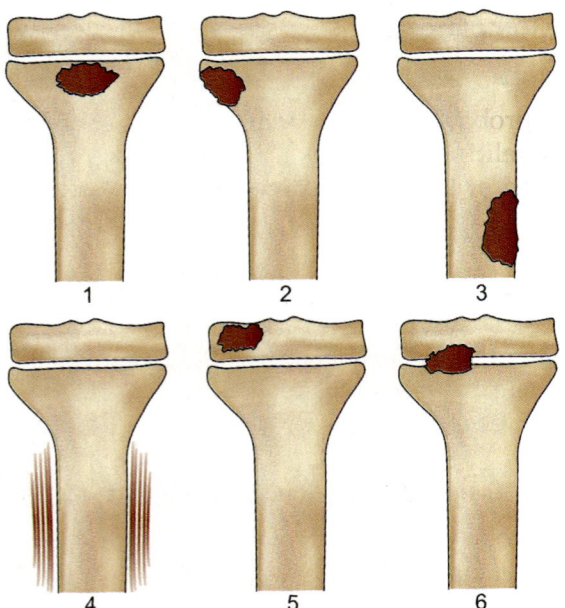

Fig. 23.5: Roberts and Drummonds classification

Treatment

For lesions that seem to be a simple abscess in the epiphysis or metaphysis, treatment is intravenous antibiotics for 48 hours followed by a 6 weeks course of oral antibiotics.

Aggressive lesions require biopsy and curettage followed by treatment with appropriate antibiotics.

BRODIE'S ABSCESS

This is a localized type of chronic osteomyelitis in which strong immune response successfully keeps the infection contained. This leads to formation of a cavity filled with pus or jelly like thick granulation tissue surrounded by a zone of sclerotic bone. Organisms of low virulence are believed to cause the lesion. *S. aureus* is cultured in 50% of patients; in 20%, the culture is negative.

Clinical Features

Brodie's abscess is usually seen in second decade of life. Upper tibial and lower femoral metaphysis are the commonest locations.

Intermittent deep boring pain of long duration is the presenting complaint. Usually pain worsens with physical exertion.

Examination reveals local tenderness and thickening over the affected area.

Imaging

On plain radiographs, a Brodie abscess generally appears as a lytic lesion with a rim of sclerotic bone, but it can have a markedly varied appearance (Fig. 23.6).

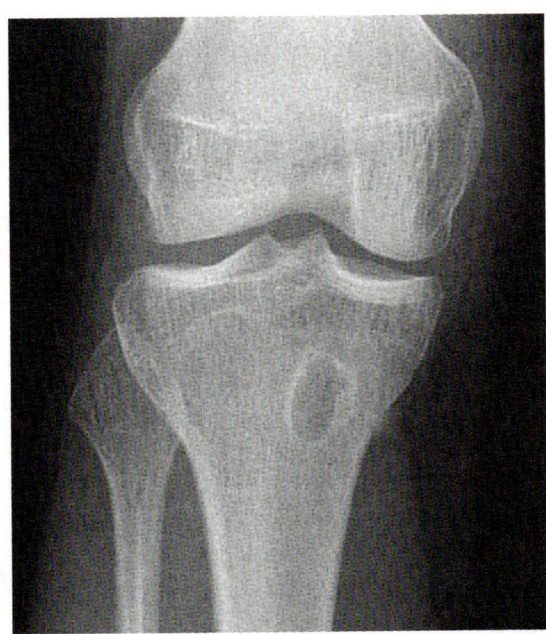

Fig. 23.6: Brodie's abscess

Treatment

This condition often requires an open biopsy for confirmation of diagnosis and to rule out malignancy. Treatment is drainage of the pus along with curettage of the cavity. The cavity if small can be left alone or can be filled with cancellous bone graft. Appropriate antibiotics should be given for 6 weeks.

CHRONIC OSTEOMYELITIS

When the infection of the bone persists for more than 6 weeks, it is called chronic osteomyelitis (Fig. 23.7). In chronic osteomyelitis, there are one or more foci in the bone that may contain purulent material, infected granulation tissue, or a sequestrum. Intermittent acute exacerbations may occur for years and often respond to rest and antibiotics. The hallmark of chronic osteomyelitis is infected dead bone within a compromised soft-tissue envelope. The infected foci within the bone are surrounded by sclerotic, relatively avascular bone covered by a thickened periosteum and scarred muscle and subcutaneous tissue.

Aetiopathogenesis

The commonest cause of chronic osteomyelitis is untreated or inadequately treated acute osteomyelitis. In acute osteomyelitis, the metaphyseal bone gets necrosed due to loss of blood supply from endosteum (thrombosis of vessels) as well as periosteum (sub-periosteal abscess). If not treated properly, infection tends to persist. The necrotic bone is converted to sequestrum. The body tries to seal off the infection by forming fibrous tissue as well as new bone. The newly formed bone surrounding the sequestrum is known as involucrum. The involucrum has multiple holes in it known as cloacae. The pus passes from pus filled cavity in the bone through cloacae outside the bone from which it drains outside the body via the discharging sinuses.

SEQUESTRUM

It is a dead piece of bone surrounded by pus and granulation tissue. The sequestrum classically has outer surface which is smooth and inner surface which is irregular (Figs 23.8 and 23.9).

Types of Sequestrum

- Bombay sequestrum—fungal, in calcaneum
- Ring sequestrum—amputations, Ilizarov
- Coarse sandy, feathery, tubular—tuberculosis, pyogenic infections
- Coke sequestrum—tuberculosis
- Ivory sequestrum—syphilis

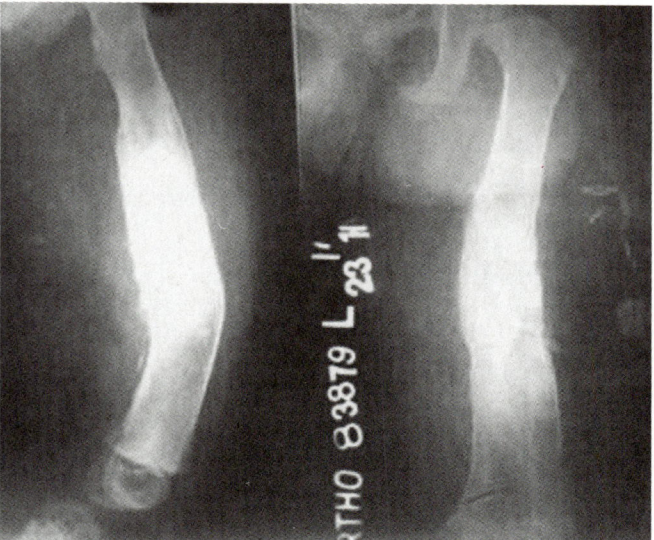

Fig. 23.7: Chronic osteomyelitis of femur in child

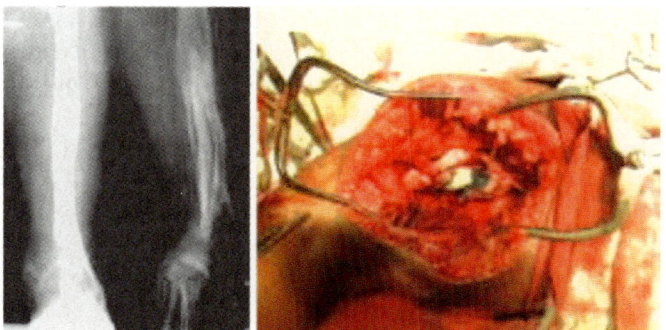

Fig. 23.8: X-ray and intraoperative picture showing sequestrum inside shaft femur—a feature of chronic osteomyelitis

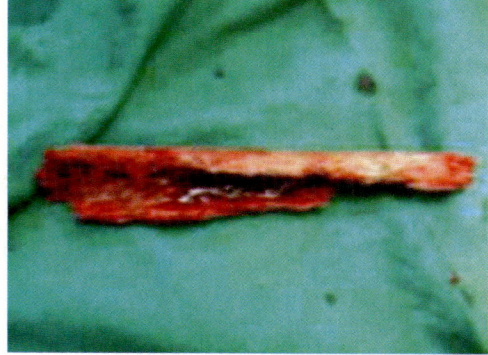

Fig. 23.9: Sequestrum

Causes of Persistence of Infection

1. The cavity in the bone which contains pus and sequestrum is noncollapsible, so cannot drain the pus effectively.
2. The sequestrum is larger than the discharging sinus, so it cannot get extruded through it.

3. Antibiotics cannot reach the infected tissue effectively as it is partly sealed off by fibrous tissue.

Cierny and Mader Classification System for Chronic Osteomyelitis (Table 23.1 and Fig. 23.10)

Table 23.1: Classification of chronic osteomyelitis		
Anatomical Type		
I	Medullary	Endosteal disease
II	Superficial	Cortical surface infected because of coverage defect
III	Localized	Cortical sequestrum that can be excised without compromising stability
IV	Diffuse	Features of I, II and III plus the mechanical instability before or after débridement
Physiological Class		
A host	Normal	Immunocompetent with good local vascularity
B host	Compromised	Local (L) or systemic (S) factors that compromise immunity or healing
C host	Prohibitive	Minimal disability, prohibitive morbidity anticipated or poor prognosis for cure

Diagnosis

Clinical Findings

- Pain
- Localised swelling
- Discharging sinus
- Irregularity of bony surface

Laboratory Investigations

- Raised ESR levels
- Raised CRP levels
- Increased leukocyte counts

Radiographs

Signs of cortical destruction and periosteal reaction strongly suggest the diagnosis of osteomyelitis. Presence of sequestrum is pathognomonic of chronic osteomyelitis (Figs 23.7 and 23.8).

Sinogram can be performed if a sinus track is present and can be a valuable adjunct to surgical planning (Fig. 23.11).

Isotope bone scanning is more useful in acute osteomyelitis than in the chronic form. Technetium-99m bone scans, which show increased uptake in areas of increased blood flow or osteoblastic activity, tend to lack specificity.

Gallium scans show increased uptake in areas where leukocytes or bacteria accumulate. A normal gallium scan virtually excludes the presence of osteomyelitis and can be useful as a follow-up examination after surgery.

Indium-111 labeled leukocyte scans are more sensitive than technetium or gallium scans and are

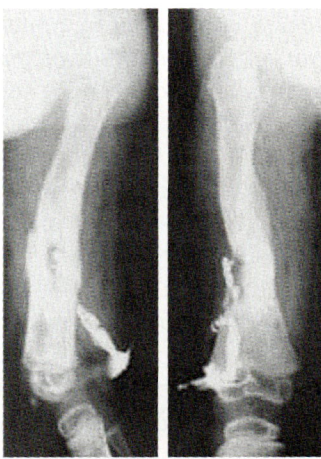

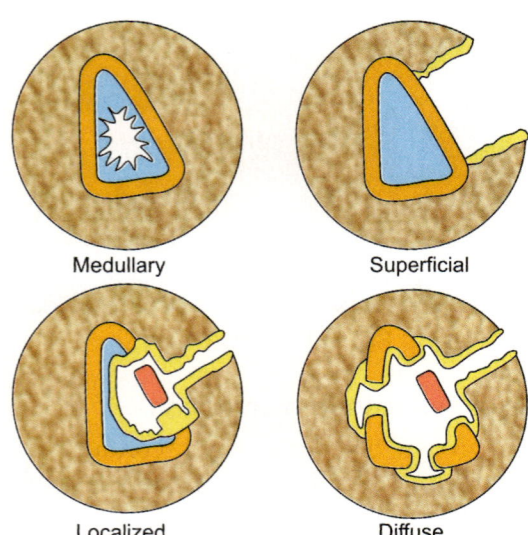

Medullary   Superficial

Localized   Diffuse

Fig. 23.10: Classification of chronic osteomyelitis

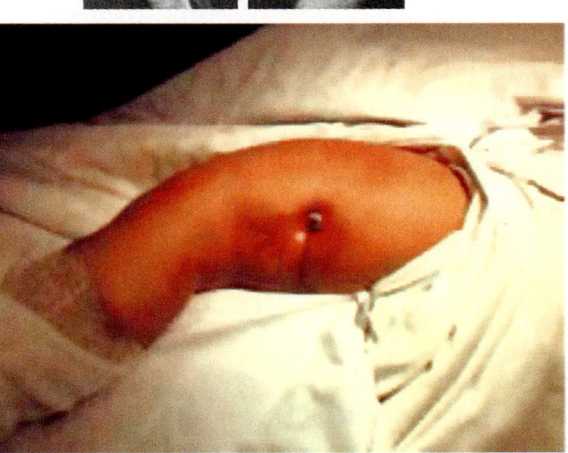

Fig. 23.11: Sinogram

especially useful in differentiating chronic osteomyelitis from neuropathic arthropathy in the diabetic foot.

CT scan provides excellent definition of cortical bone and a fair evaluation of the surrounding soft tissues and is especially useful in identifying sequestra.

In chronic osteomyelitis, MRI may reveal a well-defined rim of high signal intensity surrounding the focus of active disease (rim sign). Sinus tracks and cellulitis appear as areas of increased signal intensity on T2-weighted imaging.

Treatment

Chronic osteomyelitis generally cannot be eradicated without surgical treatment. Antibiotics alone rarely can eradicate the infection for numerous reasons. Bacteria are able to adhere to orthopaedic implants and bone matrix through various receptors. They often form a slimy coat that protects them from phagocytic cells and antibiotics. The aim of surgery for chronic osteomyelitis is:

1. To convert a noncollapsible cavity into a wide open cavity, which will help easy drainage of pus and necrotic tissue. This is known as saucerisation (Fig. 23.12)
2. Radical debridement of the infected and dead tissue including sequestrum.

Since the sequestrectomy can lead to significant instability this procedure should be done when sufficient involucrum is formed.

Adequate debridement often leaves a large dead space that must be managed to prevent recurrence and significant bone loss that may result in bony instability. Appropriate reconstruction of the bone and soft-tissue

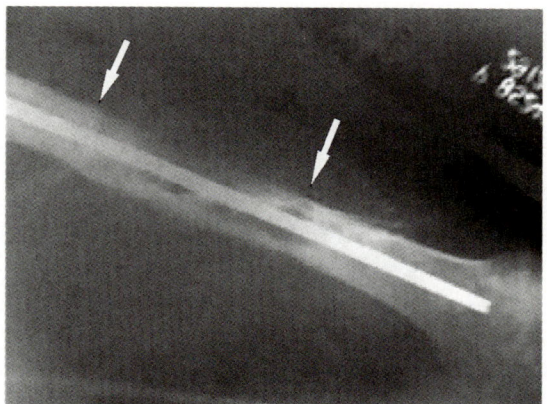

Fig. 23.13: Saucerisation—the area between the two arrows

defects may be needed after proper identification of the infecting organism and appropriate antibiotic therapy (Fig. 23.13).

Other Modalities of Treatment for Chronic Osteomyelitis

- *Papineau technique of open bone grafting:* Treatment is divided into three stages:
  1. Excision of infected tissue with or without stabilization using an external fixator or an intramedullary rod
  2. Cancellous autografting
  3. Skin closure
- Polymethylmethacrylate antibiotic bead chains
- Biodegradable antibiotic delivery systems
- Closed suction drains
- Soft-tissue transfer
- Ilizarov technique
- Hyperbaric oxygen therapy

Complications of Chronic Osteomyelitis

1. Acute excacerbations: These are very common, and may present with fever, severe pain, and sudden increase in discharge from the sinus. This needs to be managed by a course of antibiotics and local drainage.
2. *Pathological fractures:* The osteomyelitic bone is stiff and weak, thus more prone for pathological fractures (Fig. 23.14).
3. *Growth disturbances* in growing children, osteomyelitis may lead to shortening, lengthening or angular deformities due to involvement of epiphyseal growth plate.
4. *Sinus track malignancy:* A squamous cell carcinoma may develop from a long standing discharging sinus.

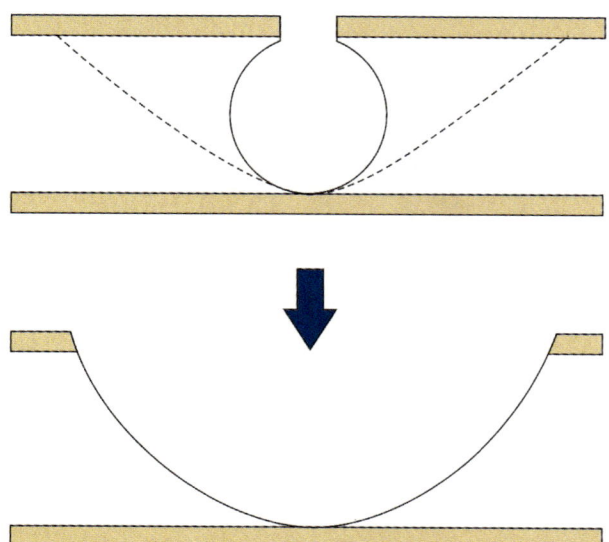

Fig. 23.12: Saucerization

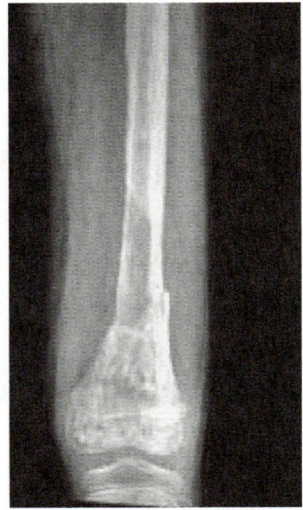

Fig. 23.14: Pathological fracture secondary to chronic osteomyelitis

SCLEROSING OSTEOMYELITIS OF GARRE

Sclerosing osteomyelitis is a chronic form of disease in which the bone is thickened and distended, but abscesses and sequestra are absent (Fig. 23.15). The disease affects children and young adults. Its cause is unknown, but it is thought to be an infection caused by a low-grade, possibly anaerobic bacteria.

Patients report intermittent pain of moderate intensity and usually of long duration. Swelling and tenderness over the affected bone may be found.

Radiographs show an expanded bone with generalized sclerosis. The erythrocyte sedimentation rate usually is slightly elevated. Biopsy specimens show only chronic, low-grade, nonspecific osteomyelitis, and cultures usually are negative.

A secondary lesion at a distant site can occur years after onset.

No treatment has been predictably helpful, but fenestration of the sclerotic bone and antibiotics are advisable.

SEPTIC ARTHRITIS

Introduction

Acute septic arthritis can occur at any age, but young children and elderly persons are most susceptible, especially if they have an already abnormal joint from previous trauma or from conditions such as haemophilia, osteoarthritis, or rheumatoid arthritis. Immune compromise for any reason and diseases such as cancer, diabetes, alcoholism, cirrhosis, and uremia increase the risk for infection.

Aetiopathogenesis

The commonest organism is *Staphylococcus aureus*. Other organisms being, Streptococci, Pneumococci and Gonococci. These organisms reach the joint via following routes (Fig. 23.16):

1. *Haematogenous:* Commonest route; primary focus being some other infection such as repiratory tract infection.
2. *Extension from acute osteomyelitis:* This is common where the metaphysis is intra-articular such as hip and shoulder.
3. Direct extension from open injuries overlying the joint.
4. *Iatrogenic:* After surgery or intra-articular injection.

Once the causative bacteria reach the joint, they get seeded and multiplied in the synovium leading to strong inflammatory reaction. This causes exudation of fluid in the joint. The exudate contains many

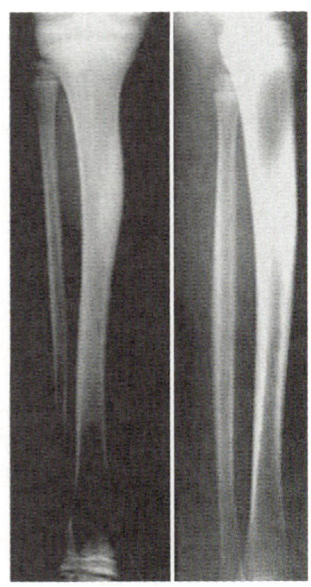

Fig. 23.15: Garre's osteomyelitis

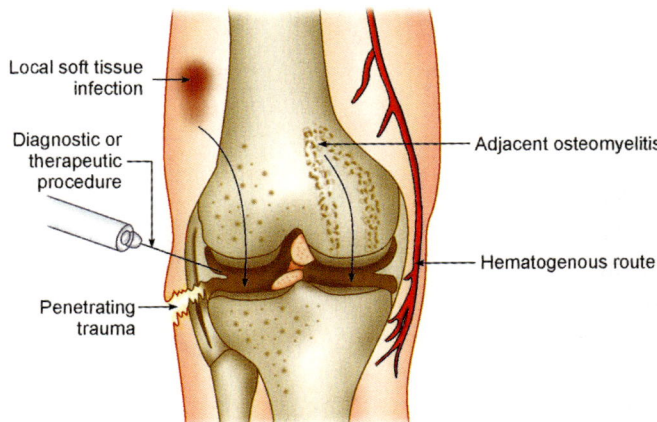

Fig. 23.16: Routes of affection of joint

proteolytic substances which cause rapid destruction of the cartilage.

Diagnosis

Clinical Diagnosis

1. Classically acute onset of generalised symptoms of septicemia such as high grade fever, malaise, child being irritable or drowsy, not feeding well.
2. Localising symptoms being severe throbbing pain, swelling and redness over the joint.
3. Local examination reveals swelling, erythema and severe tenderness over the joint. The child does not move the joint actively (pseudoparalysis). Passive movements are very painful leading to severe restriction of range of motion of the joint.
4. *Deformity:* Patient usually keeps limb in the position of ease, i.e. the position in which capacity of the joint is maximum (Fig. 23.17).

Joint	Position of ease
Hip	Flexion, abduction and external rotation
Knee	Flexion
Ankle	Plantar flexion
Shoulder	Adduction and internal rotation
Elbow	Flexion

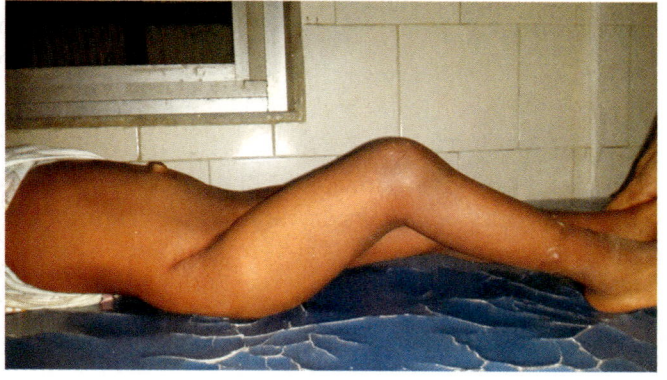

Fig. 23.17: Attitude of hip in septic arthritis

Laboratory Diagnosis

1. Complete blood count reveals leukocytosis with neutrophilia. Erythrocyte sedimentation rate and C reactive proteins are raised.
2. Blood culture is mandatory to look for causative organisms.
3. Joint fluid examination helps in diagnosis (Table 23.2).

Radiological Diagnosis

Radiographs: In the first few days of infection, radiographs usually are normal; however, they may show soft-tissue swelling, displacement of the fat pad, or joint space widening from localized oedema.

As the infection progresses, joint space narrowing from the destruction of cartilage may become evident.

Ultrasonography, in contrast to radiographs, can be used to detect even small collections of fluid deep in the joints. Non-echo-free effusions from clotted haemorrhagic collections are characteristic of a septic joint. Ultrasonography can be used to guide initial joint aspiration and drainage and to monitor the status of intra-articular compartments, joint capsules, bone surface, or adjacent soft tissues.

MRI is more sensitive and specific than ultrasonography and is very useful in the early stages of infection. It can show soft-tissue swelling, joint effusion, and abscess formation and can be used to guide joint aspiration, monitor therapy, and help select operative approaches.

Radionuclide bone scans often can detect localized areas of inflammation. Although the Technetium-99m methyldiphosphonate scan shows increases in isotope accumulation in areas of osteoblasts and increased vascularity, it may be normal in the early stages of septic arthritis. Other radiopharmaceuticals used are gallium citrate and indium-111 chloride, and gallium and indium scans are more specific and sensitive in the detection of active infection than technetium-99m methyldiphosphonate scans.

Table 23.2: Characteristics of synovial fluid in various pathologies

Feature	Normal	Noninflammatory	Inflammatory	Septic
Colour	Colourless variable	Straw yellow	Yellow	Yellow
Clarity	Transparent	Transparent	Translucent	Opaque
WBC count/cmm	<200	200–2000	2000–7500	>10,000
PMN leukocytes	<25%	<25%	>50%	>75%
Mucin clot	Firm	Firm	Friable	Friable
Glucose levels	Same as blood glucose	Near equal to blood glucose	Reduced blood glucose	Significantly reduced blood glucose

Differential Diagnosis

1. Nonarticular pathologies such as acute osteomyelitis, acute lymphadenopathy, acute bursitis, etc. These conditions can be differentiated from septic arthritis by checking joint movements which will be preserved in nonarticular conditions.
2. Articular pathologies such as rheumatoid arthritis, haemophilia, tuberculous arthritis, etc. which can be differentiated by synovial fluid analysis.

Treatment

Nade suggests three essential principles in the management of acute septic arthritis:

1. The joint must be adequately drained
2. Antibiotics must be given to diminish the systemic effects of sepsis
3. The joint must be rested in a stable position.

Prompt drainage and evaluation of purulent joint fluid seems to be crucial for preservation of articular cartilage and for resolution of the infection.

If a joint is suspected of being infected, aspiration with a large-bore needle should be done before antibiotic therapy is initiated. Careful skin preparation before aspiration is mandatory, and the fluid obtained should be sent for immediate Gram staining, culture, cell counts, and crystal analysis.

Initial antibiotic treatment is empirical based on the patient's age and risk factors. Empirical antibiotic therapy should be given until culture and sensitivity results are available, at which time definitive treatment is initiated. If no organism is isolated, empirical therapy should be continued. In general, the decision regarding duration of therapy depends on the type of infecting organism, the condition of the patient, and the response to therapy.

Complications of Septic Arthritis

1. Stiffness due to intra-articular and extra-articular adhesions.
2. *Osteoarthritis:* The articular cartilage may be damaged permanently by infection leading to osteoarthritis of the involved joint
3. *Pathological dislocation* in acute septic arthritis, the joint gets filled with pus, thus stretching the joint capsule and adjacent ligaments. This along with severe muscle spasm may lead to pathological subluxation or dislocation of the joint.

TOM SMITH ARTHRITIS

Tom Smith arthritis is a form of septic arthritis of the hip joint in infants which can destroy the whole head of the femur, being still completely cartilaginous at that age.

The diagnosis may be delayed till the child starts walking with limp. The clinical features resemble congenital dislocation of the hip.

Diagnosis

X-rays are usually normal in the early phase, although it may indicate the presence of fluid in the joint. A radionuclide bone scan using Gallium may indicate inflammation in the joint lining. MRI may confirm the presence of fluid in the joint, and inflammation of the joint lining as well.

Aspiration of the joint is helpful, especially if pus is obtained. Culture could be undertaken to identify the organism involved.

Treatment consists of drainage of the joint. Hip needs to be drained by open surgery. Intravenous antibiotics are necessary to control this severe infection.

Tuberculosis of Bones and Joints

Tuberculosis is the infection caused by *Mycobacterium tuberculosis*.

Sir Percival Pott was the first to describe tuberculosis of the spine in 1779, stating a classic description as destruction of the disc space and adjacent vertebral body, collapse of the spinal element and progressive kyphotic deformity.

Laennec (1781-1826) was the first to describe the microscopic lesion, the 'tubercle' by which name the disease is universally known at present.

Pathology of Osteoarticular Tuberculosis

Osteoarticular TB is always a secondary infection after dissemination from a primary focus. The primary focus may be active or quiescent, in lungs, lymph nodes, mediastinum, mesentery, kidney or any other viscera. The infection reaches the bone through vascular channels. Generally there is a gap of 2–3 years between appearance of primary focus and bone infection.

The bacilli invade the bone through subsynovial vessels or directly from lesions in epiphyseal region. Articular cartilage destruction begins peripherally, and this inflammatory pannus spreads below the articular cartilage. There is no evidence of formation of proteolytic enzymes as seen in septic condition. So the articular cartilage is relatively preserved till late stages in the TB of joints.

Once the bacilli reach the subchondral bone, the cartilage loses its nutrition and may be seen as free chunks in joint space, called 'rice bodies'.

Cold abscess: It is formed by collection of products of liquefaction and reactive exudation. It consists of serum, leucocytes, caseous materials, bone debris and tuberculous bacilli. This abscess penetrates the ligaments and migrates following the fascial planes along the vessels and the nerves.

Healing is usually by fibrosis leading to significant loss of joint movements and fibrous ankylosis which is a very painful condition. This fibrous ankylosis is the commonest end result of untreated TB in most places except spine where bony ankylosis is common (Fig. 24.1). The later is relatively painless condition.

Clinical Presentation

Osteoarticular tuberculosis usually occurs in first three decades of life. The characteristics are:

1. Insidious onset with gradually worsening pain, associated with night cries.
2. Mono-articular involvement.
3. Constitutional features are not common and are seen in less than 1/3rd cases as osteoarticular tuberculosis is a paucibacillary disease.

Local Signs

1. Painful restriction of movement.

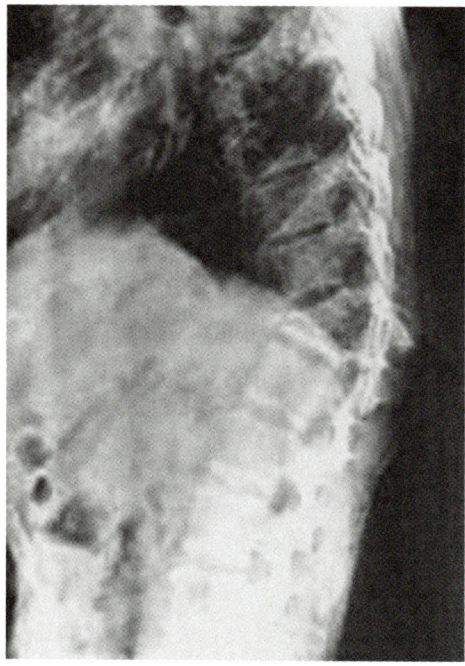

Fig. 24.1: Healing of TB spine

2. Discharging sinus characterised by pale granulation tissue, watery discharge and undermined edges.
3. Prominent muscle wasting.
4. Regional lymph nodes enlargement.

Diagnostic Investigations

1. Radiographs of the affected region.
2. Laboratory tests: Raised WBC count and ESR, reduced Hb levels.
3. Biopsy to demonstrate presence of the tubercles.
4. Isotope scintigraphy by Tc 99m.
5. ELISA test to demonstrate antibodies against *Mycobacterium tuberculosis*.
6. PCR testing is highly sensitive and specific for pulmonary TB, however the results are not that good for osteoarticular TB.
7. BACTEC—since conventional culture of TB bacilli may take more than 2 months, a newer technique called BACTEC is used which can detect growth within 14 days.
8. *Gene expert:* This is a new molecular technology detecting TB bacilli growth within hours.
9. Modern imaging techniques such as CT scan and MRI scan to delineate the extent of disease and neurological involvement.

Treatment of Tuberculosis

Tuberculosis is considered to be a medical disease, and Anti-Koch's treatment (AKT) should be started immediately after diagnosis of tuberculosis. The drugs currently used are categorized into first line, second line and newer drugs (Table 24.1).

Table 24.1: Commonly used Anti-Koch's drugs		
First line drugs	*Second line drugs*	*Newer drugs*
1. Isoniazid	1. PAS	1. Fluoroquinolones: Ciprofloxacin, Ofloxacin, Levoflox
2. Rifampicin	2. Cycloserine	2. Injectables: Amikacin, Kanamycin
3. Ethambutol	3. Ethionamide	3. Capreomycin
4. Pyrazinamide	4. Thioacetazone	
5. Streptomycin		

Multidrug resistant tuberculosis (MDR TB) is tuberculosis that is resistant to:
1. Isoniazid (INH) and
2. Rifampicin (RMP)

Extreme drug resistant tuberculosis (XDR TB) is TB that has developed resistance to ALL of the following:

1. Rifampicin
2. Isoniazid
3. Any member of the quinolone family and
4. At least one of the following second-line injectable drugs: Kanamycin, capreomycin or amikacin

XXDR TB or TDR TB (total drug resistance) is TB resistant to all the tested first line and second line drugs used in TB.

TUBERCULOSIS OF HIP

Tuberculosis of the hip is very common, the frequency of involvement is next only to spinal tuberculosis.

The initial focus of tuberculous lesion may start in the acetabular roof (1), epiphysis(2), metaphyseal region (Babcock's triangle)(3), or in greater trochanter(4) (Fig. 24.2). Rarely the disease may start in the synovial membrane and may remain as synovitis for a few months. Tuberculosis of the greater trochanter may involve the overlying trochanteric bursa without involving the hip joint for a very long time.

As the upper end of femur is entirely intracapsular, the joint gets involved rapidly from any osseous lesion situated within the capsular attachments, the disease becomes "osteoarticular", and destruction of articular surfaces of femoral head and acetabulum takes place.

When the initial focus starts in the acetabular roof, the joint involvement is late and severity of symptoms mild, therefore, by the time the patient first reports to the hospital, extensive destruction of the bone is already present.

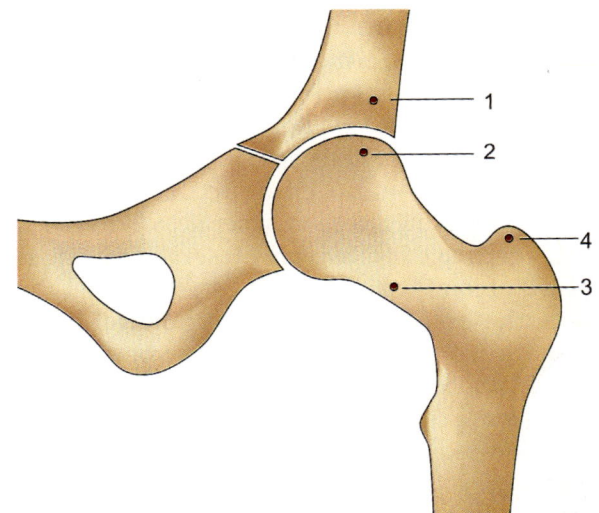

Fig. 24.2: Foci of infection in TB hip (1 to 4: *see* text)

Clinical Features

1. Pain is the most common symptom, and may be localised to the hip joint or radiate to the knee region.

Clinicoradiologic Classification of TB Hip (Table 24.2 and Fig. 24.3)

Table 24.2: Classification of TB hip		
Stages	*Clinical findings*	*Radiological features*
Synovitis	Flexion, abduction, external rotation deformity Apparent lengthening	Soft tissue swelling, haziness of the articular margins and rarefaction
Early arthritis	Flexion, adduction, internal rotation deformity. Apparent shortening	Rarefaction, osteopenia, marginal bony erosions in femoral head, acetabulum or both. No reduction in joint space
Advanced arthritis	Flexion, adduction, internal rotation deformity. True shortening	All of the above and destruction of articular surface, reduction in joint space.
Advanced arthritis with subluxation/dislocation	Flexion, adduction, internal rotation deformity. Gross shortening	Gross destruction and reduction in joint space. Wandering acetabulum

Night pain is one of the most specific symptom that is seen in TB hip and patient may get awakened from the sleep due to pain. During daytime there is protective muscle spasm which gets relieved during deep sleep at night. This leads to rubbing of the damaged articular surfaces over each other thus giving rise to night cries.

2. Limp is the earliest symptom. Patient avoids putting weight on diseased limb leading to a characteristic antalgic gait.
3. Deformity: usually there is flexion deformity which gives rise to exaggerated lumbar lordosis. There may be abduction or adduction deformities giving rise to lengthening or shortening of the limb.

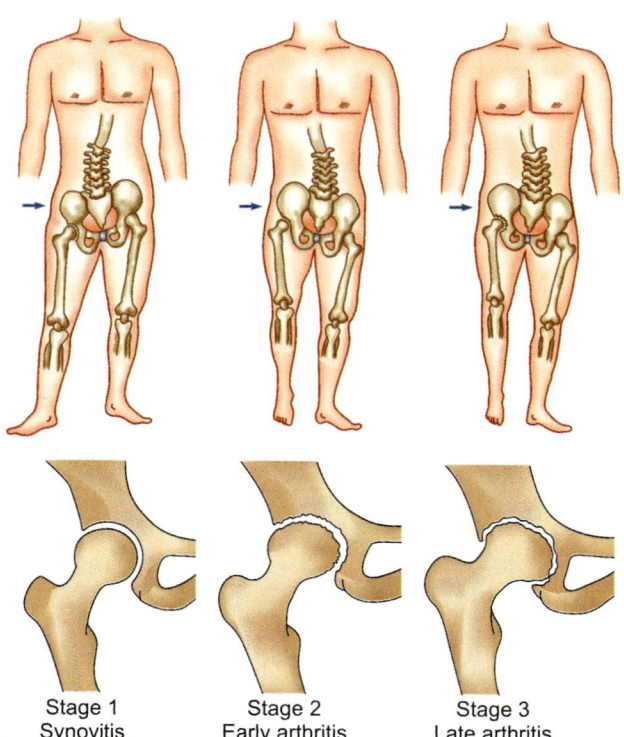

Stage 1 Synovitis   Stage 2 Early arthritis   Stage 3 Late arthritis

Fig. 24.3: Stages of TB hip

4. Discharging sinus may be present in the groin or around greater trochanter
5. Muscle wasting is prominent in gluteal and quadriceps muscles
6. Restriction of movements.

Management of Hip Tuberculosis

Diagnosis

1. Clinically, monoarticular involvement, gradually worsening pain and limp associated with night cries, significant wasting, constitutional symptoms if present go in favour of tuberculosis of hip. The clinical signs vary according to the stage of the disease.
2. *X-ray:* Pelvis with both hips AP (PBH) and both hips lateral views are the most important views. Opposite side X-rays are must for comparison especially in early course of the disease.
   • Haziness of the bones around the joint is the earliest sign on X-ray.
   • *Lytic lesion* in the acetabular roof, epiphysis, metaphyseal region (Babcock's triangle), or in greater trochanter are common
   • Reduction of joint space due to destruction of the joint space indicates stage of arthritis.
   • Acetabular changes due to arthritis or spread of infection
   • Features of sequelae

Shanmugasundaram's radiological classification of TB hip (Fig. 24.4)
Type 1: Normal type
Type 2: Travelling acetabulum
Type 3: Dislocating
Type 4: Perthes type
Type 5: Protrusio acetabuli
Type 6: Atrophic
Type 7: Mortar and pastle

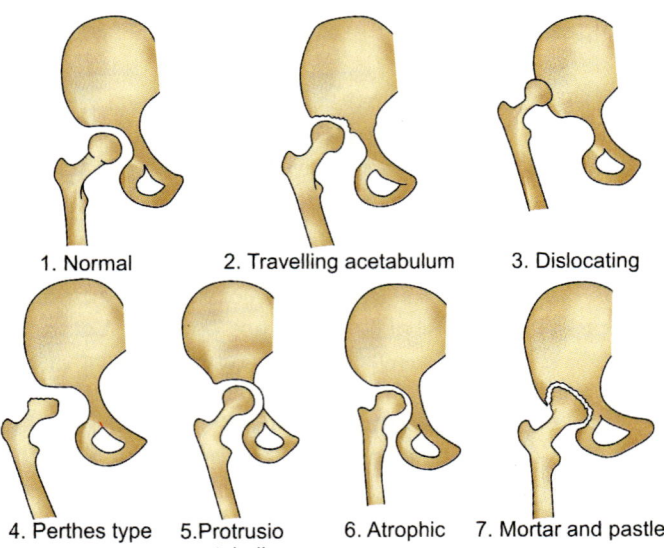

1. Normal　　2. Travelling acetabulum　　3. Dislocating

4. Perthes type　5.Protrusio acetabuli　　6. Atrophic　　7. Mortar and pastle

Fig. 24.4: Shanmugasundaram's classification

3. *MRI:* MRI can pick up TB much earlier as compared to X-rays.
4. *Synovial biopsy:* Ideally all patients suspected to have osteoarticular TB should undergo biopsy as diagnosis can be confirmed only by histopathology or culture.

Treatment of TB Hip

Up to Early Arthritis

All patients should be started with multidrug AKT.

In presence of abduction deformity (stage of synovitis), bilateral lower limb traction should be given to provide rest to the joint and prevent further abduction of affected limb.

Active assisted movements are started as soon as the pain has subsided to prevent contractures. These movements also help in fibrocartilage formation at the areas of cartilage loss.

The ambulation should be nonweight bearing for first 3 months, followed by partial weight bearing for the next 3 months. Crutches or orthosis can be discarded after a period of 1 year.

In Advanced Arthritis

Usual outcome is fibrous ankylosis, so hip spica cast should be given for 4–6 months. The ideal position will be neutral adduction or abduction, 5–10 degrees of external rotation, and 30 degrees of flexion in adults (flexion of 10 degrees is advisable in children).

Surgical Management

1. *Synovectomy and debridement:* This can be done in early stages of disease when the disease is not responding favourably to the treatment or the diagnosis is in doubt. It involves removal of the rice bodies/loose bodies, pannus, granulation tissue, debris, loose articular cartilage, and careful curettage of the hip joint.
2. *Excision/girdle stone arthroplasty:* In this surgery, the diseased portion of head and neck of the femur is removed. It gives an excellent painless and mobile joint. However, there is instability, significant shortening which needs shoe raise (Fig. 24.5).
3. *Arthrodesis:* Fusion of hip joint gives a stable and painless joint. However, movement at the hip joint is completely lost after this surgery. This is a very useful surgery for conversion of painful fibrous ankylosis into a painless bony ankylosis.
4. *Femoral corrective osteotomy:* This may be required in cases of healed tuberculosis, where the hip has healed with severe flexion adduction deformity.
5. *Replacement arthroplasty:* Total hip replacement in TB hip provides excellent functional result. However, there are chances of re-activation of the disease and thus this procedure must be done with caution. Replacement surgery can be performed when the disease has been adequately treated and has been latent for a sufficient period of time. Surgery should always be performed under cover of AKT which has been started preoperatively.

TUBERCULOSIS OF KNEE

Initial focus is haematogenous in origin. It may start in synovium, subchondral bone, or it may be juxta-articular. The synovium becomes hypertrophied, and as a rule the proliferation starts at the site of synovial reflections. Pannus may erode the margins of the articular cartilage, or grow between cartilage and subchondral bone, thus detaching the cartilage from the bone. Flakes of articular cartilage sequestrate and lie free in the joint cavity.

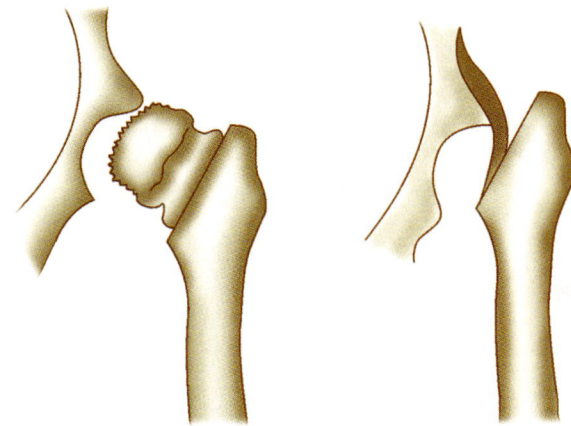

Fig. 24.5: Excision arthroplasty

Clinical Features

It initially begins with insidious onset of swelling in prepatellar and suprapatellar region. Swelling is warm and has a boggy feel due to the thickened synovium. Skin may be stretched and blanched leading to appearance called tumour alba.

Tenderness is more marked at regions of synovial reflections. For a long time there is only terminal restriction of movements. However, when arthritis sets in, the movements are grossly restricted, painful and accompanied by muscle spasms. Quadriceps wasting and regional lymphadenopathy should be checked.

In later stages, there is a classical triple deformity, consisting of flexion, posterolateral subluxation, external rotation and abduction (Fig. 24.6).

Diagnosis

X-ray: In stage of synovitis, X-rays show generalized osteoporosis, increased soft tissue swelling.

In stage of arthritis, there is loss of definition of articular margins, marginal erosions, diminution of joint space and destruction of bone. Osteolytic cavities, tuberculous sequestrum and triple deformity may be evident.

Treatment

Nonoperative treatment is given in patients with synovitis. Anti-tuberculosis drugs and traction are the mainstay of nonoperative treatment. Traction prevents flexion deformity and subluxation of the knee joint.

The patient is kept nonweight bearing for 12 weeks, and then protected ambulation can be started. Crutch free ambulation can be done only after 12 months of treatment.

Operative treatment may be required in severe cases. Various modalities available are:
1. Synovectomy and debridement
2. Knee arthrodesis
3. Interposition arthroplasty
4. Replacement arthroplasty

TUBERCULOSIS OF SHOULDER

The shoulder involvement is rare, occurring mostly in adults. The classical sites could be head of humerus, glenoid, spine of the scapula, acromioclavicular joint, coracoid process and synovial lesion. It can also be iatrogenic due to intra-articular steroid injection given for a stiff shoulder with the mistaken diagnosis of frozen shoulder, particularly in diabetics.

Clinical Features

The clinical presentation is with severe painful restriction of the shoulder movements-particularly abduction and external rotation, and gross wasting of shoulder muscles. This atrophic type of tuberculosis of the shoulder is called 'Caries sicca' (Fig. 24.7).

Differential Diagnosis

Periarthritis of the shoulder, rheumatoid arthritis and post-traumatic shoulder stiffness. Aspiration of the shoulder and fine needle aspiration biopsy might be necessary to establish the diagnosis.

Treatment

The patient responds well to anti-tuberculosis regimens. A shoulder spica in the functional position is necessary in the younger age groups. Shoulder arthrodesis is rarely necessary in severe cases.

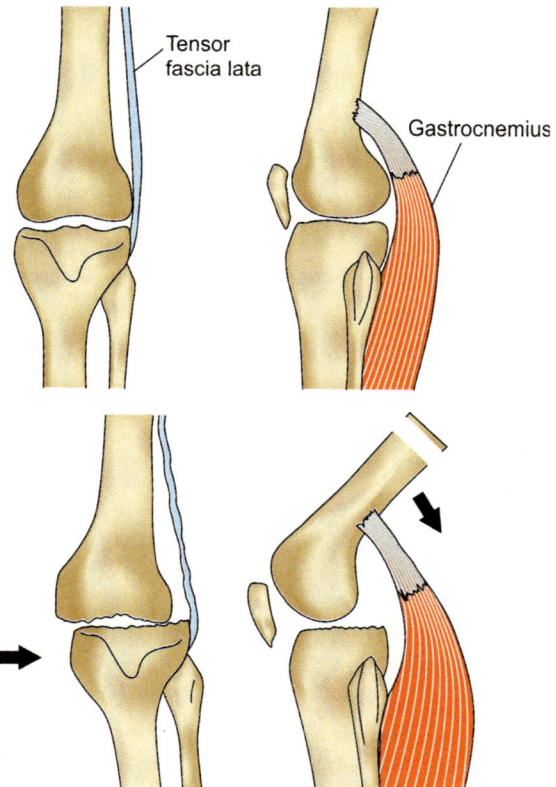

Fig. 24.6: Triple deformity

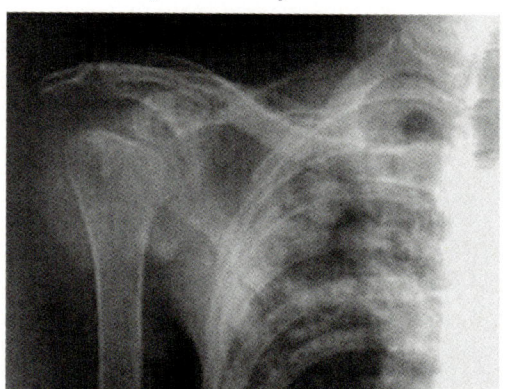

Fig. 24.7: Caries sicca of shoulder

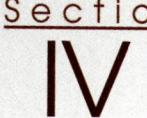

Spine

Anatomy of the Vertebral Column

Vertebral column: Consists of 33 vertebrae (Fig. 25.1).

The sacral and coccygeal vertebrae are fused, which typically allows for 24 mobile segments.

Cervical and lumbar segments: Develop lordosis as an erect posture is acquired.

Thoracic and sacral segments: Maintain kyphotic postures, serve as attachment points for the rib cage and pelvic girdle.

The length of the vertebral column averages 72 cm in men and 7 to 10 cm less in women. The vertebral canal extends throughout the length of the column and provides protection for the spinal cord, conus medullaris and cauda equina. It is important to know the topographical landmarks to identify the exact level of spine pathology (Table 25.1).

Vertebra

Consists of
1. Vertebral body and
2. Neural arch.

Neural arch: Composed of two pedicles laterally and two laminae posteriorly that are united to form the spinous process. To either side of the arch of the vertebral body is a transverse process and superior and inferior articular processes. The articular processes articulate with adjacent vertebrae to form synovial joints. The relative orientation of the articular processes accounts for the degree of flexion, extension, or rotation possible in each segment of the vertebral column. The spinous and transverse processes serve as levers for the numerous muscles attached to them (Figs 25.2 and 25.3).

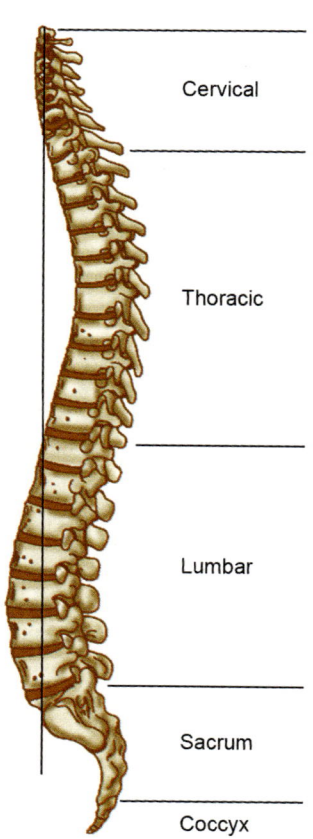

Cervical

Thoracic

Lumbar

Sacrum

Coccyx

Fig. 25.1: Anatomy of vertebral column

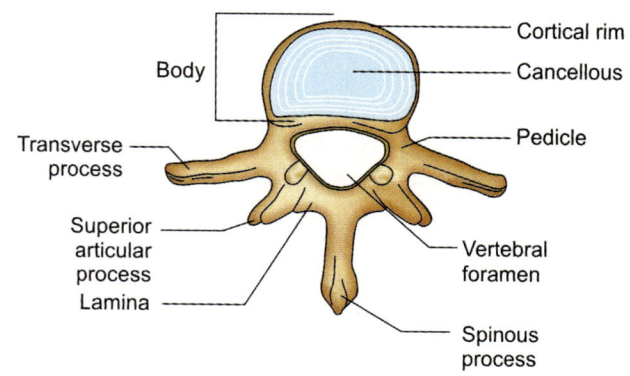

Body

Transverse process

Superior articular process

Lamina

Cortical rim

Cancellous

Pedicle

Vertebral foramen

Spinous process

Fig. 25.2: Parts of typical vertebra

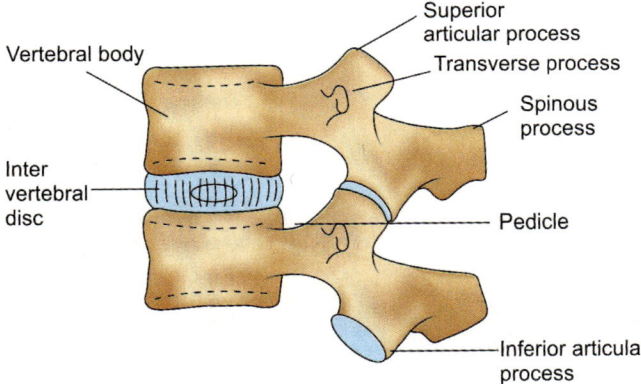

Fig. 25.3: Parts of vertebral unit

Intervertebral Discs

Between two adjacent vertebrae are specialized structures called intervertebral discs. The discs are the largest avascular structures in the body and depend on diffusion from a specialized network of end plate blood vessels for nutrition.

Function of Intervertebral Discs

1. Accommodate movement
2. Weight bearing
3. Shock absorber by being strong but deformable

Each disc contains a pair of vertebral end plates with a central nucleus pulposus and a peripheral ring of annulus fibrosus sandwiched between them. They form a secondary cartilaginous joint or symphysis at each vertebral level.

Vertebral end plates: 1 mm thick sheets of cartilage—fibrocartilage and hyaline cartilage.

Nucleus pulposus: Semifluid mass of mucoid material, 70 to 90% water, with proteoglycan constituting 65% and collagen constituting 15 to 20% of the dry weight.

Annulus fibrosus: It consists of 12 concentric lamellae, with alternating orientation of collagen fibres in successive lamellae to withstand multidirectional strain. The annulus is 60 to 70% water, with collagen constituting 50 to 60% and proteoglycan about 20% of the dry weight. With age, the proportions of proteoglycan and water decrease.

ANATOMY OF THE SPINAL CORD AND NERVES

The spinal cord is shorter than the vertebral column and terminates as the conus medullaris at the *second lumbar vertebra* in *adults* and the *third lumbar vertebra in neonates.* From the conus, a fibrous cord called the *filum terminale* extends to the dorsum of the first coccygeal segment.

The spinal cord is enclosed in three protective membranes—the pia, arachnoid, and dura mater. The pia and arachnoid membranes are separated by the subarachnoid space, which contains the cerebrospinal fluid. The spinal cord has enlargements in the cervical and lumbar regions that correlate with the brachial plexus and lumbar plexus. Within the spinal cord are tracts of ascending (sensory) and descending (motor) nerve fibres. These pathways are arranged with cervical tracts located centrally and thoracic, lumbar, and sacral tracts located progressively peripheral. This accounts for the clinical findings of central cord syndrome and syrinx.

Artery of Adamkiewicz, also called the great anterior medullary artery, makes a major contribution to the anterior spinal artery and is the *main blood supply to the lower spinal cord.* It originates from the left side in 80% of people and accompanies the ventral roots of T9–11. It originates close to the foramen and costotransverse articulation, so ligation of the segmentals should be done at the level of the vertebral bodies to avoid injury. It is the largest of the medullary arteries and is also called the *arteria radicularis magna.* It supplies the caudal two-thirds of the spinal cord.

Topographical Landmarks

Table 25.1: Topographical landmarks	
Hard palate	Arch of Atlas
Mandible	C2–3
Hyoid cartilage	C3
Thyroid cartilage	C4–5
First cricoid ring	C6
Carotid (Chassaignac tubercle)	C6 (anterior tubercle of the transverse process of C6)
Vertebra prominence	C7
Scapula spine	T3
Scapula tip	T7
Umbilicus	L3–4 disc space
Top of iliac crest	L4–5 disc space
PSIS	S2 spinous process

CHAPTER
26

Spinal Injuries

Introduction

Fractures and dislocations of the spine are serious injuries that most commonly occur in young people. The most common causes of severe spinal trauma are motor vehicle accidents, falls, diving accidents, and gunshot wounds. Spinal injury should be suspected in any patient with a head injury or severe facial or scalp lacerations. In any patient with recent trauma, complaints of neck pain or spinal pain should be considered indicative of a spinal injury until proved otherwise.

Manifestations of Spinal Shock

After a spinal cord injury, spinal shock occurs (Table 26.2). It is manifested by:
1. Flaccid paralysis
2. Hypotonia
3. Areflexia
4. An absent bulbo-cavernosus reflex (BCR)

The BCR typically returns during the first 24 to 48 hours after the injury and can be tested by squeezing the glans penis, clitoris, or pulling on a Foley's catheter and eliciting contraction of the anal sphincter.

Goals of Spine Trauma Care

1. Protect against further injury
2. Quickly identify spine injury
3. Maintain or restore spinal alignment
4. Obtain a healed and stable spinal column
5. Facilitate rehabilitation

Acute Management for SCI (Spinal cord injury)

Initial management:
1. Spine immobilization.
2. Full trauma work-up.
3. Methyl-prednisolone within the first 8 hours after injury.

Steroid (methyl-prednisolone) protocol for SCI: Maximum benefit occurs in the first 8 hours, and additional effect occurs within the first 24 hours. The dosage is as follows:
- 0 to 3 hours: 26 mg/kg loading dose, then 5.4 mg/kg for 23 hours
- 3 to 8 hours: 26 mg/kg loading dose, then 5.4 mg/kg for 48 hours
- After 8 hours: No methyl-prednisolone

Definitions of Terms Describing Spinal Cord Injury

Neurological impairment	Loss of motor and sensory function
Disability	Loss in daily life functioning
Tetraplegia	Loss of motor and/or sensory function in the cervical segments
Paraplegia	Loss of motor and/or sensory function in the thoracic, lumbar, or sacral segments
Dermatome	Area of skin innervated by sensory axons within each segmental nerve
Myotome	Collection of muscle fibers innervated by the motor axons within each segmental nerve
Incomplete injury	Partial preservation of sensory and/or motor function below the neurologic level and sensory and/or motor preservation of the lowest sacral segment (Table 26.1)
Complete injury	Absence of sensory and motor function in the lowest sacral segment
Sacral sparing	Dermatomes and myotomes caudal to the neurologic level that remain partially innervated

Diagnostic Imaging

1. *Plain radiography:* Anteroposterior and lateral views.
2. Computed tomography.
3. Magnetic resonance imaging.

Table 26.1: Descriptions of incomplete cord injury patterns		
Syndrome	Lesion	Clinical presentation
Bell's cruciate paralysis	Long tract injury at the level of decussation in brainstem	Variable cranial nerve involvement, greater upper extremity weakness than lower, greater proximal weakness than distal
Anterior cord	Anterior gray matter, descending corticospinal motor tract, and spinothalamic tract injury with preservation of dorsal columns	Variable motor, pain and temperature sensory loss with preservation of proprioception and deep pressure sensation
Central cord	Incomplete cervical white matter injury	Sacral sparing and greater weakness in the upper limbs than the lower limbs
Brown-sequard	Injury to one lateral half of cord and preservation of contralateral half	Ipsilateral motor and proprioception loss and contralateral pain and temperature sensory loss
Conus medullaris	Injury to the sacral cord (conus) and lumbar nerve roots within the spinal canal	Areflexic bladder, bowel, and lower limbs may have preserved bulbocavernosus and micturition reflexes
Cauda equina	Injury to the lumbosacral nerve roots within the spinal canal	Areflexic bladder, bowel, and lower limbs
Root injury	Avulsion or compression injury to single or multiple nerve roots (brachial plexus avulsion)	Dermatomal sensory loss, myotomal motor loss, and absent deep tendon reflexes

Most common sites for spine injuries are:
1. Craniocervical,
2. Cervicothoracic, and
3. Thoracolumbar.

Computed Tomography

CT and MRI may be useful together in determining the presence and extent of spinal column injury. MRI is superior in demonstrating spinal cord pathology and intervertebral disc herniation. CT is superior to MRI in demonstrating bony injury.

Magnetic Resonance Imaging

MRI is useful for imaging soft tissues and bone. MRI shows oedema and haemorrhage associated with acute spinal cord injury. Increased cord signal and parenchymal cord haemorrhage indicate poor prognosis for neurologic recovery. MRI is useful for assessing the craniocervical junction. MRI provides noninvasive assessment of the vertebral artery blood flow in cervical trauma, which can be frequently disrupted in cervical spine injuries.

Table 26.2: Neurogenic and hypovolaemic shock	
Neurogenic shock	Hypovolaemic shock
As a result of loss of sympathetic outflow	As a result of haemorrhage
Hypotension	Hypotension
Bradycardia	Tachycardia
Warm extremities	Cold extremities
Normal urine output	Low urine output

ATLAS FRACTURES

Atlas fractures are caused by axial loading. Neurologic injury is rare because of the wide canal diameter at this level. Fracture stability is determined by the diastasis of the lateral masses as determined by open-mouth odontoid view, but CT scan is the modality of choice. If there is spreading of the lateral masses greater than 6.9 mm, then there is transverse ligament insufficiency and instability is indicated. There are three types of atlas fractures: posterior, anterior, and combined (Jefferson fracture) (Fig. 26.1).

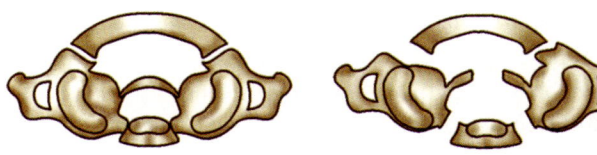

Fig. 26.1: Types of atlas fracture

Treatment

Treatment is determined on the basis of stability.
Stable fractures: Rigid cervical collar.
Unstable fractures: C1–C2 arthrodesis.

TRAUMATIC SPONDYLOLISTHESIS OF THE AXIS (HANGMAN'S FRACTURES)

The term Hangman's fracture was originally referred to neck injuries incurred during the hanging of criminals (Fig. 26.2).

Most common cause: A motor vehicle accident with hyperextension of the head on the neck.

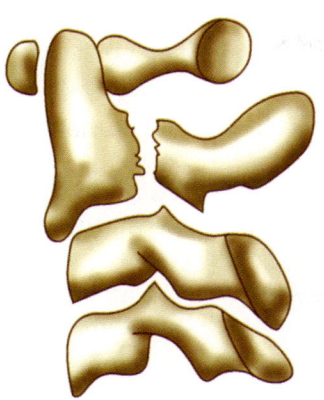 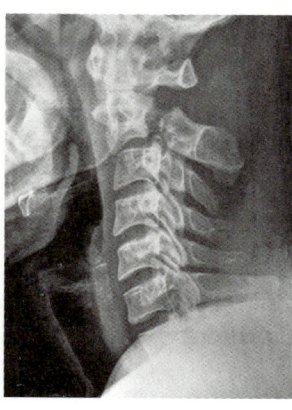

Fig. 26.2: Hangman's fracture

Diagnosis—history, clinical examination and cervical spine lateral X-rays.

Treatment: Immobilization with Philadelphia collar or hard snugly fitting collar to prevent movement at the fracture site. Unstable type of fracture requires operative stabilization.

INJURIES TO THE LOWER CERVICAL SPINE (C3–7)

Account for 40% of all cervical spine injuries where they are most commonly associated with spinal cord damage.

Management of Patient with Cervical Spine Injuries

Initial Evaluation and Emergency Care

Care for a patient with potential cervical spine injury begins in the field.

1. Manual immobilization of the head and neck should be maintained until a hard cervical collar can be applied.
2. Tracheostomy tube or an emergency crico-thyroidotomy to be done if required.
3. Airway security and haemodynamic resuscitation.

In-Hospital Resuscitation

Once the patient has arrived at the emergency room, initial assessment of the ABCs (airway, breathing, and circulation) should be performed and life-saving procedures initiated.

History and Physical Examination

An in depth examination can be executed in the awake and alert patient. In the unconscious, nonalert patient, questions about the injury mechanism may be directed toward eyewitness or emergency paramedical staff that were present at the scene.

Clinical Examination

Local Examination

1. Spinous processes should be palpated individually, noting tenderness, crepitus, or step-off. Bruising or laceration, as well as penetrating wounds, should be noted and marked.
2. Swelling and fullness in the anterior neck can suggest prevertebral haematoma.
3. Rotation of the head and neck should be noted, because patients with unilateral facet dislocations can present with their heads turned toward the nondislocated side.
4. Areas of ecchymosis on the face or scalp might be the result of a direct impact and thus suggest the direction of traumatic force delivery.

Neurological Examination

A detailed neurologic examination is performed in the awake, alert patient (Tables 26.3 and 26.4). This should include motor, sensory, and reflex testing in all myotomal and dermatomal regions. Muscle strength should be graded from 0 to 5 and accurately documented in the chart.

Perianal sensation is a sign of sacral nerve root sparing and can be a positive prognostic sign for neurologic recovery for patients with what otherwise would be classified as a complete spinal cord injury (no other motor or sensory function below the level of injury).

Muscle Grade Criteria

Motor Grade Examination Criteria

5 Able to resist full force resistance
4 Examiner able to overcome strength
3 Can overcome gravity, no resistance
2 Can move without gravity
1 Visible contraction
0 No contraction

Muscle group strength should be graded from 0 (absent) to 5 (normal).

Diagnosis

1. *Most important is cervical spine lateral X-ray:* Look for:
   a. *Alignment of the cervical vertebrae* assessed by examining longitudinal lines along vertebral bodies, lamina, and spinous processes (Fig. 26.3). The spinolaminar line (A), posterior vertebral body line (B), and anterior vertebral body line (C) are normally unbroken. On a perfect lateral view, the facet joints should appear as stacked parallelograms.

Table 26.3: Cervicothoracic nerves

Level	Nerve root	Motor effects	Sensory effects	Reflex
C1–2	C2	Clavicular head of sternocleidomastoid	Head and neck	None
C2–3	C3	Trapezius, diaphragm	Head and neck	None
C3–4	C4	Scapula, diaphragm	Lateral neck/shoulder	None
C4–5	C5	Diaphragm, deltoid, biceps (elbow flexion)	Lateral arm (axillary nerve)	Biceps
C5–6	C6	Wrist extensors, biceps (supination), triceps	Radial forearm, thumb, and index fingers (musculocutaneous nerve)	Brachioradialis
C6–7	C7	Triceps (elbow extension), wrist flexors, finger extensors Pronation	Middle finger	Triceps
C7–T1	C8	Finger flexors, interossei	Ring and little fingers (ulnar nerve), ulnar nerve, medial forearm (medial antebrachial cutaneous nerve)	None
T1–2	T1	Finger abductors (interossei)	Medial arm (medial brachial cutaneous nerve)	None

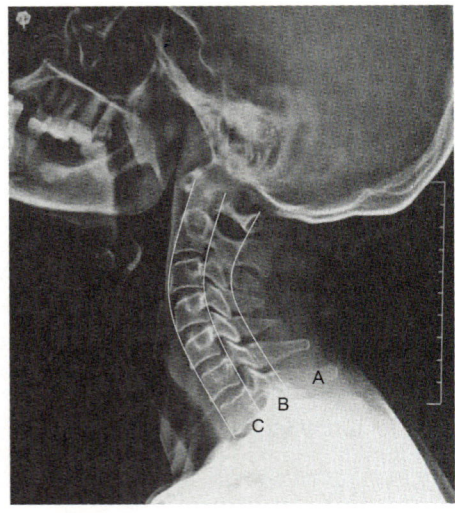

Fig. 26.3: Lateral X-ray of cervical spine

b. *Prevertebral soft tissues* can be useful as an indicator of swelling from acute haemorrhage.

The prevertebral soft tissue shadow is measured at the C2–3 and C6–7 disc spaces. More than 7 mm at the C2–3 or 21 mm at the C6–7 disc is strongly suggestive of an underlying spinal injury.

2. *MRI cervical spine:* To assess the neurological damage to spinal cord and nerves.

Treatment

Stable fractures are treated with immobilisation in a rigid cervical orthosis for 12 weeks.

Unstable fractures: Fractures with more than 3.5 mm translation or more than 11 degrees angulation.

These fractures are treated by posterior fusion. Fusion may also be considered to prevent kyphosis if there is loss of greater than 25% body height.

Vertebrobasilar artery insufficiency syndrome: This syndrome is seen in patients with cervical spine injury; the greatest risk is with flexion injuries. The brain stem, cerebellum, and occipital lobe are supplied by the vertebrobasilar (posterior) circulation. It can manifest with vertigo, visual disturbances (diplopia), facial numbness or paresthesias, dysphagia, dysarthria, and hoarseness. Physical examination may reveal nystagmus, limb ataxia, truncal ataxia (falling to the side of the lesion), contralateral deficit in pain and temperature perception, ipsilateral limb and trunk numbness, ipsilateral loss of taste, and visual field defects.

THORACOLUMBAR FRACTURES

Anatomy

Denis suggested that the spine should be divided into three columns (Figs 26.4 and 26.5):

1. Anterior column: Anterior portions of the vertebral body, disc, and anterior longitudinal ligament (ALL)
2. Middle column: Posterior portion of the vertebral body, disc, and posterior longitudinal ligament (PLL).
3. Posterior column: Pedicles and neural arch, facet joints, and associated ligaments.

Classification

They are primarily two major types:

a. Compression fractures.
b. Burst fractures.

Compression Fractures

They occur due to isolated failure of the anterior column of spine. They are mostly stable fractures and do not require operative treatment (Fig. 26.6).

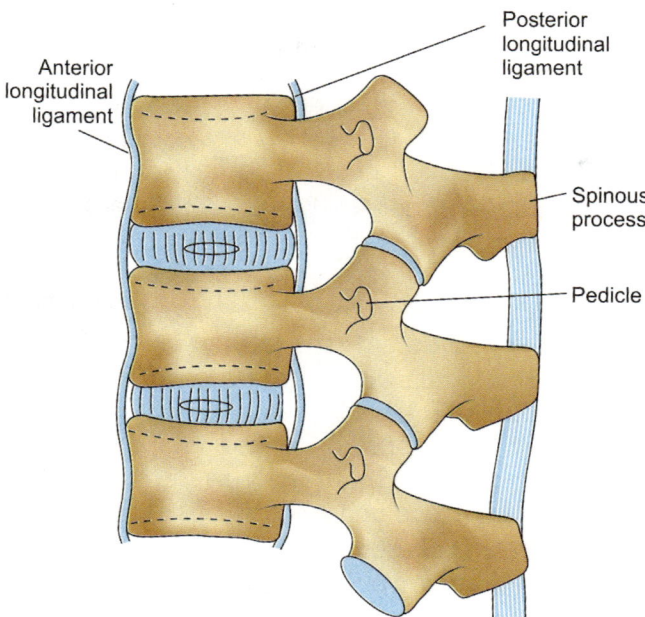

Fig. 26.4: Anatomy of thoracolumbar vertebrae

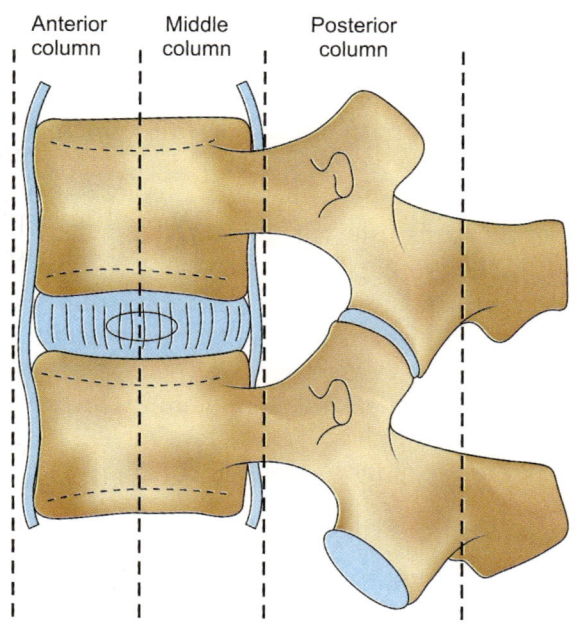

Fig. 26.5: 3-Column theory

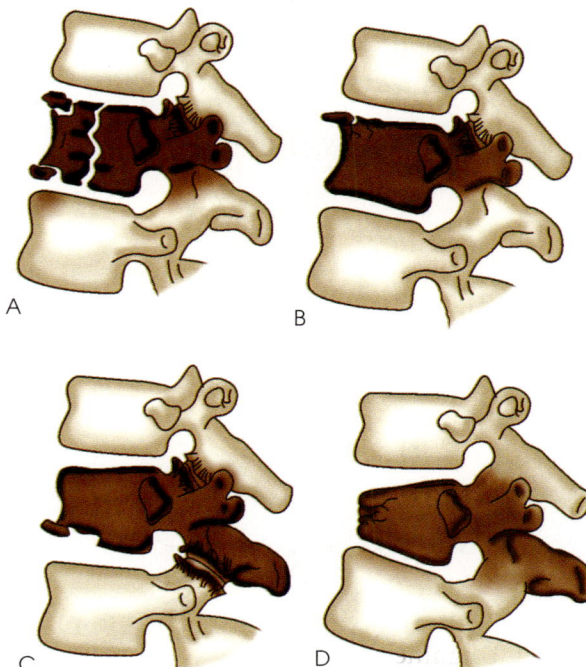

Fig. 26.6: Different types of compression fractures

the distance between the two pedicles of the same vertebra (Fig. 26.7). They are further classified as:
1. Stable burst fractures
2. Unstable burst fractures

In stable burst fractures, the anterior and middle columns fail because of a compressive load, with no loss of integrity of the posterior elements.

In unstable burst fractures, the anterior and middle columns fail because of a compressive load, with loss of integrity of the posterior elements

Chance fractures or seat-belt injuries are horizontal avulsion injuries of the vertebral bodies caused by

Factors increasing the risk of compression fracture:
1. Postmenopausal women
2. Family history of compression fracture
3. Premature menopause
4. Tobacco, smoking
5. Prolonged steroid intake

Burst Fractures

They are high energy injuries involving two or more columns of the spine with separation or widening of

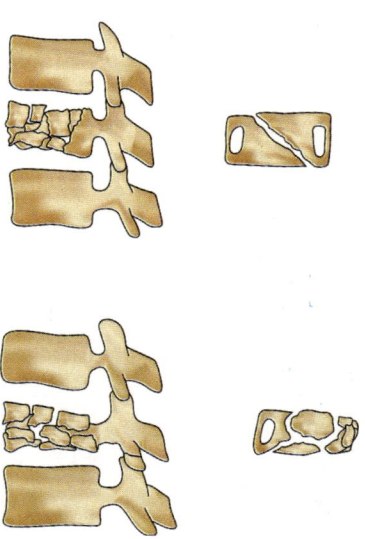

Fig. 26.7: Burst fractures

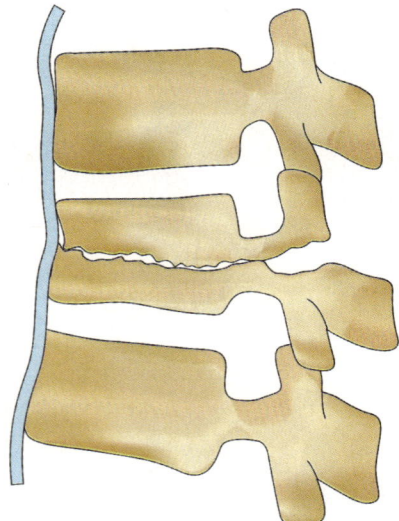

Fig. 26.8: Chance fracture

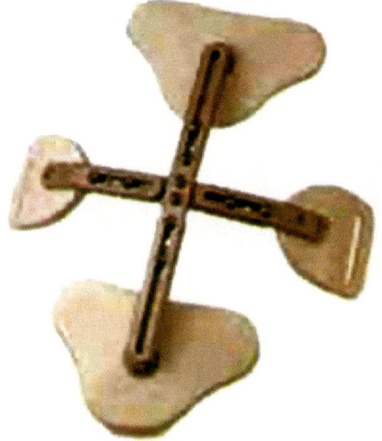

Fig. 26.10: ASH brace

flexion around an axis anterior to the anterior longitudinal ligament. The entire vertebra is pulled apart by a strong tensile force (Fig. 26.8).

Diagnosis

1. X-rays of thoracolumbar spine—anteroposterior and lateral views.
2. MRI of spine.
3. CT scan.

Treatment

Indications for non-operative treatment
1. Absence of neurological deficit.
2. Kyphosis less than 20–26 degree

Method of Non-operative Treatment

Use of specially made thoracolumbar orthoses called Taylor's brace (Fig. 26.9), ASH brace (anterior spinal hyperextension brace) (Fig. 26.10).

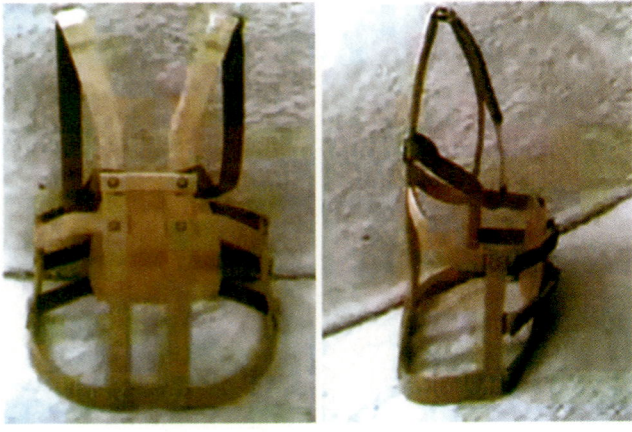

Fig. 26.9: Taylor's brace

Indication for Operative Treatment

Fracture which are:
1. Unstable
2. Cause neurological deficit
3. Cause significant kyphosis.

Method

The basic principle of treatment is to decompress the spinal cord from mechanical compression, align the spine and stabilize it with specially designed implants for the spine.

Older implants used for the spine were Hartshill's rectangle, steffi plate and Harrington rod (Fig. 26.12).

Newer implants commonly used for instrumentation of the spine are screws made of titanium inserted into the pedicle of the vertebrae called pedicle screw and rod systems which afford more stability to the spine and enhance strength and accelerate rehabilitation as compared to the older implants (Fig. 26.11).

Management of Paraplegia

Aim of Treatment

1. To prevent complications like bedsores and urinary tract infection, which can be life threatening.
2. To rehabilitate the patients to be as independent as possible.

Management includes
1. General care
2. Skin care with bedsore management
3. Bladder-bowel care
4. Muscles-joints care
5. Psychological care
6. Rehabilitation
1. *General care:* To boost immunity and overall well being

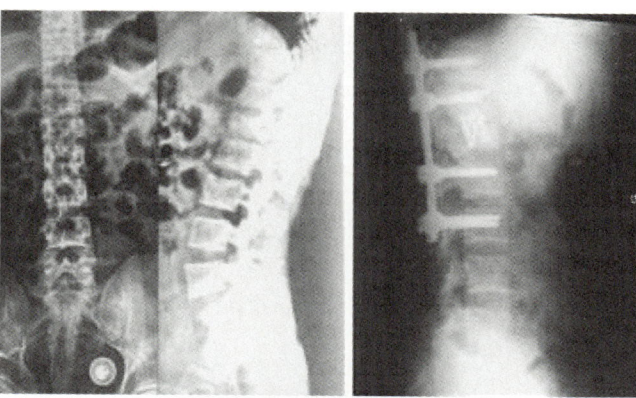

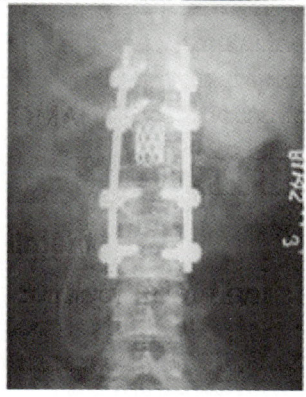

Fig. 26.11: Unstable lumbar burst fracture treated with pedicular screws and cage for stabilization

- High protein diet
- Treatment of anaemia–hematinics

2. *Skin care:* Anaesthetic skin is prone to develop pressure sores/bedsores/decubitus ulcers, e.g. sacral/trochanteric/heel area. These are localised areas of cellular necrosis resulting from prolonged excessive stresses on soft tissues.

Classification of pressure sores:

Grade I: Area of hyperaemia over pressure points

Grade II: Actual breakdown of skin

Grade III: Deep ulcer with sloughing of muscle tissue, exposing the underlying bone

Treatment of pressure sores:

- Daily dressing and debridement of devitalised tissues
- Split thickness skin grafting over healthy granulation tissue/flap surgery for grade III sores.

Pressure sores can be prevented by meticulous nursing.

- Creases in the sheets and crumbs in bed are not permitted.

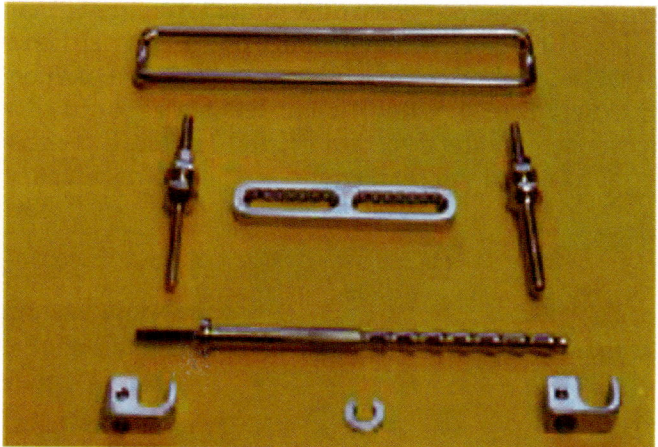

Fig. 26.12: Hartshill's rectangle, Steffi plate and Harrington rods, hooks

- Gentle roll onto side every 2 hours and careful washing of back (without rubbing), drying and powder application
- Use of water/air bed.

3. *Bladder-bowel care*
   - Use of silastic catheter—to be changed twice weekly, to prevent catheter blockage, infection.
   - Use of CSIC technique (clean self intermittent catheterisation)
   - Use of antibiotics if signs of urinary tract infection
   - Urodynamic study is advised to diagnose the status of bladder
   - Bowel training with the help of enemas, abdominal exercise.

4. *Muscles-joints care*
   - Aim is to prevent flexion contracture
   - Passive movements through full range of motion twice daily
   - Splints to maintain the position of joints.
   - Surgical intervention as necessary, if contractures develop-tenotomies/tendon transfer.

5. *Psychological care*
   - The morale of a paraplegic patient is liable to reach a low ebb and restoration of self-confidence is an essential part of management.
   - Constant encouragement and enthusiasm by doctor, nurse and therapist is very important.
   - Patients can be encouraged to develop hobbies.

6. *Rehabilitation*
   - Training for a new job at the earliest
   - Therapists can teach the patients to be as independent as possible.

Table 26.4: Tests to determine spine pathology

Sign	Pathology
I . Long Tract Signs	
Babinski: First toe dorsiflexion with fanning out of other toes when sharp instrument is rubbed on lateral border of foot from calcaneus to head of first metatarsal	Upper motor neuron (UMN) lesion; corticospinal tract.
Hoffman: Flick distal phalanx away from palm; look for pincer effect between thumb and index finger; look for asymmetry.	Cord compression; CNS dysfunction; brisk muscle stretch reflex
Tramner reflex: Elevate middle finger above other fingers and flick distal phalanx toward palm; look for pincer effect between thumb and index finger; look for asymmetry.	Cord compression; CNS dysfunction; brisk muscle stretch reflex
Inverted radial reflex: Finger flexion upon testing brachioradialis reflex	Cervical myelopathy
Finger escape: Abduction of fifth finger because of weak hand intrinsics	Cervical myelopathy
Lhermitte: Neck flexion causing lightning-like sensation radiating down back	Cervical stenosis; disc herniation; multiple sclerosis with posterior column dysfunction (original description)
Cross adductor: Stimulate patellar reflex and note contralateral thigh adductor contraction	UMN lesion
Chaddock: Laterally abduct the little toe briskly and let it slap back against the other toes or flick the third or fourth toe down rapidly; note dorsiflexion of the great toe.	UMN lesion
Jaw jerk reflex: Gently tap on patient's jaw with patient's mouth slightly open; a positive reflex is when the jaw closes	In a patient with UMN signs, a positive jaw jerk test suggests that the etiology is not in the cervical spine but that the pathology is located above the level of the pons
II. Nerve Root Compression Signs	
Spurling: Extend and bend the neck laterally and apply axial load to the top of the head; patient will report radicular pain.	Cervical nerve root compression
Straight-leg raise (SLR) with patient supine or sitting, perform SLR and patient will report pain in the distribution of the nerve root irritated; for sciatic involvement, the pain must extend distal to the knee	Nerve root compression
Contralateral SLR (Fajersztajn): Raising asymptomatic side causes pain down symptomatic side	Indicates either a central disc herniation or an axillary herniation on the symptomatic side
Lasegue: Perform SLR and then dorsiflex the ankle; it should exacerbate SLR radiculopathy; with less than 70 degrees of hip flexion is a positive Lasegue sign	Nerve root compression
Bowstring with patient supine, raise leg, flex knee, then apply pressure to popliteal fossa to elicit radicular pain	Nerve root compression
Milgram: Patient raises both legs off examining table and holds for 26 seconds; note radiculopathy	Nerve root compression
Naffziger: Compress neck veins for 10 seconds with patient supine; coughing produces radiculopathy	Nerve root compression
Hoover: Examiner places hands under patient's heel while the supine patient tries to perform SLR with the contralateral leg	If the patient is malingering or not trying, then there will be a lack of downward pressure on the hand under the heel (opposite foot not performing the SLR)
Femoral stretch with patient prone or lying on side, the hip is held in extension and the knee is flexed	Femoral neuritis or L3 or L4 radiculopathy

Degenerative Disorders of Spine

CERVICAL SPONDYLOSIS

Cervical spondylosis is a disorder in which there is abnormal wear on the cartilage and bones of the neck (cervical vertebrae). It is a common cause of chronic neck pain.

In the cervical spine the nerve root exits above its corresponding vertebra, i.e. C5 nerve root exits above C5 vertebra, whereas it is opposite in the lumbar spine, i.e the L5 nerve root exits below the corresponding vertebra, i.e. L5 (Fig. 27.1).

Cervical disc prolapse is more common in men by a ratio of 1.4:1. This is probably due to frequent heavy lifting on the job, cigarette smoking, and frequent diving from a board.

Clinical Presentation

1. Symptoms Related to Spine

Neck pain, medial scapular pain and shoulder pain are related to primary pain around the disc and spine.

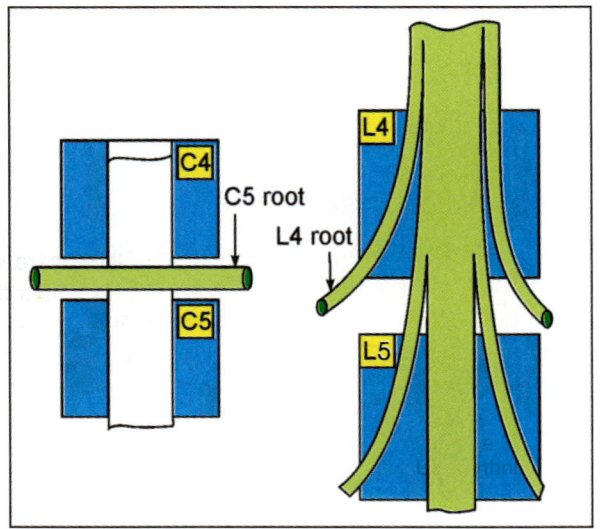

Fig. 27.1: Difference of exiting nerve roots in cervical and rest of the spine

2. Signs and Symptoms Related to Nerve

Symptoms of root compression usually are associated with pain radiating into the arm or chest with numbness in the fingers and motor weakness.

3. Signs and Symptoms of Cervical Myelopathy

Signs and symptoms of midline cervical spinal cord compression (myelopathy) are characteristic. It is associated with a generalized feeling of weakness in the lower extremities and a feeling of instability. There is spasticity and upper motor neuron signs like hyperreflexia.

4. Symptoms of Vertebral Artery Compression

Dizziness, tinnitus, intermittent blurring of vision, and occasional episodes of retro-ocular pain.

Diagnosis

1. Cervical spine X-rays—anteroposterior (AP) and lateral views.
2. Magnetic resonance imaging.

Management

Nonoperative Treatment

For patients with nonradicular neck pain only, i.e. no signs and symptoms of either nerve root or spinal cord compression, best primary treatment is short periods of rest, massage, ice, and anti-inflammatory agents with active mobilization as soon as possible.

Operative Treatment

Indications
1. Failure of nonoperative pain management,
2. Increasing and significant neurological deficit
3. Cervical myelopathy.

Technique—most commonly in the cervical spine, decompression is carried out anteriorly and then arthrodesis is done subsequently to prevent instability (Fig. 27.2).

For patients with myelopathy with more than 3 level of cervical spine involvement and maintenance of cervical lordosis-posterior decompression procedure to relieve pressure on the spinal cord can be carried out.

Back pain is the most frequent musculoskeletal complaint (Table 27.1 and Fig. 27.3).

ACUTE BACK PAIN WITH LUMBAR RADICULOPATHY

The most common cause of lumbar radiculopathy in patients younger than 40 years of age is a herniated nucleus pulposus (HNP). The nucleus pulposus may bulge into the canal. Tears of the fibres of the annulus fibrosis may allow the disc to extrude through the annulus, or the disc may sequestrate through the annulus and lie free in the spinal canal or neural foramina. Nerve root compression causes secondary inflammation of the nerve root, giving the patient subjective symptoms of pain, numbness, or tingling along the distribution of the particular nerve root. More than 95% of the ruptures of the lumbar intervertebral discs occur at L4 or L5. The most commonly affected nerve roots are L5 and S1. Pain associated with a herniated nucleus pulposus varies from mild pain along

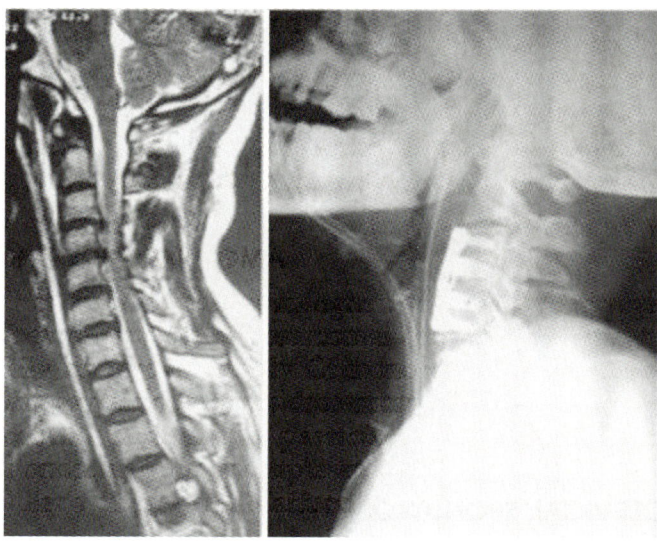

Fig. 27.2: C3–4 and C4–5 spondylosis treated with discectomy and stabilization using cage and plate

the distribution of the nerve to severe incapacitating pain.

Clinical Presentation

Symptoms

- Low back pain
- Stiffness
- Radiation of pain along a limb
- Tingling/numbness in specific areas of limb
- Weakness or sensory loss of specific dermatomal regions.
- *In severe cases:* Urinary retention (cauda equina syndrome)

Signs

- Loss of lumbar lordosis
- Restricted lumbar range of motion
- Nerve root stretch signs (given below)
- Specific sensory and motor involvement (Table 27.2)

Nerve Root Irritation Signs

1. Straight leg raising (SLR): Lasègue's sign, Lasègue test or Lazarevi's sign
   a. *Active SLR:* Patient performs action himself. Raising the affected leg of patient causes pain along the distribution of nerve. If the patient experiences sciatic pain when the straight leg is at an angle between 30 and 70 degrees, then the test is positive and a herniated disc is likely to be the cause of the pain.
   b. *Passive SLR:* When test is performed by the examiner.

Table 27.1: Differential diagnosis of low back pain

Mechanical low back or leg pain

• Congenital disease	• Lumbar strain, sprain
• Severe kyphosis	• Osteoportotic
• Severe scoliosis	compresssion fracture
• Transitional vertebrae	• Presumed instability
• Degenerative processes	• Spinal stenosis
of discs and facets, usually	• Spondylolisthesis
age related	• Spondylolysis
• Herniated disc	• Traumatic fracture
• Internal disc disruption or	
discogenic low back pain	

Nonmechanical spinal conditions

• Inflammatory arthritis	• Neoplasia
(often associated with	- Lymphoma and leukaemia
HLA-B27)	- Metastatic carcinoma
• Ankylosing spondylitis	- Multiple myeloma
• Inflammatory bowel disease	- Primary vertebral tumours
• Psoriatic spondylitis	- Retroperitoneal tumours
• Reiter's syndrome	- Spinal cord tumours

Infection

• Epidural abscess	• *Paget's disease of bone*
• Osteomyelitis	• *Scheuermann's disease*
• Paraspinal abscess	(osteochrondrosis)
• Septic discitis	

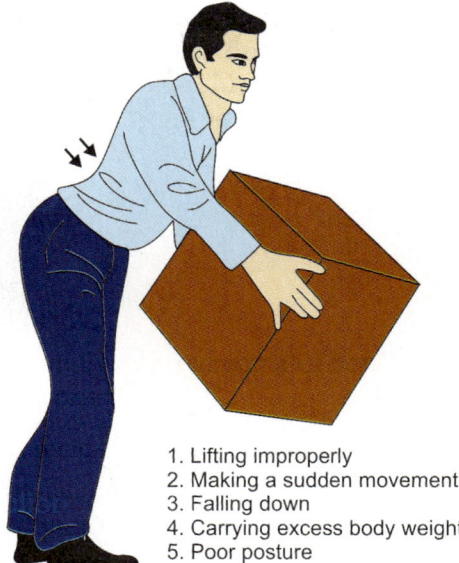

1. Lifting improperly
2. Making a sudden movement
3. Falling down
4. Carrying excess body weight
5. Poor posture

Fig. 27.3: Risk factors for back pain

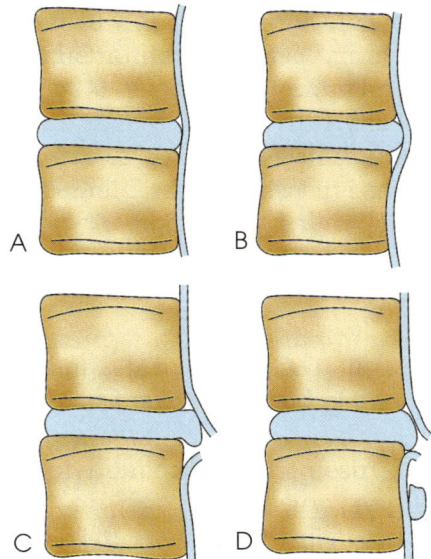

Fig. 27.4: Types of disc herniation

c. *Cross-over SLR:* Raising of the non-affected leg causes pain.

Example: For patients with back pain radiating down their right leg, perform the crossed SLR manoeuvre. If elevating their left leg passively reproduces pain down their affected right leg, this is highly predictive of a sciatic radiculopathy and disc herniation. The crossed SLR manoeuvre essentially stretches the left L4–L5–S1 nerve root and thus tugs on the right L4–L5–S1 nerve root.

2. *Bowstring test:* Patient is supine with knee flexed to 90° and his leg placed on examiner's shoulder. Place fingers in the popliteal space behind the knee and apply pressure. If test is positive there should be a tingling, burning sensation in the hip and buttocks.

Classification

Types of disc herniation (Fig. 27.4):
A. Normal bulge
B. Protrusion
C. Extrusion
D. Sequestration

Diagnosis

In addition to lumbosacral spine anteroposterior and lateral views, MRI is useful in diagnosis.

Treatment

Acute episode

1. Bedrest (1 to 2 days) with limitation or modification of activities.
2. Anti-inflammatory drugs (aspirin or non-steroidal anti-inflammatory agents).
3. Epidural steroid injections may provide short-term relief for patients with a herniated nucleus pulposus.
4. Traction, corsets or braces, and physical therapy. As the symptoms resolve, it is important to get the patient on a rehabilitation programme to prevent recurrent episodes of back pain and disability.

Table 27.2: Specific sensory and motor affection as per nerve root involvement

Nerve root	Sensory deficit	Motor weakness	Reflex change
L4	Posterolateral thigh, anterior knee and medial leg	Quadriceps Hip adductors Anterior tibial	Patellar tendon Anterior tibial tendon
L5	Anterolateral leg, dorsum of the foot, and great toe	Extensor hallucis longus Gluteus medius Extensor digitorum longus and brevis	Posterior tibial (difficult to elicit)
S1	Lateral malleolus, lateral foot, heel, and web of fourth and fifth toes	Peroneus longus and brevis Gastrocnemius-soleus complex Gluteus maximus	Achilles tendon (gastrocnemius-soleus complex)

Patients should be encouraged to increase their activity level and begin a conditioning and physical fitness programme.

Indications for Surgery

1. If the sciatica is severe and disabling
2. Nerve tension signs are positive
3. Symptoms persist without improvement for longer than 1 month
4. Clinical examination and diagnostic tests are consistent with nerve root compromise.
5. Cauda equina syndrome.

Operative treatment involves decompression of the nerve root at the involved lumbar level by performing discectomy.

CAUDA EQUINA SYNDROME

Due to massive extrusion of a disc involving the entire diameter of the lumbar canal or a large midline extrusion there is development of the triad of (a) saddle anaesthesia, (b) bilateral ankle areflexia (c) bladder symptoms. This is known as cauda equina syndrome.

Clinical Presentation (Table 27.3 and Fig. 27.5))

Pain in the back, legs, and occasionally perineum. Both legs may be paralyzed, the sphincters may be incontinent, and the ankle jerks may be absent, caused by massive intervertebral disc extrusion at any lumbar level. Cauda equina syndrome requires immediate surgical intervention. Only patients with acute cauda equina syndrome should undergo immediate diagnostic evaluation. These patients should have immediate MRI to determine the cause of the cauda

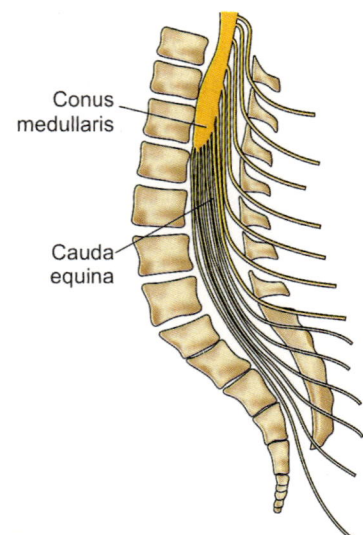

Fig. 27.5: Cauda equina and conus medullaris

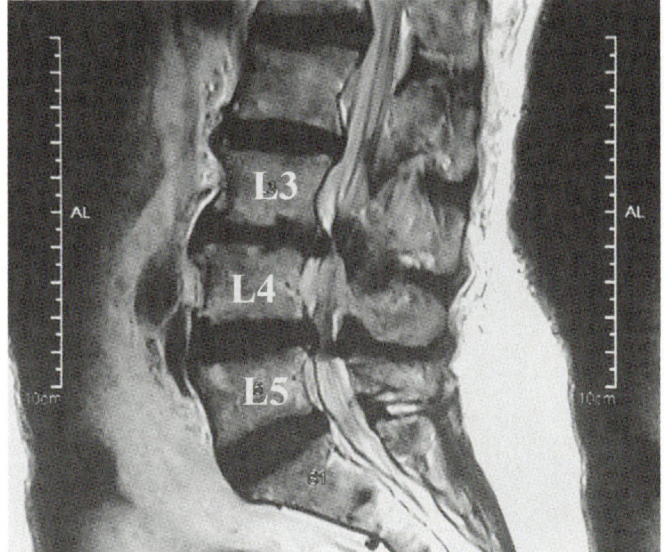

Fig. 27.6: MRI showing L3–4 and L4–5 disc herniation

equina syndrome before surgical intervention (Fig. 27.6).

Treatment

Emergency surgery: Immediate decompression of the spinal canal to reduce pressure on the cauda equina.

LUMBAR CANAL STENOSIS (LCS)

It is defined as the decrease in the diameter of spinal canal.

Classification

Based on Aetiology

- *Congenital:* Short pedicles and a medially placed facet joint with a triangular shaped canal (seen in achondroplastic dwarfs).
- *Acquired:* Degenerative changes with facet joint enlargement, thickening of the facet capsule, hypertrophy of the ligamentum flavum, herniated or bulging disc, loss of disc height, osteophyte formation, and uncinate spurring.
- *Combined:* Spondylotic changes with underlying congenital stenosis.
- Postsurgical.
- Spondylolisthesis.

Based on Location (Fig. 27.7)

- *Central stenosis:* Compression of the thecal sac producing nonspecific nerve root involvement. Etiology may include enlargement of inferior articular facet and ligamentum flavum.

Table 27.3: Symptoms and signs of conus medullaris and cauda equina syndromes

	Conus Medullaris syndrome	Cauda equina syndrome
Vertebral level	L1–L2	L2-sacrum
Spinal level	Sacral cord	Lumbosacral nerve roots
Presentation	Sudden and bilateral	Gradual and unilateral//bilateral
Reflexes	Knee jerks preserved but ankle jerks affected	Both ankle and knee jerks affected
Radicular pain	Less severe	More severe
Low back pain	More	Less
Sensory symptoms and signs	Numbness tends to be more localized to perianal area; symmetrical and bilateral; sensory dissociation occurs	Numbness tends to be more localized to saddle area; asymmetrical, may be unilateral; no sensory dissociation
Motor strength	Typically symmetric, hyperreflexic distal paresis of lower limbs that is less marked; fasciculations may be present	Asymmetric areflexic paraparesis that is more marked; fasciculations rare; atrophy more common
Impotence	Frequent	Less frequent; erectile dysfunction that includes inability to have erection, inability to maintain erection, lack of sensation in pubic area (including glans penis or clitoris), and inability to ejaculate
Sphincter dysfunction	Urinary retention and atonic anal sphincter cause overflow urinary incontinence and fecal incontinence; tend to present early in course of disease	Urinary retention; tends to present late in course of disease

- *Lateral recess stenosis:* Thecal sac to medial wall of the pedicle. It produces compression of the traversing nerve root from impingement. Etiology may include superior facet enlargement and facet capsular thickening with or without disc bulging.
- *Foraminal stenosis:* Lateral to medial wall of pedicle. Produces exiting nerve root impingement. Etiology may include enlarged medial border of the superior facet, uncinate spur, and a far lateral disc herniation.

Clinical Presentation

- Back pain
- Stiffness
- Radiculopathy—in patients with foraminal stenosis
- *Neurogenic claudication:* Seen in 50% of cases. It is described as pain radiating proximally and

extending distally into legs, typically worse with walking and better with forward flexion (Table 27.4).

Physical examination: Limited extension and loss of lordosis.

Typically, there may be no neurologic deficit and a negative straight leg raising test(SLR). Bowel and bladder symptoms are rare.

Diagnosis

1. Lumbosacral spine X-ray—AP and lateral view
2. MRI/CT scans

Treatment

Conservative treatment: It includes physical therapy, NSAIDs, bracing, and either epidural or transforaminal steroid injections.

Operative

Indications: Persistent significant pain after non-operative treatment or progressive weakness. There are two operations that are performed:

- Laminectomy and decompression of compressed nerve roots
- Laminectomy with fusion arthrodesis (with or without instrumentation), performed in cases with degenerative spondylolisthesis or scoliosis or spinal instability.

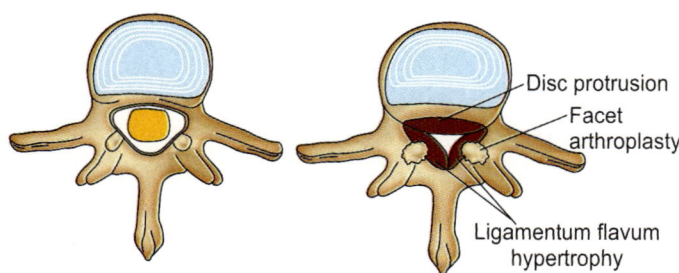

Fig. 27.7: Pathology of lumbar canal stenosis

Table 27.4: Neurogenic versus vascular claudication

Activity	Vascular (Pseudo) claudication	Neurogenic claudication
Walking	Distal to proximal leg and calf pain; relieved with standing still	Proximal to distal thigh pain; relieved with sitting or flexion
Walking distance	Constant	Variable
Uphill walking	Symptoms develop sooner	Symptoms develop later
Bicycling	Symptoms develop	Symptoms do not develop
Lying flat	Relief	May exacerbate symptoms
Distal pulses	Weak	Normal

LUMBAR SPONDYLOLYSIS/SPONDYLOLISTHESIS

Definition

Spondylolysis: Term referring to a defect in the pars interarticularis. The defect may be unilateral or bilateral and may be associated with spondylolisthesis (Figs 27.8 and 27.9).

Spondylolisthesis refers to the anterior displacement (translation) of a vertebra with respect to the vertebra caudal to it (Figs 27.8 and 27.10).

Isthmic Spondylolisthesis

This condition is secondary to spondylolysis which weakens the pars and leads to forward slipping of one vertebra over the other and hence low back pain and symptoms of radiculopathy due to foraminal stenosis.

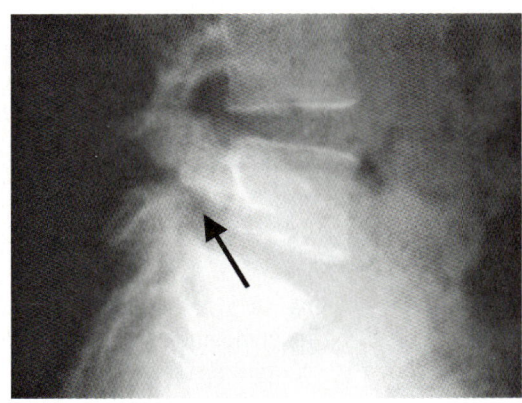

Fig. 27.9: Lumbosacral spine lateral X-ray showing L5 spondylolysis

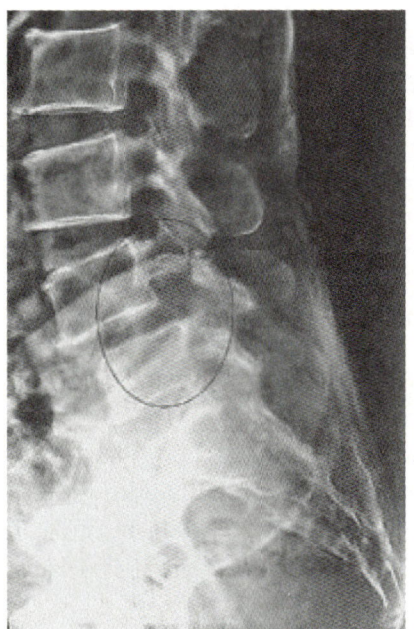

Fig. 27.10: Spondylolisthesis at L4–L5

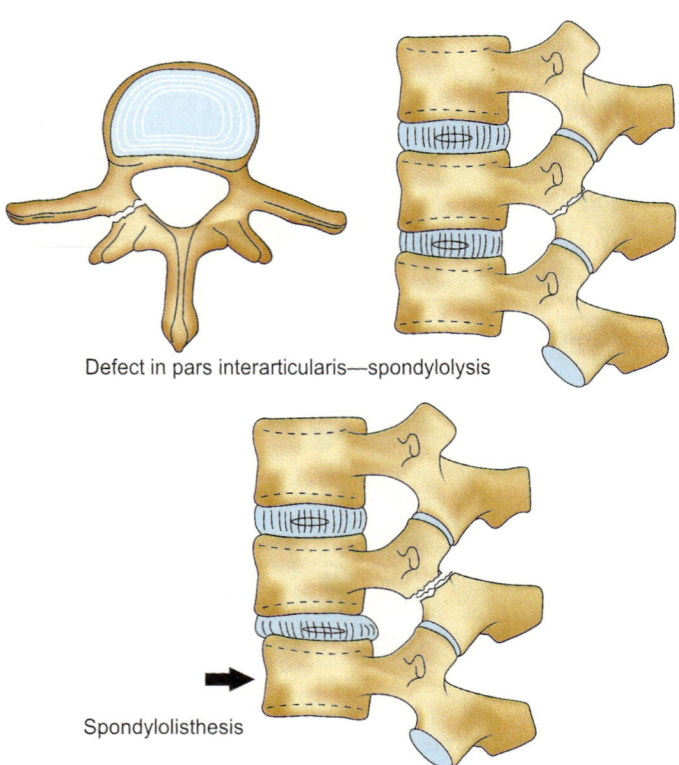

Defect in pars interarticularis—spondylolysis

Spondylolisthesis

Fig. 27.8: Spondylolysis and spondylolisthesis

Clinical Presentation

Spondylolysis is one of the more common causes of low back pain in children, adolescents, and young adults. It is thought to be a fatigue fracture in the pars interarticularis due to shear stress on the pars from the repetitive hyperextension.

Physical examination reveals limited extension and pain with extension.

Diagnostic Imaging

1. X-rays of lumbosacral spine—AP (anteroposterior) and lateral view (Fig. 27.9).
   Oblique X-rays are important to see for the pars interarticulars defect, the typical "Scottie dog" appearance (Fig. 27.11)
2. MRI will demonstrate nerve root compression if spondylolisthesis is present.

Classification

Meyerding classification (Fig. 27.12): The severity of the slip has been classified by Meyerding on the basis of the degree of anterior translation (relative to the adjacent caudal vertebral width).

Treatment

Initial treatment is typically nonoperative: Physical therapy with flexion exercises, NSAIDs, bracing, and activity modification.

Surgical indications and treatment for isthaemic spondylolisthesis: Indications for operative treatment are significant pain after failure of conservative treatment and/or slip progression or significant associated neurological compression.

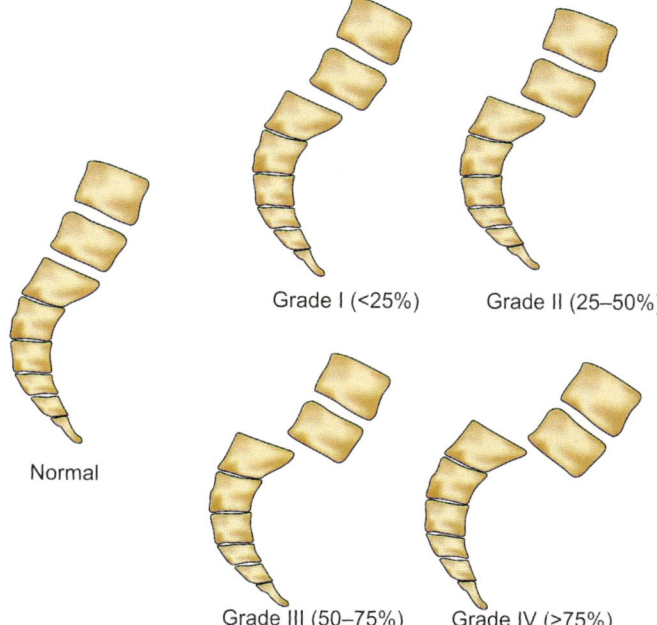

Fig. 27.12: Grades of spondylolisthesis

Grade I or II (<50% translation) slips: *In situ* posterior fusion.

Grade III or IV (>50% translation): Reduction before fusion may be required in some high grade spondylolisthesis to restore the physiological spino pelvic balance. Decompression is considered if leg pain is a major component of symptoms (Fig. 27.13).

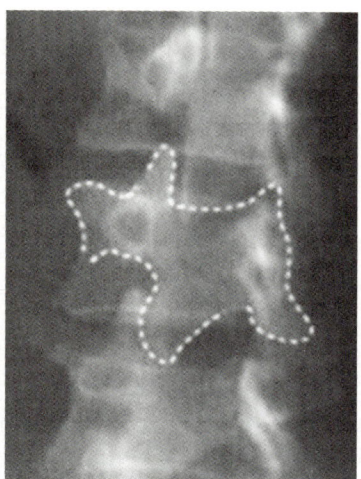

Fig. 27.11: Scottie dog appearance on oblique X-ray of lumbar spine

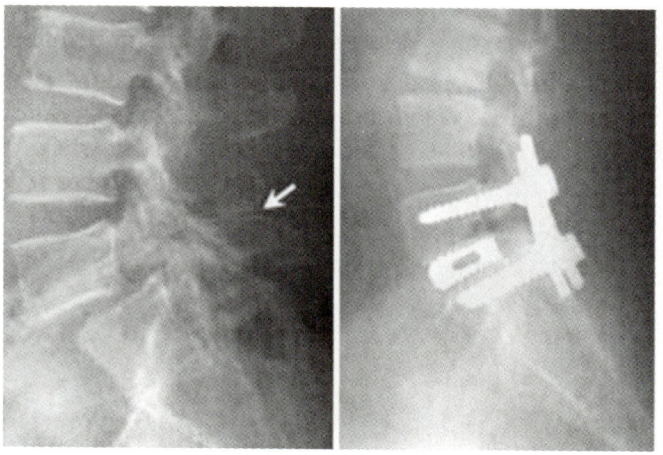

Fig. 27.13: Posterior lumbar interbody fusion (PLIF)

Spinal Deformities

SCOLIOSIS

Definition

It is an abnormal lateral curvature of the spine as viewed in the coronal plane (Fig. 28.1).

Classification (based on aetiology)

I. Idiopathic scoliosis
A. Infantile (under 3 years of age)
B. Juvenile (from 3 to 10 years of age)
C. Adolescent (from 10 years of age to skeletal maturity)
D. Adult

II. Neuromuscular scoliosis
A. Neuropathic
 1. Upper motor neuron
  a. Cerebral palsy
  b. Charcot-Marie-Tooth disease
  c. Syringomyelia
  d. Spinal cord trauma
 2. Lower motor neuron
  a. Poliomyelitis
  b. Spinal muscular atrophy
  c. Myelomeningocele

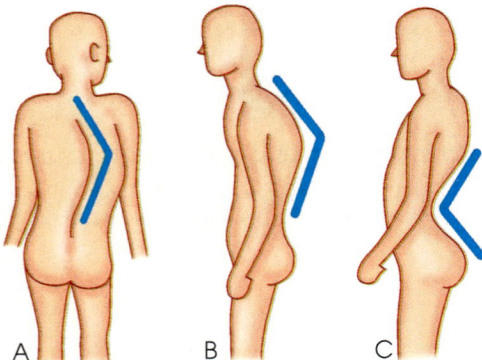

Fig. 28.1: Different spinal deformities. (A) Scoliosis, (B) Kyphosis, (C) Lordosis

B. Myopathic
 1. Arthrogryposis
 2. Muscular dystrophy

III. Congenital scoliosis
A. Failure of formation
B. Failure of segmentation
C. Mixed failure of formation and segmentation

IV. Neurofibromatosis

V. Connective tissue disorders
A. Marfan's syndrome
B. Ehlers-Danlos syndrome

VI. Osteochondrodystrophy
A. Diastrophic dwarfism
B. Mucopolysaccharidosis
C. Spondyloepiphyseal dysplasia
D. Multiple epiphyseal dysplasia
E. Achondroplasia

VII. Metabolic disorders

VIII. Nonstructural scoliosis
A. Postural, hysterical
B. Secondary to nerve root irritation

Diagnosis

1. History and physical examination
2. Age when the deformity was first noted
3. Perinatal history
4. Developmental milestones
5. Other illnesses
6. Family history of scoliosis or other diseases that may affect the musculoskeletal system.

In children and adolescents, the curvature is generally not painful. If the patient complains of pain, appropriate diagnostic tests should be performed to determine whether the curvature is secondary to the presence of a bony or spinal tumour, herniated disc, or other abnormality.

Clinical Examination

The patient's skin, habitus, and back should be carefully inspected. The presence of café au lait spots, skin tags, or axillary freckles is suggestive of neurofibromatosis. The presence of hairy patches or dimples over the spine is suggestive of spinal dysraphism. Numerous clinical syndromes are associated with scoliosis. Tall, long-limbed patients may have Marfan's syndrome and should be examined for high-arched palate, cardiac murmur, and dislocated lenses. Dwarfs have a high incidence of spinal deformity, both kyphosis (*see* section on kyphosis) and scoliosis, as well as spinal instability.

In patients with scoliosis, the shoulders or pelvis are not level, and there is waist asymmetry (Fig. 28.2). Most commonly, these patients have scapular prominence, with rotational deformity and rib prominence. The rib hump, or the lumbar prominence of a lumbar curve, can be accentuated by having the patient lean forward from the waist, permitting the arms to hang down; the examiner then views the spine from above or below. The rib hump can be quantified by direct measurement of its height or by using a scoliometer, which permits measurement of angular deformity.

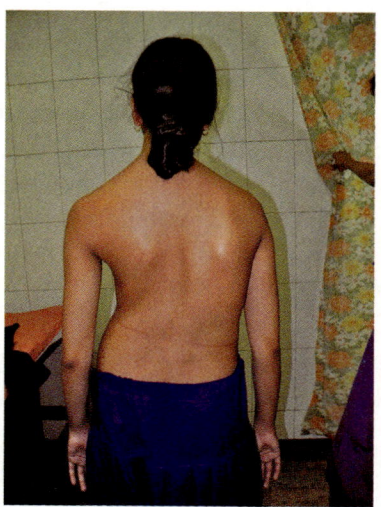

Fig. 28.2: Dorsolumbar scoliosis with convexity to right

Neurological Tests

Patients should demonstrate a normal gait and be able to walk on their toes and heels. Motor and sensory testing of the lower extremities should be performed, and testing of the upper extremities should also be done if the curve pattern is atypical or if a neuromuscular condition is suspected. Reflexes should be tested, and the presence of asymmetry or a pathologic reflex (e.g., clonus, positive Babinski sign, or positive Hoffmann sign) should be noted and suggest a nonidiopathic aetiology.

Imaging Studies

AP and lateral radiographs of the entire length of the spine should be taken, and this generally requires the use of an extra-long X-ray cassette. When the radiographs are taken, the patient should be in the standing position. If neuromuscular problems make it impossible for the patient to stand, radiographs can be taken with the patient sitting. Curves are measured using the Cobb's method, as shown in Fig. 28.3.

Cobb's angle: Lines are drawn along the endplates of the upper and lower vertebrae that are maximally tilted into the concavity of the curve. Next, a perpendicular line is drawn to each of the earlier-drawn lines. The angle of intersection is the Cobb's angle.

Treatment

Conservative Treatment

- Mild curves (less than 20 degrees) managed conservatively.
- In an adolescent who has less than 2 years of skeletal growth remaining, has not demonstrated progression, and has a curve that is still less than 30 degrees.

Long-term braces designed to arrest progression must be custom moulded for the patient, with pads placed to exert appropriate pressure to reduce deformity. Depending on the anatomic level of the curvature, they may be positioned under the arm or may extend to the neck (Milwaukee brace). This type of brace is usually worn 24 hours a day (Fig. 28.4).

All braces must be modified or replaced to accommodate growth. In general, bracing is only effective with flexible curvatures in growing children.

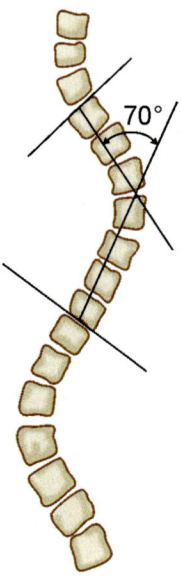

Fig. 28.3: Calculation of Cobb's angle

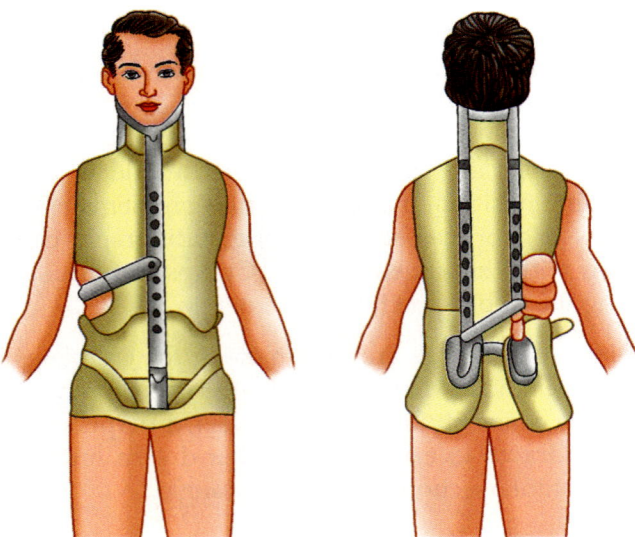

Fig. 28.4: Milwaukee brace

Surgical Treatment

Surgical intervention is indicated for curvatures that progress despite adequate conservative treatmen. It is also required when spinal compression is imminent or when a curvature is so severe that bracing is impossible and future progression is likely.

Surgical Principles

Surgery involves two separate stages: Correction and stabilization. After posterior exposure of the spine, correction is achieved with a variety of mechanical internal fixation devices. These are usually rods with hooks, screws, wires, or other mechanisms to distract, compress, or bend spinal segments. Once correction is obtained, the cortex of spine is removed and bone graft is placed over the raw bone. Subsequently, solid fusion occurs within 6 months, permanently stabilizing the spine (Fig. 28.5).

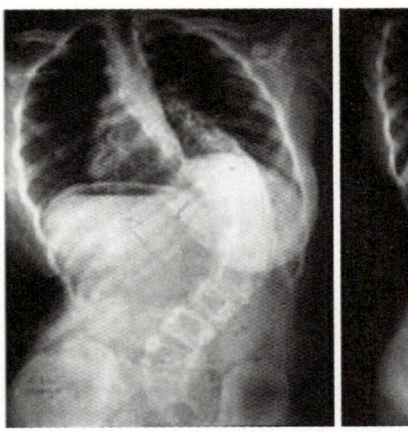
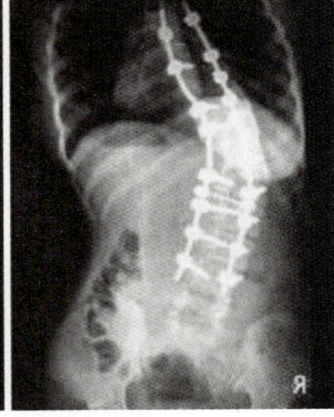

Fig. 28.5: Preoperative and postoperative X-ray showing surgical treatment of scoliosis

SCHEUERMANN KYPHOSIS

This is condition is seen in skeletally immature adolescents. It has a strong hereditary component, with an unknown etiology.

Criteria for Diagnosis

- Thoracic kyphosis greater than 45 degrees
- Thoracolumbar kyphosis greater than 30 degrees (thoracolumbar spine normally straight)
- Wedging greater than 5 degrees of 3 adjacent vertebrae.

Diagnosis

Standing lateral radiographs.

Associated features include vertebral endplate irregularities, Schmorl node (erosion of endplates), and scoliosis (in one-third of patients); the apex is usually located at T7 and T8.

Treatment

Nonoperative treatment: Bracing and hamstring stretching. Curves less than 50 degrees do not progress after skeletal maturity.

Operative treatment
Indications for surgical interventions are:
- Kyphosis greater than 75 degrees,
- Persistent pain after nonoperative treatment, and
- Rigid kyphosis greater than 55 degrees.
  Procedures: Anterior release, interbody and posterior fusion, and posterior instrumentation.

ANKYLOSING SPONDYLITIS

Ankylosing spondylitis (AS, from Greek ankylos—stiff; spondylos—vertebrae), also known as Bekhterev's disease, Bekhterev syndrome, and Marie-Strümpell disease is a chronic inflammatory disease of the axial skeleton with variable involvement of peripheral joints and nonarticular structures. AS is a form of spondyloarthritis, a chronic, inflammatory arthritis and autoimmune disease mainly affecting joints in the spine and the sacroiliac joint in the pelvis, and can cause eventual fusion of the spine resulting in a complete rigidity of the spine, a condition known as "bamboo spine".

Ankylosing spondylitis is one of a cluster of conditions known as seronegative spondyloarthropathies, in which rheumatoid factor tests are negative and the characteristic pathological lesion is an inflammation of the enthesis (the insertion of tensile connective tissue into bone). Other seronegative spondyloarthropathies are:

- Reiter's arthritis
- Psoriatic arthritis
- Ulcerative colitis
- Crohn's disease.

Clinical Presentation

Usually affects males, between 20 and 40 years. Symptoms are typically chronic pain and stiffness in the middle part of the spine or sometimes the entire spine, often with pain referred to one or other buttock or the back of thigh from the sacroiliac joint.

In 40% of cases, ankylosing spondylitis is associated with an inflammation of the eye (iritis and uveitis), causing redness, eye pain, vision loss, floaters and photophobia. This is thought to be due to the association these two conditions have with inheritance of HLA-B27.

Other Symptom

Fatigue, nausea, aortitis, apical lung fibrosis. When the condition presents before the age of 18, it is relatively likely to cause pain and swelling of large limb joints, particularly the knee. In prepubescent cases, pain and swelling may also manifest in the ankles and feet, where calcaneal spurs may also develop.

Pain is severe at rest, but improves with physical activity.

Diagnosis

Clinical examination, MRI and X-ray studies of the spine, which show characteristic spinal changes and sacroiliitis, in a patient who tests positive for HLA-B27.

Rome Criteria for Diagnosing Ankylosing Spondylitis

Clinical criteria

1. Low back pain and stiffness for more than 3 months which is not relieved by rest
2. Pain and stiffness in the thoracic region
3. Limited motion in the lumbar spine
4. Limited chest expansion
5. History or evidence of iritis or its sequelae

Radiological criteria: X-ray showing bilateral sacroiliac changes and 'Bamboo spine' characteristic of ankylosing spondylitis (Fig. 28.6).

New York Criteria for Ankylosing Spondylitis

1. Limitation of motion of the lumbar spine.
2. History or the presence of pain at the dorsolumbar junction or in the lumbar spine.
3. Limitation of chest expansion to 1 inch (2.5 cm) or less, measured at the level of the fourth intercostal space.

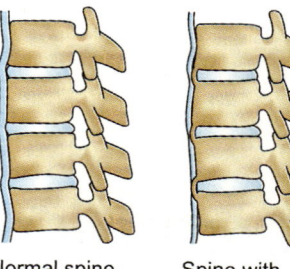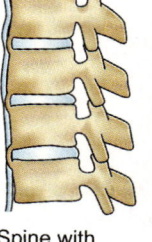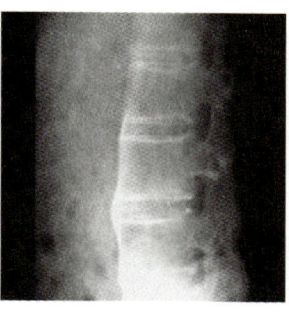

Normal spine   Spine with ankylosing spondylitis

Fig. 28.6: Bamboo spine appearance in ankylosing spondylitis

Treatment

Physiotherapy and physical exercises along with medical treatment to reduce the inflammation and pain.

Three major types of medications used to treat ankylosing spondylitis are:

- NSAIDs—non-steroidal anti-inflammatory drugs like ibuprofen, phenylbutazone, diclofenac, indomethacin, naproxen and COX-2 inhibitors, which reduce inflammation and pain. Some patients require opioid analgesics, which are very effective in alleviating the type of chronic pain commonly experienced by those suffering from AS, especially in extended-release formulations.
- DMARDs—disease modifying antirheumatoid drugs such as cyclosporin, methotrexate, sulfasalazine, and corticosteroids, used to reduce the immune system response through immunosuppression.
- TNF blockers (antagonists) such as etanercept, infliximab, golimumab and adalimumab (which are biologics), are indicated for the treatment of and are effective immunosuppressants in AS as in other autoimmune diseases. They are very costly.

Surgery

- Joint replacement (arthroplasty) for fused hip and knee joints is carried out (Fig. 28.7).
- Corrective osteotomy is indicated for severe spine deformity.

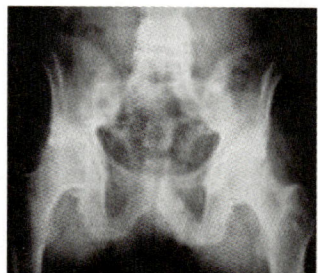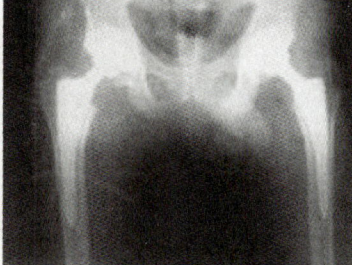

Fig. 28.7: Bilateral total hip arthroplasty for ankylosed hips

Tuberculous Spondylodiscitis (Pott's Spine)

Introduction

Tuberculosis of the spine, also called Pott's disease, is the commonest site of bone and joint tuberculosis, forming 40–45% of the total incidence of skeletal tuberculosis. The lower thoracic and upper lumbar vertebrae are the areas of the spine most often affected. Pott's disease results from haematogenous spread of tuberculosis from other sites, often pulmonary. It is the most dangerous form of musculoskeletal tuberculosis because it can cause bone destruction, deformity, and paraplegia.

Sites of Vertebral Tuberculosis (Fig. 29.1A)

1. Paradiscal-most common site
2. Central
3. Anterior
4. Posterior
5. Facet joint

Spondylodiscitis is the most common and facet joint involvement the rarest.

Pathophysiology

Spinal tuberculosis is always secondary to haematogenous spread of infection from primary elsewhere in the body, such as lungs, gastrointestinal tract or genitourinary tract.

1. Central type of vertebral body involvement, skip lesions in the vertebral column and vertebral disease associated with TB meningitis are due to spread of infection along Batson's perivertebral plexus of veins.
2. Typical paradiscal lesions are due to spread by way of arteries that supply the areas of two adjacent vertebra along with the intervening disc, developing from single sclerotome (Fig. 29.1B).
3. Anterior type of involvement of vertebral bodies seems to be due to extension of an abscess beneath the anterior longitudinal ligament and periosteum.

Infection may spread up and down stripping the anterior and posterior longitudinal ligaments and periosteum from the front and sides of the vertebral

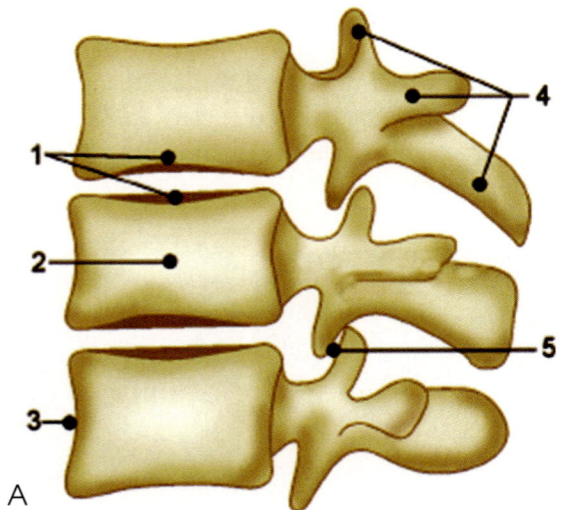
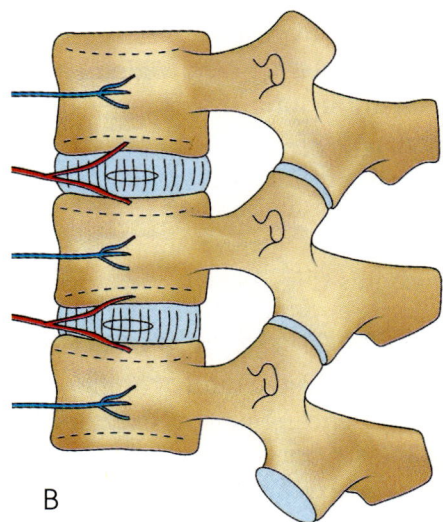

Fig. 29.1A and B: Types of Pott's spine, spread as per blood supply

bodies. This results in loss of periosteal blood supply and destruction of anterolateral surface of many contiguous vertebral bodies. The vertebral bodies slowly collapse with anterior wedging, leading to angular kyphosis. Pressure on the neural structure is more likely in the thoracic spine, where the caliber of the vertebral canal is very small. The histological changes in the bone are typical of tuberculous lesions elsewhere. Bone debris, caseous material, serum leukocytes and tuberculous bacilli together form the cold abscess.

Clinical Presentation

- Back pain
- Fever
- Weight loss
- Neurological abnormalities occur in 50% of cases and can include spinal cord compression with paraplegia, paresis, impaired sensation, nerve root pain, and/or cauda equina syndrome.
- Cervical spine tuberculosis is a less common presentation but is potentially more serious because severe neurologic complications are more likely.
  - This condition is characterized by pain and stiffness.
  - Patients with lower cervical spine disease can present with dysphagia or stridor.
  - Symptoms can also include torticollis, hoarseness, and neurological deficits.

Spinal tuberculosis seems to be more common in persons infected with HIV.

Physical Examination

The examination should include the following:

- Sinuses over the skin
- Assessment of spinal alignment:

  Presence of spine deformity like knuckle, gibbus or kyphos.

  Knuckle: One vertebra involved

  Gibbus: Three vertebrae involved

  Kyphos: More than three vertebrae involved

- *Abdominal evaluation for subcutaneous flank mass:* Large cold abscesses of paraspinal tissues or psoas muscle may protrude under the inguinal ligament and present as fluctuant mass.
- *Meticulous neurological examination:* Neurological deficits may occur early in the course of Pott's disease. Signs of such deficits depend on the level of spinal cord or nerve root compression and may pesent as single nerve palsy to hemiparesis or quadriplegia.

Complications

- Vertebral collapse resulting in kyphosis
- Spinal cord compression
- Sinus formation
- Paraplegia (so called Pott's paraplegia).

POTT'S PARAPLEGIA

10–30% Koch's spine patients develop paraplegia due to pressure effects on the neural tissues within the canal especially at the dorsal spine level as the canal is the narrowest. This is called Pott's paraplegia.

Types

In pre-antitubercular era, Pott's paraplegia had been classified as follows:

Group A: Early onset—in active stage of disease, within 2 years of the onset.

Group B: Late onset—many years (more than 2 years) after the disease has persisted in the vertebral column.

Pathology

The compression on the spinal cord can be due to extrinsic/mechanical or intrinsic causes.

Extrinsic

- Tubercular debris
- Extradural granuloma/tuberculoma
- Sequestra from vertebral body and disc
- Internal gibbus
- Vertebral canal stenosis

Intrinsic

- Infarction of the spinal cord
- Syringomyelia changes
- Prolonged stretching of the spinal cord
- TB meningomyelitis
- Pathological dislocation of spine
- Spinal tumour syndrome

  (Diffuse extradural granuloma/tuberculoma in the spinal cord and perineural fibrosis that mimics spinal tumour)

Classification (based upon motor weakness)

Stage I (negligible): Patient unaware of the neural deficit, physician detects plantar extensor and/or ankle clonus.

Stage II (mild): Patient aware of deficit but manages to walk with support.

Stage III (moderate): Nonambulatory because of paralysis (in extension), sensory deficit <50%.

Stage IV (severe): III + Flexor spasms/paralysis in flexion/flaccid/sensory deficit more than 50%/sphincters involved.

Diagnosis

Blood Tests

- Anemia
- Lymphocytosis
- Hypoproteinaemia
- Increase in ESR
- Mantoux test is helpful in children below 2–3 years of age but is not diagnostic

Radiodiagnosis
- X-ray of affected region of spine is very important to identify the following changes (Fig. 29.2)

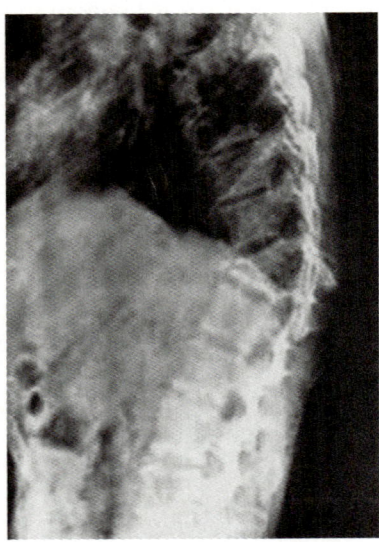

Fig. 29.2: Characteristic X-ray of Pott's spine showing kyphosis

- Earliest changes—disc space narrowing and loss of disc space in common paradiscal lesions
- Late changes
  - Anterior wedge compression in anterior vertebral involvement
  - Late cases show kyphosis and severe deformities.
  - Central vertebral bridge collapse also called concertine collapse in central involvement
  - Posterior element destruction in posterior involvement
- *Paravertebral shadow* if seen on X-ray indicates abscess formation
- *Skip lesions:* Bone lesions may occur at more than one level.

MRI: This is very useful investigation as it picks up disease activity earlier. Apart from bone destruction it also shows cord compression (Fig. 29.3)

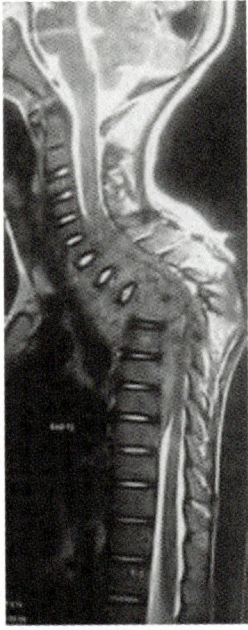

Fig. 29.3: Characteristic MRI of Pott's spine showing prevertebral abscess, vertebral destruction and kyphosis

Gallium scanning: Useful in disseminated TB

Biopsy: Whenever possible it is recommended to have biopsy of lesion as it not only confirms the diagnosis but gives opportunity to get sample for culture of the organism. Culture and antituberculous drug sensitivity is essential because of high prevalence of multidrug resistant (MDR) TB.

USG: Helps in diagnosis and USG guided drainage of soft tissue abscess such as psoas abscess.

Management

Before initiating treatment of Koch's spine, definitive diagnosis is must which is obtained by:
- Biopsy and histopathological examination
- Culture of organism

Nonsurgical

General Treatment

- *Aim:* Build up general resistance of patient with protein rich diet, haematinics, adequate exposure to sunlight
- Rest, usually for 4 to 8 weeks is advised for pain relief and to prevent collapse of the involved vertebrae.

Local Treatment

- Aim: To prevent, correct or decrease deformities using braces.
- Tubercular soft tissue abscesses resolve with antituberculous/anti-Koch's treatment (ATT/AKT).

- Aspiration of abscess is recommended if tensed.
- Physiotherapy to avoid joint stiffness, chest infections and decubitus ulcers.

Antituberculous/Anti-Koch's Treatment (ATT/AKT)

This is the mainstay of treatment. As soon as disease is diagnosed, four drugs AKT is started along with Vit B6. Most of the cases can be treated successfully using AKT and bedrest followed by mobilization using brace. Following drugs are commonly used.

1st line	2nd line
P: Pyranzinamide	C. Capriomycin
R. Rifampicin	A: Amikacin
L: Isoniazide	K: Kanamycin
S: Streptomycin	E: Ethionamide
E: Ethambutol	C: Cycloserine
	A: Aminosalicylic acid (PAS)

Operative Treatment

Indications for Surgical Treatment

Absolute indications

1. Progressive neurological deficit even after starting AKT
2. Paraplegia or quadriplegia with bowel and bladder affection (Pott's paraplegia)
3. Large prevertebral abscess in cervical spine causing respiratory distress

Strong indications

1. No improvement/nonsatisfactory improvement in neurological recovery with conservative treatment
2. Plateau neurological recovery after initial improvement
3. Severe bony destruction which is likely to lead to severe deformity
4. Multi drug resistant tuberculosis

Relative indications

1. Soft tissue abscesses not responding to AKT
2. To obtain tissue from deep structures for biopsy where percutaneous or CT guided biopsy is difficult.

Aim of Surgical Treatment

- Excise infected tissue
- Decompress the intraspinal neural elements
- Obtain sample for histopathology and culture
- Provide stability by fixation and fusion

Tuli Middle Path Regime

Most widely accepted protocol for management of TB spine. This regime starts with conservative manage-

ment such as AKT along with complete bed rest. Patient is regularly assessed clinically as well as with X-rays and ESR. If patient improves then gradual mobilization with brace is started usually after 4 to 8 weeks of bedrest. If patient fails to improve with conservative management then he is offered surgery under cover of AKT.

Surgical Techniques

Minimal debridement

1. Such as drainage of abscess, curettage of abscess walls

Radical debridement

1. ALD (anterolateral decompression) (Fig. 29.6)
   - Surgery of choice for Pott's paraplegia
   - Remove solid and liquid debris

Advantage: Technically easy

2. *Anterior decompression* (via thoracotomy/laparotomy) (Fig. 29.5)

   Advantage: Allows direct visualization and complete cord decompression

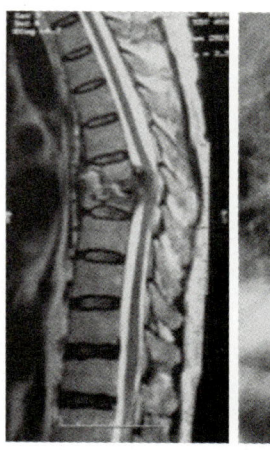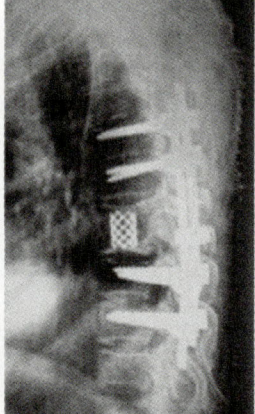

Fig. 29.4: Posterior approach: D6–D7 Koch's spine treated by debridement and reconstruction using cage and pedicular screws

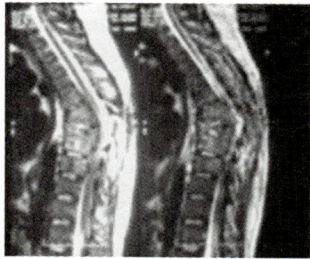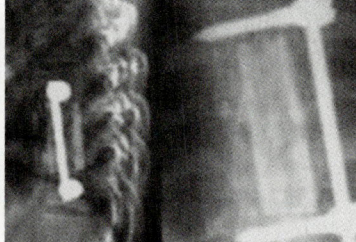

Fig. 29.5: Anterior approach—radical debridement, bone graft and instrumentation

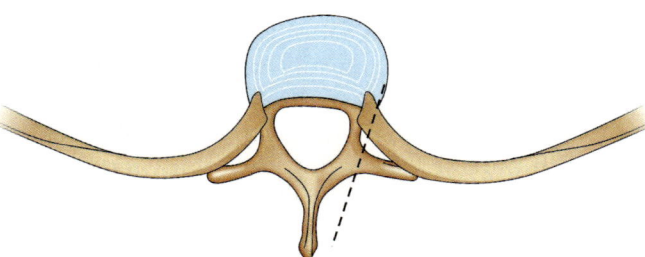

Fig. 29.6: Anterolateral decompression

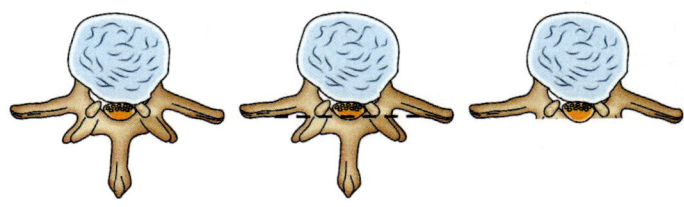

Fig. 29.7: Laminectomy

Disadvantages:
- Technically demanding
- High morbidity

3. *Laminectomy* (Fig. 29.7)

This is indicated for posterior element involvement

Advantage: Technically simple

4. Posterior decompression and spinal fusion (Fig. 29.4)

Most widely performed surgery

Advantages
- Technically easy
- Less morbidity

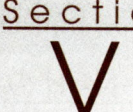

Tumours

CHAPTER
30

Bone Tumours: General Principles

Introduction

Tumours of the musculoskeletal system are heterogeneous group of neoplasms consisting of many benign types of neoplasms and numerous malignant conditions (Table 30.1). The tumours arise from embryonic mesoderm and are categorized according to their differentiated or adult histology.

Benign tumours—behave in a nonaggressive fashion with little tendency to recur locally or to metastasize.

Malignant tumours or sarcomas such as osteosarcoma and synovial cell sarcoma, cause invasive, locally destructive growth with a tendency to recur and to metastasize. Sarcomas are more common in older patients, with 15% affecting patients younger than 15 years and 40% affecting persons older than 55 years. Tumours inflict a tremendous emotional and financial toll on individuals and society alike.

Table 30.1: Common benign and malignant bone tumours

Benign	Malignant
Bone-producing lesions	Osteogenic sarcoma
Osteoid osteoma	Parosteal osteogenic sarcoma
Osteoblastoma	Periosteal osteogenic sarcoma
Fibrous lesions of bone	Malignant fibrous
Fibrous dysplasia	histiocytoma (MFH)
Nonossifying fibroma	Adamantinoma
Giant cell tumour	
Cartilage-producing lesions	Chondrosarcoma (dediffe-
Osteochondroma	rentiated chondrosarcoma)
(multiple exostoses)	
Enchondroma (multiple	
enchondromatosis)	
Chondromyxoid fibroma	Mesenchymal
Chondroblastoma	chondrosarcoma
Tumours of vascular or	
uncertain histogenesis	
Aneurysmal bone cyst	Ewing's sarcoma

The most common site for bone tumours is about the knee, especially the distal femur.

Aetiology

Tumorigenesis is a complex multiple-step process by which healthy tissue progressively transforms from a normal phenotype into an abnormal colony of proliferating cells.

How bone or soft-tissue tumours develop?

One must have a basic understanding of the cell cycle during which cell division occurs. The cell cycle is divided into four distinct phases:
1. G1 (gap 1)—majority of cell growth takes place during G1
2. S (DNA synthesis)—DNA synthesis occurs during the S phase
3. G2 (gap 2)
4. M (mitosis)—chromosomal separation and cell division

The mature state for mesenchymal tissues is normally in a resting, nonproliferative phase designated G0. It is the factors that affect the exit of the cell from G0, with entrance into G1, that is the hallmark of neoplastic disease.

Evaluation of Patient of Bone Tumour: History and Physical Examination

When evaluating a new patient with a possible tumour, the work-up must commence with a thorough history and physical examination as follows:
1. *The patient's age:* Certain tumours are relatively specific to particular age groups (Fig. 30.1).
2. *Duration of complaint:* Benign lesions generally have been present for an extended period (years). Malignant tumours usually have been noticed for only weeks to months.

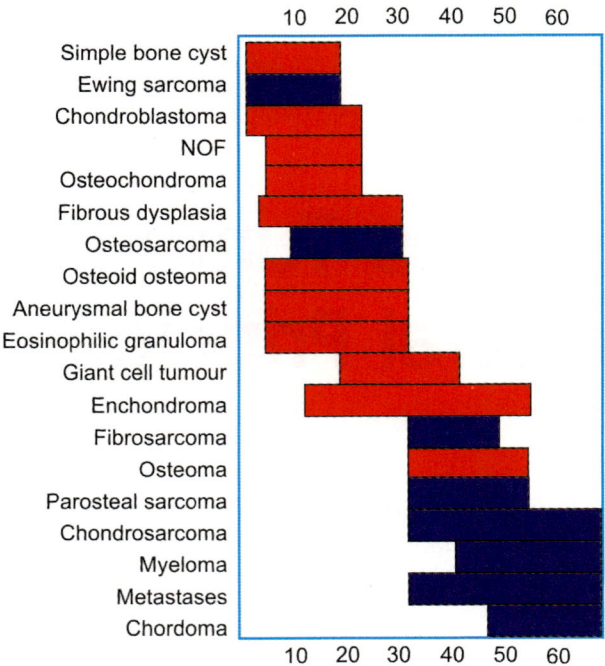

Fig. 30.1: Tumour distribution by age. Red: Benign, Blue: Malignant

3. *Rate of growth:* A rapidly growing mass, as in weeks to months, is more likely to be malignant. Growth may be difficult to assess by the patient if it is deep seated, as can be the case with bone. Deep lesions may be much larger than the patient thought ("tip-of-the-iceberg" phenomenon).

4. *Pain associated with the mass:* Benign processes are usually asymptomatic. Osteochondromas may cause secondary symptoms because of encroachment on surrounding structures. Malignant lesions may cause pain.

5. *History of trauma:* With a history of penetrating trauma, one must rule out osteomyelitis. With a history of blunt trauma, healing fracture must be entertained, as differential diagnosis.

6. *Personal or family history of cancer:* Adults with a history of prostate, renal, lung, breast, or thyroid tumours are at risk for developing metastatic bone disease. Children with neuroblastoma are prone to bony metastases. Patients with retinoblastoma are at an increased risk for osteosarcoma. Secondary osteosarcomas and other malignancies can result from treatment of other childhood cancers. Furthermore, certain benign bone tumours can run in families (e.g. hereditary multiple exostoses).

7. *Systemic signs or symptoms:* Generally there should be no significant findings on the review of systems with benign tumours. Fevers, chills, night sweats, malaise, change in appetite, weight loss, and so on,

should alert the physician that an infectious or neoplastic process may be involved.

Examination of a Mass/Lump

1. Skin colour
2. Warmth
3. Location
4. *Swelling:* Swelling, in addition to the primary mass effect, may reflect a more aggressive process.
5. *Neurovascular examination:* Changes may reflect a more aggressive process.
6. *Joint range of motion* of all joints in proximity to the region in question, above and below.
7. *Size:* A mass greater than 5 cm should raise the suspicion of malignancy.
8. *Tenderness:* Tenderness may reflect a more rapidly growing process.
9. *Firmness:* Malignant tumours tend to be firmer on examination than benign tumours. This applies more to soft-tissue tumours than osseous ones.
10. *Lymph nodes:* Certain sarcomas (e.g., rhabdomyo-sarcoma, synovial sarcoma, epithelioid, and clear cell sarcomas) all have increased rates of lymph node involvement.

Imaging

X-rays: In every patient, anteroposterior and lateral X-rays should be taken.

Location of tumour (Fig. 30.5)
- *Epiphyseal:* Usually benign
- *Metaphyseal:* Malignant primary sarcoma, eg. osteosarcoma.
- *Diaphyseal:* Round cell tumour, e.g. Ewing sarcoma, multiple myeloma, lymphoma
- *From surface of long bones:* Osteochondroma, low-grade sarcoma, parosteal osteosarcoma

Appearance/Patterns of Destruction (Fig. 30.2)

- Geographic or well circumscribed implies that the lesion has a distinct boundary and is sharply marginated, suggesting a benign tumour (Fig. 30.3).
- Permeative or moth eaten. It is a poorly defined, infiltrative process and reflects a more aggressive process such as a malignancy, although some benign processes can have this radiographic quality (Fig. 30.4).

An exception to this rule is multiple myeloma, which is a malignant tumour but demonstrates a punched-out, well-demarcated appearance in multiple locations.

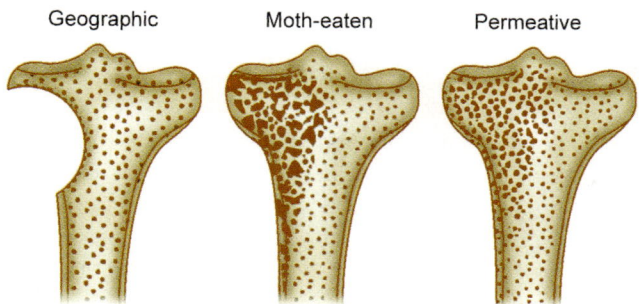

Geographic   Moth-eaten   Permeative

Fig. 30.2: Radiological appearances of bone tumours

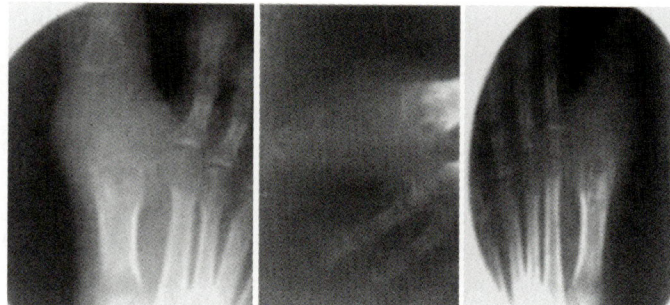

Fig. 30.4: Permeative appearance: Osteosarcoma

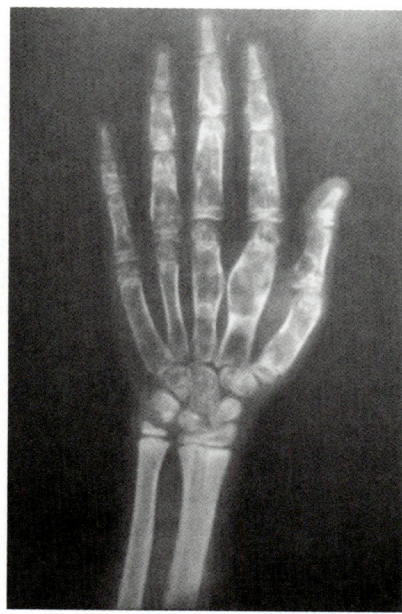

Fig. 30.3: Geographic appearance: Enchondroma

Computed Tomography and Magnetic Resonance Imaging

Computed tomography (CT) remains a standard imaging procedure.

CT chest/brain: For evaluation of patients with sarcoma for possible lung/brain metastases

CT abdomen: For detection of primary tumours in cases of bony metastasis.

CT pelvis: For tumours involving pelvis and sacrum.

PET-CT: For evaluation of both the structure and function of tumour cells and tissues in the body.

MRI is the imaging modality of choice for evaluating bone marrow involvement as well as noncalcific soft-tissue lesions. MRI can also demonstrate the normal anatomy of soft structures, including nerves and vessels, thereby nearly eliminating the need for arteriography and myelograms. Dynamic/enhanced MRI estimates tumour blood flow by examining the rate of contrast uptake and clearance, it serves as a

predictor of clinical outcome, or tumour response to chemotherapy.

Isotope Bone Scanning

Technetium-99 radioisotope scans are used to assess the degree of osteoblastic activity of a given lesion. They are excellent screening tools for remote lesions (staging). The best indication for a bone scan is suspected multiple bony lesions, such as those commonly seen in metastatic carcinomas and lymphomas of bone. Isotope bone scanning is far simpler to perform, less expensive, and requires less total body irradiation than skeletal surveys. Serial isotope scans are used to follow patients with suspected metastatic disease and at the same time evaluate the effectiveness of their systemic therapy programme.

Laboratory Studies

Biopsy

Needle biopsies, either core or fine needle, are used for lesions that are easily diagnosed, such as metastatic carcinomas or round cell tumours. Core biopsies allow the surgeon to sample various areas of the tumour to avoid sampling error in a heterogeneous tumour. In cases of deep pelvic lesion or a spinal lesion, a CT-guided needle biopsy is ideal because it avoids excessive multicompartmental contamination.

Excisional biopsies are done where the lesion is particularly small (less than 2–3 cm) or in an area where a cuff of healthy uninvolved tissue of at least 1 cm can be removed as well. This technique ideally avoids a second procedure to remove the entire biopsy site if the lesion turns out to be malignant.

The biopsy should usually be the final staging procedure. The imaging studies aid the surgeon in selecting the best site for a tissue diagnosis. In most cases, the best diagnostic tissue is found at the periphery of the tumour, where it interfaces with normal tissue. For example, in the case of a malignant bone tumour, soft-tissue invasion is usually evident outside the bone, and this area can be sampled without violating cortical bone and thus avoiding a fracture at the biopsy site. If a medullary specimen is needed, a small round or oval hole should be cut to decrease the chance of fracture. If the medullary specimen is malignant, the cortical hole should be plugged with bone wax or bone cement to reduce soft-tissue contamination following the procedure.

Special Studies

Special studies such as immune histochemistry, cytogenetics, flow cytometry, and electron microscopy can be done on the biopsy specimen.

Molecular diagnostics is on the verge of revolutionizing sarcoma diagnostics.

Specific translocations are found in a variety of tumours.

Staging of the Tumour

Staging refers to an assessment of the grade of the tumour and the extent to which the disease has spread. They have the purpose of helping the physician plan a logical treatment programme and establish a prognosis for the patient.

Enneking System for Staging Benign and Malignant Musculoskeletal Tumours

Benign

1. Latent
2. Active
3. Aggressive

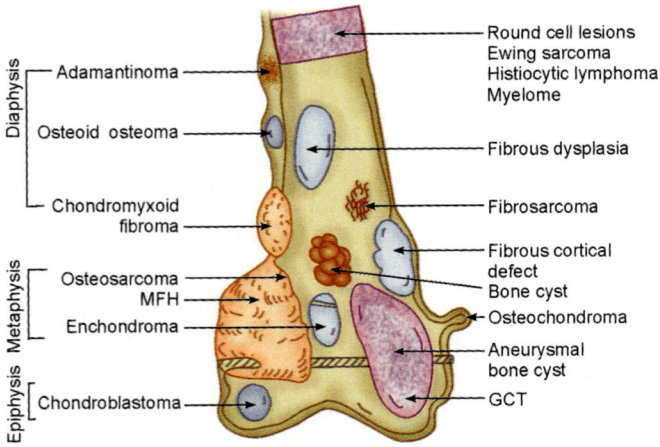

Fig. 30.5: Common bone tumours at various sites

Malignant (Table 30.2)

Table 30.2

Stage	Grade	Site	Metastases
IA	Low	Intracompartmental	None
IB	Low	Extracompartmental	None
IIA	High	Intracompartmental	None
IIB	High	Extracompartmental	None
III	Any	Any	Regional or distant metastases

American Joint Committee on Cancer System for Staging Soft-Tissue Sarcomas (Table 30.3)

Table 30.3

Stage	Grade	Size	Depth	Metastases
I	Low	Any	Any	None
II	Low	<5 cm	Any	None
	High	>5 cm	Superficial	None
III	High	>5 cm	Deep	None
IV	Any	Any	Any	Regional or distant

American Joint Committee on Cancer System for Staging Bone Sarcomas (Table 30.4)

Table 30.4

Stage	Grade	Size	Metastases
I-A	Low	<8 cm	None
I-B	Low	>8 cm	None
II-A	High	<8 cm	None
II-B	High	>8 cm	None
III	Any	Any	Skip metastasis
IV-A	Any	Any	Pulmonary metastases
IV-B	Any	Any	Nonpulmonary metastases

Solitary Lytic Bone Lesion

Differential Diagnosis (Mnemonic = **FOGMACHINES**)

F—Fibrous dysplasia

O—Osteoblastoma

G—Giant cell tumour

M—Metastasis/myeloma

A—Aneurysmal bone cyst

C—Chondroblastoma

H—Hyperparathyroidism (brown tumours)/ hemangioma

I—Infection

N—Non-ossifying fibroma

E—Eosinophilic granuloma/enchondroma

S—Solitary bone cyst

Benign Bone Tumours

Introduction

Benign bone tumours are more common than malignant. The usual presentation is a palpable mass or lump, pain or occassionally a pathological fracture. Their X-rays show geographic, well defined pattern with sclerotic reactive margins that suggest a long-standing process and a slow growth potential.

In many cases, further studies such as MRI or bone isotope studies are not necessary for a typical benign tumour, such as fibrous dysplasia, enchondroma, or nonossifying fibroma.

Staging

Stage 1 Latent lesions: They generally are asymptomatic and should be observed.

Stage 2 Active lesions: They show progressive growth but are limited by natural barriers. They frequently require surgical intervention with aggressive treatment. Recurrence is not infrequent.

Stage 3 Aggressive lesions: They show progressive destruction, are not limited by natural barriers. Treatment often requires wide en bloc resection.

Treatment

Excision of tumour (Table 31.1).

OSTEOCHONDROMA/ OSTEOCARTILAGINOUS EXOSTOSIS

Introduction: Oesteochondroma is the most common benign tumour of bone. It represents an error in epiphyseal plate/embryonal cartilage anlage or the restraining periosteum and ring of Ranvier. Osteochondroma may be considered as anomaly of normal growth.

Age: Any age, but most commonly present in adolescents during a growth spurt, because at this time

Table 31.1: Various types of tumour excision

Margin	Surgical procedure	Disadvantage
Intralesional	Piecemeal debulking or curettage	Leaves macroscopic disease
Marginal	Shell out en bloc through capsule or reactive zone	Leaves "satellite" or "skip" lesions
Wide	Intracompartmental -en bloc with cuff of normal tissue	May leave "skip" lesions if not recognized by prior imaging
Radical	Extracompartmental - en bloc entire compartment	No residual local disease

like the epiphyseal plate, they undergo enchondral ossification and rapidly enlarge.

Site: Metaphyseal ends of any bone, lie adjacent to epiphyseal plate. Most commonly involved bones are:
- Distal femur, proximal tibia.
- Proximal humerus.
- Proximal femur, distal tibia.

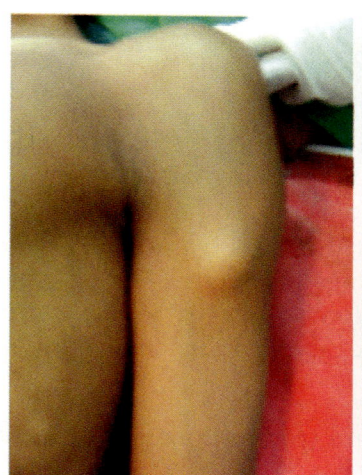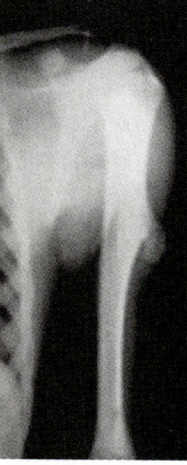

Fig. 31.1: Osteochondroma

Diagnosis

Clinical presentation: Painless, bony hard swelling arising from ends of bones (Fig. 31.1).

Radiology (Fig. 31.1)
- Sessile/pedunculated/stalked excrescence arising form metaphysis.
- Projecting away from the joint.
- Cortex of underlying bone continuous with cortical margin of exostosis.
- Occasionally cartilage cap becomes calcified, appearing as punctate or small rounded opacities.

Malignant potential of osteochondroma is extremely rare (<< 1%).

Treatment: Small exostosis need no treatment.

Indications for surgery
- Malignant transformation (increased activity on bone scan).
- Painful, tender swelling, bursitis.
- Pressure on adjacent neurovascular structure.
- Limitation of motion of an adjacent joint, especially around hip.
- Pathological fracture of narrow stalk.

Surgical principles
- Removal of only cartilaginous cap or entire lesion down to its juncture with host bone.
- Removal of perichondrium and overlying bursa
- In areas like pelvis/scapula: Removal of segment of bone underlying exostosis.

Recurrence: Rare

Hereditary Multiple Exostosis

It is a major genetic disorder of skeleton with autosomal dominant transmission with high degree of penetrance and frequent mutations.

Pathogenesis: Two theories
- Periosteal envelope is defective in infancy (permitting spill of embryonal cartilage cells into periosteal space, i.e. diaphyseal aclasis).
- Lesions represent pull-offs from the epiphyseal plate/defects in rings of Ranvier. With advancing age and termination of growth, lesions becomes quiescent. Cartilage cap thins but does not disappear.

Clinical presentation
- Shortness of stature (proportionate to number of lesions present)
- Varus/valgus deformity

- Limitation of movements around the joints especially ankle
- Shortening and bowing of ulna and ulnar club hand and pronation/supination limitation
- Alteration in vertebral column, sometimes causing pressure on cord/cauda
- Distortion of femoral neck–disorder of function of hip

Indication for surgery: Same as for solitary osteochondroma.

Malignant potential: Conversion to low grade, well differentiated chondrosarcoma significantly higher than solitary osteochondroma.

ENCHONDROMA

Introduction: Enchondroma is a benign bone tumour mostly occurring due to genetic error with retention of protion of embryonic cartilage anlage or physis within the shaft of small, long or flat bone in place of normal marrow.

Age: Any age, but mostly in people aged 10–40. The tumour grows during period of active skeletal growth, but once maturity is reached, there is little or no growth.

Site: Centrally placed within diaphysis or metaphysis. Only rarely, epiphyseal in growing child or subchondral in adults. Most commonly involves phalanges of hands and feet, metacarpals, metatarsals.

Clinical presentation: Usually asymptomatic, but may enlarge and become painful.

Radiology (Fig. 31.2)
- Centrally located osteolytic lesion with symmetric expansion and thinning of cortical bone
- Calcific masses may be present within the lesion

Malignant potential: 5% or more especially if large or centrally placed.

Treatment

Asymptomatic: No treatment
Symptomatic: Curettage and bone grafting

Patients with multiple enchondromas (Ollier's disease) and especially multiple enchondromatosis with venous malformations (Maffucci's syndrome) have a much higher risk (25–30%) of chondrosarcoma.

CHONDROBLASTOMA

Chondroblastoma is rare and occurs most commonly among people aged 10 to 20. Arising in the epiphysis,

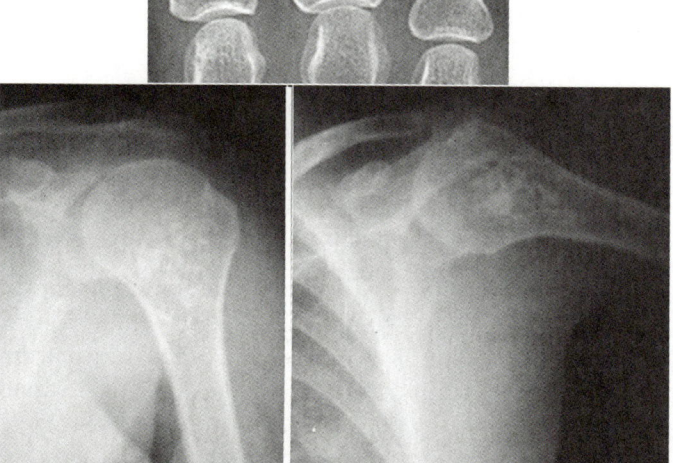

Fig. 31.2: Enchondroma

this tumour may continue to grow and destroy bone and the joint. It appears on imaging studies as a sclerotic marginated cyst containing spots of punctate calcification (Fig. 31.3). MRI can help in diagnosis by showing characteristic changes well away from the lesion.

The tumour must be surgically removed by curettage, and the cavity must be bone grafted. Local recurrence rate is about 10 to 20%, and recurrent lesions often resolve with repeat curettage and bone grafting.

CHONDROMYXOID FIBROMA

Chondromyxoid fibroma is very rare and usually occurs before age 30. The X-ray shows a lesion, which is usually eccentric, sharply circumscribed, lytic, and located near the end of long bones (Fig. 31.4). Treatment after biopsy is surgical excision or curettage.

OSTEOID OSTEOMA

Introduction

Age: Osteoid osteoma is a unique lesion of uncertain aetiology and characteristic clinical picture. It affects young people (commonly aged 10 to 30). It can occur in any bone but is most common among long bones, like femur and tibia. There is prediliction for certain locations like medial side of neck of femur and foot, especially talus.

Clinical features: The classical presentation is sharp, dull, boring, deep or intense pain that is worse at night, reflecting increased nocturnal prostaglandin-mediated inflammation. Pain is typically relieved by mild analgesics (particularly aspirin or other NSAIDs) that target prostaglandins. In growing children, the inflammatory response and associated hyperemia, if close to the open growth plate, may cause overgrowth and limb length discrepancy. Physical examination may reveal atrophy of regional muscles because the pain causes muscle disuse.

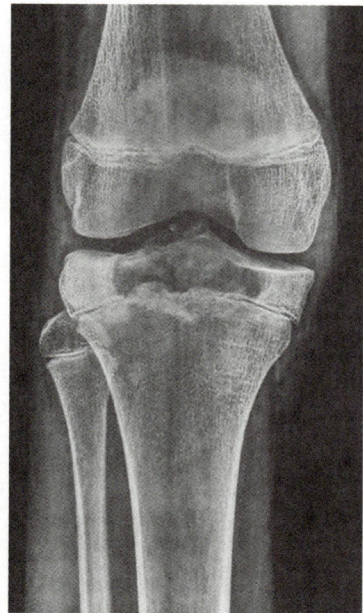

Fig. 31.3: Chondroblastoma

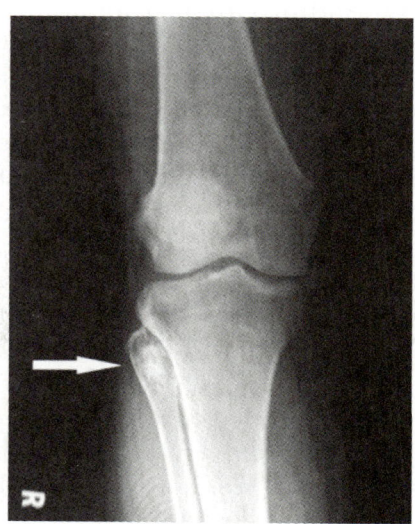

Fig. 31.4: Chondromyxoid fibroma

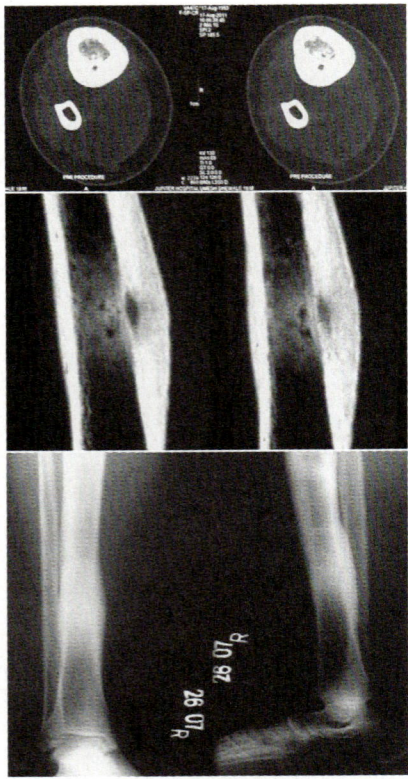

Fig. 31.5: X-ray and CT appearance of osteoid osteoma

Imaging: Characteristic appearance on imaging studies is a small radiolucent zone surrounded by a larger sclerotic zone (nidus). This appearance on CT scan is called "Bull's eye" appearance. CT with fine image sequences is also done and is most helpful in distinguishing the lesion.Technetium-99 bone scan demonstrates intense focal increase in uptake in the nidus resembling a "headlight in the fog" (Fig. 31.5).

Treatment: Removal of the small radiolucent zone with percutaneous radiofrequency ablation provides permanent relief. Less often, osteoid osteomas are surgically curetted or excised. Surgical removal may be preferred when the osteoid osteoma is near a nerve or close to the skin (e.g. spine, hands, feet) because the heat produced by radiofrequency ablation may cause damage.

NONOSSIFYING FIBROMA
(FIBROUS CORTICAL DEFECT)

Nonossifying fibroma (fibrous cortical defect, fibroxanthoma) is a benign fibrous lesion of bone that appears as a well-defined lucent cortical defect on X-ray. A very small nonossifying fibroma is called a fibrous cortical defect. These lesions are developmental defects in which parts of bone that normally ossify are instead filled with fibrous tissue. They commonly affect the metaphyses, and the most commonly affected sites are, in order, the distal femur, distal tibia, and proximal tibia. They can progressively enlarge and become multiloculated. Nonossifying fibromas are common among children. Most lesions eventually ossify and undergo remodelling, often resulting in dense, sclerotic areas. However, some lesions enlarge.

Clinical presentation: Small nonossifying fibromas are asymptomatic. However, lesions that involve nearly 50% of the bone diameter tend to cause pain and increase the risk of pathological fracture.

Imaging: Nonossifying fibromas are generally first noted incidentally on imaging studies (e.g. after trauma). They typically are radiolucent, single, < 2 cm in diameter, and have an oblong lucent appearance with a well-defined sclerotic border in the cortex. They can also be mutiloculated (Fig. 31.6).

Treatment: Small nonossifying fibromas require no treatment and limited follow-up. Lesions that cause pain or are close to 50% of the bone diameter may warrant curettage and bone grafting to decrease risk of a pathological fracture through the lesion.

GIANT CELL TUMOUR (GCT)

Introduction: GCT comprises 5% of all bone tumours. It was first described by Sir Astley Cooper, who called it a 'Fungous exostosis of the medullary membrane'.

Giant cell tumour may be benign, latent or aggressive.

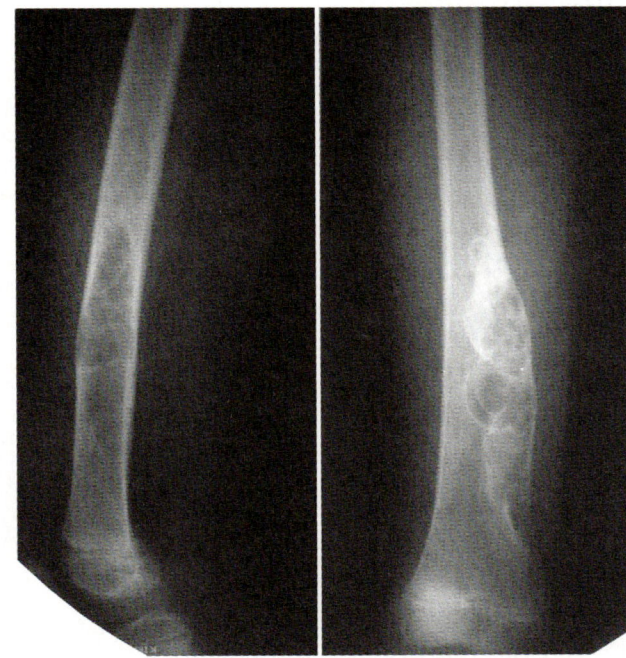

Fig. 31.6: Nonossifying fibroma

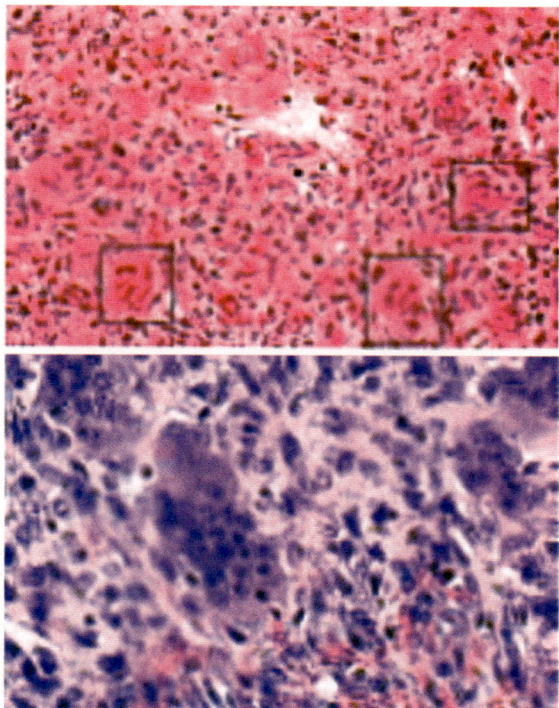

Fig. 31.7: Giant cells of GCT

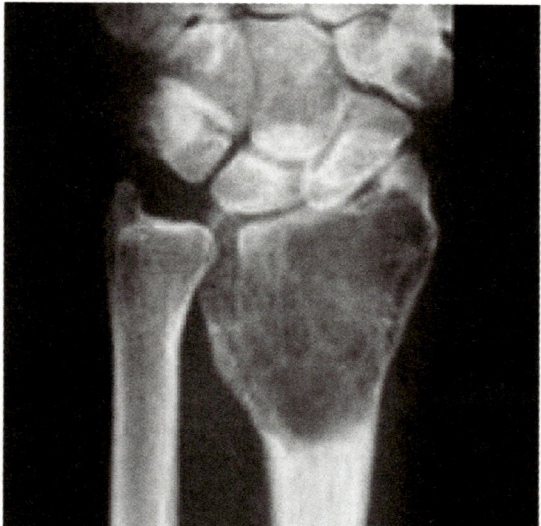

Fig. 31.8: Giant cell tumour of distal radius

GCTs are notorious for their tendency to recur. Rarely GCT may metastatize to the lung, even though it remains histologically benign.

Age: > 20 years, appear after physeal closure, Peak: 3rd decade.

Site: Metaphysis and epiphysis of 3 common sites
• Distal femur
• Proximal tibia
• Distal radius
Sometimes the tumour extends to and through subchondral bone.

Clinical presentation
• Pain
• Pathological fracture
• Tenderness/local heat/atrophy of muscles around the involved joint
• Extra-osseous mass felt occasionally.

Radiology

X-ray
• Radiolucent lesion in metaphysis/epiphysis without intralesional densities (Fig. 31.8).
• Narrow transitional zone, producing a geographic pattern of destruction.
• No reactive rim of bone at periphery
• Cortical destruction and extraosseous extension often present

• Periosteal reactive bone formation minimal unless there is a pathological fracture
• 'Soap bubble appearance' is classical

Bone scan: GCT is often present as a multicentric disease, hence bone scan is an excellent way to evaluate the entire skeletal system.

CT/MRI

More accurate to know the exact intraosseous extent, cortical erosion and soft tissue extension.

Pathology

Gross
• Reddish brown/yellow brown/whitish grey
• Friable and vascular
• Presence of blood filled cavities within the tumour

Histopathology
• Stromal cells and large number of multinucleated giant cells
• Numerous vascular channels present.

Treatment
  I. *Surgery:* Mainstay of treatment
  i. Curettage and autogenous bone graft packing
    Disadvantage: Recurrence rate ~ 60%
  Adjuvant to curettage:
• Freezing of adjacent margin of bone with liquid nitrogen
• Phenol irrigation: No proved effect
• Use of PMMA (polymethyl methacrylate bone cement): It markedly reduces the incidence of local recurrence

Mechanism of action: Monomer is toxic and may kill microscopic tumour at the periphery. Residual tumour cells are killed by the heat of exothermic reaction associated with polymerisation.

II. Resection of local area

III. Radiotherapy: Rarely indicated in sacral GCTs.

IV. Resection arthrodesis: Occasionally in tumour around knee

V. Resection and reconstruction using fibula in distal radius GCT.

ANEURYSMAL BONE CYST (ABC)

ABCs occur in bone primarily or in association with other tumours, such as giant cell tumour, chondroblastoma, and osteosarcoma.

Age: This lesion is a nonneoplastic reactive condition found in the first 3 decades of life.

Site: They usually occur in the metaphyses of long bones, especially in the femur and tibia, but are also seen in the posterior spine.

Clinical features: Patients often present with pain and swelling lasting months to years.

Imaging: The classic radiographic finding is an eccentric, lytic, ballooning expansion within the metaphysis (Fig. 31.9). Lesions frequently have a delicate rim of expanded cortical bone which may be best seen on CT scan. Fluid-filled levels are frequently seen.

Typical histologic features are blood-filled spaces without endothelial lining.

Treatment: Not all lesions require treatment because they sometimes reach an inactive state.

Treatment is curettage and bone grafting with local recurrence as high as 25%. Haemorrhage from these lesions can be significant, and embolization should be considered when treating lesions of the spine and pelvis. Recently, percutaneous sclerotherapy with injection of polidocanol 2–4 mg/kg body weight has been found to be useful especially in ABC of pelvis and sacrum where surgery is associated with considerable morbidity.

Radiographic differential diagnosis includes:

1. Simple bone cyst
2. Giant cell tumour of bone
3. Telangiectatic-osteosarcoma
4. Angiosarcoma

SIMPLE/UNICAMERAL BONE CYST

Introduction: Simple bone cyst, or unicameral bone cyst is an extremely common lesion that either represents anomaly in the veins of affected bone or arises from some pre-existing lession like fibrous dysplasia.

Age and site: It presents in the first 2 decades of life. Simple bone cysts are the most frequent cause of pathological fracture in children. They are typically asymptomatic until fracture and occur almost exclusively in the metaphyses of long bones, especially in the proximal humerus, proximal femur, and proximal tibia.

Imaging (Fig. 31.10): Radiographically, they appear as a central lytic area with symmetric cortical thinning. The

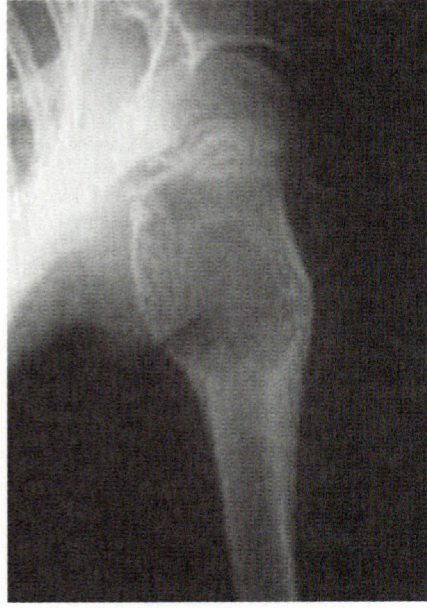

Fig. 31.9: Aneurysmal bone cyst of proximal humerus

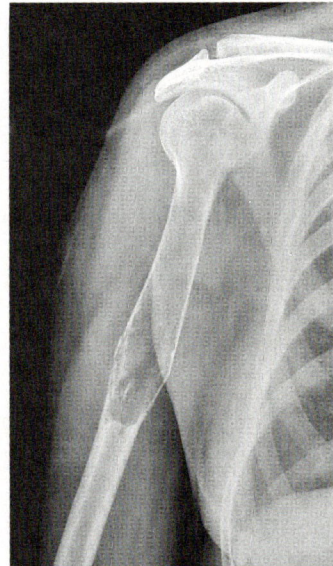

Fig. 31.10: Simple bone cyst with pathological fracture (fallen leaf sign)

bone is often expanded. Unlike the ABCs, they are rarely greater than the width of the adjacent physeal plate. The "fallen leaf" or the "fallen fragment" sign, signifying a piece of cortical bone that fell into the intramedullary cyst as a result of fracture, is often seen (Fig. 31.10).

Treatment: Simple bone cysts usually heal on their own by skeletal maturity, allowing for observation in most cases. In a weight-bearing location, such as the proximal femur, lesions should be treated more aggressively. These lesions can be treated with repeated aspiration and injection with methylprednisolone, bone marrow and bone substitute, or with curettage and bone graft.

FIBROUS DYSPLASIA

Introduction: Fibrous dysplasia occurs as a result of intrinsic defect of endochondral bone maturation that results in incomplete or immature ossification pattern.

Histologically, it shows benign fibrous stroma stippled with bony islands of metaplastic bone.

Age: Most common between 3 and 15 years of age.

Site: Two types: Monostotic (involving single bone): usually ribs.

Polyostotic (involving multiple bones): Femur, tibia, maxilla.

Clinical presentation: 85% of fibrous dysplasia patients develop pathological fracture. The disease process becomes inactive at puberty, but can be reactivated by pregnancy.

• *Deformity of long bones:* Most common is 'Shepherd Crook' deformity of femur, resulting from multiple stress fractures of upper femur during growing years (Fig. 31.11).
• Bone pain

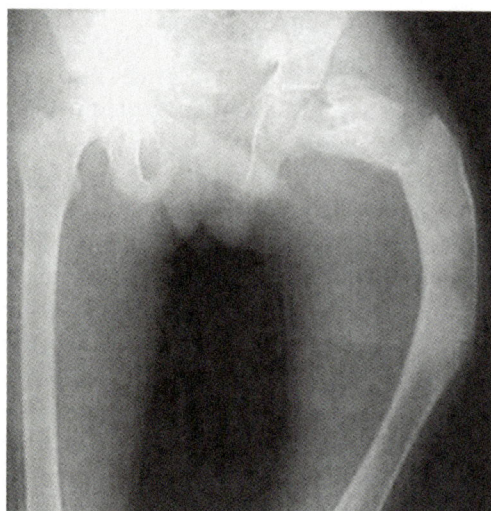

Fig. 31.11: Shepherd crook deformity

Malignant potential is <1%

'Albright syndrome' is polystotic fibrous dysplasia along with endocrine abnormality (increased secretion of hypothalamic hormones).

Treatment

1. Observation, bracing for prevention of deformity and fracture.
2. Pathological fracture managed by standard methods according to the site of fracture.

Surgical treatment—principles

1. Recurrent fracture require internal fixation with intramedullary rods and bone graft.
2. Severe angular deformities-treated with closing wedge osteotomies, bone grafting, and internal fixation. (Sheekh Kabab Osteotomy)
3. Leg length discrepancy-treated with epiphysiodesis of contralateral limb at an appropriate age.

HEMANGIOMA

Benign lesions characterized by vascular spaces lined with endothelial cells.

50% of osseous hemangiomas are found in the vertebral bodies (especially thoracic) and 20% in the calvarium.

The remaining lesions are found in the tibia, femur and humerus.

The radiological appearance can be quite striking and depends on the location of the lesion.

The lesions are often poorly defined, appearing as a somewhat localized area of abundant, dilated vessels, some of which may be on the surface of the bone. Vertically striated appearance due to thickening of bony trabeculae give the typical 'corduroy' appearance of vertebral body hemangioma (Fig. 31.12). CT scan shows the 'polka dotted' or 'salt and pepper' appearance.

Asymptomatic hemangiomas rarely develop into symptomatic lesions. Symptomatic hemangiomas usually respond well to conservative surgical procedures. Selective arterial embolization is safer and more effective treatment than radiation. Anterior resection and fusion are reserved for pathological collapse and neural compromise or refractory cases.

JOINT TUMOURS

Tumours rarely affect joints, unless by direct extension of an adjacent bone or soft-tissue tumour.

However, two conditions—synovial chondromatosis and pigmented villonodular synovitis—occur in the lining (synovium) of joints. These conditions are benign but locally aggressive. Both usually affect one joint, most often the knee and sometimes hip and can cause

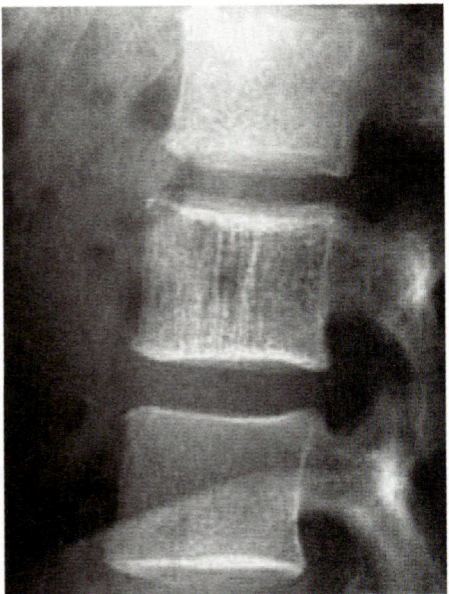

Fig. 31.12: Haemangioma of vertebra: Prominent vertical striations

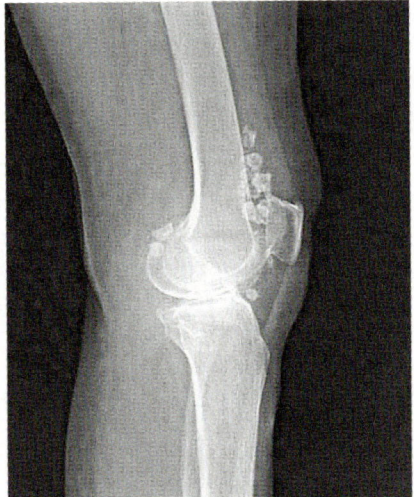

Fig. 31.13: Synovial chondromatosis

pain and effusion. Both are treated by synovectomy and removal of any intra-articular bodies.

SYNOVIAL CHONDROMATOSIS

Synovial chondromatosis (previously called synovial osteochondromatosis) is considered metaplastic. It is characterized by numerous calcified cartilaginous bodies in the synovium, which often become loose. Each body may be no larger than a grain of rice, in a swollen, painful joint. Malignant change is very rare. Recurrence is common. Diagnosis is by imaging, usually CT or MRI. Treatment may be symptomatic, but if mechanical symptoms are prominent, arthroscopic or open removal of the bodies or synovium is warranted (Fig. 31.13).

PIGMENTED VILLONODULAR SYNOVITIS

Pigmented villonodular synovitis is considered neoplastic condition. The synovium becomes thickened and contains hemosiderin, which gives the tissue its blood-stained appearance and characteristic appearance on MRI (Fig. 31.14). This tissue tends to invade adjacent bone, causing cystic destruction and damage to the cartilage. Pigmented villonodular synovitis is usually monoarticular but may be polyarticular. Late management, especially after recurrence, may require total joint replacement. On rare occasions after several synovectomies, radiation therapy is sometimes used.

Benign Conditions that Mimic Malignant Tumours

- Heterotopic ossification (myositis ossificans) and exuberant callus formation after fracture can cause

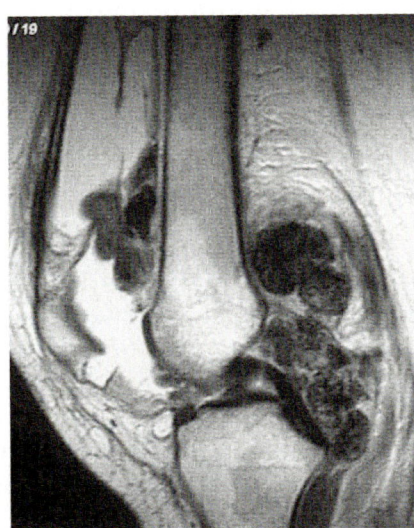

Fig. 31.14: MRI appearance of pigmented villonodular synovitis

mineralization around bony cortices and in adjacent soft tissues, mimicking malignant tumours.
- Langerhans' cell histiocytosis (histiocytosis X, Letterer-Siwe disease, Hand-Schüller-Christian disease, eosinophilic granuloma) can cause solitary or multiple bone lesions that are usually distinguishable on X-ray. In solitary lesions, there may be periosteal new bone formation, suggesting a malignant bone tumor.
- Osteopoikilosis (spotted bones) is an asymptomatic condition of no clinical consequence but can simulate osteoblastic bone metastases of breast cancer. It is characterized by multiple small, round, or oval foci of bony sclerosis, usually in the tarsal, carpal, or pelvic bones or the metaphyseal-epiphyseal regions of tubular bones.

Malignant Bone Tumours

MULTIPLE MYELOMA

Multiple myeloma (from Greek Myelo-bone marrow), also known as plasma cell myeloma or Kahler's disease (after Otto Kahler), is a cancer of plasma cells, a type of white blood cell normally responsible for producing antibodies. In multiple myeloma, collections of abnormal plasma cells accumulate in the bone marrow, where they interfere with the production of normal blood cells. Most cases of myeloma also feature the production of a paraprotein an abnormal antibody which can cause kidney problems.

It is the most common primary tumour of bone, accounts for 45% of all malignant bone tumours. It is the second most common haematopoietic malignancy. An estimated 90% of cases are in patients older than 40 years.

Signs and Symptoms

Because many organs can be affected by myeloma, the symptoms and signs vary greatly. A mnemonic sometimes used to remember the common tetrad (four parts) of multiple myeloma is CRAB: C = Calcium (elevated), R = Renal failure, A = Anaemia, B = Bone lesions.

Bone Pain

Myeloma bone pain usually involves the spine and ribs, and worsens with activity. Persistent localized pain may indicate a pathological bone fracture. Involvement of the vertebrae may lead to spinal cord compression. Myeloma bone disease is due to the over expression of Receptor Activator for Nuclear factor ~ B Ligand (RANKL) by bone marrow stroma. RANKL activates osteoclasts, which resorb bone. The resultant bone lesions are lytic in nature and are best seen in plain radiographs, which may show "punched-out" resorptive lesions (including the "pepper pot" appearance of the skull on radiography). The breakdown of bone also leads to release of calcium into the blood, leading to hypercalcemia and its associated symptoms.

Infection

The most common infections are pneumonias and pyelonephritis. Common pneumonia pathogens include *S. pneumoniae*, *S. aureus*, and *K. pneumoniae*.

Renal Failure

Renal failure may develop both acutely and chronically. It is commonly due to hypercalcemia. It may also be due to tubular damage from excretion of light chains, also called Bence Jones proteins, which can manifest as the Fanconi syndrome (type II renal tubular acidosis). Other causes include glomerular deposition of amyloid, hyperuricemia, recurrent infections (pyelonephritis), and local infiltration of tumour cells.

Anaemia

The anaemia found in myeloma is usually normocytic and normochromic. It results from the replacement of normal bone marrow by infiltrating tumour cells and inhibition of normal red blood cell production (haematopoiesis) by cytokines.

Neurological Symptoms

Common problems are weakness, confusion and fatigue due to hypercalcemia. Headache, visual changes and retinopathy may be the result of hyperviscosity of the blood depending on the properties of the paraprotein. Finally, there may be radicular pain, loss of bowel or bladder control (due to involvement of spinal cord leading to cord compression) or carpal tunnel syndrome and other neuropathies (due to infiltration of peripheral nerves by amyloid). It may give rise to paraplegia in late presenting cases.

Investigations

- Anaemia, high ESR, kidney dysfunction.
- Raised beta-2 microglobulins
- High serum protein (raised globulin or immuno-globulin)

Protein electrophoresis of the blood and urine, will show the presence of a paraprotein (monoclonal protein, or M protein) band, with or without reduction of the other (normal) immunoglobulins (known as immune paresis) (Fig. 32.1). One type of paraprotein is the Bence Jones protein which is a urinary paraprotein composed of free light chains. Quantitative measurements of the paraprotein are necessary to establish a diagnosis and to monitor the disease. The paraprotein is an abnormal immunoglobulin produced by the tumour clone. Very rarely, the myeloma is nonsecretory (not producing immunoglobulins).

Plasma Cells

The osteolytic lesions are caused by increased osteoclastic resorption that is stimulated by cytokines released by the plasma cells (Fig. 32.2).

Diagnosis of case of multiple myeloma includes a skeletal survey. This is a series of X-rays of the skull, axial skeleton and proximal long bones. Myeloma activity sometimes appear as "lytic lesions" (with local

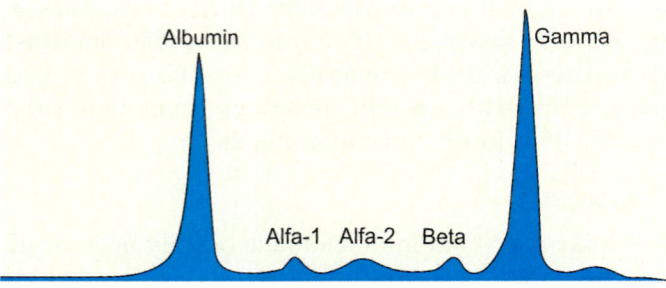

Fig. 32.1: Serum electrophoresis showing paraprotein peak

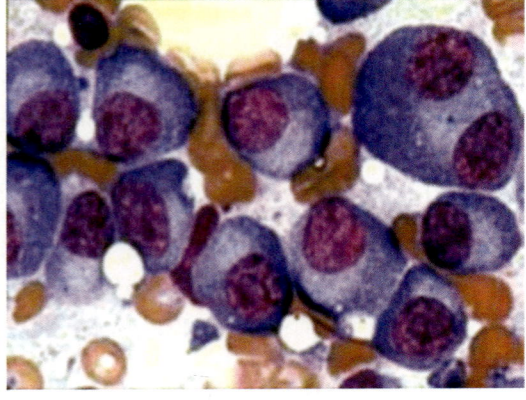

Fig. 32.2: Plasma cells

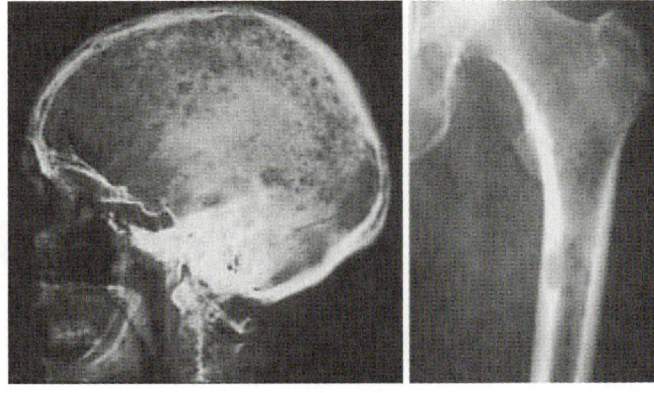

Fig. 32.3: Multiple lytic lesions of multiple myeloma

disappearance of normal bone due to resorption), and on the skull X-ray as "punched-out lesions" (pepper pot skull) (Fig. 32.3).

A bone marrow biopsy is usually performed to estimate the percentage of bone marrow occupied by plasma cells. This percentage is used in the diagnostic criteria for myeloma.

Immunohistochemistry (staining particular cell types using antibodies against surface proteins) can detect plasma cells which express immunoglobulin in the cytoplasm and occasionally on the cell surface; myeloma cells are typically CD56, CD38, CD138 positive and CD19 and CD45 negative.

Treatment

Treatment is aimed to decrease the clonal plasma cell population and consequently decrease the signs and symptoms of disease.

Bisphosphonates (e.g. pamidronate or zoledronic acid)—prevent fractures; they have also been observed to have direct anti-tumour effect even in patients without known skeletal disease.

If needed, red blood cell transfusions or erythropoietin can be used for management of anaemia.

New Chemotherapy Regimens

1. Treatment with bortezomib, melphalan, and prednisone.
2. Lenalidomide plus low-dose dexamethasone.

Treatment of related hyperviscosity syndrome is required to prevent neurologic symptoms or renal failure.

Renal failure in multiple myeloma can be acute (reversible) or chronic (irreversible). Acute renal failure typically resolves when the calcium and paraprotein levels are brought under control. Treatment of chronic renal failure is dependent on the type of renal failure and may involve dialysis.

Prognosis

With high-dose therapy followed by autologous stem cell transplantation, the median survival has been estimated to be approximately 4.5 years.

OSTEOSARCOMA

Introduction: Osteosarcoma (osteogenic sarcoma) is the 2nd most common primary bone tumour and is highly malignant.

Age: It is most common among people aged 10 to 25, although it can occur at any age.

Site: Osteosarcoma usually develops around the knee (distal femur more often than proximal tibia) or in other long bones, particularly the metaphyseal-diaphyseal area, and may metastasize, usually to lung or other bone.

Clinical features: Pain and swelling are the usual symptoms.

Pathology

Gross
- Greyish-white
- Hard and fleshy/soft and vascular with areas of haemorrhage

Microscopic
- Presence of malignant osteoid
- Stromal cells are spindle shaped osteoblasts with excessive mitosis, pleomorphism and hyperchromatism

Classification (Table 32.1)

Table 32.1: Classification of osteosarcoma	
Central (medullary)	*Surface (peripheral)*
• Conventional central telangiectatic (intermediate grade)	• Parosteal (low grade)
• Interosseous/intramedullary well differentiated (low-grade)	• Periosteal (low to high grade) surface osteosarcoma
• Small cell osteosarcoma	

Imaging: Findings on imaging studies vary and may include sclerotic or lytic features. There are mottled areas of rarefaction with areas of osteosclerosis. Osteosarcoma produces malignant osteoid (immature bone) from tumour bone cells. When the tumour spreads beyond the cortex, the periosteum is raised and new bone formation occurs in lines at right angles to the cortex. This is seen as 'Sun ray' appearance in the X-ray (Fig. 32.4).

A Codman triangle is a type of periosteal reaction seen with aggressive bone lesions. With aggressive

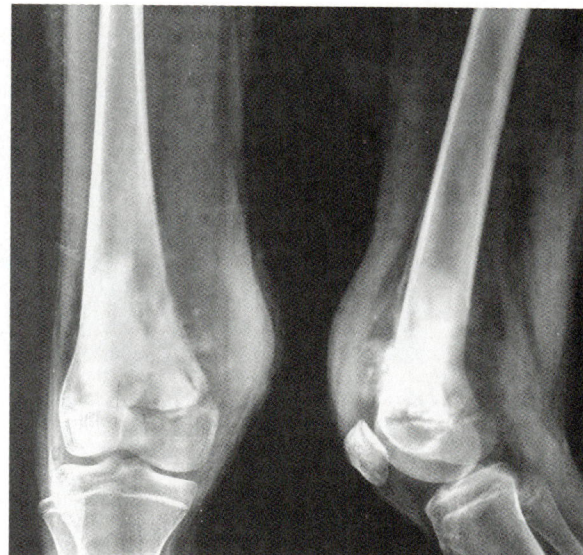

Fig. 32.4: X-ray appearance: Periosteal reaction with formation of "sunray" appearance

lesions, the periosteum does not have time to ossify with shells of new bone (e.g. as seen in single layer and multilayered periosteal reaction), so only the edge of the raised periosteum will ossify.

The Codman triangle may be seen with aggressive lesions:
- Osteosarcoma
- Ewing sarcoma
- Osteomyelitis
- Active aneurysmal bone cyst
- Giant cell tumour
- Metastasis
- Chondrosarcoma (especially juxtacortical chondrosarcoma)
- Malignant fibrous histiocytoma

Patients need a chest X-ray and CT to detect lung metastases and a bone scan to detect bone metastases.

Laboratory findings: Serum alkaline phosphatase may be significantly increased.

Treatment: Treatment is a combination of chemotherapy and surgery. After several courses of chemotherapy (over several months), limb-sparing surgery and limb reconstruction can proceed.

In limb-sparing surgery, the tumour is resected en bloc, including all surrounding reactive tissue and a rim of surrounding normal tissue; to avoid microscopic spillage of tumour cells, the tumour is not violated. More than 85% of patients can be treated with limb-sparing surgery without decreasing the long-term survival rate. Continuation of chemotherapy after surgery is usually necessary.

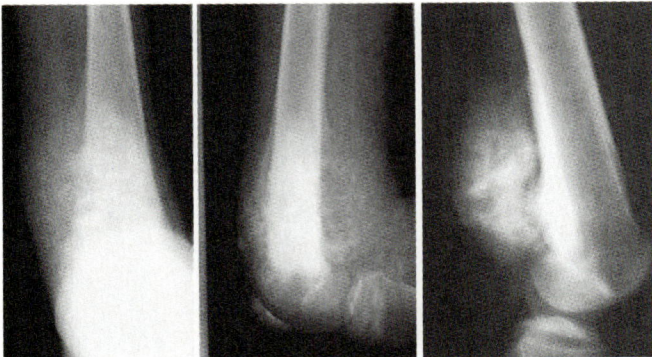

Fig. 32.5: Parosteal OGS

Chemotherapeutic drugs for OGS are:
1. High-dose methotrexate
2. Doxorubicin
3. Ifosfamide/MESNA
4. Cisplatin
5. Doxorubin
6. Bleomycin
7. Cyclophosphamide
8. Datinomycin

Variants of conventional osteosarcoma: Parosteal osteosarcoma (Fig. 32.5) and periosteal osteosarcoma (Table 32.2).

Table 32.2: Differentiation between paraosteal and periosteal osteosarcoma

Paraosteal osteosarcoma	Periosteal osteosarcoma
Involve posterior cortex of distal femur	Involve mid-shaft of femur
Well differentiated	Poorly differentiated
Comparative less chance of metastasis	High chance of metastasis
Require surgical en bloc resection but no chemotherapy	Treated similar to conventional osteosarcomas with chemotherapy and surgical en bloc resection.

FIBROSARCOMA

Fibrosarcomas have similar characteristics to osteosarcomas but produce fibrous tumour cells (rather than bone tumour cells), affect the same age group, and pose similar problems. Treatment and outcome for high-grade lesions are similar to osteosarcoma.

MALIGNANT FIBROUS HISTIOCYTOMA

Malignant fibrous histiocytoma is clinically similar to osteosarcoma and fibrosarcoma, although malignant fibrous histiocytomas have been classified as different from the osteosarcoma group because of a different histology (no tumour bone production). Malignant fibrous histiocytomas tend to occur in children and adolescents but can also occur in older adults as secondary lesions in bone infarcts and radiation fields. Treatment and outcome are similar to that of conventional osteosarcoma.

CHONDROSARCOMA

Chondrosarcomas are malignant tumours of cartilage. They differ from osteosarcomas clinically, therapeutically, and prognostically. Of chondrosarcomas, 90% are primary tumours. Chondrosarcomas arise in other pre-existing conditions, particularly multiple osteo-chondromas and multiple enchondromatosis (e.g. in Ollier's disease and Maffucci's syndrome).

Age: Chondrosarcomas tend to occur in older adults.

Site: They often develop in flat bones (e.g. pelvis, scapula).

X-rays: Reveal punctate/popcorn calcification calcifications, cortical bone destruction and loss of normal bone trabeculae (Fig. 32.6).

Technetium-99m bone scintigraphy is a helpful screening study; all cartilaginous lesions show increased uptake on the scan.

Biopsy: For diagnosis and can also determine the tumour's grade (probability of metastasizing) and appearance.

Treatment: Low-grade chondrosarcomas (grade 1/2) - treated intralesionally (wide curettage) with addition of an adjuvant (often freezing liquid nitrogen, argon beam, heat of methyl methacrylate, radiofrequency, or phenol). Other tumours are treated with total surgical resection. When surgical resection with maintenance of function is impossible, amputation may be necessary.

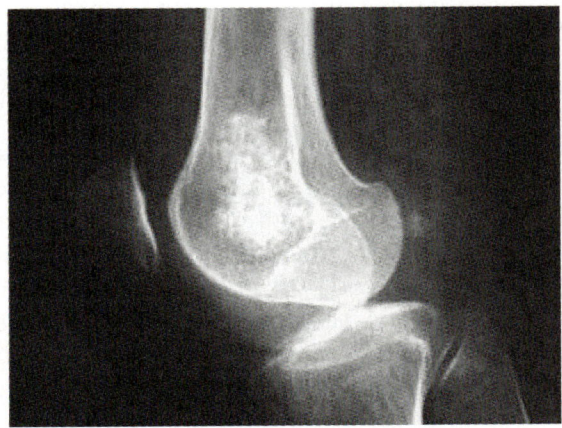

Fig. 32.6: Chondrosarcoma: Popcorn calcification

Meticulous care is taken to avoid spillage of tumour cells into the soft tissues during a biopsy or surgery, otherwise recurrence is likley. If no spillage occurs, the cure rate depends on the tumour grade. Low-grade tumours are nearly all cured with adequate treatment. Because these tumours have limited vascularity, chemotherapy and radiation therapy have little efficacy.

EWING'S SARCOMA

Introduction: Ewing's sarcoma of bone is a round-cell malignant bone tumour.

Age: Peak incidence between 10 and 25 years.

Site: Most tumours develop in the extremities, but any bone may be involved. Ewing's sarcoma tends to be extensive, sometimes involving the entire bone shaft, most often the diaphyseal region (Fig. 32.7). About 15 to 20% occur around the metaphyseal region.

Clinical features: Pain and swelling are the most common symptoms.

Imaging: Lytic destruction, particularly a permeative infiltrating pattern without clear borders, is the most common finding on imaging (Fig. 32.7), but multiple layers of subperiosteal reactive new bone formation may give an "onion-skin appearance".

X-rays do not usually reveal the full extent of bone involvement, and a large soft-tissue mass usually surrounds the affected bone.

MRI better defines disease extent, which can help guide treatment.

Many other benign and malignant tumours can appear very similarly, so diagnosis is made by biopsy. At times this type of tumour may be confused with an infection. Accurate histologic diagnosis can be accomplished with molecular markers, including evaluation for a typical clonal chromosomal abnormality.

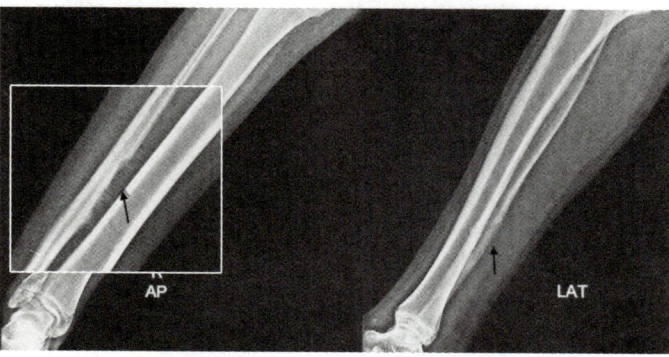

Fig. 32.7: Ewing's sarcoma of fibula

Treatment: Treatment includes various combinations of surgery, chemotherapy, and radiation therapy. Currently, > 60% of patients with primary localized Ewing's sarcoma may be cured by this multimodal approach. Cure is sometimes possible even with metastatic disease. Chemotherapy in conjunction with surgical en bloc resection, if applicable, often yields better long-term results.

MALIGNANT GIANT CELL TUMOUR

Malignant giant cell tumour (GCT) is a rare tumour usually located at the extreme end of a long bone.

X-ray reveals classic features of malignant destruction (predominantly lytic destruction, cortical destruction, soft-tissue extension, and pathologic fracture) (Fig. 32.8). A malignant giant cell tumour that develops in a previously benign giant cell tumour is characteristically radioresistant. Treatment is similar to that of osteosarcoma, but the cure rate is low.

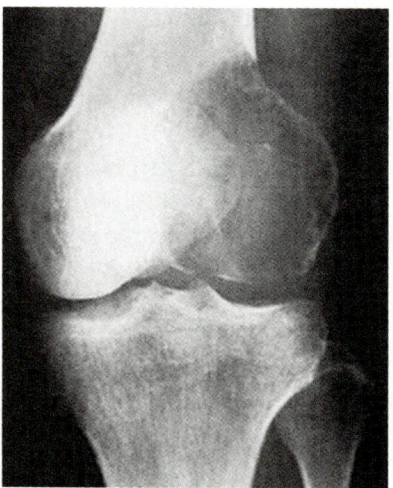

Fig. 32.8: Malignant GCT

CHORDOMA

Chordoma, develops from the remnants of the primitive notochord, and it is a rare tumour.

Site: It tends to occur at the ends of the spinal column, usually in the middle of the sacrum or near the base of the skull (Fig. 32.9).

Clinical features: A chordoma in the sacrococcygeal region causes nearly constant pain. A chordoma in the base of the skull can cause deficits in a cranial nerve, most commonly in nerves to the eye. Symptoms may exist for months to several years before diagnosis.

Diagnosis: A chordoma appears on imaging studies as an expansile, destructive bone lesion that may be

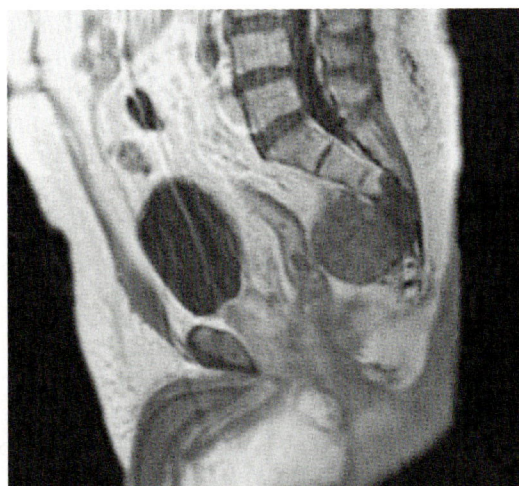

Fig. 32.9: Chordoma of sacrum

associated with a soft-tissue mass. Metastasis is unusual, but local recurrence is not. Chordomas in the sacrococcygeal region may be cured by radical en bloc excision. Chordomas in the base of the skull are usually inaccessible to surgery but may respond to radiation therapy.

METASTATIC BONE TUMOURS

Any cancer may metastasize to bone, but metastases from carcinomas are the most common, particularly those arising in the following areas:

- Breast
- Lung
- Prostate
- Kidney
- Thyroid
- Colon

Prostate cancer in men and breast cancer in women are the most common types of cancers. Lung cancer is the most common cause of cancer death in both sexes. Breast cancer is the most common cancer to metastasize to bone. Any bone may be involved with metastases.

Symptoms and signs: Metastases manifest as bone pain. Bone metastases may cause symptoms before the primary tumour is suspected or may appear in patients with a known diagnosis of cancer.

Diagnosis: Metastatic bone tumours are considered in all patients with unexplained bone pain, but particularly in patients who have

- Known cancer
- Pain at more than one site
- Findings on imaging studies that suggest metastases

X-ray
Prostate cancer-blastic,
Lung cancer-lytic, and
Breast cancer-blastic or lytic.

- CT and MRI are highly sensitive for specific metastases.
- Bone scan is more sensitive for early and asymptomatic bone metastases than plain X-rays and can be used to scan the entire body.
- Positron emission tomography (PET) for almost whole-body scanning is now often used for some tumours; it is more specific for bone metastases than is radionuclide bone scan and can identify many extra skeletal metastases.
- Needle biopsy of the lesion is often done to confirm the diagnosis of a metastasis.

If bone metastases are suspected because multiple lytic lesions are found, assessment for the primary tumour can begin with clinical evaluation for primary cancers (particularly focused on the breast, prostate, and thyroid), chest X-ray, mammography, and measurement of prostate-specific antigen level. Initial CT of the chest, abdomen, and pelvis may also reveal the primary tumour. However, bone biopsy, especially fine-needle or core biopsy, is necessary if metastatic tumour is suspected and the primary tumour has not been otherwise diagnosed. Biopsy with use of immunohistologic stains may give clues to the primary tumour type.

Treatment
- Usually radiation therapy.
- Surgery to stabilize bone at risk of pathologic fracture.
- Kyphoplasty or vertebroplasty for certain painful vertebral fractures.

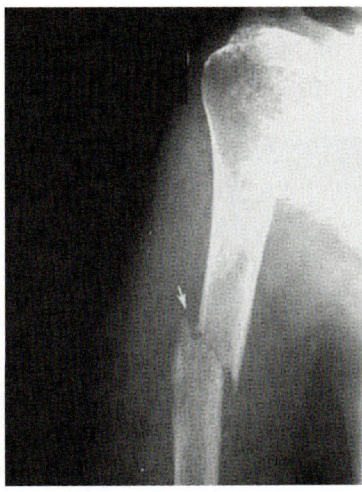

Fig. 32.10: Pathological fracture due to metastasis

Treatment depends on the type of tissue involved (which organ tissue type). Radiation therapy, combined with selected chemotherapeutic or hormonal drugs, is the most common treatment modality. Early use of radiation (30 Gy) and bisphosphonates (e.g., zoledronate, pamidronate) slows bone destruction. Some tumours are more likely to heal after radiation therapy; e.g., blastic lesions of prostate and breast cancer are more likely to heal than lytic destructive lesions of lung cancer and renal cell carcinoma. Drugs used to treat receptor activator of nuclear factor kappa-B ligand (RANKL) are now being used to reduce bone destruction.

If bone destruction is extensive, resulting in imminent or actual pathologic fracture (Fig. 32.10), surgical fixation or resection and reconstruction may be required to provide stabilization and help minimize morbidity. When the primary cancer has been removed and only a single bone metastasis remains (especially if the metastatic lesion appears 1 year after the primary tumour), en bloc excision sometimes combined with radiation therapy, chemotherapy, or both rarely may be curative. Insertion of methyl methacrylate (bone cement) into the spine (kyphoplasty or vertebroplasty) relieves pain and expands and stabilizes compression fractures that do not have epidural soft-tissue extension.

Important Points

- Carcinomas of breast, lung, and prostate are the most common sources of metastatic bone tumours.
- Bone metastases should be suspected in patients with known cancer, when pain is at more than one site, and/or when findings on imaging studies suggest metastases.
- Bone biopsy is needed if the primary tumour is unknown after clinical and radiographic evaluation.
- Most often, radiation therapy and bisphosphonate are used to slow bone destruction.
- Pathologic fractures may require treatment with surgery, kyphoplasty, or vertebroplasty.

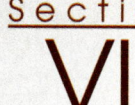

Congenital and Developmental Disorders

TORTICOLLIS

Latin word, meaning, 'twisted neck'.

Definition: Torticollis is an asymmetric deformity of head and neck, caused by unilateral contracture or spasm of sternocleidomastoid muscle.

Aetiology: Mainly of 2 types:
Congenital (Wryneck)
- Congenital muscular torticollis of infancy
- Vertebral anomalies/failure of segmentation
- Klippel-Feil syndrome

Acquired (painful/painless)
- Paroxysmal torticollis
- Hysterical
- Associated with ligament laxity (Down's syndrome)
- Traumatic: C1/C2 (atlantoaxial) subluxation
- Tumours of CNS: Posterior fossa tumours, eosinophilic granuloma
- Cervical spine: Osteoid osteoma, osteoblastoma
- Calcified cervical disc

Most common variety is congenital muscular torticollis, which is likely to result from local venous occlusion/ischaemia resulting from intrauterine malposition and local compartment syndrome, producing fibrotic muscle.

Clinical features
- More common in first born/breech and difficult forceps delivery
- Common association with DDH, metatarsus adductus, hip abduction contracture and pelvic obliquity.
- The head is tilted towards the contracted muscle and the chin is rotated towards the contralateral shoulder—'cock robin' appearance (Fig. 33.1).
- A non-tender, fusiform mass/knot (tumour) may be felt in the first month in the sternal and clavicular

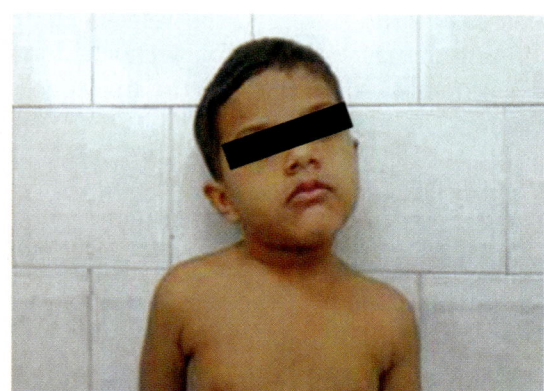

Fig. 33.1: Torticollis

head of sternocleidomastoid. The mass enlarges gradually over 2–3 months; it may regress and disappear at 4–6 months, or may be replaced by a readily palpable fibrous contracted band within sternocleidomastoid.
- Contralateral flexion and ipsilateral rotation is restricted.
- Secondary deformities of face and head:
  – Plagiocephaly—flattening of face due to external pressure on the facial bones due to position of infant while sleeping in prone position
  – Levels of eyes and ears become uneven, child may complain of eyestrain.
  – Cervicodorsal scoliosis with concavity to affected side.

Diagnosis
Mainly clinical
Radiological examination of cervical spine is required to rule out higher vertebral abnormalities.

Treatment
Conservative: Massage and stretching exercise by rotating infant's chin to the ipsilateral shoulder and

simultaneously tilting the head towards contralateral shoulder. Also, positioning toys and other manoeuvres to stimulate active rotation towards involved side, is successful in around 90%.

Surgical

Indications
- Child > 12–18 months
- Restriction of range of motion > 30 degrees
- Older child >6 yrs with facial asymmetry

Surgical techniques
- *Unipolar release–distal:* Partial excision of clavicular attachment and Z-lengthening of sternal attachment, to maintain normal V-contour of neck.
- *Bipolar release (by Ferkel):* Distal release along with sectioning of mastoid origin of sternocleidomastoid
  Complications of surgery: Injury to spinal accessory nerve.

SPRENGEL'S DEFORMITY/ CONGENITAL ELEVATION OF SCAPULA

Introduction: It is a condition in which the scapula lies more superiorly than it should, in relation to the thoracic cage and is usually hypoplastic and misshapen (Fig. 33.2).

Associated anomalies
- Cervical ribs/malformation of ribs.
- Anomalies of cervical vertebrae (Klippel-Feil syndrome).
- Partial/complete absence of one or more scapular muscles.

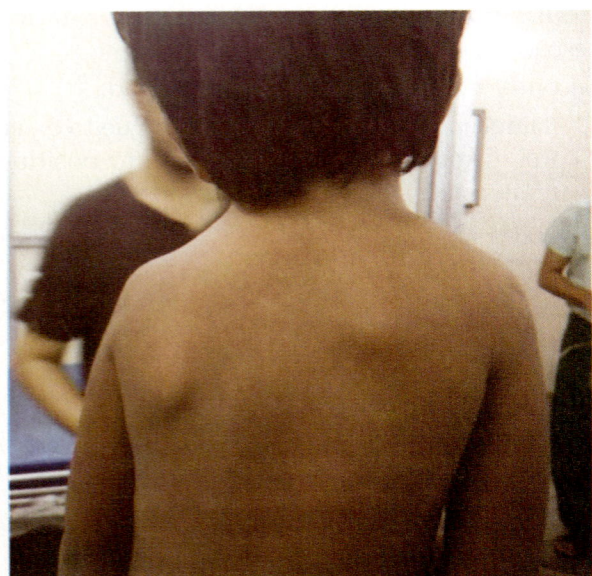

Fig. 33.2; Sprengel's deformity

Clinical features

Mild: Scapula only slightly higher and a bit smaller, minimal restriction of shoulder motion.

Severe: Scapula very high, may touch the occiput, size very small, motion severely restricted.

Omovertebral bar: In 1/3rd of patients, a rhomboid plaque of cartilage or bone lies in a strong fascial sheath, extending from superior angle of scapula to the spinous process, lamina or transverse process of one or more lower cervical vertebrae.

Treatment
- *Mild:* No treatment
- *Severe:* Surgery to bring the scapula inferiorly to its near normal position (matching the level of scapula spine)
- *Ideal time for surgery:* After 3 years of age, at the earliest.

Surgical techniques
1. *Green:* Surgical release of muscles from the scapula, excision of supraspinatus portion of scapula and any omovertebral bone. The scapula is then moved inferiorly to the desired level and muscles are reattached.
2. *Woodward:* Transferring the origin of trapezius muscle to a more inferior position of the spinous process.

Complications: Brachial plexus palsy: To avoid this, morcellation of the clavicle (cutting clavicle into small pieces) on the ipsilateral side is done as a first step, in cases of severe deformity.

LIMB DEFICIENCY

Limb deficiency can be transverse or longitudinal.

Transverse deficiencies include those deformities in which there is complete absence of parts distal to some point on the extremity, producing amputation like stumps.

Longitudinal deficiency includes all failure-of-formation anomalies that are not considered transverse deficiencies.

Phocomelia: Where intercalated segment is absent, e.g. hand suspended from the body near the shoulder.

Radial club hand/radial deficiency: Where there is longitudinal failure of formation of parts along the pre-axial or radial border of upper limb, i.e. absent/deficient thenar muscles, a shortened unstable or absent thumb, a shortened or absent radius (Fig. 33.3).

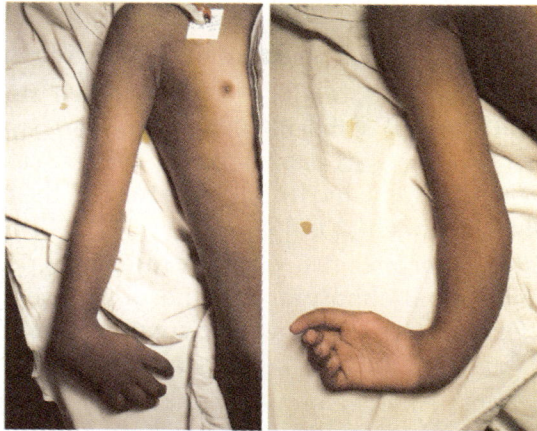

Fig. 33.3: Radial clubhand

Cleft hand/central deficiency: Where there is a longitudinal failure of formation of the 2nd/3rd or 4th ray.

Ulnar clubhand/ulnar deficiency: Where there is longitudinal failure of formation of parts along the postaxial or ulnar border of upper limb.

Tibial hemimelia: Where there is longitudinal failure of formation of parts along the preaxial or medial border of lower limb.

Fibular hemimelia: When there is longitudinal failure of formation of parts along the postaxial or lateral border of lower limb.

Proximal focal femoral deficiency: Where there is partial skeletal defect in the proximal femur with a variably unstable hip joint, shortening and associated other anomalies (Fig. 33.4).

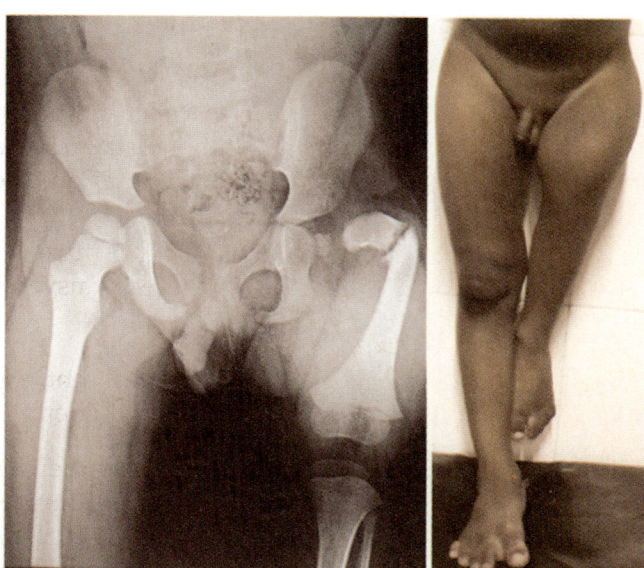

Fig. 33.4: Proximal focal femoral deficiency

SYNDACTYLY (WEBBED FINGERS/TOES)

Introduction: Syndactyly is the most common congenital anomaly of the hand, occurring due to the failure of the fingers to separate during embryonic development.

Classification

1. *Complete/Incomplete:* When the fingers are joined from the web to the fingertip, it is called complete syndactyly (Fig. 33.5).

   When the fingers are joined from the web to a point proximal to the fingertip, it is called incomplete syndactyly.

2. *Simple/complex:* When only skin or other soft tissue bridges the fingers, it is called simple syndactyly.

   When there are common bony elements shared by involved fingers, it is called complex syndactyly (Fig. 33.6).

Most commonly affected fingers

- Long and ring fingers 3rd web (in > 50%), next 4th web
- Syndactyly is bilateral in about 50% patients

Treatment

- *At birth and in infants:* Massaging the web in an attempt to stretch the intervening skin, is recommended
- When digits of different sizes are completely involved, early separation between ages of 6 and 12 months is recommended, because it may lead to angular, rotational and flexion deformity.
- Steps of surgery:
  - Separation of digits
  - Commissure reconstruction
  - Resurfacing of intervening border.

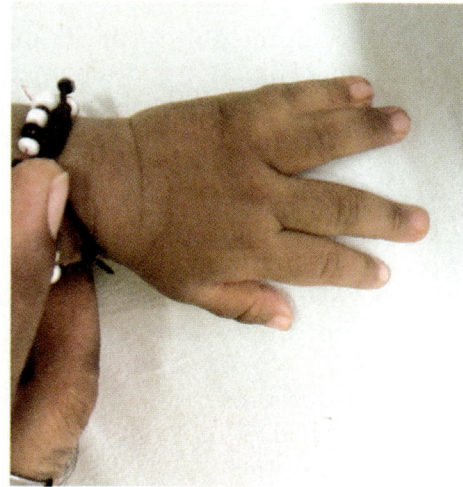

Fig. 33.5: Complete syndactyly

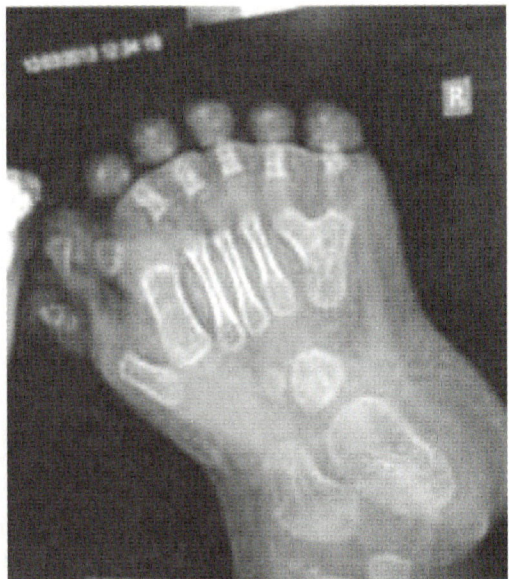

Fig. 33.6: Complex syn-polydactyly

- Simultaneous release of the radial and ulnar sides of a finger is contraindicated and may jeopardize the viability of the finger.

POLYDACTYLY

Polydactyly refers to presence of extra digit.

The extra digit is usually a small piece of soft tissue that can be removed. Occasionally it contains bone without joints; rarely it may be a complete, functioning digit. The extra digit is most common on the ulnar (little finger) side of the hand, less common on the radial (thumb) side, and very rarely within the middle three digits. These are respectively known as postaxial (little finger), preaxial (thumb), and central (ring, middle, index fingers) polydactyly.

DEVELOPMENTAL DYSPLASIA OF HIP

Introduction: Developmental dysplasia of the hip (DDH) is a spectrum of hip disorders ranging from hip instability, to subluxation, frank dislocation or only acetabular dysplasia, occurring before, during or just after birth.

Aetiology

1. *Congenital or developmental*
- Mechanical factors: Greater incidence in first born child related to an unstretched uterus, taut abdominal muscles, oligohydramnios and increased likelihood of breech presentation in primigravida (45% incidence of DDH in frank breech with hip flexion and knee extension)

- Genetic influences:
  - When a sibling is affected, the risk to subsequent siblings is 6%
  - When one parent is affected, the risk to the child is 12%
  - When a parent and a child are affected, the risk to subsequent child is 36%
2. *Teratologic or prenatal:* As seen in arthrogryposis, chromosomal abnormalities and other congenital malformations (common association with torticollis, metatarsus adductus)
3. *Syndromic:* Association with syndromes like Larsen syndrome, diastrophic dysplasia, Freeman-Sheldon syndrome, etc.
4. *Neuromuscular:* Due to spasticity, muscle imbalance or paralysis as seen in CP, MMC, Poliomyelitis, etc.
5. *Postnatal:* Due to infant positioning such as swaddling with hip and knee in extension.

Epidemiology

- Frank dislocation: 1 to 1.5 per 1000
  Hip instability: 1 per 100
  Most cases of hip instability resolve in the first few weeks after birth.
- Incidence lower in Chinese, Africans and Native Americans. Highest among white races due to different handling practice.
- F:M= 6:1 (influence of maternal hormones—relaxin, progesterone)

Pathoanatomy and obstacles to reduction: Various pathological changes occur within and around hip joint in DDH. They act as obstacles to reduction and need to be released during surgery (Fig. 33.7).

I. *Intra-articular*

Capsule: Thickened, elongated, adhesions with acetabulum.

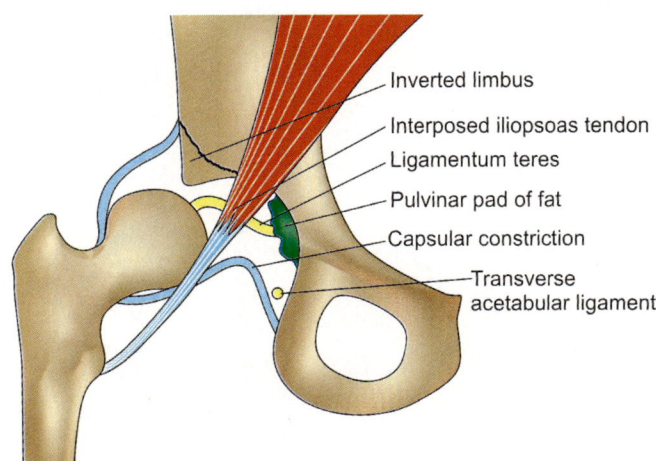

Inverted limbus
Interposed iliopsoas tendon
Ligamentum teres
Pulvinar pad of fat
Capsular constriction
Transverse acetabular ligament

Fig. 33.7: Pathoanatomy of DDH

Ligamentum teres: Hypertrophic and elongated.

Limbus: Hypertrophic fibrocartilaginous labrum.

Pulvinar pad of fibrofatty tissue: Lining the base of acetabular socket.

Inferior acetabular ligament: Blocks entry into lower part of acetabulum.

II. *Extra-articular*

Iliopsoas: Forms an hourglass constriction of capsule.

Pelvifemoral muscles: Adductors, abductors, hamstrings, hip flexors.

Diagnosis and clinical assessment

I. *Neonatal period:* Up to 4–6 months
- Barlow test and Ortolani sign (Fig. 33.8)

Ortolani sign

- Described in 1936 by Ortolani (paediatrician) as a palpable sensation of hip gliding in and out of the acetabulum
- Initially noted by a mother who used to feel the clunk at the time of baby's diaper change.
- This test is performed in a relaxed, supine baby on a firm table.
- *Method:*
  – Pelvis is stabilized with one hand.
  – Other hand is used to hold the lower limb with hip flexed to 90°.
  – Index and middle fingers are kept on greater trochanter, thumb is kept medially on thigh.

– On gentle abduction of hip, as the femoral head glides into the acetabulum, 'clunk of entry' is felt (Fig. 33.8a).

– Next, while adducting the hip, femoral head is displaced out of the acetabulum with a palpable clunk, 'clunk of exit' (Fig. 33.8b).

Barlow test

- Provocative manoeuvre to check whether hip is dislocatable
- *I part:* In position of 90° flexion of hip and knee, hip is adducted and pushed, leading to dislocation of hip (Fig. 33.8a).
- *II part:* Now, hip is abducted and pulled, causing 'clunk' indicating reduction of hip (Fig. 33.8b).

II. Older child

- Limitation of abduction
- *Galeazzi sign/Allis sign:* Appears as lowering of knee on affected side in a lying child with hip and knee flexed (Fig. 33.9).
- Asymmetrical thigh and gluteal folds
- Positive telescopy
- Positive Trendelenburg's test
- Positive vascular sign of Narath
- Apparent shortening of limb
- *Bilateral dislocation:* Waddling gait, lumbar hyperlordosis.

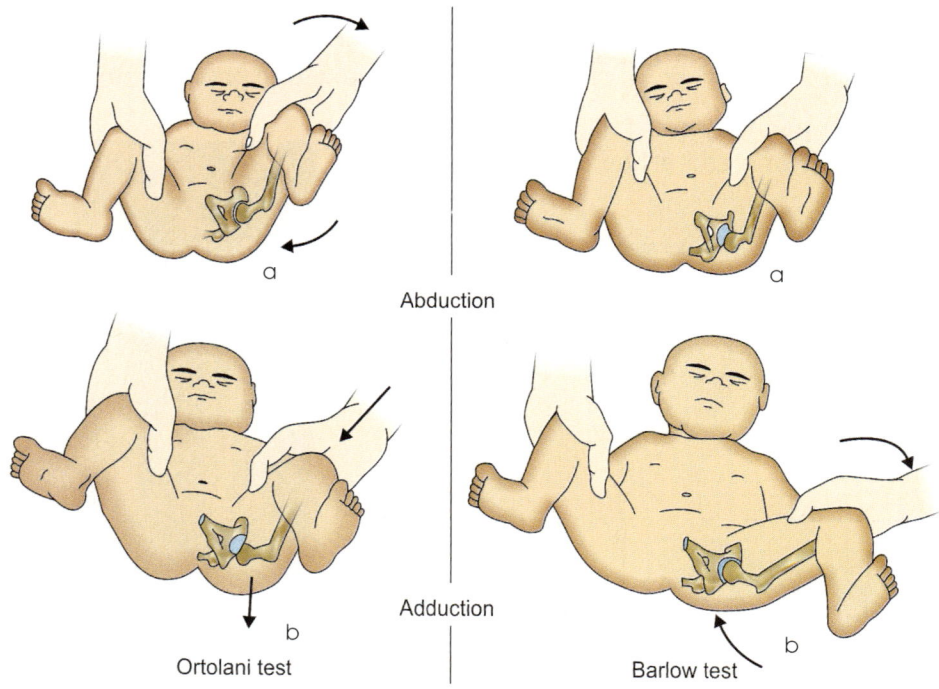

Abduction

Adduction

Ortolani test

Barlow test

Fig. 33.8: Ortolani and Barlow test

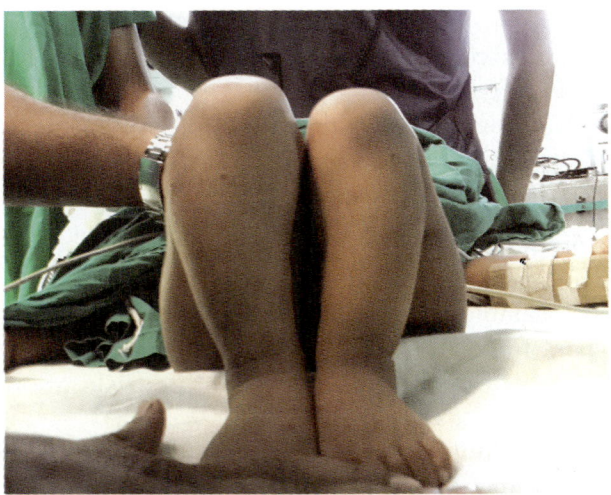

Fig. 33.9: Galeazzi sign

Radiological features

I. X-rays

- *In neonate:* X-rays are not very helpful as femoral head and acetabulum are largely unossified.
- X-rays are most reliable after the age of 3–6 months when ossific nucleus is present in capital femoral epiphysis.

In Von Rosen/True AP pelvic radiograph, following parameters should be noted (Fig. 33.10):
- *Perkin's (P) line:* Vertical line drawn at the outer border of acetabulum.
- *Hilgenreiner's line:* Horizontal line at the level of triradiate cartilage.
- *Shenton's line:* Smooth curve along inferior border of femoral neck and superior margin of obturator foramen.
- *Acetabular index:* Acetabular index is the angle between the Hilgenreiner's line and a line drawn from the triradiate epiphysis to the lateral edge of the acetabulum
- *CE (centre-edge) angle of Wiberg:* Normal—15°–30°

In DDH (Fig. 33.11)
- Femoral head does not lie in lower and inner quadrant formed by 'H' and 'P' lines.
- Shenton's line is broken.
- Delayed appearance and retarded development of ossification of femoral head.
- Shallow acetabulum: Acetabular index increased
- Widened teardrop.

II. Ultrasound: Primary imaging and screening tool to assess hip in neonates and young infants. There are two commonly used techniques.
- *Static non-stress technique by Graf of Austria:* Alpha angle (depth of socket) and beta angle (labral eversion) assessed.
- *Dynamic stress technique by Hareke and Clarke:* Imaging in transverse and coronal planes while applying stress.

Ultrasound screening at birth is recommended only in high risk infants.

III. Arthrography
- Performed by using radio-opaque contrast medium like urograffin (sodium diatrizoate 76%) with aseptic technique via anterior or medial approach.
- Very useful imaging modality especially intra-operatively to assess the adequacy/concentricity of hip reduction in infants.
- Typical arthrographic findings in DDH are:
  - Medial dye pool >7 mm.

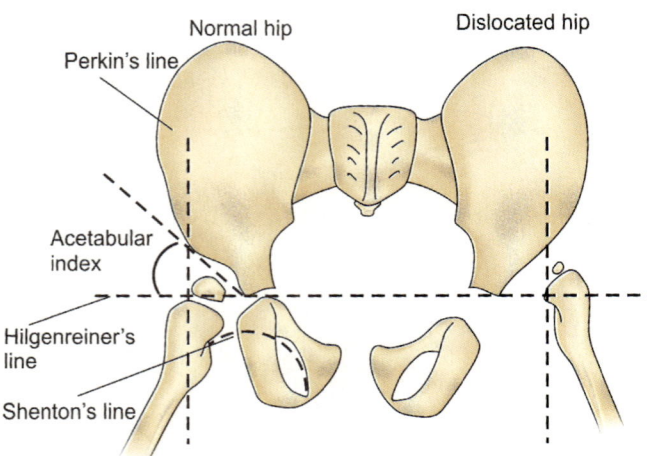

Fig. 33.10: Radiological parameters of DDH

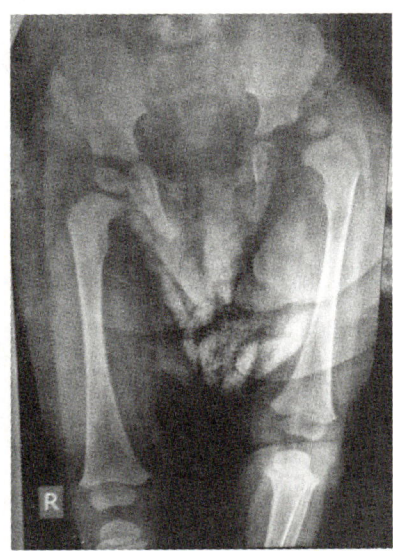

Fig. 33.11: X-ray picture of DDH

– Hourglass constriction of capsule
– Filling defects in the floor of acetabulum
– Blunting of rose-thorn sign outlining the limbus.

IV. MRI: Important non-invasive modality to understand obstacles to reduction and also helpful in revision surgeries.

V. CT Scan and 3D reconstruction: Useful in older age group and late diagnosed cases.

Treatment

Goal:
- Concentric reduction
- Maintenance of reduction
- Prevent proximal femoral growth disturbance
  The treatment depends on age of patient

I. Birth to 6 months
- *Pavlik harness:* Flexion–abduction orthosis with an anterior flexion strap and posterior abduction strap, tightened enough to maintain reducible hip in stable range. Ultrasound is useful to confirm the reduction. Once this is confirmed, the harness is kept for 4–6 wks and then gradually weaned over next 4 wks (Fig. 33.12).
- Other splints: Von Rosen splint/Frejka pillow

II. 6 months–18 months
- Traction/gentle closed reduction under anaesthesia, after adductor tenotomy.
- Confirmation of concentric reduction by arthrography.
- Maintenance in hip spica cast, in 'human position' of flexion >100° and abduction between 45 and 60° for 3 months.
- Avoid excess abduction and internal rotation to avoid avascular necrosis and proximal femoral growth disturbance.
- After removal of spica, maintenance of reduction in abduction orthosis for 6–12 months.
- If there is failure of closed reduction, open reduction is recommended.

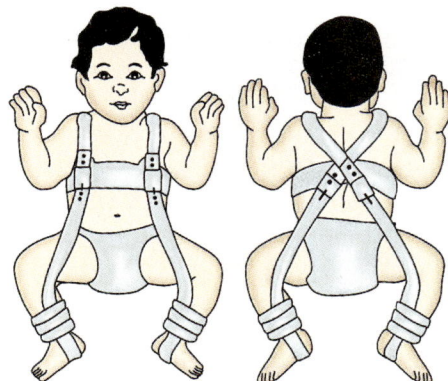

Fig. 33.12: Pavlik harness

III. 18 months–3 years
- Open reduction through anterior or medial approach
- Capsulorrhaphy
- Concomitant femoral varus de-rotation osteotomy (VDRO)/acetabular (Salter's) osteotomy, if indicated (Figs 33.13 and 33.14).

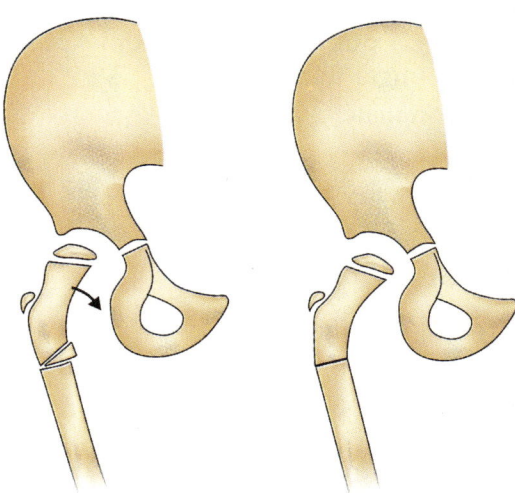

Fig. 33.13: VDRO

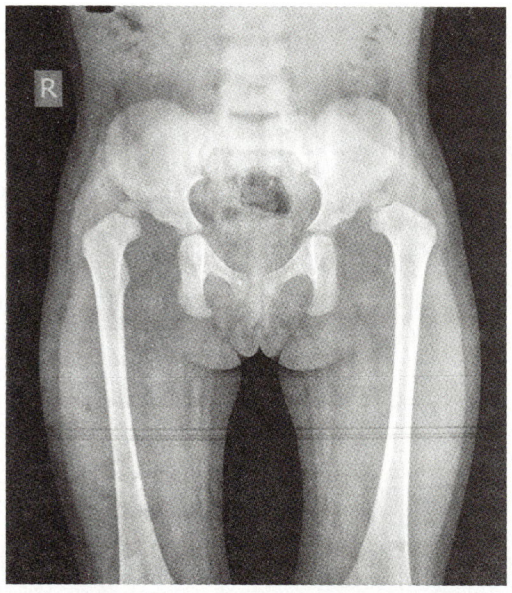

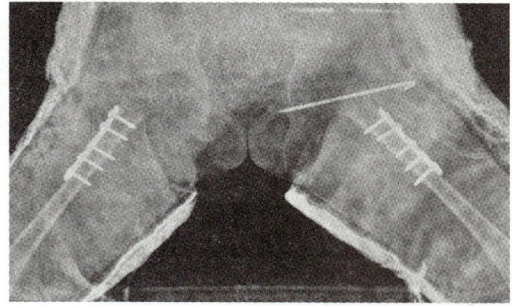

Fig. 33.14: Pre-operative and post-operative x-ray of bilateral DDH treated by open reduction and femoral osteotomy

IV. >3 years

- May need femoral shortening

Types of Pelvic Osteotomies in DDH

With concentric reduction:

Redirectional

- *Salter:* Require an intact hinge, i.e. triradiate cartilage or symphysis pubis. Therefore, only possible in children younger than 8 years.
- Triple innominate
- Ganz

Reshaping

- Dega
- Pemberton

Without concentric reduction:

- Shelf
- Chiari

Complications in DDH

- Residual femoral/acetabular dysplasia
- Subluxation/redislocation
- Stiffness
- AVN and proximal femoral growth disturbance

CONGENITAL DISLOCATION OF KNEE

Introduction: Congenital abnormalities of the knee include three grades of severity

- Congenital hyperextension
- Congenital hyperextension with anterior subluxation of tibia on femur
- Congenital hyperextension with anterior dislocation of tibia on femur (Fig. 33.15)

Aetiology

- Abnormal fetal position where feet become locked beneath the mandible or in axilla

- Congenital absence or hypoplasia of cruciate ligaments
- Common association with skeletal abnormalities elsewhere in the extremity mainly DDH, CTEV, Larsen's syndrome, Ehler-Danlos syndrome.

Pathology

- Contracture of anterior capsule of knee and quadriceps
- Hypoplasia or absence of patella
- Fibrosis of vastus lateralis
- In severe cases, hamstrings and collateral ligaments are subluxed anteriorly.

Treatment

- Newborn with mild to moderate hyperextension / subluxation: Conservative treatment—serial casting into flexion and bracing.
- Older children with severe deformity: surgery:
  - Anterior capsular release
  - Lengthening of intramuscular adhesions
  - Reduction of tibia on femur.

CONGENITAL PSEUDOARTHROSIS OF TIBIA (CPT)

Definition: Congenital pseudoarthrosis of tibia is a complex affection in which there is dysplasia of bone with failure of normal bone formation in its distal half and consequent segmental weakening of bone, anterolateral angulation of tibia and pathological fracture. Hamartomatous tissue forms at fracture site and pseudoarthrosis results, as normal callus does not form.

Incidence: Very rare, 1 per 250,000

Etiology: Exact cause not known. 50–90% associated with stigmata of neurofibromatosis.

Classification: By Boyd (Figs 33.16 and Fig. 33.17)
Type I: Anterior bowing and a defect in tibia present at birth.

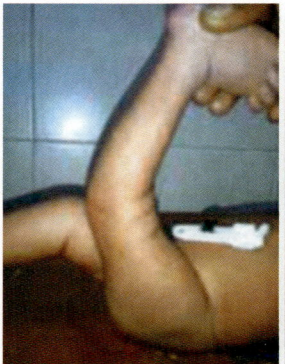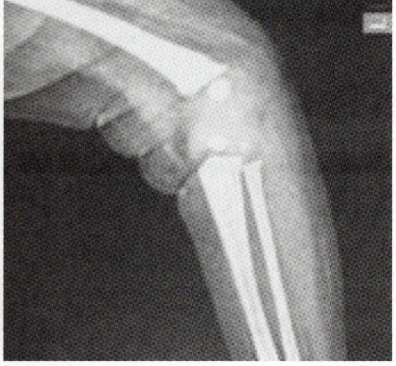

Fig. 33.15: Grade III—congenital dislocation of knee

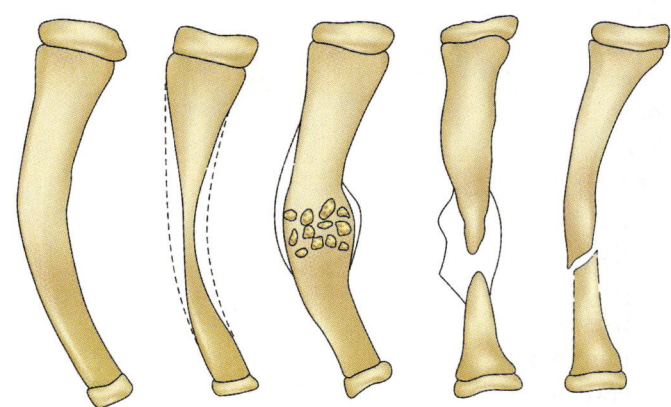

Fig. 33.16: Different types of CPT

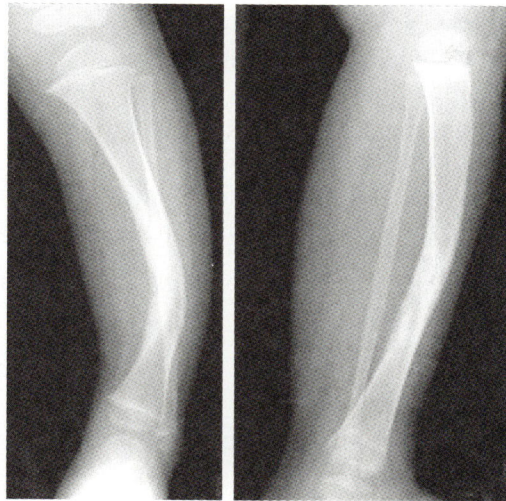

Fig. 33.17: X-ray CPT

Type II: Anterior bowing and an hourglass constriction of tibia present at birth.

- Spontaneous fracture or fracture following minor trauma occurs before 2 years of age, hence called 'high risk' tibia
- Often associated with neurofibromatosis
- Poorest prognosis

Type III: Pseudoarthrosis develops in congenital cyst near middle and distal third junction. Anterior bowing may precede or follow the development of fracture.

Type IV: Pseudoarthrosis originates in a sclerotic segment of bone in the classic location without narrowing of tibia. An 'Insufficiency' or 'Stress' fracture develops in the cortex and gradually extends through the sclerotic bone.

Type V: Pseudoarthrosis of tibia occurs with a dysplastic fibula.

Type VI: Pseudoarthrosis occurs in an intraosseous neurofibroma or schwannoma. Extremely rare.

Treatment

- Treatment of CPT is one of the most challenging problems in orthopaedics as it is difficult to obtain and maintain union and multiple surgeries may be necessary.
- Treatment depends on age of the patient and type of pseudoarthrosis.
- Principles of treatment
  - Excision of pseudoarthrosis with abnormal periosteum and surrounding hamartomatous tissue
  - Removal of dead sclerotic bne ends till bleeding ends appear
  - Bone grafting

  - Stabilisation: Internal/external
  - Correction of angular deformity and limb length discrepancy
- Type III: Prophylactic curettage and autologous iliac crest bone grafting + immobilization in plaster until union + bracing till skeletal maturity.

CTEV/CLUB FOOT

Congenital Talipes Equinovarus

Introduction: Clubfoot is one of the most common congenital orthopaedic anomalies, characterized by equinus of ankle and foot, inversion of foot, adduction of forefoot and internal rotation of tibia (Fig. 33.18).

Types

1. *Idiopathic:* Most common

   When club foot is the isolated skeletal anomaly, it is called idiopathic clubfoot
2. *Non-idiopathic/secondary:* Clubfoot associated with
   - Genetic syndromes: Larsen's/constriction ring syndrome.
   - Neurological disorders and neural tube defects e.g. MMC, spinal dysraphism.
   - Paralytic disorder (muscle imbalance), e.g. polio, spina bifida.
   - Arthrogryposis multiplex congenita (AMC)

Pathoanatomy: Clubfoot is congenital talo calcaneo-navicular joint dislocation. The true clubfoot is characterized by:

- Equinus at ankle, talocalcaneo-navicular joint and forefoot .
- Varus at hindfoot and forefoot
- Cavus involving forefoot.

Bone and joint abnormalities

- Talus has broadening of anterior part of trochlea, medial deviation and foreshortening of neck and flattening of head

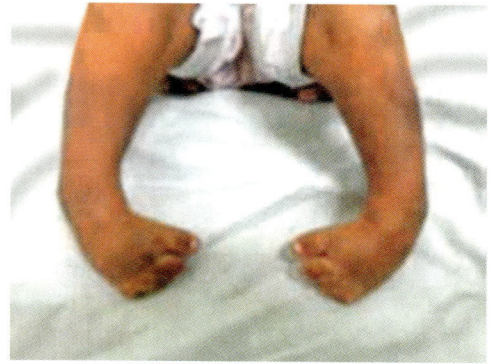

Fig. 33.18: Bilateral CTEV

- Calcaneus has flattened facet on its superior surface
- Navicular and cuboid are displaced medially.

Soft tissue contractures (muscles, tendons, ligaments, capsule)

Posterior
- Tendo Achilles
- Tibiotalar (ankle) and talocalcaneal (subtalar) capsule
- Posterior talofibular and calcaneofibular ligaments

Medial
- Tibialis posterior tendon
- Talonavicular capsule
- Deltoid ligament and spring ligament
- 'Master knot of Henry'(fibrous thickening of tendon sheaths of FHL and FDL) overlying navicular tuberosity.

Subtalar
- Talocalcaneal interosseous ligament
- Bifurcated Y ligament

Plantar
- Abductor hallucis
- Plantar fascia
- Intrinsic toe flexors

Theories of aetiology
- *Mechanical theory:* Clubfoot results from elevated intrauterine pressure during pregnancy
- *Neuromuscular theory:* Increase in type I:II muscle fibre ratio suggesting neural basis.
- *Histological theory:* Abnormal peroneus brevis
- *Primary germ plasm defect:* In talus
- *Arrested fetal development:* In equinovarus stage
- Genetic basis

None of the theories are satisfactorily proven and current theory suggests it to be a multifactorial problem, involving all/any of the above theories.

Clinical features
- Bilateral in 50%
- Bean shaped foot, with convex lateral and concave medial border.
- Characteristic deformity
- Increased crease/cleft medially and plantar ward
- In older, untreated children, callosities on lateral border due to abnormal walking
- Associated abnormalities: In hips/spine especially non-idiopathic type.

Radiology
- If teratological aetiology is suspected, X-rays are taken at 3–4 months.
- AP/lateral stress views: Various angles are measured (Fig. 33.19).
- Kite's index: Combined talocalcaneal angles in AP and Lateral views <40° is diagnostic of clubfoot.

Scoring system: To know severity and response to treatment
- Pirani
- Dimeglio

Treatment: It should always begin at birth or as early as possible.

In newborn and < 1 month old child: Gentle, repeated manipulation by mother to stretch the tight structure.

Ponseti technique of manipulation and casting
- Serial/weekly above-knee casts with a special technique and gradually correcting every component of deformity (Fig. 33.20).
- Before the final cast of 3 weeks, percutaneous TA (tendo Achilles) tenotomy may be required to get adequate dorsiflexion
- Incorrect technique can lead to rocker bottom deformity (spurious correction), with dorsiflexion at midfoot joint.
- Once correction is achieved, the feet are maintained in Dennis-Brown splint/modified foot abduction orthosis (Steenbeck type) given for 23 hours in initial 3 months and gradual weaning of orthosis (Fig. 33.21).

Brace wear is important to prevent relapse.

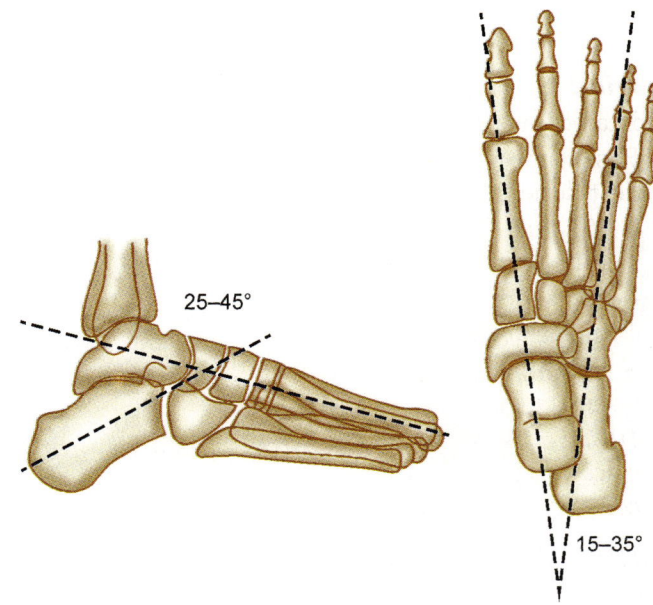

25–45°

15–35°

Fig. 33.19: Talocalcaneal angles in AP and lateral views

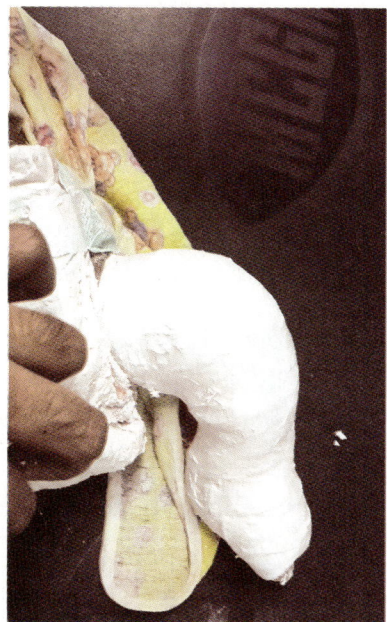

Fig. 33.20: Corrective cast for CTEV

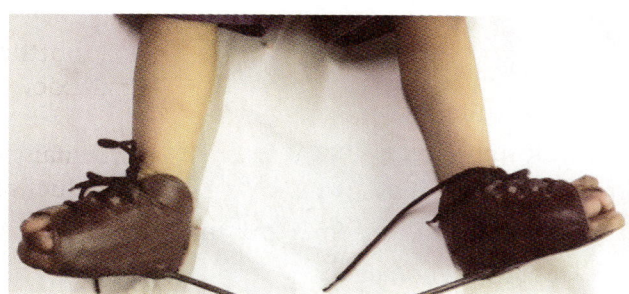

Fig. 33.21: CTEV orthosis

Surgical

Indicated in resistant/relapse/neglected cases

- Posteromedial soft tissue release: (Turco/Cincinnati) best done at young age (6 months–3 years)
- *4–10 years:* Lateral column shortening procedures required
  - Dilwyn-Evan's procedure: Resection and fusion of calcaneocuboid joint
  - Lichtblau's procedure: Shortening of calcaneal neck proximal to calcaneocuboid joint
- *10–12 years:* Triple arthrodesis—Talocalcaneal, calcaneocuboid and talo-navicular joints fused after corrective osteotomy.

External fixator: JESS (Joshi's external stabilisation system), Ilizarov for gradual correction of deformity (Fig. 33.22).

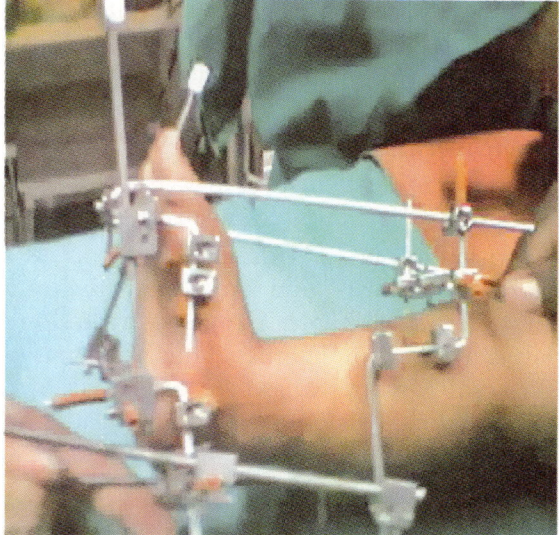

Fig. 33.22: Dr. B.B. Joshi's fixator for CTEV

Complications

- Recurrence
- Under/over correction/spurious correction
- Stiffness of ankle, foot

CONGENITAL VERTICAL TALUS/ ROCKER BOTTOM FOOT

Definition: It is a congenital deformity of the foot, characterized by convex plantar surface with apex of convexity at the talar head. The talus is so distorted plantarward and medially as to be almost vertical.

Clinical features (Fig. 33.23)

- The heel (calcaneus) is fixed in equinus and valgus
- The forefoot is dorsiflexed at the midtarsal joints and lies in valgus externally rotated position.
- The navicular lies on the dorsal aspect of head of talus, where it abuts the anterior tibial surface at the front of ankle joint.

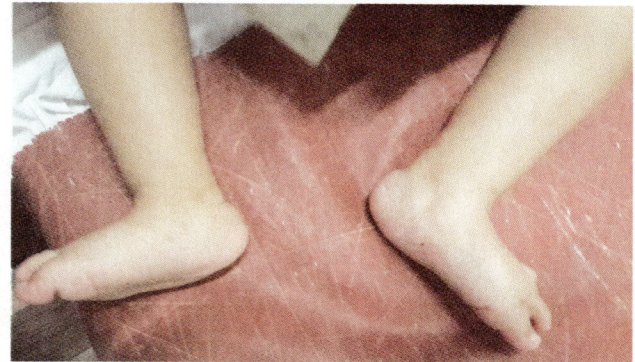

Fig. 33.23: Rocker bottom feet

- All the capsules, ligaments and tendons on the dorsum of the foot including peroneals and anterior tibialis tendon become contracted.

Radiological features

- Radiographs are important to differentiate congenital vertical talus from severe pes planus.
- AP and lateral/lateral plantar flexion stress view: In normal plantar flexion stress view, the long axis of first metatarsal passes plantar ward to long axis of talus. In congenital vertical talus, long axis of first metatarsal remains dorsal to long axis of talus, indicating dorsal dislocation of mid foot and forefoot (Fig. 33.24).

Treatment: Difficult to correct and tend to recur.

Conservative: Gentle manipulation and casting only to stretch the tight skin and soft tissue. Reduction of talonavicular joint is rarely possible by conservative treatment alone.

Surgery

- *1 to 4 years:* Open reduction and realignment of talonavicular and subtalar joints.

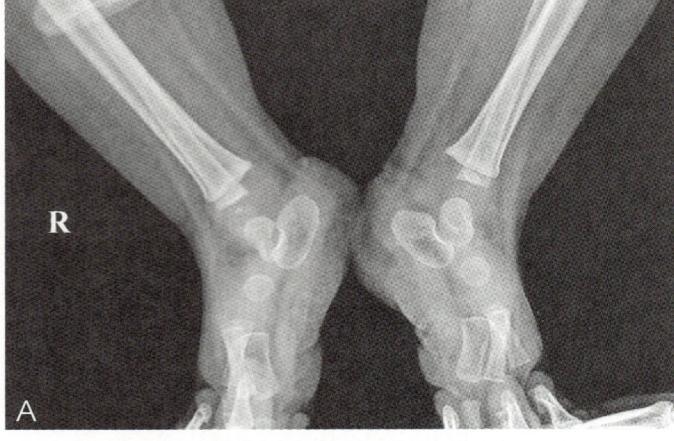

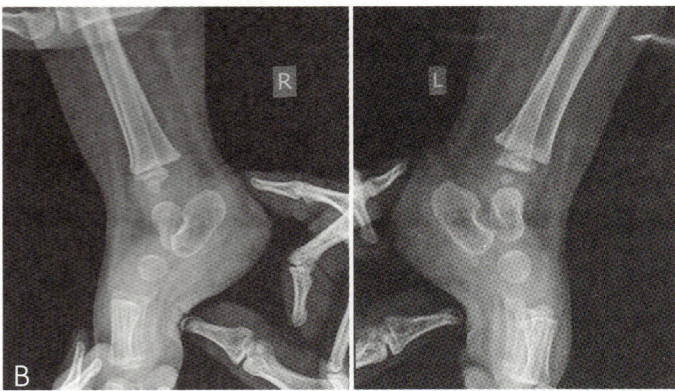

Fig. 33.24: (A) X-ray showing bilateral vertical talus, (B) stress plantar flexion lateral X-ray of CVT

- *4 to 8 years:* Open reduction, soft tissue procedures with extra-articular subtalar arthrodesis.
- *>12 years:* Triple arthrodesis.

OSTEOPETROSIS/ALBERS-SCHONBERG DISEASE

Also called marble bone disease/chalk bones.

Introduction: A development abnormality characterized by dense/brittle bone and insufficient bone marrow development, and encroachment of cranial foramina, leading to fatal complications.

Aetiology: Exact aetiology not known
- Associated with consanguinity of parents
- Recessive/dominant inheritance

Pathology: Immune disorder with thymic defect, osteoclast abnormality, continuous deposition of new bone on unresorbed calcified cartilage, failure of remodelling
- Marked widening of metaphysis and club-shaped appearance of long bones.
- Brittle, white bone solid on cross-section with medullary canal obliteration.

Clinical presentation

Three types,

 I. *Infantile malignant form*
- Onset in infancy
- Autosomal recessive
- Failure to thrive
- Myelophthisic anaemia and thrombocytopenia
- Hepatosplenomegaly
- Lymphadenopathy
- Spontaneous bruising, abnormal bleeding
- Multiple fractures
- Usually death due to overwhelming infection, haemorrhages, anaemia within 2 years.

 II. *Intermediate form*
- Presents in first decade of life
- Autosomal recessive
- Milder presentation as compared to infantile form

 III. *Mild form*
- Autosomal dominant
- Repeated fractures and subsequent deformities like coxa vara
- Normal life expectancy

Investigations: X-rays are diagnostic
- Entire long bone including epiphysis uniformly dense and without proper medullary and cortical differentiation (Fig. 33.25)

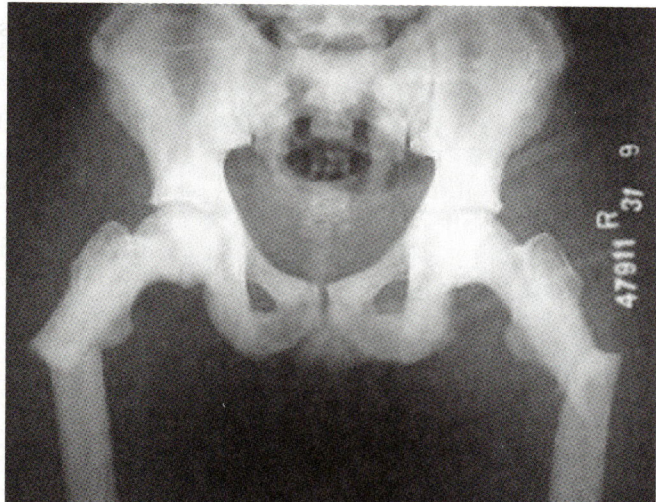

Fig. 33.25: Osteopetrosis

- With intermittent activity of disease process, alternate dense and clear bands on bones.
- Greatest density of skull and the base
- Air sinuses absent and dense.

Treatment: Bone marrow transplant from HLA–matched donor is the new hope in treatment of malignant/severe type.

OSTEOGENESIS IMPERFECTA

Introduction

Also known as Lobstein's disease/Vrolik's disease/Brittle bone disease.

It is a genetic disorder of connective tissue characterized by bone fragility, blue sclera, deafness due to otosclerosis and abnormal teeth (dentinogenesis imperfecta).

Pathology

The basic defect is failure of maturation of type I collagen beyond reticulin fibre stage, with a defect in cross-linking. Formation of both, intramembranous and endochondral bones is disturbed. Type I collagen is one of the major component of fibrillar connective tissue in skin ligaments, sclera and teeth also thereby affecting all these structures.

Classification

Looser Classification

Type I: OI congenita: Fractures occurring in perinatal period.

Type II: OI tarda: Fractures occurring after perinatal period.

Silence Classification

I	Autosomal dominant:
	A (blue sclera)
	B with dentinogenesis imperfecta
II	Autosmal recessive
	Severe bone fragility, usually perinatal death
III	Autosomal recessive
	Moderate bone fragility, death by 3rd decade
IV	Autosomal dominant:
	A (normal sclera)
	B with dentinogenesis imperfecta

Clinical features

Bones and Joints (Fig. 33.26)

- Due to osteopenia and fragility, multiple fractures occur right from the perinatal period
- Any fracture pattern may be seen
- Fractures heal at a normal rate, many times abundant callus formation may be seen
- Bones usually fracture repeatedly because of deformity causing malalignment, atrophy due to disuse and joint stiffness
- Frequency of fractures decreases after puberty or adolescence
- Hyperlaxity of ligaments, with hypermobility of joint is common

Muscles: Usually hypotonic

Skin: Thin and translucent. Capillary fragility may lead to subcutaneous haemorrhage.

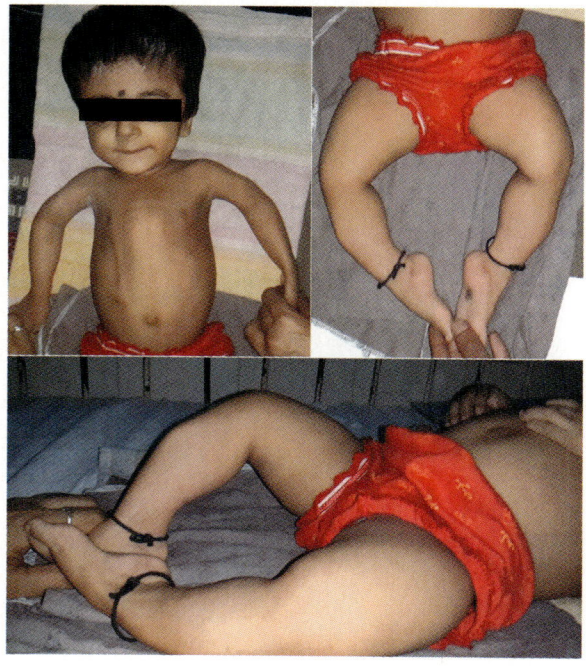

Fig. 33.26: Osteogenesis imperfecta

Forehead: Broad, triangular, elfin-shape of face. Described as 'soldier's helmet head'

Sclera: Due to thinness of collagen layer, intraocular pigment which varies from deep sky blue to bluish white is easily evident, giving rise to classical blue sclera.

'Saturn's ring' appearance may be seen due to white sclera immediately surrounding cornea.

Teeth: Dentinogenesis imperfecta
- Deficient dentin, affecting both milk and permanent teeth.
- Teeth break easily and are prone to caries.
- Yellowish brown or translucent bluish grey tinge is common

Deafness: Usually arises in adult life.

May be conduction type due to otosclerosis or nerve type due to pressure on auditory nerve as it emerges from skull.

Spine: Severe kyphoscoliosis may occur.

Metabolic features: Excessive sweating and intolerance to heat
- Malignant hyperthermia may occur during general anaesthesia.

Radiological features (Fig. 33.27)
- In severe form, the long bones are short, wide and thin. There may be fractures in different stages of healing, malunions, deformities

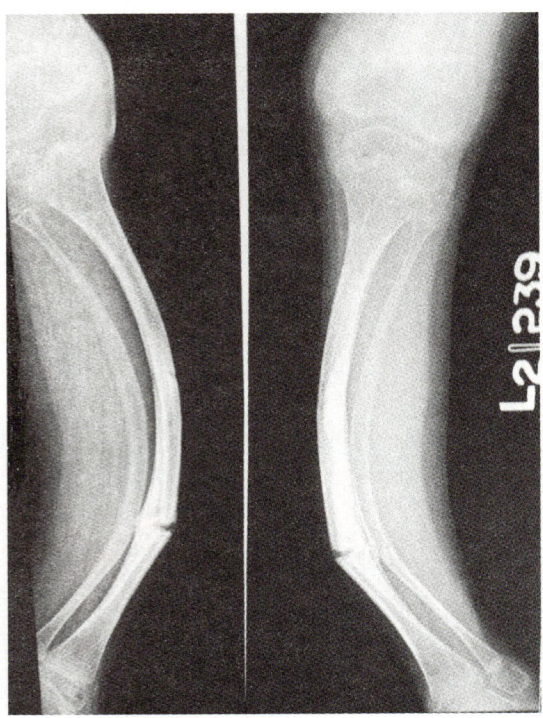

Fig. 33.27: Osteogenesis imperfecta

- Skull: Mushroom appearance with thin calvarium
- Wormian bones: These are detached portions of primary ossification centres of adjacent bones, 4 mm × 6 mm > 10 such bones arranged in mosaic pattern are considered to be significant
- Popcorn calcification and whorls of radiodensities may be evident
- Spine shows marked osteoporosis with biconcave vertebrae.

Diagnosis/Investigations
- *Blood investigations:* Alkaline phosphatase levels may be elevated
- *Prenatal diagnosis:* By measurement of inorganic pyrophosphate in the fluid obtained by amniocentesis. It is usually elevated 3–4 times normal for that gestational age.
- Chorionic villi biopsy at 8–12 weeks can demonstrate synthesis of abnormal pro chains.
- *Genetic:* Molecular defect in type I procollagen can be detected by incubating skin fibroblasts with radioactive amino acids and then analyzing the pro X chains by electrophoresis.

Treatment
- No specific treatment is available to treat the basic pathology of OI.
- Recently, uses of bisphosphonate (pamidronate/zolendronate) have shown to improve BMD and reduce bone pain and fracture frequency.
- Orthoses: To protect the limbs and reduce fracture frequency.
- Surgery: Multiple osteotomies, realignment and intramedullary rod fixation (Sofield-Millar technique) for severe deformities of long bones interfering with orthoses fit. Recently, extensible intramedullary rods are also being used to allow elongation of the rod as the bone elongates.

Prognosis
- In severe variety, perinatal death is common.
- In mild to moderate cases, children remain short statured, prognosis is variable according to frequency of fracture.

ACHONDROPLASIA

Introduction: It is the most common form of dwarfism, inherited as autosomal dominant trait. However, 80–90% cases are sporadic, due to mutation in gene coding for fibroblast growth factor reception 3 (FGFR-3), which plays role in endochondral cartilage growth to regulate linear growth.

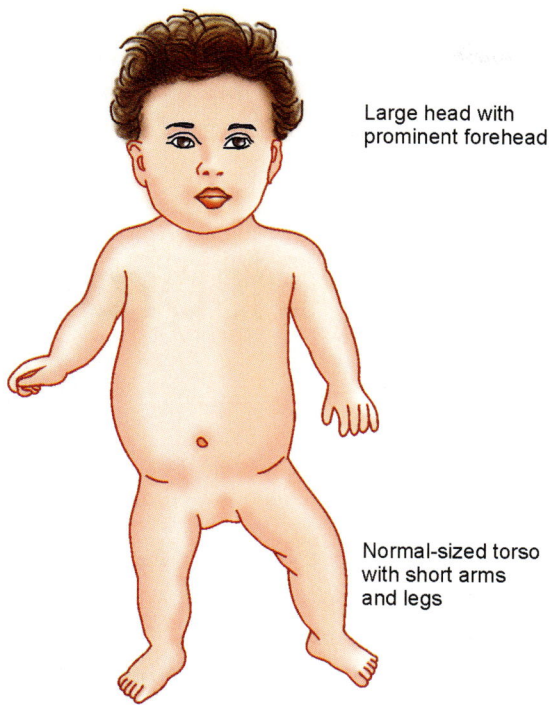

Large head with prominent forehead

Normal-sized torso with short arms and legs

Fig. 33.28: Clinical features of achondroplasia

Clinical features

- Short stature, more severe in proximal limbs (rhizomelic) Trunk height is usually normal, but arm span and standing height is less (Fig. 33.28).
- Ultimate height is about 4 feet 4 inches (131 cm) for males and 4 feet 1 inch (124 cm) for females.
- Skull is usually large with frontal bossing, depressed saddle-shaped nose, small maxilla and prominent mandible.
- Intelligence is usually normal
- *Hands:* Short/broad. Middle finger is shorter than usual, resulting in all the digits being of equal length (Starfish hand).There is separation between middle

and ring finger described as trident hand or main en trident

- *Spine:* Excessively lordotic back and prominent buttocks. Shortening of pedicles may lead to lumbar canal stenosis and disc prolapse in adulthood.
- *Limbs:* Legs bowed, elbows bent.

Radiological features

- Long, tubular bones are short with apparent increase in bony diameter and density
- Epiphyses are normal, physis are V or U shaped, metaphyses are widened.
- Broad pelvis with squared iliac wings giving rise to 'champagne glass' appearance (Fig. 33.29).
- Spinal canal narrows and interpedicular distance reduces from L1 to L5.

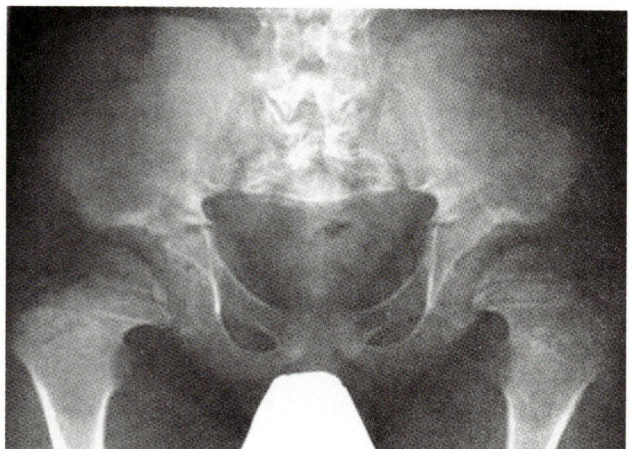

Fig. 33.29: X-ray pelvis in achondroplasia

Treatment

- Increase in height can be obtained by limb lengthening operations.
- Orthopaedic and neurological complications may require specific treatment.

Common Paediatric Disorders

SLIPPED CAPITAL FEMORAL EPIPHYSIS (SCFE)

Introduction

During a period of rapid growth in adolescence, weakening of upper femoral physis and shearing stress from excessive body weight may cause the femoral capital epiphysis to displace from its normal relation to the femoral neck, this is called SCFE.

Incidence

2 per 1, 00,000

- More common in males, and left side
- Blacks more commonly affected
- Higher risk with endocrine and metabolic abnormalities.

Classification (Table 34.1)

I. *Temporal classification* (according to onset of symptoms)
   Acute: Prodromal symptoms < 3 wks.
   Chronic: > 3 wks.
   Acute on chronic: Prodromal symptoms > 3 weeks with sudden exacerbation of pain.

II. *Functional classification* (according to patient's ability to bear weight)
   Stable: Able to wear weight
   Unstable: Unable to wear weight

III. *Morphological classification* (according to the extent of displacement of the femoral epiphysis relative to the neck). Measure femoral head-shaft angle on lateral view (Fig. 34.1).
   Mild (<30°)
   Moderate (30–60°)
   Severe (>60°)

Aetiology

Unknown in majority of patients.

Predisposing Factors

- Obese/hypogonadal male (adiposogenital syndrome)
- Hypothyroidism
- Growth hormone deficiency
- Chronic renal failure (secondary hyperparathyroidism)
- Pan hypopituitarism
- *Mechanical factors:*
  – Thinning of the perichondrial ring complex with maturation
  – Retroversion of femoral neck
  – Obliquity of physis

Pathology

Upward/anterior movement of femoral neck on capital epiphysis causes anterosuperior portion of neck to form a 'hump' or ridge of bone, that impinges on the rim of acetabulum. Usually slip occurs through the hypertrophic zone of physis.

Clinical Presentation

Stable

- Dull/vague pain in the region of groin may be referred to medial aspect of thigh and knee. Pain is continuous/intermittent, exacerbated by physical activities like running or sports.
- Antalgic gait, externally rotated lower limb, thigh atrophy, shortening, limitation of flexion, abduction, internal rotation.

Unstable

- Sudden onset of severe, fracture-like pain in the hip, usually as the result of a relatively minor fall or twisting injury.
- Unable to bear weight.

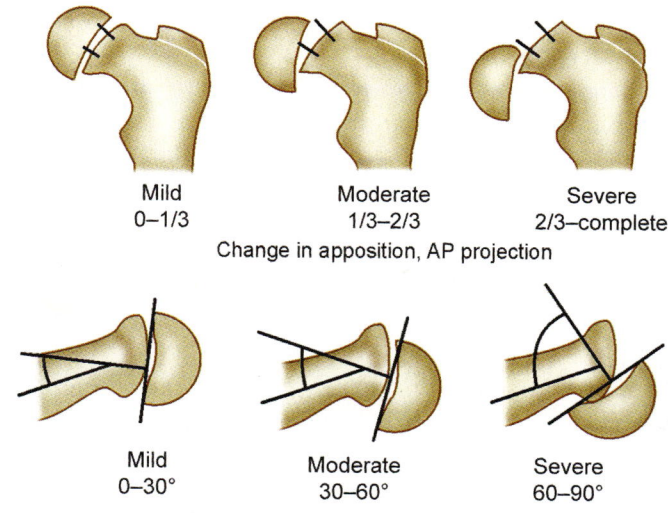

Mild
0–1/3

Moderate
1/3–2/3

Severe
2/3–complete

Change in apposition, AP projection

Mild
0–30°

Moderate
30–60°

Severe
60–90°

Slip angle, true lateral projection

Fig. 34.1: Grades of SCFE

Radiological Investigations

X-rays

- *Earliest sign:* Widening and irregularity of the physis with rarefaction in its juxta-epiphyseal portion (pre-slip stage)
- *Trethowan's sign:* The line drawn tangential to the superior femoral neck on AP view will intersect a very small/no portion of the epiphysis (Fig. 34.2).
- *Metaphyseal blanch sign of steel:* A crescent shaped area of increased density overlying the metaphysis, adjacent to the physis (due to overlapping of femoral neck and posteriorly displaced epiphysis).
- *Lateral view:* Shows the direction of slip.

CT Scan

- To detect decreased upper femoral neck anteversion or true retroversion.
- For more accurate measurement of head-neck angle
- For assessing deformity of upper femur.

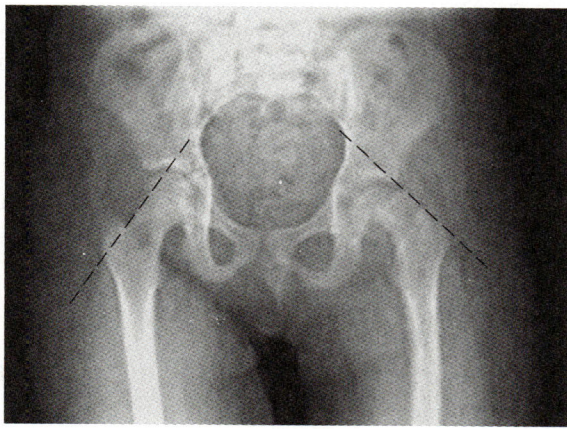

Fig. 34.2: X-ray showing SCFE: Trethowan's sign

Treatment

Goal: To restore the normal relation of femoral head and neck and delay the onset of degeneration.

Time	Mild < 30	Moderate 30–60	Severe > 60
Preslip	Pin *in situ*	-	
Acute < 3 wks	Pin *in situ*	Reduce and pin or pin *in situ*	Reduce and pin
Acute–on -chronic < 3 wks >3 wks	Pin *in situ* Reduce/pin	Reduce and pin or pin *in situ*	Reduce and pin Osteotomy
Chronic > 3 wks	Pin *in situ*	Osteotomy or pin *in situ*	Osteotomy

Table 34.1: Classification and treatment of SCFE severity (degrees)

PERTHES' DISEASE
(LCPD: LEG CALVE PERTHES' DISEASE)

Introduction

LCPD is a childhood osteochondritis of the hip which occurs secondary to avascular necrosis of the capital femoral epiphysis.

Aetiology and Epidemiology

The key feature in the pathogenesis of LCPD is ischemia of femoral head, which may result from a single or repeated vascular insult. Between 4 and 7 years of age, the main blood supply of femoral head is from lateral epiphyseal vessels which are vulnerable to stretching and pressure from an effusion.

Predisposing Factors

- Coagulopathy involving protein C and S and hypofibrinolysis, sickle cell disease, thalassemia
- Abnormal growth and development (delay in bone age relative to patient's chronological age and growth hormone abnormality)
- Trauma, especially in 'predisposed' child
- Hereditary influence (genetic component)
- Environmental influences especially nutritional factors
- Sequelae of synovitis.

Pathogenesis

Perthes' disease is a self-limiting disorder and revascularization of the epiphysis occurs spontaneously over 2–4 years. However, the femoral head may become deformed while revascularisation is occurring and this may lead to osteoarthritis in adult life.

I Stage: Stage of AVN and synovitis. Hypertrophy of articular cartilage of femoral head and acetabulum.

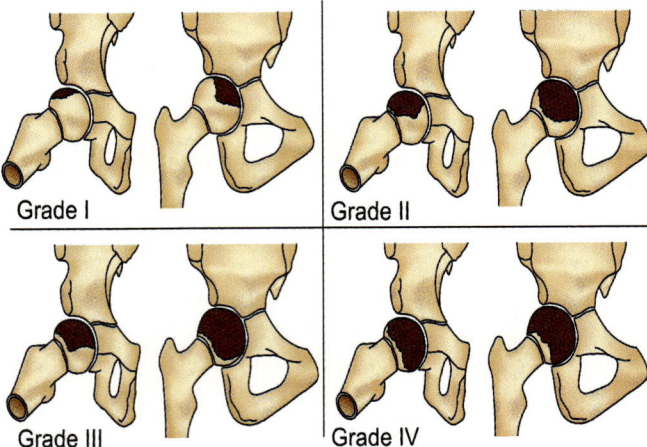

Grade I   Grade II

Grade III   Grade IV

Fig. 34.3: Classification of Perthes' disease

Maximum hypertrophy occurs medially and displaces femoral head laterally.

II Stage: Fragmentation stage. Collapse of necrotic trabeculae of the infarcted zone. Perthes' disease is classified based on extent of involvement of femoral head (Fig. 34.3).

III Stage: Regeneration stage. Immature woven bone replaces infarcted trabeculae.

This 'biologically plastic' bone is vulnerable to deformation by weight bearing stress and muscular forces.

IV Stage: Residual/healed stage. There are residual changes in femoral head–neck in the form of:
- Coxa magna: Enlarged femoral head
- Coxa breva: Short neck
- Coxa irregularis: Distorted contour of femoral head
- Coxa vara: Due to trochanteric overgrowth, there is reduction in neck-shaft angle.

Clinical Presentation
- Onset
  Between 1½ yrs and skeletal maturity
  Majority between 4 and 12 yrs.
- M:F = 4.5:1
- Bilateral in 10–12% patients

Symptoms
- Limp—increased by activity and relieved by rest
- Pain—anterior/groin/around greater trochanter
- H/o antecedent trauma

Signs
- Abductor limp, combination of antalgic and Trendelenburg's gait.
- Positive Trendelenburg's test

- Restricted range of motion, especially abduction and internal rotation
- *Caterall's sign:* When the hip is flexed, it may go into obligatory external rotation.
- Slight atrophy of femoral muscles.

Radiological Features

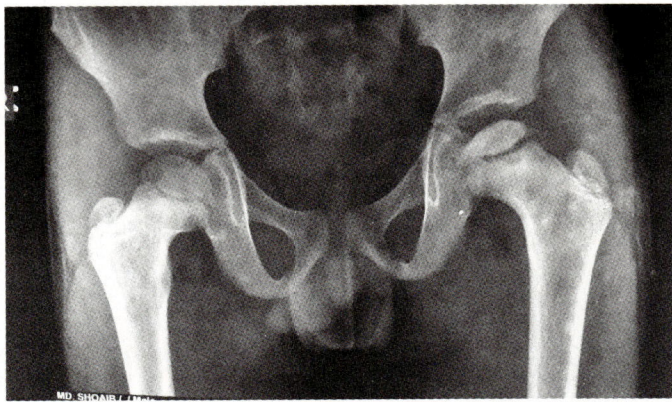

Fig. 34.4: X-ray showing Perthes' affection of hip

Epiphyseal Changes
I. *Avascular necrosis* (Fig. 34.4)
  - Small, denser, flatter capital epiphysis
  - Increased medial joint space
  - Some lateral extrusion of epiphysis
II. *Fragmentation*
  - Radiolucent lines in epiphysis associated with resorption of dead bone
  - Fragmentation of ossific nucleus
III. *Regeneration/revascularization*
  - New bone appears on medial and lateral edges of epiphysis and grows gradually towards centre.
  - Takes 2–4 yrs.
IV. Healed.

Metaphyseal Changes
- Osteoporosis
- Cysts
- Widening of femoral neck

Bone scan: 'Cold area' in region of epiphysis

MRI: Accurate for early diagnosis.

Arthrography
- For shape of femoral head and extrusion of head
- Preoperative and intraoperative use

Treatment
Two methods of treatment
1. Symptomatic/weight relief
  - Rest

- Traction
- Anti-inflammatory drugs.
2. Containment of extruded femoral head: by femoral/acetabular/combined osteotomy. Most commonly done surgery is VDRO: Varus Derotation Osteotomy (Fig. 34.5)

Best result are obtained if containment is done in early fragmentation stage.

Prognosis

Depends on the following factors.
1. *Age of onset:* Best if treated <6 yrs.
   >10 yrs: Almost all develop osteoarthrosis
2. *Extent of epiphyseal involment:* Poor prognosis if >50% epiphysis is involved
3. Lateral extrusion of femoral head
   If > 20 %: Poor prognosis

TRANSIENT SYNOVITIS OF THE HIP

Introduction

It is a condition characterized by acute onset of mono-articular hip pain and limp in a child without any systemic illness, with gradual and complete resolution of symptoms over time in majority of cases.

Other names: Observation hip, irritable hip, toxic synovitis.

Aetiology

Exact aetiology not known. Usually associated with,
- Nonspecific upper respiratory tract infection (70%)
- Local trauma (20–30%)
- Allergic predisposition (16–25%)

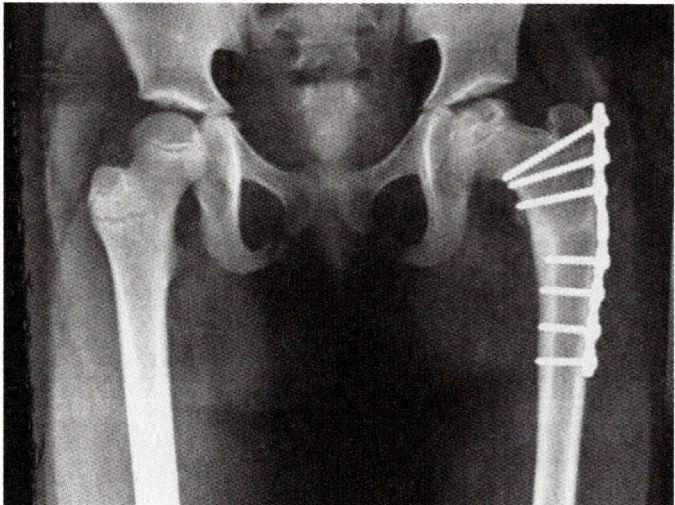

Fig. 34.5: Femoral osteotomy for containment of hip

Clinical Presentation

- Age of presentation: 3–18 yrs. Average: 6 yrs.
- H/o respiratory infection may be present
- Acute onset pain in groin
- Limp, antalgic gait
- Flexion contracture and adductor spasm
- Restricted movements of hip, especially abduction and internal rotation
- Low grade fever may be present

Investigations

Diagnosis of transient synovitis is a diagnosis of exclusion
- X-ray/USG: Mild effusion present in 70%
- MRI: Altered signal in bone marrow
- Other investigations like CBC, urine, RA factor, Mantoux test, etc. are done to exclude other hip pathologies that may mimic transient synovitis in early stages.

Differential Diagnosis

- Septic arthritis
- Perthes' disease
- Koch's hip
- Osteomyelitis of femoral neck/pelvis
- Slipped capital femoral epiphysis
- Tumour

Natural History

Complete resolution of symptoms and signs usually occurs within 10 days. In long term, recurrence noted in up to 17% cases. Coxa magna occurs in about 32% patients.

Treatment

- Strict bed rest and nonweight bearing till synovitis resolves
- Avoid strenuous activites of hip.
- Traction with hip in 30–40° flexion, if spasm persistent.
- Anti-inflammatory medication for symptomatic relief
- No role of routine hip aspiration

GENU VALGUM (KNOCK KNEE)

Introduction

Valgus alignment of lower limb is normal in the child between 2 and 8 years of age with maximum amount of physiological valgus between 2 and 4 years. Beyond 8 years, there should be little/no change in lower limb

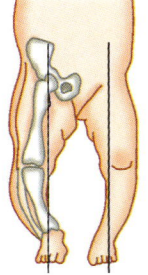
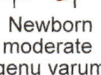
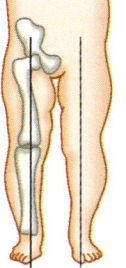
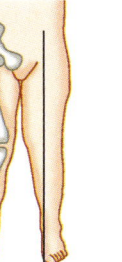
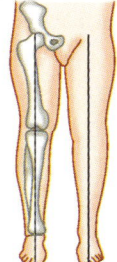

Newborn moderate genu varum — 1½ to 2 years legs straight — 2 to 6 years physiologic genu valgum — 6 to 8 years legs straight

Fig. 34.6: Evolution of lower limb alignment from varus to valgus

alignment. An outward deviation of the longitudinal axis of lower limb with apex at medial knee is called genu valgum (Fig. 34.6).

Aetiology

- Physiological (75% cases)
- Idiopathic (most common)
- Post-traumatic
- Metabolic (rickets) (Fig. 34.7)
- Spondyloepiphyseal dysplasis/metaphyseal dysplasia
- Enchondromatosis/fibrous dysplasia/Multiple exostosis

Clinical Presentation

- Knock-knee with increased intermalleolar distance (Fig. 34.7)
- Knee discomfort
- Difficulty in running
- Gait disturbance
- Patellar malalignment
- Ligament laxity
- Cosmetic concern
- Plumb line test: Normally a line drawn firm ASIS to middle of the patella, if extended down strikes the medial malleolars. In genu valgum the medial malleolus is outside this line.
- Knee flexion test: To detect the site of deformity. On flexion of the knee, if the deofrmity disappears, the cause lies in the lower end of femur. But if the deformity in flexion persists, the cause lies in upper tibia.

X-Ray

Standing alignment X-ray from hip to ankle with patella facing forward to measure the valgus angle and cause of deformity (Fig. 34.8A and B).

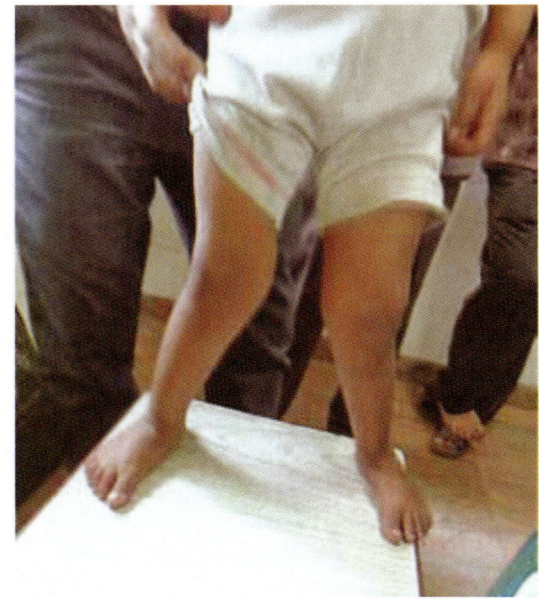

Fig. 34.7: Bilateral genu valgum

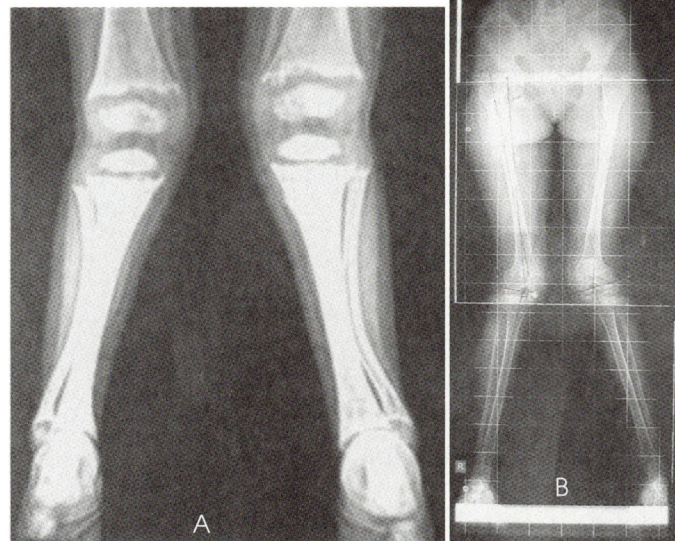

Fig. 34.8: (A) X-ray showing bilateral genu valgum secondary to rickets, (B) Standing alignment X-ray

Treatment

- *Younger child (boys <12 yrs, girls <10 yrs):* Reversible/ transient hemiepiphysiodesis of distal medial femoral condyle using '8' plate.
- *Older children near/after skeletal maturity:* Corrective medial closed wedge osteotomy in distal femur (Fig. 34.9).

GENU VARUM (BOWLEGS)

It is a very common paediatric deformity, defined as lateral angulation of the knee.

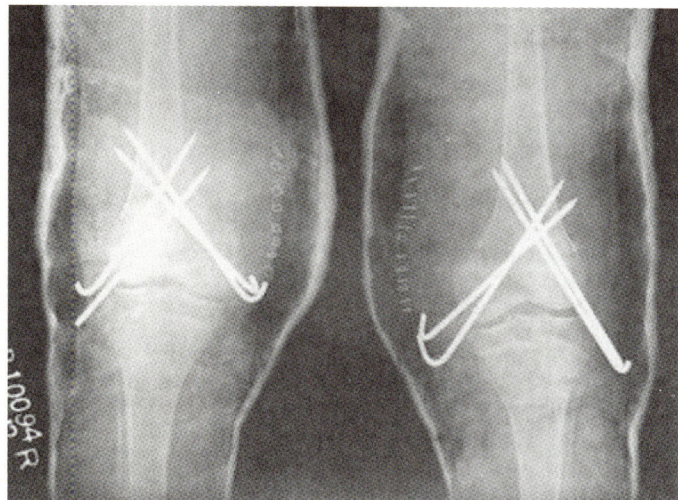

Fig. 34.9: Genu valgum corrective osteotomy

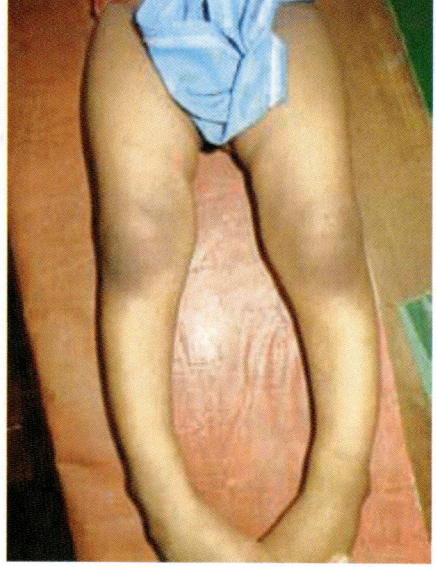

Fig. 34.10: Bilateral genu varum

Physiologic Genu Varum

A deformity with

- A tibiofemoral angle of at least 10° varus
- A radiologically normal appearing growth plate
- Medial bowing of proximal tibia and often of the distal femur.

The legs of most new borns typically are bowed with 10–15° varus angulation. When the infant begins to stand and walk, the bowing may appear more prominent with weight bearing. The presence of genu varum beyond 2 yrs, can be considered abnormal.

Etiology

Unilateral

- Due to growth abnormalities/trauma/tumour of upper tibial or distal femur epiphysis
- Infection like osteomyelitis

Bilateral

- Development/congenital causes
- Metabolic/endocrine disorders. Most common cause is rickets
- Idiopathic
- Degenerative disorders in adults (like OA knee)
- Blount's disease (tibia vara)

Clinical Presentation

- Bowlegs with increased intercondylar distance (Fig. 34.10).
- In-toeing of both feet.
- Ligament laxity.

X-Ray

- Apparent delay in ossification of medial side of distal femur and proximal tibial epiphyses (Fig. 34.11).
- Flaring of medial distal femoral metaphysis.

Treatment

- Physiological genu varum resolves spontaneously. Regular follow up is necessary to ensure resolution.
- Lateral hemiepiphysiodesis for skeletally immature and corrective lateral closed wedge or medial open wedge osteotomy nearing/after skeletal maturity (Fig. 34.12).

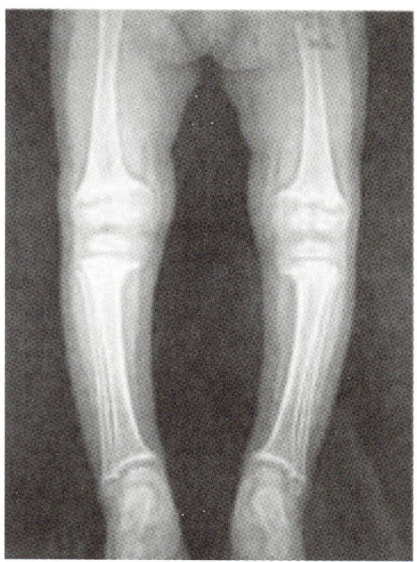

Fig. 34.11: X-ray of bilateral genu varum secondary to rickets

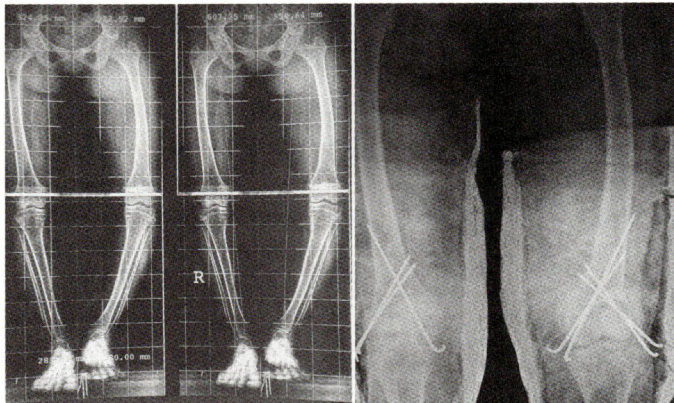

Fig. 34.12: Genu varum treated with corrective osteotomy

FLAT FOOT/PES PLANUS

Introduction

Pes planus/flat foot refers to loss of the normal medial longitudinal arch.

Pathoanatomy

- *Hindfoot:* Valgus
  Calcaneus eversion at subtalar joint
- *Midfoot:* Lateral angulation /abduction at midtarsal joint (talonavicular and calcaneocuboid)
- *Forefoot:* Supinated relative to hind foot

Types

- *Flexible:* On non-weight bearing, a rather normal appearing medial longitudinal arch develops.
- *Fixed/rigid:* Even on non-weight bearing, arch does not appear.

Aetiology

Rigid

- Tarsal coalition: Calcaneo-navicular(C-N), talo-calcaneal (T-C) (Fusion between various tarsal bones)
- Accessory navicular
- Peroneal spastic flatfoot

Flexible: Ligament laxity

Clinical Presentation

- Majority asymptomatic
- Large bony prominence medially may interfere with footwear.
- Vague foot pain, especially dorsolaterally, difficulty walking on uneven surfaces, foot fatigue, painful limp.

- Accessory navicular: Bursitis
- Tibialis posterior tendinitis
- Synchondritis (between accessory and main navicular)
- Tarsal coalition: Peroneal muscle tightness and associated pain

Radiological Features (Fig. 31.13)

X-ray: AP/lateral/45° oblique views

- Look for bony bar C-N/T-C
- Plantar flexion of talus, 'sag' at T-N/N-C joints/both
- Increased talocalcaneal divergence
- Accessory navicular

CT scan: Helpful in c/o small tarsal coalition.

Treatment

- *Asymptomatic child < 3 yrs:* No treatment.
- *Symptomatic child with flexible pes planus:* Medial arch support in shoes.
- *Symptomatic accessory navicular child <10–12 yrs:* Excision and rerouting tibialis posterior into more plantar position.
- *Symptomic flat feet:* Soft tissue balancing procedure/calcaneal osteotomy/triple arthrodesis.
- *Rigid flatfeet with tarsal coalition:* Resection of bony bar with fat or muscle interposition or triple arthrodesis.

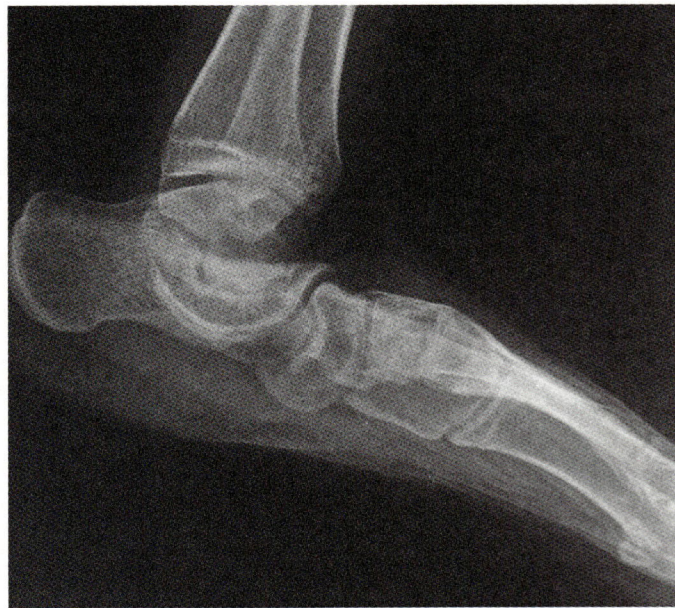

Fig. 34.13: X-ray foot showing 'Sag' at talonavicular joint in pes planus

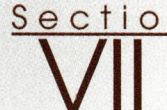

Other Orthopaedics Disorders and Special Subjects

Neurological Disorders

POLIOMYELITIS

Definition: Poliomyelitis is a viral infection of the anterior horn cells of spinal cord or motor nuclei of brainstem, causing paralysis of muscles of limbs and spine.

Pathogenesis

There are 3 types of causative viruses.
- Brunhilde (Type I)
- Lansing (Type II)
- Leon (Type III)

Transmission: Faeco oral route

The virus travels through nerve and blood to reach and damage anterior horn cells of spinal cord/motor nuclei of brainstem. This causes lower motor neuron type of paralysis of corresponding muscle/muscle group. The changes in neuron cells are reversible to a certain extent and hence marginal recovery of some paralysed muscles is possible.

Clinical Presentation (Figs 35.1 and 35.2)

Stage I (Acute stage)

Pre-paralytic:
- Marked tenderness of involved muscles
- Fever/headache
- Ache/spasm of back muscles

Paralytic:

Acute flaccid asymmetrical paralysis without any sensory/bladder-bowel involvement.
- *Spinal form:* Muscles of extremities and trunk affected.
- *Bulbar form:* Cranial nerves affected.

Stage II (Recovery/Convalescent)

Gradual recovery of paralysed muscles over 3–6 months, may be up to 2 years.

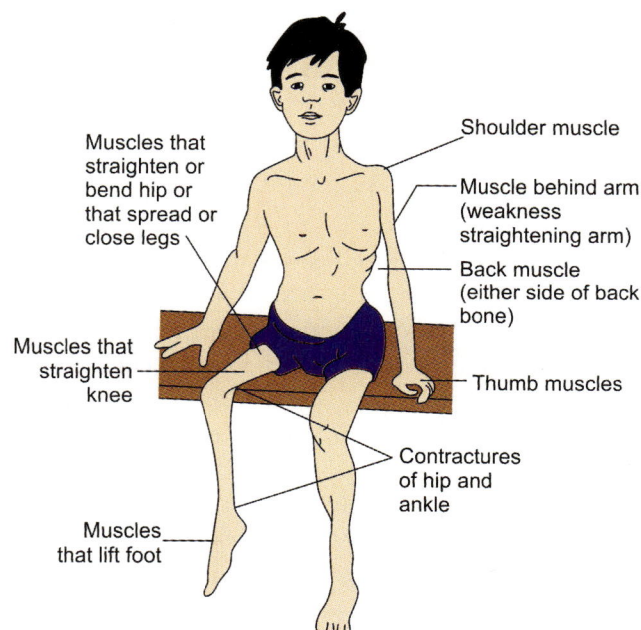

Muscles that straighten or bend hip or that spread or close legs

Muscles that straighten knee

Muscles that lift foot

Shoulder muscle

Muscle behind arm (weakness straightening arm)

Back muscle (either side of back bone)

Thumb muscles

Contractures of hip and ankle

Fig. 35.1: Commonly involved muscles in poliomyelitis

Stage III (Residual paralysis stage)
- Post polio residual paralysis (PPRP, beyond 2 years of onset of disease)
- Deformity occurs due to muscle imbalance.

Common Deformities
- *Hip:* Flexion, abduction, external rotation
- *Knee:* Flexion, triple deformity, genu valgum
- *Foot:* Talipes equinovarus

Management

Acute stage: Medical management of fever and meningeal irritation.

Recovery stage: To prevent deformities and assist natural recovery
- Physiotherapy
- Splinting

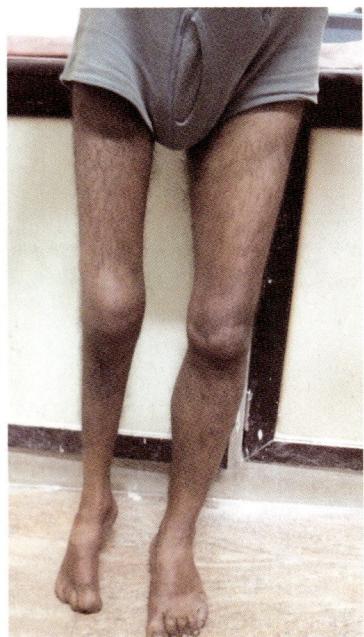

Fig. 35.2: PPRP

Stage of PPRP: After thorough assessment, various types of soft tissue/bony surgeries are advocated

- Release of flexion/abduction contracture of hip, flexion contracture of knee and equinus contracture of ankle.
  - *Ober-Yount's procedure:* Release of iliotibial band contracture
  - *Soutter's release:* Muscle originating from anterosuperior iliac spine released.
- Osteotomies to correct knee deformity.
- Improvement of muscle balance by tendon transfer surgeries.
- Arthrodesis, e.g. triple arthrodesis in foot.

ARTHROGRYPOSIS MULTIPLEX CONGENITA (AMC)/AMYOPLASIA CONGENITA/MULTIPLE CONGENITAL CONTRACTURE (MCC)

Introduction

AMC is a non-progressive syndrome characterized by contractures of multiple joints in the body right from birth.

Aetiology

Two main types:

1. *Neurogenic:* More common—
   - Due to degeneration or reduced number of anterior horn cells, peripheral nerves and motor end plates.
   - Characterized by weakness of muscles.

2. *Myogenic*
   - 10%
   - Myodystrophy with replacement of muscle by fibrofatty tissue.

Eight different forms of AMC are encountered.

Common variety is quadriplegic type: Scoliosis may be present in 20%.

Clinical Features (Fig. 35.3A and B)

- Rigid and deformed joints
- Common deformities:
  - *Foot:* Equinovarus/planovalgus
  - *Knee:* Flexion/fixed extension
  - *Hip:* Flexion, abduction, external rotation
  - *Wrist:* Flexion

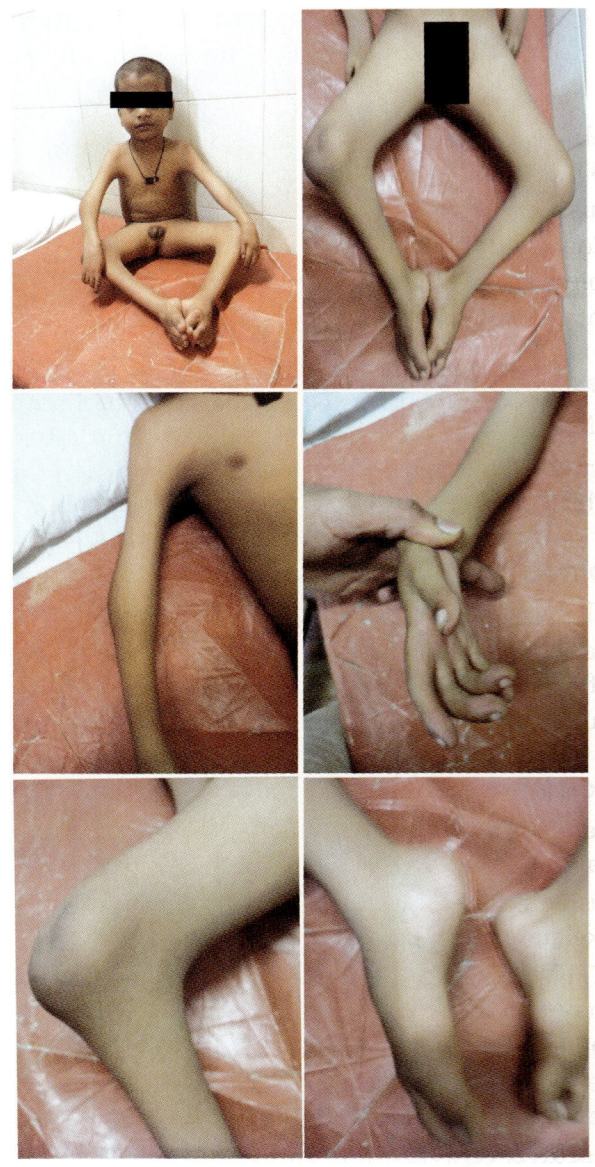

Fig. 35.3A: Clinical features of AMC

Typical Baby with Arthrogryposis

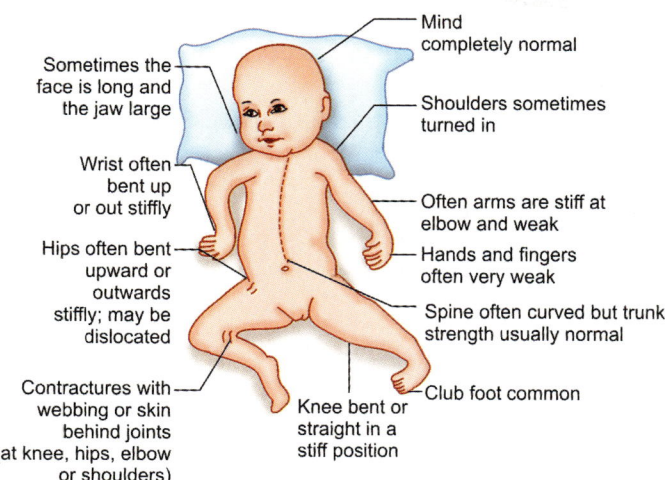

Fig. 35.3B: Clinical features of AMC

- – *Elbow:* Extension
- – *Shoulder:* Internal Rotation
- Absent/weak atrophic muscles
- Diminished joint creases and subcutaneous tissue
- Fusiform, cylindrical, cone-shaped extremity
- Contracture of capsule and periarticular structures
- Joints may be dislocated, e.g. hip
- Intact sensation and intellect

Investigations

- EMG/nerve conduction study
- X-ray for dislocation, scoliosis
- MRI

Treatment

Goal is to make the patient ambulatory.

- Passive stretching exercise/serial casting or splinting of limb.
- Surgical correction

Principles of Surgery

- Tenotomies to be accompanied by capsulotomy or capsulectomy
- Osteotomies to be done only after completion of skeletal growth (to prevent recurrence)
- CTEV (congenital talipes equinovarus) correction may require talectomy
- DDH (developmental dysplasia of hip) may not reduce by closed method and may require open reduction.
- Recurrence is common due to inelastic nature of muscles.

MYELOMENINGOCELE (MMC)

Introduction

MMC is a sac-like structure containing CSF and neural tissue. The hernial protrusion of the spinal cord and its meninges through a defect in the vertebral canal results in variable neurological defects depending on the location and severity of lesion.

Pathogenesis

The nervous system develops by formation of a tubular structure (neurulation) and closure of this tube is due to closure of cranial and caudal neuropores at about days 24 and 26 of gestation (Fig. 35.4).

True MMC results from failure of fusion of neural folds during this process.

Associated Neurological Conditions

- *Hydrocephalus:* 80–90% association
- *Arnold-Chiari malformation*
- Tethered spinal cord
- *Hydromyelia:* Accumulation of fluid in enlarged central spinal canal.

Common Orthopaedic Problems in MMC

- Club foot
- Hip dislocation
- Kyphosis
- Scoliosis

Classification and Clinical Presentation

Based on neurological level of lesion.

Group I: Thoracic and high lumbar level

- No quadriceps function
- Community ambulation difficult

Meningomyelocele

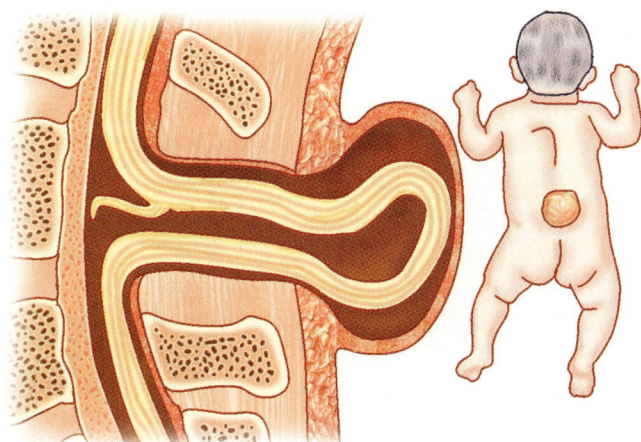

Fig. 35.4: MMC

Group II: Low lumbar level (Fig. 35.5)
- Quadriceps and medial hamstrings good
- No gluteus medius function
- Most children require AFO for support and crutches for trunk stability.

Group III: Sacral level
- Functioning quadriceps and gluteus medius
- Most children can walk without support

Investigations
- X-ray LS spine
- CT scan/MRI
- Early diagnosis: Maternal serum AFP (alpha feto protein)
- Amniotic fluid for AFP
- Ultrasound scan

Treatment
Goal: To achieve a stable posture
- In spite of the best medical and surgical care, about 40% of children with MMC will not walk as adults.
- Most children achieve maximum level of ambulation around 4 yrs of age.

Non-operative treatment
- Aimed at obtaining effective mobility with minimal restriction.
- Depending on level of affection, various types of orthoses like AFO, KAFO, HKAFO (hip knee ankle foot orthosis) are used.

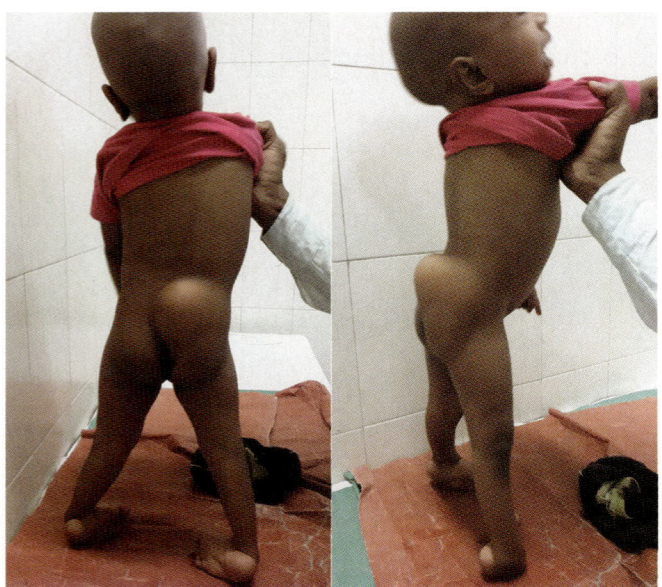

Fig. 35.5: MMC low lumbar level

Operative treatment
Principles
- Multiple procedures preferred under single anaesthesia.
- Possible complication to be kept in mind
  - Increased chance of disuse osteoporosis and pathological fracture.
  - Decreased sensation
  - Increased danger of infection secondary to urinary problems.

Common Surgeries
- Radical posteromedial release with excision rather than lengthening of tendons for CTEV
- Radical release for knee flexion contracture.
- Release surgery for hip contracture.
- Surgery for spine deformity correction.

Prevention
All pregnant women should take folic acid during pregnancy to prevent occurrence of MMC.

DUCHENNE'S MUSCULAR DYSTROPHY (DMD)

Introduction
Muscular dystrophy is defined as a group of chronic disease with most prominent characteristic being progressive degeneration of skeletal muscles leading to weakness, atrophy, contractures, deformity and progressive disability.

Aetiology
Majority cases of muscular dystrophy are inherited. Two common types of muscular dystrophy are Duchenne and Becker.

DMD: 30% occur as spontaneous gene mutation

Becker's: Begins later in life and slowly progressive.

Genetic pattern: Sex linked dystrophy where mother is the carrier. Almost never found in a female child.

Clinical Features (Figs 35.6A and B)
- Normal at birth
- H/o delay in walking
- Toe walking, flat foot or clumsiness
- By 3–5 years, difficulty in climbing stairs and arising from a sitting position.
- *Gower's sign:* While getting up from floor, the child has to take support of his hands on knees, as if the child climbs on himself.

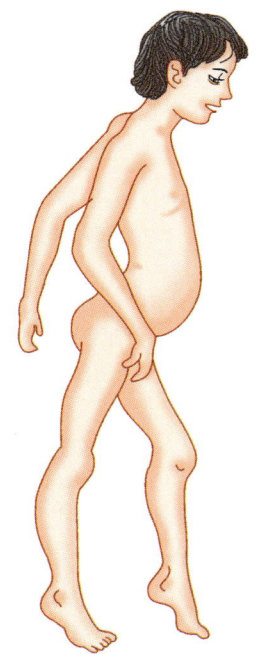

Fig. 35.6A: Clinical features of DMD

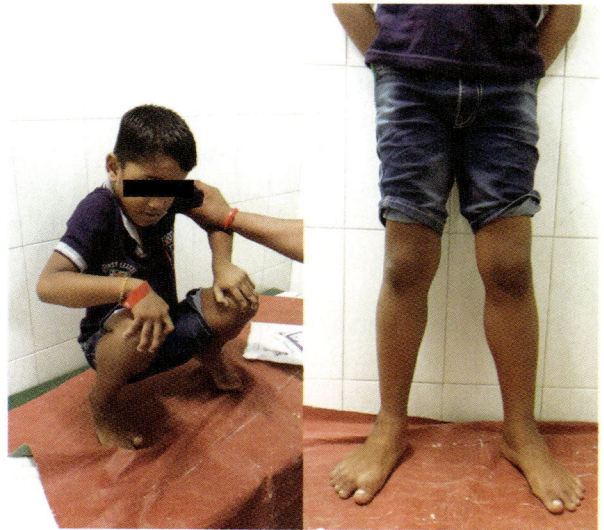

Fig. 35.6B: Gower's sign and pseudohypertrophy of calf

- Pseudohypertrophy of muscles especially calf (muscles replaced by fibrous tissue and fat infiltration).
- Progressive weakness from proximal to distal in axial and limb musculature with eventual unstable gait and frequent falls.
- Progressive deformity of spine.
- 80% children develop cardiomyopathy, mild congestive heart failure and fatal pneumonia.

Investigations
- Sr. CPK levels markedly raised
- Muscle biopsy
- 2-D echo to detect cardiomyopathy
- Early diagnosis—genetic counselling to prevent at risk births by following tests.
  - Amniotic fluid analysis
  - USG to know probability of male offspring.

Treatment
Three stages:
1. *Ambulation:* From birth till child is a household and community walker.
2. *Transition:* Community ambulation becomes difficult.
3. Wheel-chair confinement.

Aim of treatment is to maintain walking by prevention and treatment of contractures. Later orthoses can be applied.

Recently, role of stem cell therapy is being investigated for DMD.

CEREBRAL PALSY/LITTLE'S DISEASE

Definition
It is a non-progressive upper motor neuron lesion arising in childhood, affecting the locomotor system.

Causes
Prenatal/natal/postnatal

Prenatal
Genetic factors
- Kernicterus
- Developmental defect in CNS

Natal
- Birth asphyxia
- Prematurity

Postnatal
- Head injury
- Encephalitis/meningitis
- Cardiovascular accidents (stroke)

Classification
Topographic: Diplegia/hemiplegia/paraplegia/quadriplegia/monoplegia

Clinical: Spastic/athetoid/ataxic/rigid/mixed
   Spastic type is the commonest (70%).

SPASTIC CEREBRAL PALSY

Pathology

Part of the motor cortex of the brain is replaced by areas of gliosis. There is degeneration of pyramidal tracts.

Clinical Features (Fig. 35.7)

- Delayed milestones
- *Weakness:* Marked muscle imbalance
- *Spasticity:* Muscles are stiff and resist passive movements
- Exaggerated deep tendon reflexes/clonus
- *Lack of voluntary control:* When a patient attempts to move a single group of muscle, other group contracts at the same time.
- *Deformity:* When spasm and muscle imbalance are pronounced, fixed deformity develops.
- Commonest deformity of upper limb:
  – Flexion at elbow
  – Pronation of forearm
  – Flexion of wrist
  – Adduction of thumb
- *Commonest deformity of lower limb:*
  Flexion adduction of hip
  Flexion at knee
  Equinus of ankle
- *Mental deficiency:* Usually intelligence is normal
  Impairment in speech
  Defective vision, deafness

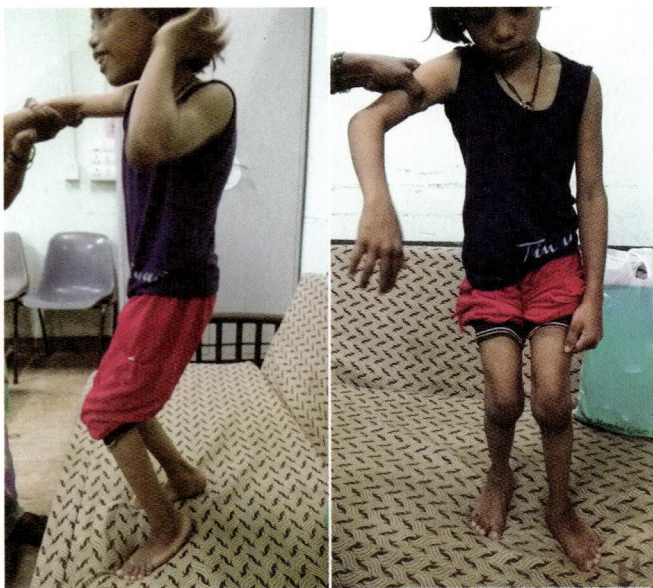

Fig. 35.7: CP child with crouch

Prognosis

Complete cure is impossible, but improvement can occur with regular therapy, surgical treatment.

Treatment

Multidisciplinary approach is important including orthopaedic surgeons, neurologists, physiotherapist, occupational therapist, speech therapist.

The aim of treatment is to achieve maximum functional ability and skill that child can acquire.

1. *Muscle training:* By therapist
   Principle
   - To teach the child to relax spastic muscles
   - To develop use of individual muscle group
   - To improve coordination
   - To train in ADL (activities of daily living)
2. *Splints:* After correction of deformity by gradual stretching of contracted muscle/manipulation under anaesthesia/surgical release, plaster is given for 6–8 weeks and later splints are given for maintenance and prevention of recurrence.
3. *Surgical treatment*
   - Tendon division or elongation, e.g.
     – Adductor tenotomy
     – Fractional lengthening of hamstring
     – Gastrocnemius aponeurotic lengthening
   - *Tendon transfer:* Muscle which is aggravating deformity may so modify muscle's action that it acts beneficially instead of as a deforming farce, e.g. hamstring transfer in fixed flexion deformity of knee.
   - *Arthrodesis:* When skeletal growth is complete, it is sometimes done to eliminate persistent deformity from pull of spastic muscle, e.g. wrist arthrodesis.
   - *Osteotomies*, e.g. extension osteotomy in supracondylar femur region for fixed flexion deformity of knee.
   - *Neurectomy:* To divide part or whole of the nerve that supplies an overactive spastic muscle, e.g. anterior branch of obturator nerve for adduction deformity of hip.
4. *Botox injection:* This anticholinergic agent acts at neuromusclular junction, inhibits stretch reflex thereby reducing spasticity. The action lasts for 3–6 months and dose is adjusted according to individual muscle and weight of the patient.

The injection can be repeated if required.

Metabolic Disorders

SCURVY

Introduction

Scurvy is a metabolic bone disorder, occurring due to lack of vitamin C, characterized by dysfunction of osteoblasts and failure to produce osteoid tissue and form new bone.

Normal requirement of vitamin C: Varies as per age 20–40 mg/day for normal function of collagen tissue in children.

Natural sources: Citrus fruits, green vegetables, cow's milk, human milk.

Clinical Presentation

2 types

I. Infantile Scurvy

- Presentation between 6 months and 2 years.
- Painful walking, tender lower limb and irritability (pseudoparalysis) due to subperiosteal haemorrhage.
- Joints swollen and tender
- Tender costochondral beading due to depression of sternum (different from rounded beading in rickets).
- Bleeding from various sites:
  Gums: Bluish discolouration and loose teeth.
  Retro-orbital: Proptosis
  Microscopic haematuria
  Malena
- Low grade fever, anaemia

II. Adult Scurvy

- Not very frequent
- Non-specific weakness, anorexia, weight loss, fatigue
- Haemorrhage and ecchymosis of skin, subcutaneous tissue and gums.
- Haemarthrosis
- Osteoporosis especially in spine—biconcave vertebrae

Investigations

Radiological (Fig. 36.1)

Diagnostic features are seen especially at sites of rapid bone growth, e.g. knee, wrist, proximal humerus and costochondral junction.

- Generalised osteoporosis
- Ground glass appearance and pencil thin contex: due to lack of formation of osteoid tissue and normal osteoclastic resorption activity.
- White line of Frankel at metaphysis
- Ringing of epiphysis (due to calcification of normal chondroitin tissue)
- Calcified sub-periosteal haemorrhage.
- Subluxation of epiphysis may occur due to weak zone of provisional calcification.
- Zone of rarefaction under white line of Frankel: Characteristic of scurvy.
- *Corner/angle sign:* Peripheral metaphyseal cleft due to defect in spongiosa and cortex just adjacent to provisional zone of calcification, seen as spur on X-ray.

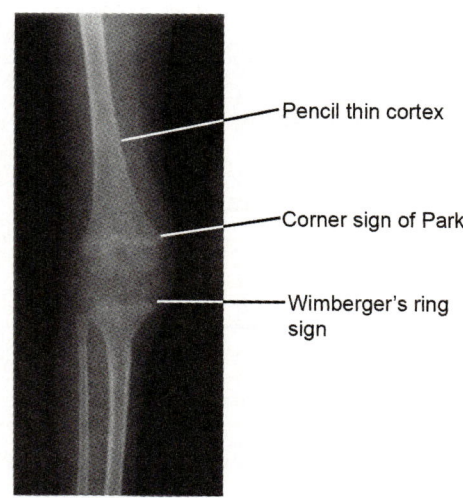

Pencil thin cortex

Corner sign of Park

Wimberger's ring sign

Fig. 36.1: Radiological features of scurvy

Laboratory Investigations

- Fasting Sr. Vitamin C < 6 mg/L
- Anaemia
- Microscopic haematuria

Differential Diagnosis (Pseudoparalysis)

- Poliomyelitis
- Congenital syphilis

Treatment

- Vitamin C oral/parenteral 100–200 mg daily.
- Prognosis is excellent and complete recovery is possible.

RICKETS AND OSTEOMALACIA

Introduction

Rickets and Osteomalacia are metabolic bone disorders of growing and mature bones respectively, occurring due to deficiency of calcium and/or phosphorus leading to defective mineralization of bone and softening.

Metabolic Control of Ca Metabolism

Note the metabolic control of calcium metabolism (Fig. 36.2) and normal metabolism of vitamin D (Fig. 36.3). Various types of rickets according to aetiology:

I. Nutritional/Vit. D Deficiency Rickets

- Dietary deficiency
- Impaired skin production
- Malabsorption—liver/pancreatic disease
  Coeliac disease
  Postgastrectomy
- Rickets of prematurity

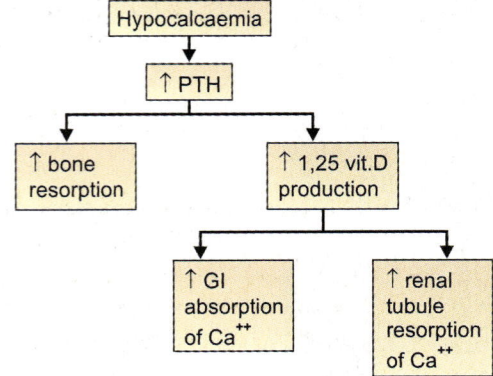

Fig. 36.2: Metabolic control of calcium metabolism

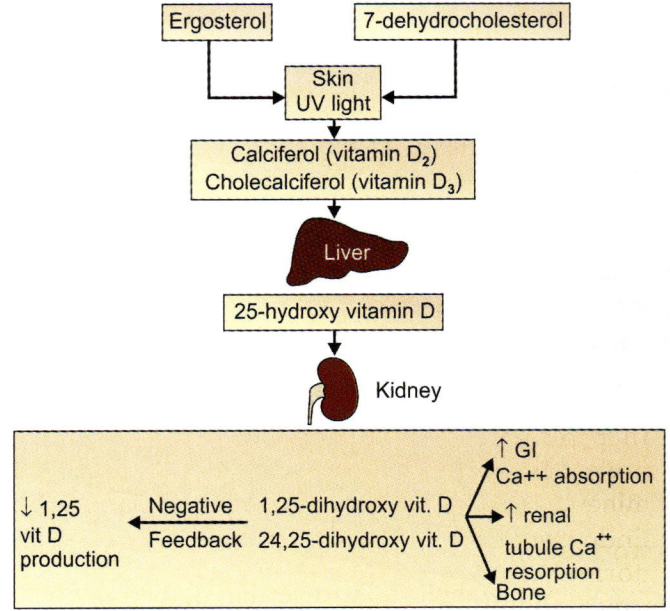

Fig. 36.3: Normal metabolism of vitamin D

Vitamin D deficiency → failure of absorption of calcium and phosphorus → hypocalcaemia and hypophosphatemia → release of PTH.

II. Familial Hypophosphatemic Rickets (Renal Tubular Rickets)

A group of disorders in which normal dietary intake of vitamin D is insufficient to achieve normal mineralization of bone.

a. Vitamin D resistant (Fanconi, oncogenic rickets, renal tubular acidosis):

Kidney excretes fixed bases and wastes bicarbonates leading to wasting of Na^+ and Ca^{2+}.

Renal tubules' inability to retain phosphorus leads to phosphate diabetes and hypophosphatemia.

b. Vitamin D dependent type I (inability to hydroxylate):

Failure of kidney to perform second hydroxylation of vitamin D.

c. Vitamin D dependent type II (receptor insensitivity)

III. Renal Osteodystrophy (Renal Glomerular Rickets)

Congenital renal disease, leading to damage of glomeruli and inability of glomeruli to excrete phosphorus, hence hyperphosphatemia → decreased production of vitamin D → hypocalcaemia → secondary PTH increase.

Pathology

- Primary disturbance is failure of calcification of cartilage and osteoid tissue.

Table 36.1: Biochemical features of various types of rickets

Condition	Ca	Phos.	Alk Phos.	PTH	25 (OH) Vit D	1.25 (OH)$_2$ Vit D
Nutritional	N/↓	N/↓	↑	↑	↓↓	↓
Vitamin D resistant	N	↓	↑	N	N	N
Vitamin D dependent (Type I)	↓	↓	↑	↑	↑↑	↓↓
Vitamin D dependent (Type II)	↓	↓	↑	↑	N/↑↑	↑↑↑↑
Renal osteodystrophy	N/↓	↑	↑	↑↑	N	↓↓

In proliferative zone, chondrocytes multiply normally, but zone of calcification is poorly mineralized.

Endosteal and periosteal osteoblastic activity is normal, forming abundant osteoid, which is irregularly placed.

Osteoclastic resorption of uncalcified osteoid does not occur, hence wide osteoid seams are formed leading to thin, weak new trabeculae.

With just loading, metaphysis becomes wide, cortices are thin and prone for stress fracture/deformity.

Clinical Features (Fig. 36.4A and B)

Generalised muscle weakness, lethargy, listlessness, irritability

Delayed motor milestones

Protuberant abdomen with separation of recti

Craniotabes/box shaped large head, open fontanelle, frontoparietal bossing (hot cross bun)

Metaphyseal widening of ankle (double malleoli), wrist, knee

Rachitic rosary (enlargement of costochondral junction causing beaded ribs)

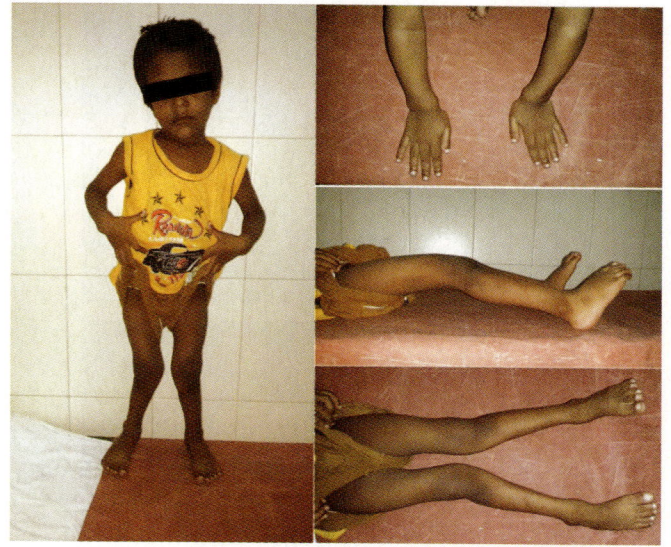

Fig. 36.4B: Clinical picture of rickets

- Harrison's groove: Lateral indentation of chest due to pull of diaphragm on ribs
- Pectus carinatum (forward projection of sternum)
- Short stature
- Limb deformities (genu varum/valgum, coxa vara)
- Kyphoscoliosis
- Delayed dentition with irregular, soft, decaying teeth.
- Pale skin, flabby subcutaneous tissue
- Waddling gait (in osteomalacia) due to pseudo-fractures.

Radiological Features (Fig. 36.5)

- Bowing of diaphysis with thinning of cortices
- Cupping, fraying, splaying of metaphysis.
- Osteopenia
- Looser's zone in 20%

  Looser's zone are thin transverse bands of rarefaction due to incomplete stress fracture which heals with callus, seen especially in shafts of long bones.
- Cod fish (biconcave) vertebra and trefoil/champagne glass appearance of pelvis.

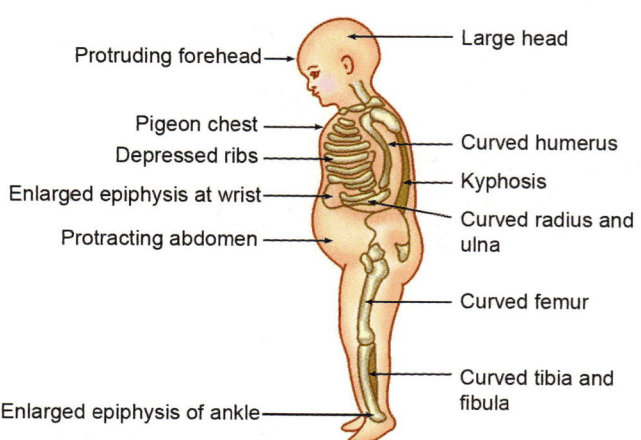

Protruding forehead

Pigeon chest

Depressed ribs

Enlarged epiphysis at wrist

Protracting abdomen

Enlarged epiphysis of ankle

Large head

Curved humerus

Kyphosis

Curved radius and ulna

Curved femur

Curved tibia and fibula

Fig. 36.4A: Clinical features of rickets

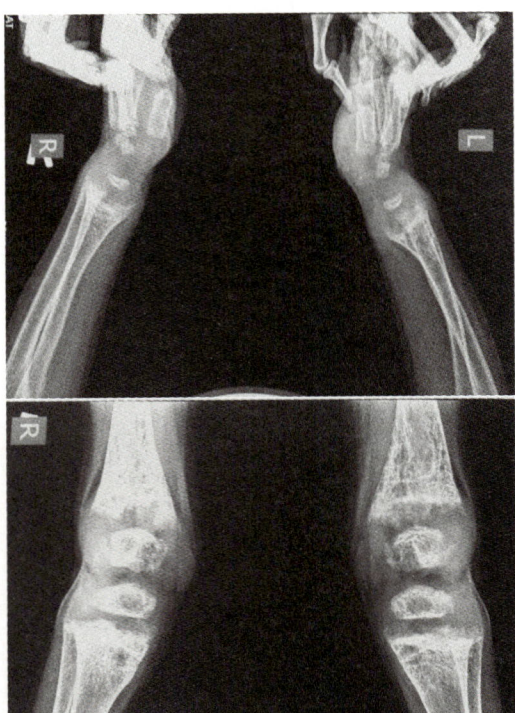

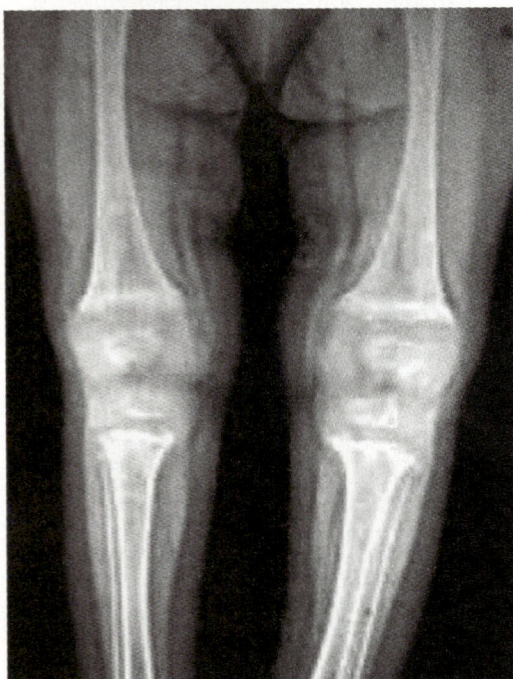

Fig. 36.5: Radiological features of rickets

Investigations/Biochemical Abnormalities

- Most types of rickets and osteomalacia are characterized by diminished levels of Sr. Ca and P, raised levels of alkaline phosphatase and diminished urinary excretion of calcium (Table 36.1).
- Renal function tests: BUN, Sr. creatinine.
- USG kidney.

Management

Dietary advice, exposure to sunlight.

Medical Treatment

- Single oral dose of 6 lakh IU vitamin D
- If no signs of healing in 3–4 weeks, then second dose can be given.
- In severe cases, maintenance dose of 400–600 IU daily may be required.
- Prevention of deformity by avoiding weight bearing, giving rest and splints for the legs.

Surgical Treatment

- Corrective osteotomy for established genu varum/valgum deformity of lower limb in mature child.
- Growth modulation plate in skeletally immature children.

OSTEOPOROSIS

Definition: Osteoporosis is defined as reduction in the mass per unit volume of bone, leading to increased risk of fracture. According to WHO, it is defined as a bone density that falls 2.5 standard deviation (SD) below the mean for young healthy adults of same race and gender (T score–2.5). This occurs when the rate of bone resorption exceeds that of bone formation.

Predisposing Factors

- Sedentary lifestyle
- Early menopause
- Steroid therapy
- Asthenic build
- Family history
- Smoking/alcohol
- Low calcium diet

Causes

- *Primary/age related/involutional*
  Normal blast activity (unassociated with disease)
  - Type I: Postmenopausal in females (>45 yrs.)
  - Type II: Senile (males > females) > 55 yrs.
  - Type III/idiopathic: Child/young men and premenopausal women
- *Secondary/active/pathological:*
  (Associated with disease)
  - Endocrine
  - Metabolic
  - Nutritional
  - Drug induced
  - Postimmobilization
  - Association with congenital and heritable disorders.

Clinical Features

- Asymptomatic until complicated by fracture, occurring as a result of trivial trauma.
- May be associated with dull vague bone pain, low back pain, weakness, slow movements.

Common Sites of Fracture

- Neck of femur
- Distal radius
- Wedge compression fracture dorsolumbar spine

Investigations

Radiological: Minimum of 30% loss of bone mass is essential for detection of osteoporosis on X-ray.

Vertebrae: Loss of small horizontal trabeculation with prominence of vertical striations is the earliest change.
- Ground glass appearance
- Loss of vertical height of vertebrae due to collapse, especially anterior part (Fig. 36.6).
- Wedge compression fracture (Fig. 36.7).

Femur: Singh's osteoporosis index is based on femoral head and neck trabecular pattern (Fig. 36.8).

It is one of the most accurate diagnostic and prognostic scales of assessment.

Grades

VI: Normal/minimal thinning of secondary trabeculae.

V. Loss of secondary compression and tension trabeculae.

IV. Thinning of primary tension trabeculae.

III. Fragmentation of primary tension trabeculae.

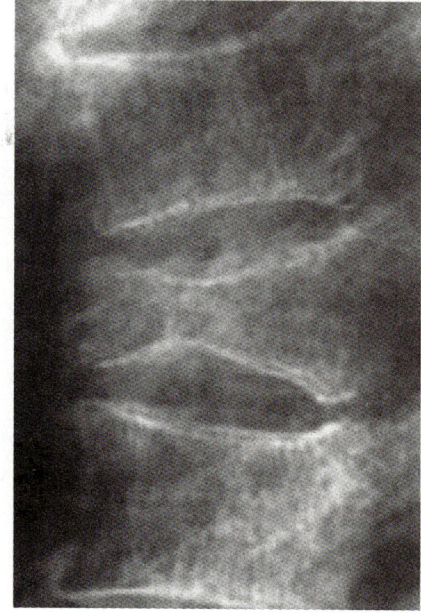

Fig. 36.7: Osteoporotic compression fracture of vertebra

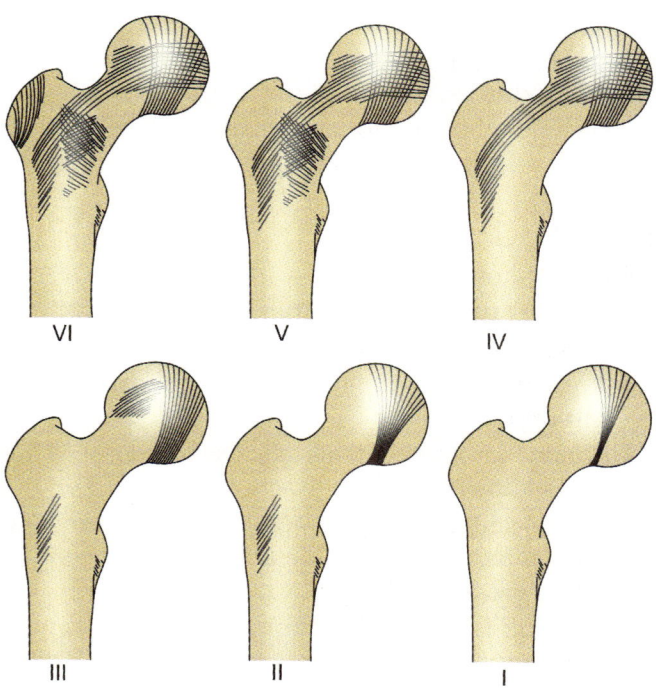

Fig. 36.8: Singh's index

II. Complete absence of primary tension trabeculae.

I. Thinning and fragmentation of primary compression trabeculae.

Pathological/stress fracture can occur in femur neck if Singh's index is low.

Metacarpal index and vertebral index: Combined thickness of both cortices is <45% of bone width.

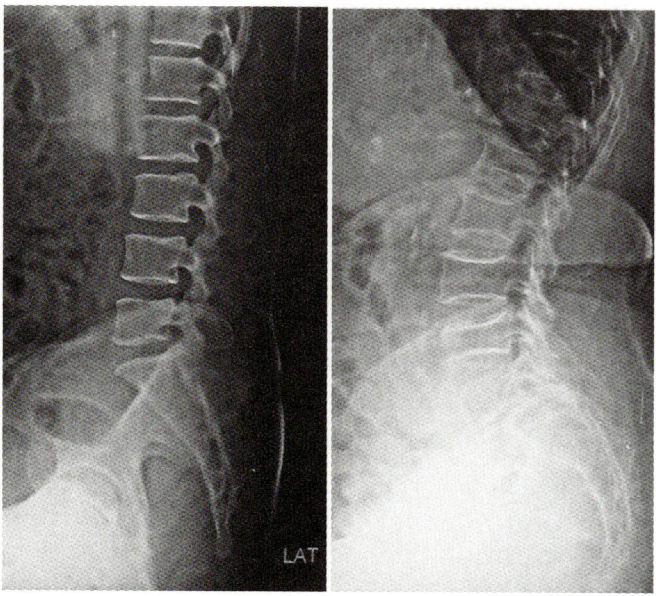

Fig. 36.6: Normal and osteoporotic bone

Laboratory Investigations

- Serum Ca/P/Alk phosphatase is usually normal
- Urine hydroxyproline: Increased excretion
- Urine hydroxypyridium compounds: More specific for increased resorption.
- Sr. Osteocalcin: Specific marker for decreased bone formation.
- Investigations for cause of secondary osteoporosis: Sr. BUN/creatinine/hormonal assay.

Other Investigations

1. *DEXA/Bone mineral density analysis:* For knowing T-score (matched with young adults) and Z-scores (age matched).

   T score – 1 or more: Normal

   –1 to –2.5 : Osteopenia

   Less than – 2.5: Osteoporosis
2. Neutron activation analysis.

Treatment

General measures

- High protein and calcium rich diet.
- Use of spinal brace-like ASH (anterior spinal hyperextension) or Taylor's brace to prevent compression of vertebrae and kyphotic deformity.
- Regular exercise of back, postural exercise and walking.

Drugs

1. Bisphosphonate:
   - Inhibits osteoclast activity and bone resorption.
   - Dose of alendronate: 10 mg/day
   - Newer drugs: Etidronate, ibandronate, risedronate
2. Hormone replacement therapy: Oestrogen 0.625 mg. daily is known to reduce fracture rate by 75%
3. SERM (selective estrogen receptor modulator) like reloxifen reduces other side effects of estrogen like uterine/breast cancer.
4. *Calcitonin:* Given as injection (50–100 IU/day) or nasal spray (200 IU/day).

   It reduces pain and slows down bone loss by inhibiting osteoclastic activity.
5. *Calcium supplement:* 1000 to 1500 mg/day and Vit. D analogue 0.5 mcg/day or vitamin D (600–2800 IU/day).

Surgical

- Use of locking plates while treating fractures in osteoporotic bones.
- Vertebroplasty (bone cement insufflation) for restoring vertebral body height and reducing back pain.

FLUOROSIS

Skeletal fluorosis is a bone disease caused by excessive consumption of fluoride. In advanced cases, skeletal fluorosis causes pain and damage to bones and joints. Fluorosis is of two types:

1. Dental fluorosis
2. Skeletal fluorosis

Common Causes of Fluorosis

1. Consumption of fluoride from drinking water derived from deep bore wells. Over half of ground water sources in India have fluoride above recommended levels.
2. Inhalation of fluoride dusts/fumes by workers in industry, use of coal as an indoor fuel source which is a common practice in China.
3. Consumption of fluoride from the drinking of tea, particularly brick tea.

   Skeletal fluorosis can be caused by cryolite (Na_3AlF_6, sodium hexafluoroaluminate).

Symptoms

- Limitation of joint movement
- Calcification of ligaments of neck, vertebral column
- Crippling deformities of the spine and major joints
- Muscle wasting
- Neurological defects/compression of spinal cord
- Increased frequency of fractures.
- Most patients suffering from skeletal fluorosis show side effects from the high fluorine dose such as gastritis and nausea.
- Fluorine can also damage the parathyroid gland leading to hyperparathyroidism.

Treatment

No established treatments for skeletal fluorosis patients.

Patients with fractures are treated accordingly.

Arthritis

OSTEOARTHRITIS (OA)

Definition

Osteoarthritis (more rightly, osteoarthrosis) is a degenerative, non-inflammatory, slowly progressive disease of diarthrodial (synovial) joints, characterized by destruction of articular cartilage and formation of new bone at the joint surface and margins.

Types

- *Primary/idiopathic:* Cause unknown.
- *Secondary:* Joint cartilage altered by various conditions.

Predisposing Factors

1. **Age:** By 55–65 years of age, approximately 85% have radiological evidence of the disease.
2. **Sex:** Beyond 55 years, more severe and more generalized in women.
3. **Heredity:** Genetic tendency in OA knee twice as strong as in OA hip.
4. **Obesity:** Prevalence of OA twice in obese individuals.

Secondary Osteoarthritis

- *Trauma:* Major trauma, repetitive stress, meniscal and cruciate ligament injury.
- *Congenital/developmental disorders:* Perthes' disease, developmental dysplasia of hip, slipped capital femoral epiphysis, bone dysplasia
- *Inflammatory:* Rheumatoid arthritis
- *Metabolic disorders:* Gout, ochronosis, haemochromatosis.
- *Endocrine disorders:* Diabetes mellitus, hypothyroidism, hyperparathyroidism, acromegaly.

Joints Commonly Involved

- Any synovial joint may be affected, but most severe degeneration occurs in joints subjected to weight bearing like hips, knees, lower spine and the joints affected by strong, repetitive muscle force, e.g. 1st metatarsophalangeal and 1st carpometacarpal joint and midcervical joints.
- Other common affections are in hands (Fig. 37.1):

  Distal interphalangeal joint *(Heberden's nodes)*

  Proximal interphalangeal joint *(Bouchard's nodes)*
- *Less common sites:* Glenohumeral, acromioclavicular, tibiotalar joint.

Pathogenesis (Fig. 37.2)

- Focal degeneration of articular cartilage.
- Alteration of the physicochemical characteristics, diminishing the cartilage resistance to compressive and tensile force.
- Development of fibrillations, deep clefts, shredding.
- Formation of marginal osteochondral outgrowths *(osteophytes)*.
- Eventual joint deformity. In the knee, the degenerative process usually begins in the anteromedial compartment, leading to varus deformity.

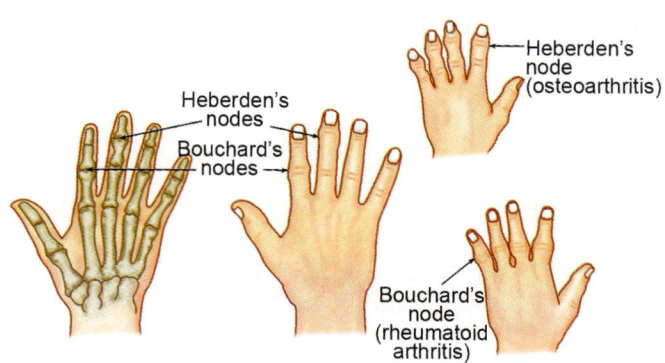

Fig. 37.1: Osteoarthritis of DIP and PIP joints

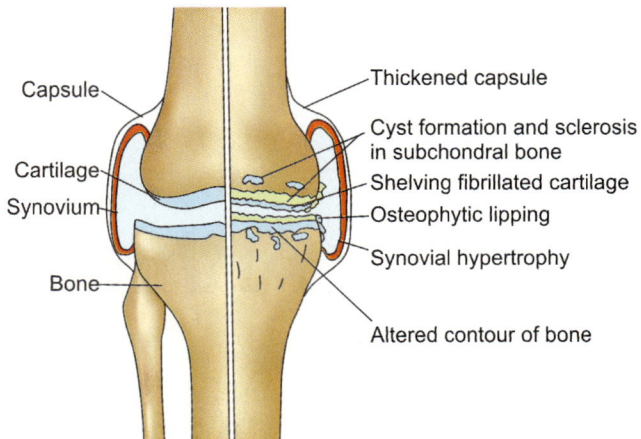

Fig. 37.2: Pathology of osteoarthritis

Clinical Features

- Pain is the predominant clinical symptom. It is insidious in onset, continuous, mild, aching.
- Stiffness occurring with rest, pain felt after rising in the morning
- Swelling and deformity may occur due to effusion
- Deformity may be evident in advanced cases
- Limited range of motion associated with grating sensation
- *Muscle spasm and wasting:* Quadriceps is the main muscle involved in OA knee

Investigations

- *Blood investigations:* ESR/RA test/Sr. uric acid for knowing underlying cause.
  Hypothyroid state in 10–30% of patients
- *X-ray:* Weight bearing X-rays are important (Fig. 37.3). In the early stage, X-rays are normal, but gradually, joint space narrowing develops.

- *Advanced stage*
  - Marked narrowing of joint space.
  - Sharp articular margin.
  - Subchondral cysts/sclerosis.
  - Loose bodies and deformities.
- *Synovial fluid examination:* Non-inflammatory parameters.

Treatment

Conservative: 50% patients respond to conservative line of treatment in the form of:

Rest: During an acute inflammatory attack

Physiotherapy:
- Moist heat
- Range of motion exercise
- Isometric exercise

Drugs
Analgesic, anti-inflammatory during acute stage.
Chondroprotective: Glucosamine, chondroitin sulphate tablets (during early stage).
Viscosupplementation: Intra-articular hyaluronate injection in the knee for improving joint lubrication
Use of knee brace/walking aids
Management of predisposing factors like obesity

Surgical
- Total joint replacement: TKR/THR (Fig. 37.4)
- Chondral resurfacing procedure
- Arthroscopic lavage
- Corrective high tibial osteotomy (HTO) for OA knee

Indications for Surgery

- Pain refractory to conservative treatment
- Deformity

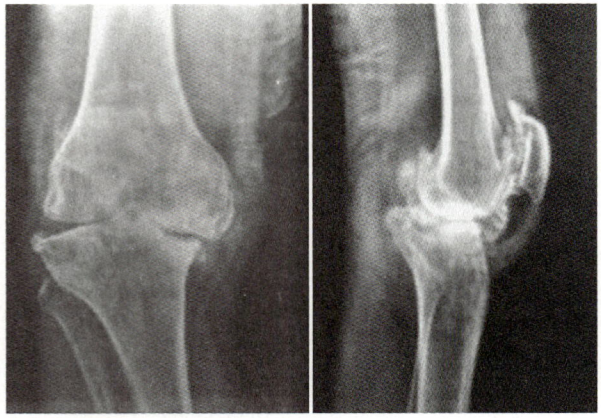

Fig. 37.3: X-ray knee AP and lateral showing severe osteo-arthritis

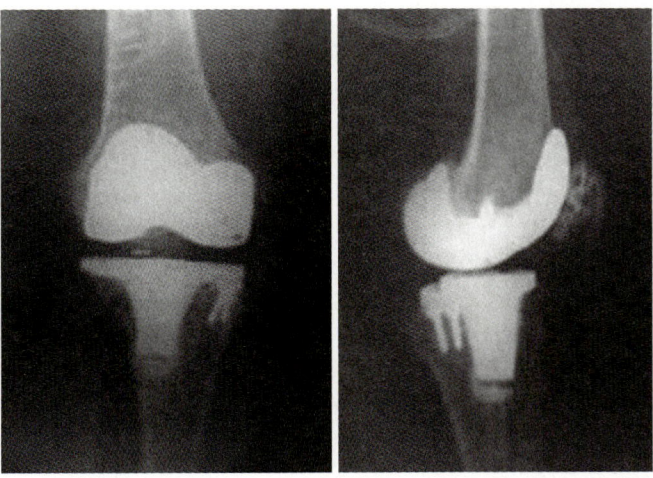

Fig. 37.4: X-ray features of OA knee treated with total knee arthroplasty

- Joint instability
- Progressive limitation of motion

RHEUMATOID ARTHRITIS (RA)

Introduction

Rheumatoid arthritis is an immunologically mediated chronic multisystem disease of young or middle aged adults, characterized by persistent inflammatory synovitis involving peripheral joints in a symmetrical distribution.

Joints involvement: Usually symmetrical affection of synovial joints.

Commonly involved:
- Wrist, MCP, PIP joint
- Elbow, knee, ankle, MTP joint

Less commonly involved:
- Hip joint
- Upper cervical spine facet joint with atlantoaxial dislocation.

Not involved:
- DIP joint
- Lumbar spine

Pathogenesis (Fig. 37.5)

The most widely held theory of pathogenesis is that an immunological response takes place in the synovial tissue.

Exogenous antigen(Ag) attacks lymphocytes.

↓

Transformation into larger plasma cells

↓

Formation of antibody (Ab)

↓

Ag + Ab complement form complex

↓

Lysosomes of phagocytic cells engulf and destroy the complex partially

↓

Some lysosomes escape from phagocytic cells and their protease attacks the cartilage and synovium

↓

Self-perpetuating cycle of destruction → debris → phagocytic response → further destruction.

- 'Pannus' is the granulomatous mass formed by inflamed synovium that grows over and destroys cartilage, tendons and ligaments.
- In response to human IgG, auto-antibodies are synthesized as *rheumatoid* factor.

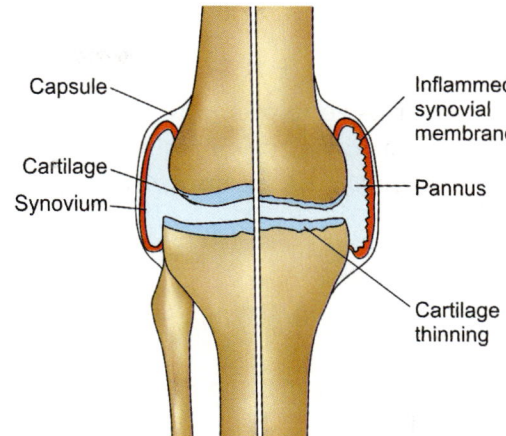

Fig. 37.5: Pathogenesis of RA

- The typical microscopic lesion is an area of fibrinoid necrosis surrounded by fibroblasts arranged radially to the surface of necrosis. Eventual result is fibrous ankylosis.

Clinical Features

- 80% affection in females.
- Mean age of onset: 40 years
- Usually insidious onset with stiffness and aching of various joints. Later there is pain, swellings, warmth, tenderness, and limited motion of joints with typical fusiform appearance
- Order of involvement: Hands-feet-knee-wrist

Characteristic Deformities of Hands/Feet (Fig. 37.6)

- **Z-deformity:** Radial deviation of wrist and ulnar drift of the digits with palmar subluxation of the digits with palmar subluxation of proximal phalanx
- **'Swan-neck' deformity:** Hyperextension at PIP joint and flexion at DIP joint.
- **Boutonnière deformity:** Flexion at PIP and extension at DIP joint
- Hind **foot** eversion, plantar subluxation of metatarsal heads, splaying of forefoot, hallux valgus, and hammer toes.

The course is one of remissions and exacerbations.

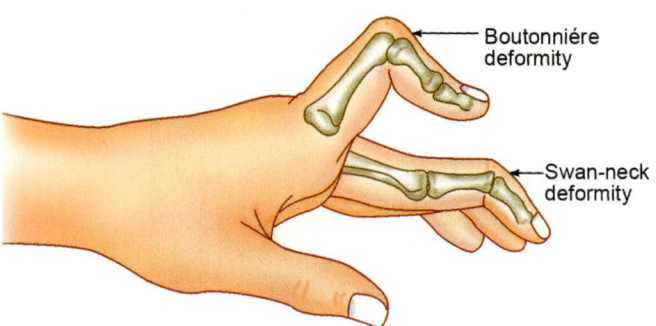

Fig. 37.6: Hand deformities in RA

Diagnosis

Radiological Features (Fig. 37.7)

- Juxta-articular osteoporosis, cortical thinning
- Symmetrical narrowing of joint interval in later stage
- Finally, bony trabeculations bridge and obliterate the joint space.

Laboratory Findings

1. Raised ESR (even up to 100 mm) especially in active stage.
2. Hypochromic, normocytic anaemia
3. Positive RA factor.

   RA factor
   - It is IgM auto Ab reactive with IgE
   - Found in 2/3rd patients of RA
   - Not specific for RA
   - Found in 5% of healthy persons and many other conditions like tuberculosis and leprosy.
   - Not useful as screening procedure, but more of prognostic value.
   - High titres of RA is suggestive of poor prognosis.
4. Anti-CCP antibody titres: Highly specific for rheumatoid arthritis.

1987 Revised Criteria for RA

According to the American College of Rheumatology, at least 4 out of 7 criteria should be present for diagnosis of RA, patients with 2 or more criteria are not excluded.

Criteria 1 to 4 must be present for at least 6 weeks.

1. Morning stiffness > 1 hour before maximum improvement.
2. Arthritis of 3 or more joint areas (observed by a physician simultaneously) having soft tissue swelling or joint effusion, not just bony overgrowth.

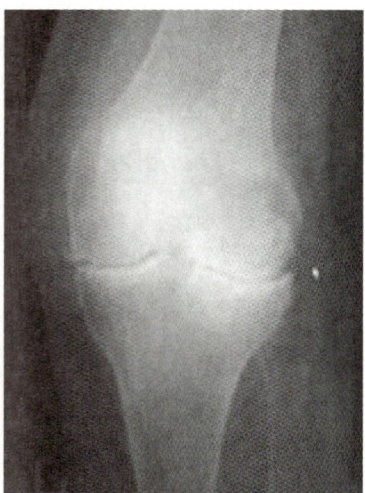

Fig. 37.7: X-ray features of RA

3. Arthritis of hand joints, e.g. wrist, MP or PIP.
4. Symmetrical changes: bony erosion or unequivocal bony decalcification, periarticular osteoporosis and narrowing of joint space.
5. Rheumatoid nodules.
6. Serum rheumatoid factor demonstration.
7. X-ray changes: Periarticular osteopenia/erosion.

Treatment

Aim of treatment: To keep the inflammatory process at a minimum, thereby preserving joint motion and preventing secondary joint stiffness and deformity.

Medical Treatment

- NSAID (nonsteroidal anti-inflammatory drugs)
- DMARDS (disease modifying anti rheumatic drugs)
  - Methotrexate
  - Antimalarial, e.g. chloroquine
  - Sulfasalazine
  - Gold compounds
  - D-Penicillamine
- Glucocorticoid therapy, e.g. in vasculitis and systemic manifestations
- Immunosuppressive therapy
- Anti-cytokine (TNF neutralizing) agent, e.g. infliximab, etanercept.

Physiotherapy

- Rest
- Splints to immobilize inflamed joint
- Exercise to maintain joint motion
- Lifestyle modification

Surgical Management

- *Synovectomy:* Open/arthroscopic
- Total joint replacement, e.g. knee/hip/hand joints (Fig. 37.8)

Prognosis

- Median life expectancy is shortened by 3–7 years
- Raised mortality in severe articular disease attributed to cardiovascular disease, bleeding or infection.

JUVENILE RHEUMATOID ARTHRITIS (JRA)

Still's Disease

It is a generalized multisystem disease that can result in severe sequelae, like crippling joint deformities, heart disease, amyloidosis and permanent blindness.

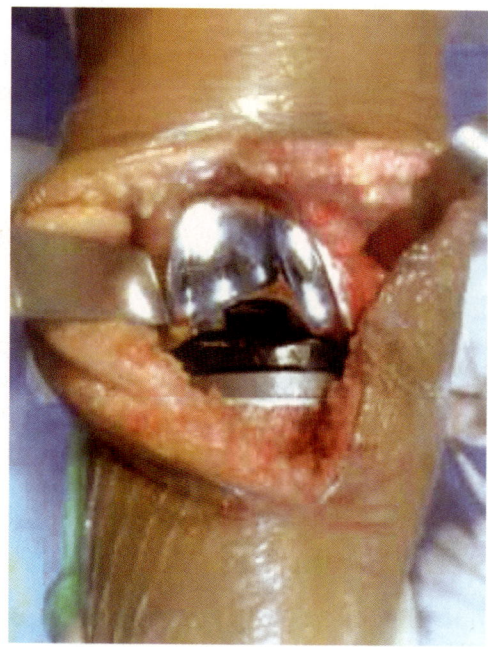

Fig. 37.8: Intraoperative picture of TKR

Features that are Different from Adult RA

- High fever
- Characteristic rash
- Lymphadenopathy
- Splenomegaly
- Chronic iridocyclitis, may lead to blindness
- Pericarditis
- Only 50% polyarticular involvement
- RA factor positive in 15–20%
- More common in females, F:M = 7:3
- Average age of onset: 6 years
- Systemic corticosteroids indicated in JRA when other treatment fails, cases of iridocyclitis and life threatening complications.

GOUT

Introduction

Gout is a disorder of purine metabolism characterized by hyperuricaemia, deposition of mono-sodium urate crystals in and around joints, causing repeated attacks of acute synovitis (Fig. 37.9).

Also known as podagra when it involves the big toe.

Epidemiology

Age: Male >30 years, female—after menopause
Sex: M: F~20:1

The risk of developing clinical features and complications of gout increases with increasing levels of serum uric acid.

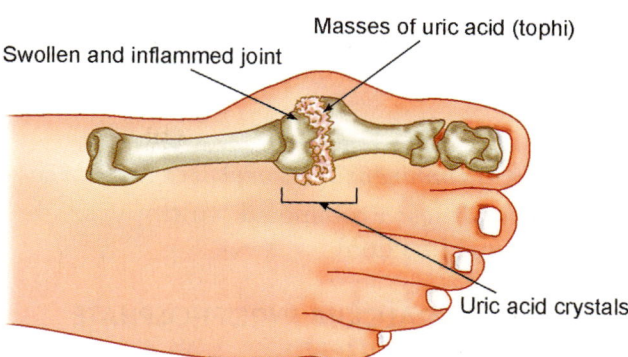

Fig. 37.9: 1st MTP gout arthritis

Pathology

Monosodium urate crystals get deposited in small clumps forming the classical gouty 'tophi' (porous stones). They can ulcerate through skin or destroy the cartilage and periarticular tissue. The nodular deposits can be found in articular cartilage (especially small joints of hands and feet), tendon, bursae, synovium, subcutaneous tissue, ligaments, periarticular tissue, pinna of ear, kidney.

Clinical Features

- Sudden onset of severe joint pain, usually following minor trauma, unaccustomed exercise, illness or alcohol consumption
- Common sites: MTP joint of big toe, ankle, finger joints, olecranon bursa.
- The overlying skin is red, shiny, swollen, hot and very tender mimicking a septic arthritis or cellulitis
- Acute attack may last for a week or two.

Diagnosis

- Negatively birefringent urate crystals in the synovial fluid examined by polarizing microscope are diagnostic.
- Serum uric acid: May or may not be elevated during an acute attack. A low serum uric acid level rules out gout, but hyperuricemia is not diagnostic as it is often seen in normal middle aged men.
- *X-ray:* Acute attack: Soft tissue swelling
  - *Chronic:* Characteristic punched out cysts or deep erosions with overhanging bony edges (*Martel's or 'G' sign*)
  - *Advanced stage:* Joint space reduction and secondary OA.

Treatment

Acute Attack

- Rest/elevation/ice packs

- NSAID (except aspirin)
- Colchicine/glucocorticoids.

Chronic

- *Allopurinol (xanthine oxidases inhibitor):* Drug of choice
- *Uricosuric drugs:* Probenecid/sulfinpyrazone (if normal renal function)

PSEUDOGOUT—CALCIUM PYROPHOSPHATE DIHYDRATE DISEASE (CPPD)

A disorder characterized by deposition of positively birefringent, rectangular shaped calcium pyrophosphate crystals, usually associated with hyperparathyroidism, haemochromatosis, hypophosphatasia, hypomagnesemia, chondrocalcinosis.

Joints affected: Larger joints like knee, wrist, shoulder, ankle, elbow and hands, temporomandibular joints.

Clinical Features (Fig. 37.10)

- Middle aged women
- Moderate pain
- Joints swollen and tense.

Diagnosis

- *X-rays*

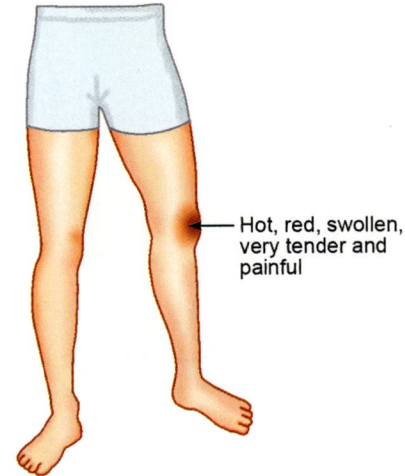

Hot, red, swollen, very tender and painful

Fig. 37.10: Clinical presentation of pseudogout

- CT scans and MRIs show calcific masses (usually within the ligamentum flavum or joint capsule).
- Synovial fluid shows calcium pyrophosphate crystals.

Treatment

- Non-steroidal anti-inflammatory drugs (NSAIDs)
- Intra-articular corticosteroid injection
- Systemic corticosteroids
- Colchicine

Miscellaneous Disorders

AVASCULAR NECROSIS (AVN)

Definition

AVN is defined as a group of conditions associated with aseptic infarction of the bone usually due to interference with the blood supply.

Aetiology

- Traumatic: Fractures or dislocations resulting in vascular damage
- Idiopathic
- Secondary to systemic anomalies:
  - Physical: Burns/electric injury/Caisson's disease
  - Metabolic: Diabetes mellitus, SLE, pancreatitis, etc.
  - Pregnancy
  - Sickle cell disease
  - Alcoholism
  - Iatrogenic: During fracture reduction or internal fixation
- High dose systemic steroid therapy or local steroids

Commonly Affected Bones

- Femur neck
- Scaphoid: Proximal end
- Talus body
- Lunate
- Femoral condyles
- Head of humerus
- Capitellum

Pathogenesis

Arterial insufficiency/venous occlusion/intravascular capillary occlusion → Necrosis/infarction of bone.

AVN Hip

Clinical Presentation

- Pain (sudden or gradual onset)
- Restricted range of motion and stiffness
- Limp
- Stiffness of hip
- Development of fixed deformity in advanced cases

Ficat and Arlet Staging

Stage I: Preclinical diagnosis on MRI, bone scans and bone biopsy as X-ray normal.

Stage II: Painful with some limitations. Density change in femoral head on X-ray.

- A: Sclerosis or cysts, normal joint line, normal head contour
- B: Flattening (crescent sign)

Stage III: Profound symptoms. Loss of sphericity and collapse on X-ray.

Stage IV: Marked collapse and degenerative arthritis.

Investigations

- *X-ray:* May be normal in early stages (1–3 months), later changes according to the stage of AVN (Fig. 38.1).
- Tc 99m bone scan: Cold spots in stage I
  Increased uptake in later stages
- MRI : Decreased signal intensity

Treatment

- Immobilization, non-weight bearing
- Physiotherapy
- Biphosphonates have definite role in slowing down progression of AVN.
- Core decompression in stages I and II
- Revascularisation—using bone graft/core decompression in femur

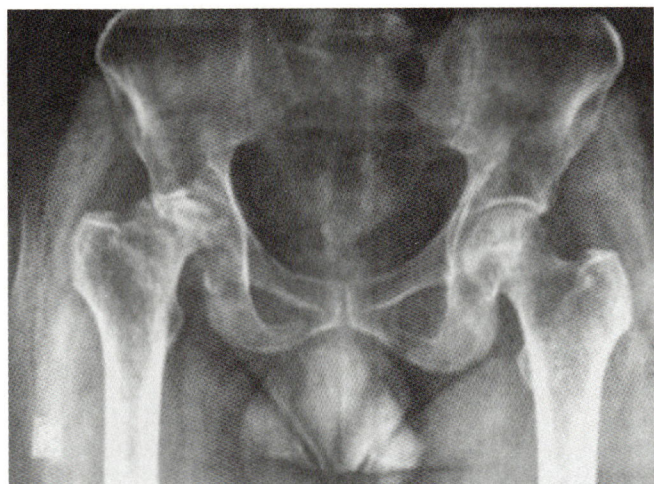

Fig. 38.1: AVN of right femur head

- Realignment osteotomy (e.g. trochanteric osteotomy) in patient > 45 yrs.
- Excision followed by prosthetic replacement in neck femur fracture.
- Total joint replacement arthroplasty or arthrodesis.

OSTEOCHONDRITIS DISSECANS

Definition

A condition characterized by separation of a segment of articular surface of bone and overlying articular cartilage, forming a loose body as a result of ischaemic necrosis.

Site: Usually medial femoral condyle

Pathology: Avascularity of subchondral bone

↓

Softening of overlying cartilage

↓

Line of demarcation from normal bone formed

↓

Separation of fragment as a loose body.

Clinical Presentation

- Adolescent/young adult
- Pain, discomfort, occasional swelling in knee, especially after exercise.
- Knee effusion
- Locking may be present due to loose bodies.

X-Ray (Fig. 38.2)

- Defect in articular surface
- Separated articular fragment seen in place or as a loose body.

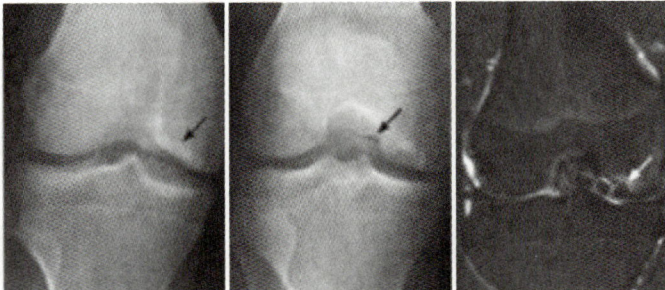

Fig. 38.2: Classical osteochondritis dissecans

Arthroscopy

Diagnostic and therapeutic

Treatment

Developing stage

- Support knee with crepe bandage.
- Avoid strenuous activities.
- Small lesions may heal spontaneously.

In established case

- Arthroscopic excision.

OSTEOCHONDRITIS

Introduction

Osteochondritis describes certain obscure affection of the developing ossific nuclei in children and adolescents.

Classification

1. Crushing Osteochondritis/Juvenile Osteochondritis

Ossific nucleus undergoes avascular necrosis and is crushed under pressure.

Various terminologies for osteochondritis at different sites.

Ossific nucleus of lunate—Kienböck's disease.

Ossific nucleus of navicular—Köhler's disease.

Head of 2nd metatarsal—Freiberg's disease.

Base of 5th metatarsal—Iselin's disease.

Epiphysis of head of femur—Legg-Calvé-Perthes' disease.

Ring epiphysis of vertebra—Scheuermann's disease.

2. Osteochondritis Dissecans/ Splitting Osteochondritis

Due to avascularity, part of epiphysis becomes separated and forms an intra-articular loose body.

- Femoral condyle in knee especially medial condyle

- Capitellum in elbow
- Talus in ankle

3. Pulling/Traction Osteochondritis

Due to pull by tendon attached to a bone
- Tibial tubercle: Osgood-Schlatter's disease
- Calcaneal apophysis: Sever's disease.

Treatment

Established stage: (Clear line of demarcation)
- Arthroscopic removal
- Defect fills with fibrocartilage/osteochondral transplant
- Large fragment may be fixed with pin.

LOOSE BODIES

Introduction

Loose bodies are mainly seen in the knee joint. Depending on their constitution, there are various causes of loose bodies.

Types

1. Osteocartilagenous: May arise from
   - Osteochondral fracture
   - Osteophytes (osteoarthritis)
   - Osteochondritis dissecans (most common)
   - Synovial chondromatosis (multiple)
   These can be detected on X-rays.
2. *Cartilagenous:* Usually traumatic, arising from articular surface of tibia, femur, patella.
   These are radiolucent, not detected on X-rays.
3. *Fibrous:* From synovium due to trauma or chronic inflammatory conditions like Koch's.
4. *Others:* Intra-articular pathologies like nodular synovitis, tumours, foreign body.

Clinical Features

- Pain/swelling
- Locking
- Restricted range of motion

Treatment

Removal of loose bodies through open technique/arthroscopy.

STENOSING TENOSYNOVITIS/DE QUERVAIN'S DISEASE

Definition

Inflammation of the synovial lining of a tendon sheath is called 'tenosynovitis'.

de Quervain's disease is the chronic inflammation, thickening and eventual stenosis of the common sheath of the tendons of abductor pollicis longus and extensor pollicis brevis.

Aetiology

- Unaccustomed overuse
- Degeneration
- Infection

Clinical Features

- Usually women > 40 years
- Pain, swelling, restricted movement of hand.
- Tenderness present at radial styloid
- Swelling
- *Finkelstein's test:* Ask the patient to make a fist, with thumb in palm and fingers superimposing over thumb. Now, push the hand passively to the ulnar side. Severe pain is experienced by the patient at the radial styloid and pain may radiate down the thumb or up to elbow. This is positive Finkelstein's test.

Diagnosis

Clinical

Treatment

- Rest
- Splinting the wrist
- Anti-inflammatory, analgesics
- Local ultrasonic therapy
- If above measures fail → local injection of hydrocortisone
- In resistant cases → surgical release of stenosing tendon sheaths.

GANGLION

Definition

A ganglion is a cystic swelling, overlying a joint or a tendon sheath, most frequently occurring about the wrist.

Aetiology

Two theories:
1. Mucinous degeneration of connective tissue of joint capsule/tendon sheath → formation of multiple small cysts containing mucin → coalesce to form a large cyst
2. Defect in capsule or tendon sheath permits protrusion of synovial tissue.

Pathology

Cyst unilocular/multilocular
- Cyst fluid is thick, sticky, clear, colourless and of a soft jelly consistency.

Clinical Features

- H/o trauma may or may not be present.
- More common in females 20–50 years.
- Sudden or gradual occurrence of swelling may be associated with pain.
- Swelling may diminish in size and may even disappear, only to recur.
- Most common sites are dorsum of wrist, volar aspect of wrist, tarsal area of foot, lateral joint interval of knee in front of biceps and anterolateral aspect of ankle.
- Dorsal wrist ganglion becomes tense on flexing the wrist.
- When it is connected with a tendon sheath, a sense of weakness is experienced in affected finger.

Treatment

Non-operative: The cyst may be aspirated and injected with steroid or sclerosing agent.

Operative: Through a transverse incision, the cyst is dissected free from the origin—capsule or tendon sheath and the resultant defect is tightly sutured to prevent recurrence.

Complication

Recurrence.

TRIGGER FINGER/THUMB

Definition

It is a condition characterized by stenosing tenovaginitis of flexor tendons, leading to characteristic snap—'triggering' while moving the finger.

Aetiology

- Unaccustomed activity
- Rheumatoid arthritis
- Collagen disease
- Gout
- Diabetes mellitus
- Repeated trauma/acute trauma

Pathology (Fig. 38.3)

Repeated trauma → thickening of tendon sheath (especially A1 pulley) → constriction of tendon → bulbous enlargement of tendon, especially at

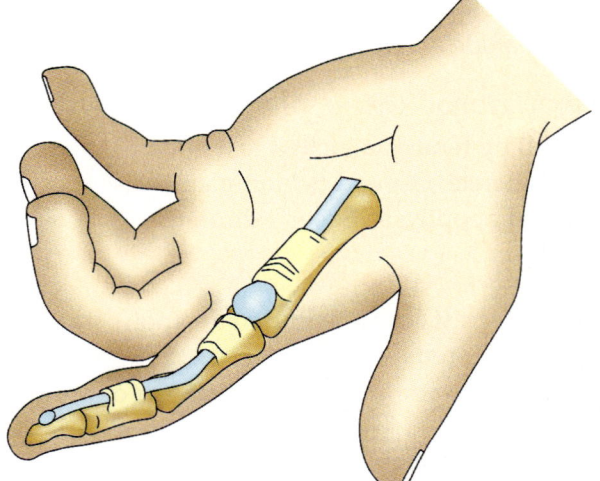

Fig. 38.3: Pathology of trigger finger

metacarpophalangeal (MCP) joint → momentary obstruction when passing through stenosed sheath → movement through narrowed canal of the thickened tendon leads to characteristic 'thump' or snap → triggering.

Clinical Features

- Common involvement of ring and middle finger, also thumb.
- Catching/locking of affected finger after forceful flexion, may require opposite hand to passively extend the finger.
- Triggering more pronounced in the morning
- Tender nodule may be felt at MCP joint

Congenital Trigger Digits

- Most common in thumb
- Bilateral in 25%
- Child present within first 2 years with relatively fixed flexion posture of interphalangeal joint and even with force, it is not possible to fully extend the interphalangeal joint of thumb.
- No classical clicking/ snapping like in adults.

Treatment

- Rest
- Anti-inflammatory drugs
- Local injection of corticosteroid into tendon sheath and immobilization in cast for a few weeks
- Surgical release of A1 pulley

For Congenital Trigger Digits

- Spontaneous resolution occurs in 30%
- If not, by 2 years—release of first annular pulley

TENNIS ELBOW/LATERAL EPICONDYLITIS

Definition

It is a condition characterised by pain and tenderness on the lateral side of the elbow, resulting from repetitive stress. It not only occurs in tennis players but also in other sports or may be occupation related (activities involving forceful repetitive wrist extension like hammering).

Pathology

Not exactly known.
- Single or multiple small tears within common extensor origin (especially ECRB—extensor carpi radialis brevis) or capsule or radial collateral ligament (Fig. 38.4).
- Periostitis due to repeated strains

Clinical Features

- Usually seen in age group 30–40 years.
- Pain localized to lateral epicondyle, aggravated by movements like turning a door handle, wringing clothes, pouring out tea, lifting with pronated forearm.

Special Tests

Cozen's test: To perform the Cozen's test, hold the patient's elbow with one hand while the patient is asked to pronate the forearm and extend and radially deviate the wrist against manual resistance of the clinician. The test is considered positive if it produces pain or reproduction of other symptoms in the area of the lateral epicondyle.

Mill's Maneuver: The patient's wrist is passively flexed when his forearm is pronated. This causes tremendous pain at the site of the attachment of the common extensor tendons.

Treatment

- Rest, anti-inflammatory drugs, tennis elbow splint
- Local steroid injection

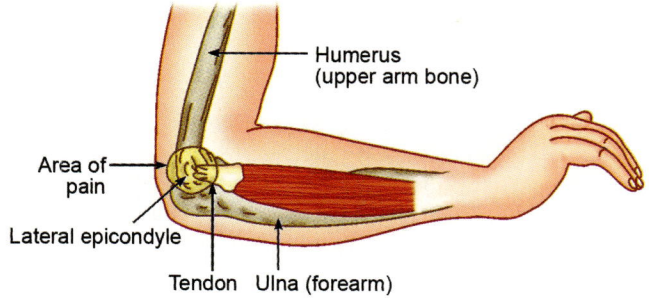

Fig. 38.4: Pathology of tennis elbow

- Refractory cases: Detachment of common extensor origin.

GOLFER'S ELBOW

Medical epicondylitis, involving common flexor pronator origin (Fig. 38.5).

Similar presentation and management as Tennis elbow.

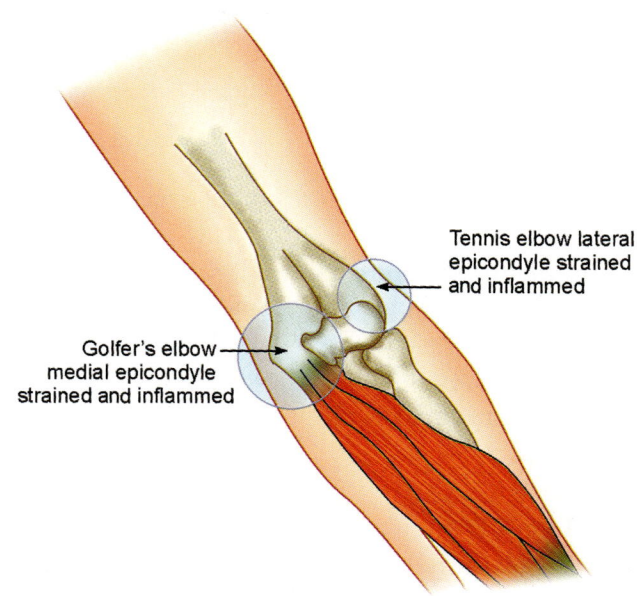

Fig. 38.5: Pathology of Golfer's elbow

CARPAL TUNNEL SYNDROME (TARDY MEDIAN NERVE PALSY)

Definition

A condition resulting from compression of the median nerve within the carpal tunnel.

Anatomy of Carpal Tunnel (Fig. 38.6)

Aetiology

Conditions that crowd or reduce the capacity of carpal tunnel.
1. *Trauma:* Colles' fracture: Acute compression of median nerve occurs due to immobilization of wrist in extreme palmar flexion and ulnar deviation.
2. Oedema from inflammation
3. Tumour or tumorous conditions: Like ganglion, lipoma or xanthoma
4. *Systemic conditions:* Like obesity, diabetes mellitus, thyroid disorders.
5. *Habit:* Habitual sleeping posture at night in which the wrist is kept acutely flexed.

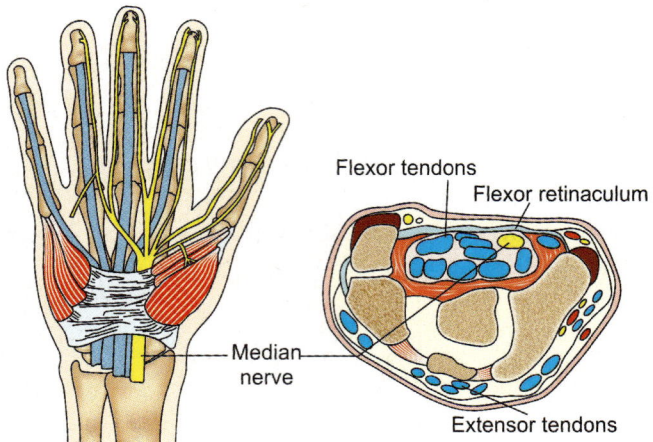

Fig. 38.6: Anatomy of carpal tunnel

6. *Occupation:* Labourers using vibrating machinery, office workers especially typists and data entry clerks, who spend long hours with wrist flexed.
7. Pregnancy related oedema around wrist
8. *Vascular :* Thrombosis of median artery
9. Idiopathic

Clinical Features

- Age: 30–60 years
- *Sex:* M:F=1:5

Symptoms

Paraesthesia over the sensory distribution of the median nerve, especially at night, awakening the patient and relieved by exercise—shaking the hand.

Signs

- *Tinel's sign:* Percussion of median nerve at the wrist leads to tingling and numbness in the median nerve distribution.
- *Atrophy of median nerve innervated thenar muscles* in 50% cases
- *Phalen's test:* Acute flexion of the wrist for 60 seconds increases paraesthesia.
- *Carpal compression test:* Direct compression of median nerve for 30 seconds with thumb leads to numbness, pain or paraesthesia in median nerve distribution.

Diagnosis

Electromyography and nerve conduction (EMG-NC) study.

Treatment

Carpal tunnel release.

DUPUYTREN'S CONTRACTURE

Introduction

Dupuytren's contracture is a condition caused by proliferative fibroplasia of the subcutaneous palmar tissue, occurring in the form of nodules and cords, causing secondary flexion contracture of the finger joints.

Epidemiology

Age: 50–70 yrs.
Sex: M: F=10:1
Bilateral involvement: 45%

More common and severe in alcoholics and epileptics.

Aetiology

Exact cause not known. Possible causes are:
- Heredity
- Vascular insufficiency
- Cigarette smoking

Pathogenesis/Clinical Features

Proliferation of myofibroblasts → contracture of various fascial cords → gradual contracture of MCP and PIP joints
- Lesion usually begins in the ring finger at distal palmar crease and progresses to involve ring and little fingers (Fig. 38.7).
- Thinning of overlying subcutaneous fat, adhesion of skin to the lesion and later pitting or dimpling of skin.

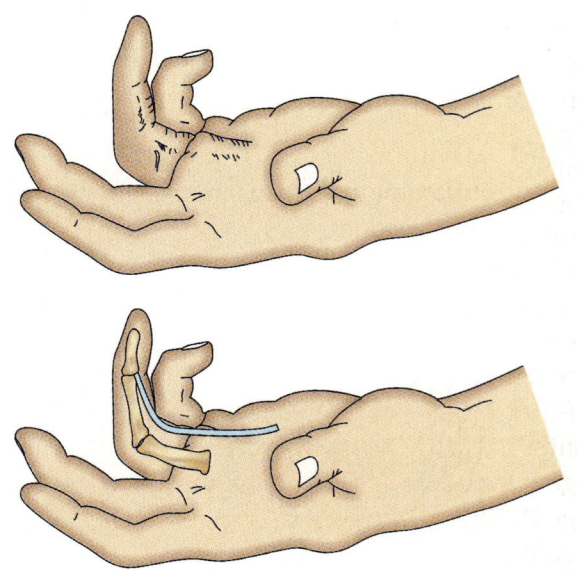

Fig. 38.7: Pathology of Dupuytren's contracture

Treatment

- No treatment in the absence of contracture, keep the patient under observation every 3 months.
- Surgery indicated if sufficient discomfort, pitting , formation of palmar nodule.

Types of Surgery

- Subcutaneous fasciotomy
- Partial fasciectomy
- Complete fasciectomy
- Fasciectomy with skin grafting
- Amputation.

FROZEN SHOULDER

Also known as periarthritis shoulder/adhesive capsulitis.

Definition

A condition characterized by pain and limitation of movement of shoulder joint, probably due to loss of resilience of joint capsule and development of adhesions, without inflammatory or destructive changes.

Pathogenesis

Various theories:

- Overuse, minor tears, acute supraspinatus and bicipital tendinitis/coracoacromial impingement, etc. can lead to chronic tendinitis.
- Autoimmune response to products of local tissue breakdown causes capsulitis.
- Changes in microvascular blood supply.

Clinical Features

- *Age:* 40–60 yrs.
- Common in females and diabetics
- H/o trauma may be present. Pain occurs especially at night, associated with stiffness.
- Pain and tenderness felt on anterolateral aspect of shoulder, radiating along outer side of arm, forearm and hand.
- Pain subsides over months followed by stiffness. Abduction, extension and external rotation earliest to be restricted.
- Self-limiting disease divided into 3 stages of 3–8 months each.
  Stage I: Increasing pain and stiffness
  Stage II: Decreasing pain but persistent stiffness
  Stage III: Painless return of movement.

X-ray: Juxta-articular osteopenia

Treatment

Stage I

- Reassurance (very important)
- NSAIDs
- Physiotherapy: Heat and SWD

Stage II

In addition to stage I regime,

- Physiotherapy: Pendulum exercise.
- If severe constant pain persists, manipulation under general aneasthesia (MUGA)+ intra-articular injection of steroid with local anaesthetic.

Stage III

In addition to stage I and satge II regime,

- Distension arthrography if severe restriction of range of motion or saline distension
- MUGA, if slow recovery.

PAINFUL ARC SYNDROME/IMPINGEMENT SYNDROME

Definition

It is a condition characterized by pain in the shoulder and upper arm during mid-range of glenohumeral abduction (Fig. 38.8).

Etiology

- Subacromial bursitis
- Partial/complete supraspinatus tear

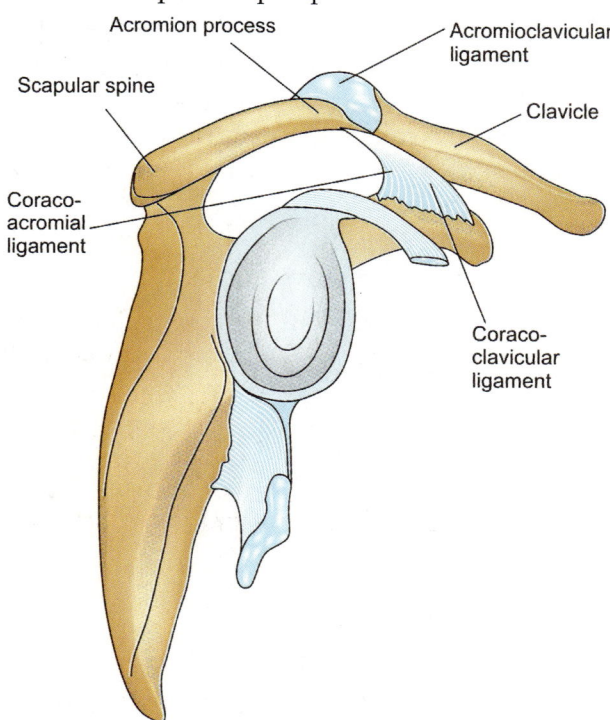

Fig. 38.8: Anatomy of coracoacromial arch

- Supraspinatus calcific tendinitis
- Greater tuberosity injury

Predisposing Factors

- Excessive overhead activities
- Shoulder dislocation
- Anterior prominent hooked acromion

Mechanism: Since the functional arc of abduction and elevation is in the anterolateral plane, nipping of a lesion between anterior 1/3rd of undersurface of acromion and superior aspect of greater tuberosity during mid-range of abduction causes pain (Fig. 38.9).

Clinical Features

- Mainly affects elderly individuals and young athletes involved in sports with overhead motions (e.g. tennis, swimming)
- Pain around greater tuberosity and upper arm. May radiate to arm, chest, back. Pain worse at night.
- Impairment of daily activities like combing, reaching on overhead objects, lifting objects.
- *Impingement sign:* Passive elevation in forward plane of abduction causes pain in midrange between 60 and 120°. If impingement sign is positive, subacromial injection of 10 cc lignocaine leads to reduction in pain and improved mobility.

Neer's Stages of Impingement Syndrome

1. Oedema stage
2. Tendinitis and fibrositis
3. Rotator cuff tear and rupture of biceps tendon
4. Bony changes.

X-ray: May show calcific deposits in supraspinatus

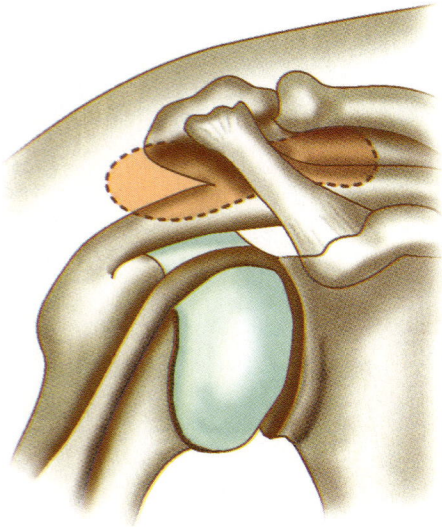

Fig. 38.9: Pathoanatomy of impingement syndrome

Treatment

Conservative: 90% effective

- NSAIDs
- Heat, massage
- Local hydrocortisone
- Subacromial steroid injection—active and passive exercise.
- Rarely, surgery may be required in the form of:
  - Excision of calcific deposits
  - Excision of adhesions
  - Manipulation of shoulder.

ROTATOR CUFF TEAR

Introduction

Fine adjustments of the humeral head within the glenoid is maintained by four muscles arising from scapula-supraspinatus, infraspinatus, teres minor, teres major which are together called rotator cuff.

Aetiology

- Age>40 yrs.
- M : F = 2:1
- Excessive overhead activities
- Overhead sports like tennis, throw ball, swimming
- Degenerative tears

Classification

Depending on size of tear.

- Small (< 1 cm.)
- Medium (1–3 cm)
- Large (3–5 cm)

Clinical Features

- Symptoms like frozen shoulder or painful arc syndrome.
- Limitation of active shoulder movement in presence of preserved passive movement is hallmark of rotator cuff tear.
- In complete tear, there is inability to initiate active abduction. The patient shrugs his shoulder or bends to one side to achieve the initial 15–20° of abduction, normally done by supraspinatus, and later deltoid takes over.
- Drop sign—when patient lowers the arm, it suddenly drops in terminal range (Fig. 38.10).

Investigations

1. X-ray of shoulder
   - Reduced subacromial space (<6 mm)
   - Sclerotic inferior acromion (eyebrow sign)

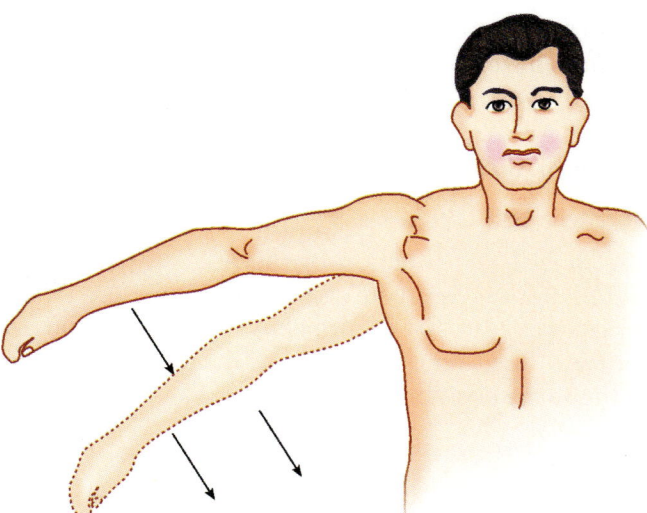

Fig. 38.10: Drop arm test

- Hooking of acromion
- Humeral head degeneration
2. *Arthrogram:* Diagnostic
3. *MRI:* Accurate but expensive (Fig. 38.11)

Treatment

Conservative treatment as given in "painful arc syndrome".

Failure of conservative treatment, especially in young, active person with significant loss of shoulder function—surgery

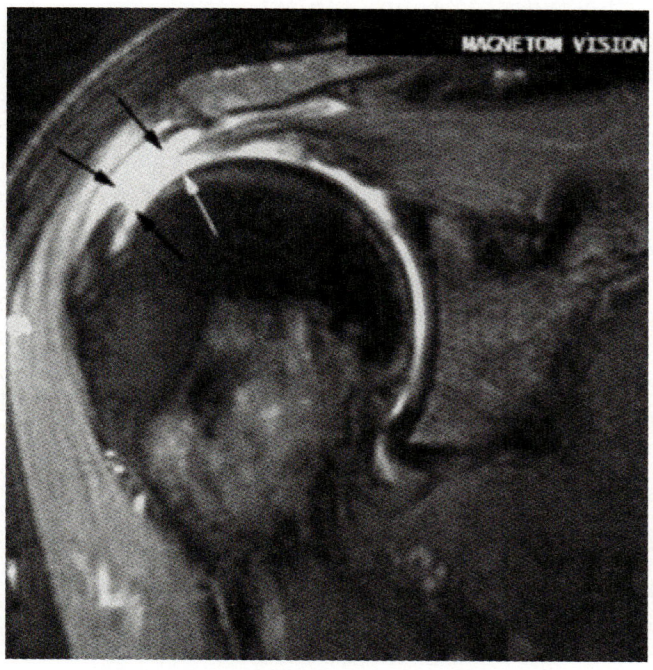

Fig. 38.11: MRI showing rotator cuff tear

Surgery

- Arthroscopic surgery in small, partial tears.
- Open repair in major tears.

MERALGIA PARAESTHESIA

It is a condition in which lateral cutaneous nerve of thigh is entrapped in the fascia of thigh medial to anterior superior iliac spine. The patient develops paraesthesia, tingling or burning sensation in anterolateral aspect of thigh.

Treatment

Usually responds well to analgesics and neurotropic drugs such as methylcobalamine, pregabaline, etc. Local steroid injection or surgical decompression is rarely required.

PLANTAR FASCIITIS/PAINFUL HEEL

Introduction

It is a common orthopaedic problem characterized by pain beneath the anteromedial prominence of the calcaneal tuberosity.

Aetiology/Pathogenesis

Exact cause not known, possible theories are:
- Degenerative changes in the elastic adipose tissue of heel pad.
- Traction on the origin of plantar fascia, causing microscopic tears.
- Pull of flexor digitorum brevis (FDB) on calcaneal tubercle—fatigue fracture. Calcification in FDB in order to heal the fracture—formation of 'Spur' seen in X-ray.

Clinical Features

- Age: 40–70 years
- Obesity is the predisposing factor.
- Pain beneath the heel, which is worse in the morning or on getting up after sitting for a long time. After a few steps, the pain decreases. Patient comfortable during the day, discomfort is more of an aching, which is relieved by non-weight bearing (Fig. 38.12).
- Localized tenderness at inferomedial aspect of calcaneal tuberosity.

X-ray
Calcaneal spur in 50% patients (Fig. 38.13).

Treatment

- NSAID
- Shoe modification/ inserts (silicone cups/pads)

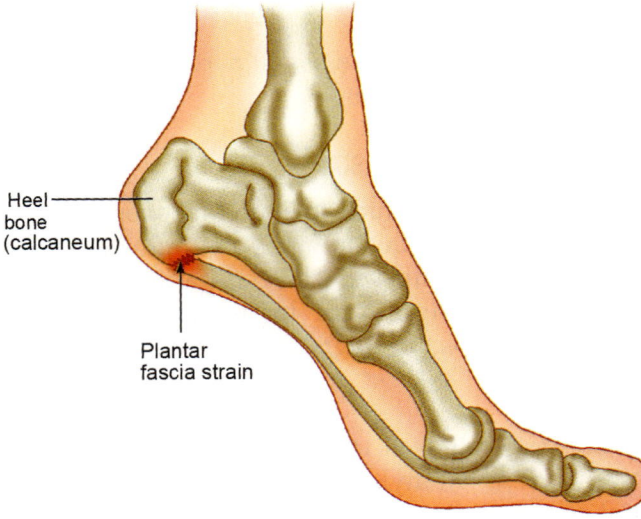

Fig. 38.12: Plantar fasciitis

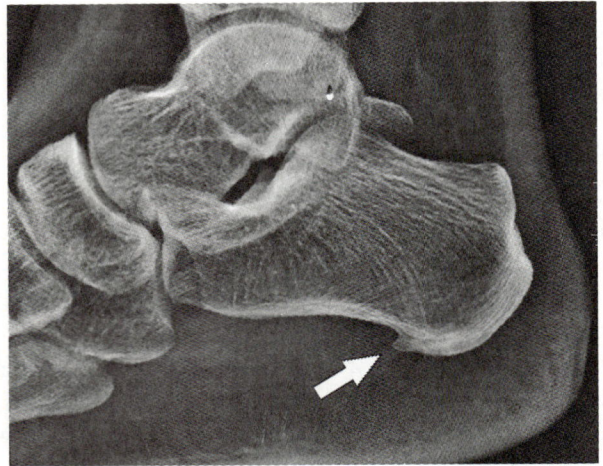

Fig. 38.13: Heel spur

- Local steroid injection
- *Physiotherapy:* Ultrasound/wax therapy.
- Rarely surgical release of plantar fascia.

NORMAL GAIT AND GAIT ABNORMALITY

Normal Gait Cycle

The most basic function of the lower extremities is ambulation. A complete gait cycle is considered to be a series of events that occurs between the time one foot contacts the ground and the time the same foot returns to the same position.

Phases of Normal Gait Cycle

Although ambulation is a continuous process, a gait cycle is arbitrarily said to begin when one foot strikes the ground (Fig. 38.14).

1. *Heel strike:* Because first contact normally is made with the heel, this point in the gait cycle is described as heel strike.
2. *Foot flat:* As the individual continues to move forward, the forefoot makes contact with the ground. The point at which both the forefoot and the heel are in contact with the ground is called foot flat.
3. *Midstance:* At the same time, the opposite foot is pushing off the ground and beginning to swing forward. The point at which the swinging limb passes the weight bearing limb is the point of midstance for the weight bearing limb. This is an extremely helpful point in the gait cycle to look for abnormalities, because the limb that is in midstance is temporarily bearing all the weight of the individual's body.
4. *Push off:* As the opposite limb continues to move forward, weight is transferred from the swinging limb, and the standing limb begins to push off.

The portion of the gait cycle just described, from heel

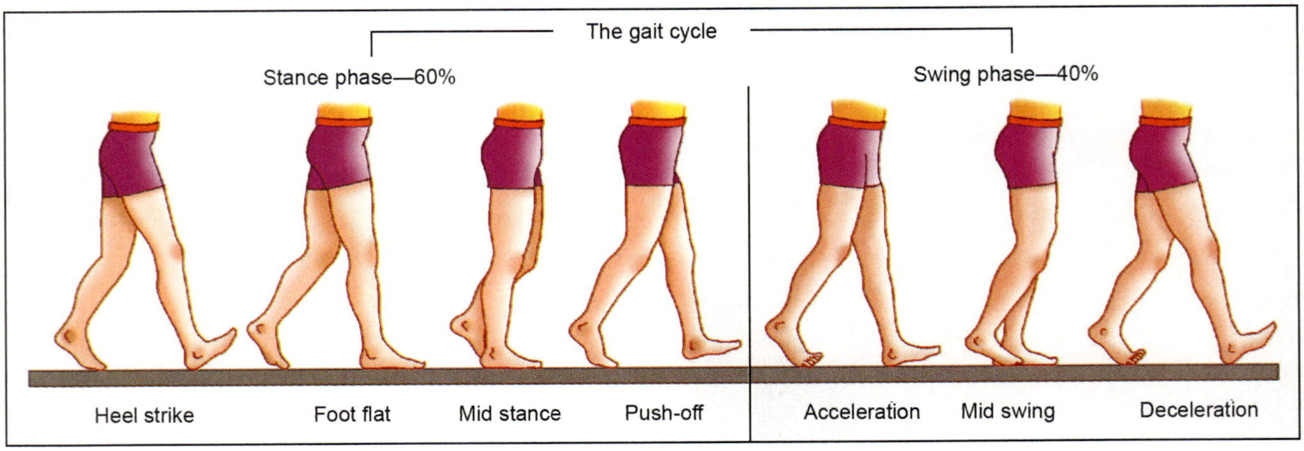

The gait cycle

Stance phase—60%   Swing phase—40%

Heel strike   Foot flat   Mid stance   Push-off   Acceleration   Mid swing   Deceleration

Fig. 38.14: Phases of normal gait cycle

strike to toe off, is known as the stance phase of gait. After toe-off, the limb passes through the swing phase of gait as it is advanced forward towards the next heel strike.

5. *Acceleration:* The process of push off provides much of the propulsive energy used for ambulation. It is sometimes divided into heel-off, the point at which the heel leaves the ground, and the toe-off, the point at which the forefoot leaves the ground.

6. *Deceleration:* During this time, the opposite limb is progressing through the same components of stance phase just described. When the first heel strikes the ground again, one entire gait cycle has been completed.

Each lower limb spends about 60% of their gait cycle in stance phase because there is a portion of the cycle during which both feet are in contact with the ground. The portion of the cycle during which both lower limbs are weight bearing is called double leg stance, whereas the portions during which only one limb is weight bearing is called single leg stance.

Abnormal Gait Patterns

Antalgic Gait

An antalgic gait is an intuitive, self-protective adaptation to pain generated during the stance phase of gait. Pain that is induced by weight bearing anywhere in the lower extremity can produce a similar pattern. In an antalgic gait, the stance phase on the affected limb is shorter than on the normal limb because the patient attempts to remove weight from the affected limb as quickly as possible. To effect this change, the normal limb is brought forward more quickly, and the time it spends in swing phase is thus decreased. The result is a shorter stride length on the uninvolved side, decreased walking velocity, and a decreased cadence, that is, fewer steps per minute. An antalgic gait can be seen in arthritic conditions involving the ankle, the subtalar joint, or the midfoot; plantar fasciitis; infections or any other painful conditions.

Short Limb Gait

A short limb gait may develop in response to a leg length discrepancy. Again, this pattern is not specific for leg length discrepancies arising from the lower leg, ankle, or the foot. A patient with one leg shorter than the other may develop a lateral shift to the affected side, with the pelvis tilting downward toward the same side. The patient may supinate the foot on the affected side or even toe walk in an attempt to lengthen the shorter limb. The unaffected limb may demonstrate exaggerated hip or knee flexion to help compensate for the limb length discrepancy. Finally, the patient may demonstrate hip hiking on the unaffected side during swing phase to allow the foot of the longer limb to clear the ground.

Trendelenburg's Gait

In humans, the gluteus medius and minimus muscle counteract the tendency of the pelvis to fall toward the opposite side by pulling it towards the greater trochanter of the weight bearing limb. This precariously balanced system can break down in several ways. If the gluteus medius and minimus are not quite strong enough to counterbalance the patient's upper body weight, the pelvis tends to droop toward the floor when the patient is bearing weight on the weak limb. This results in an exaggerated up-and-down motion of the pelvis during ambulation known as Trendelenburg's gait (Fig. 38.15).

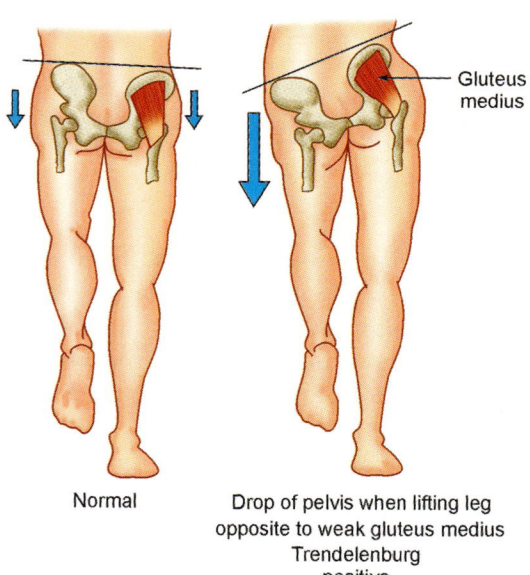

Normal   Drop of pelvis when lifting leg opposite to weak gluteus medius Trendelenburg positive

— Gluteus medius

Fig. 38.15: Trendelenburg's gait

FIBROMYALGIA

Definition

Fibromyalgia is a clinical syndrome of diffuse pain (present at rest but exacerbated by activity), fatigue and sleep disturbance. The American College of Rheumatology defined two criteria for diagnosing fibromyalgia in 1990.

1. A history of widespread pain
2. Pain in at least 11 of 18 defined tender point sites on digital palpation with a force of 4 dyne/cm^2 (Fig. 38.16)

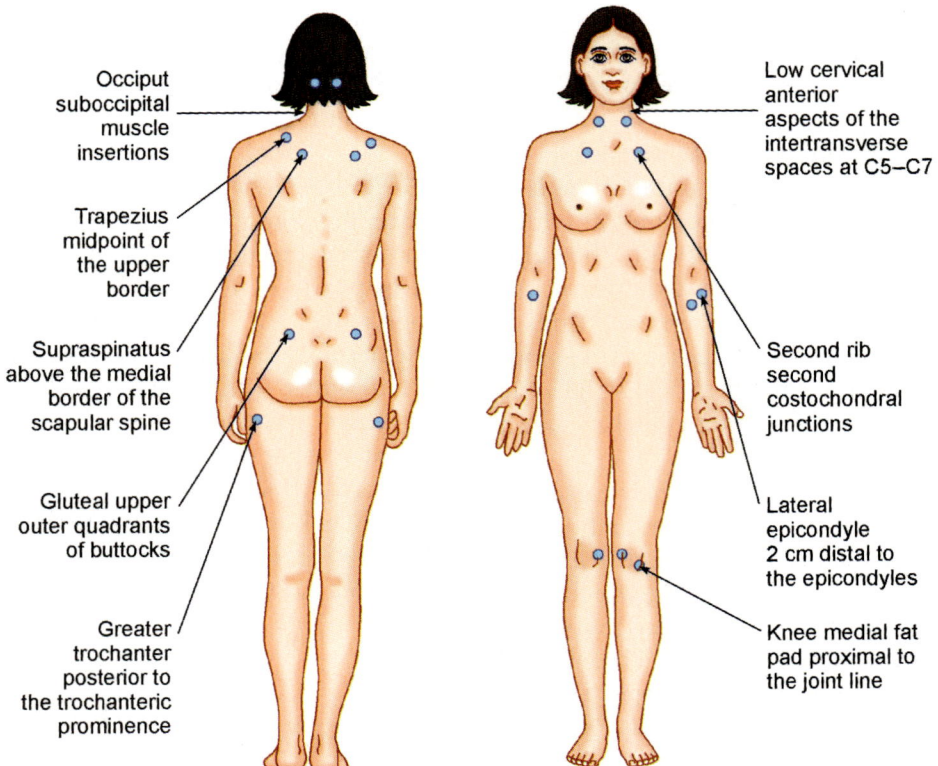

Fig. 38.16: Tender points of fibromyalgia

Clinical Presentation

Fibromyalgia predominantly occurs in females (>90%) with a positive family history and begins in teenage.

The usual symptoms are 'hurting all over', stiffness, tingling, numbness of hands and feet. In severe cases there is allodynia i.e. even gentle pinching of skin is painful.

Pathogenesis (Fig. 38.17)

Progressive failure of inhibitory neurons in spinal cord to focus afferent sensory impulses appropriately, leading to 'central sensitization'.

There is no primary physiological abnormality of muscles.

Management

Radiological/ laboratory findings: Normal

Three aspects of treatment:
1. Patient education.

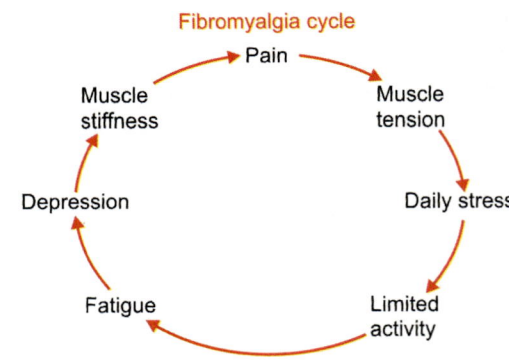

Fig. 38.17: Fibromyalgia cycle

2. Therapeutic exercise.
3. *Drug treatment:* Tricyclics, e.g. amitryptyline to achieve sound sleep.

Analgesics have minor role in case of severe symptoms.

Orthopaedic Appliances

TRACTIONS

Introduction

When a limb is painful as a result of injury or inflammation, the controlling muscles go into spasm and produce deformity. When traction is applied to such a limb, it can overcome the effect of the original deforming force.

Uses of Traction

- Reduction of fracture and dislocation and maintenance of alignment and stability by immobilization.
- Immobilization of painfully inflamed and diseased joints of the limb.
- Reduce pain and oedema of affected limb by elevation
- Correction and prevention of deformities, angulation and contractures.

Types of Traction

a. Skin/surface traction
b. Skeletal traction
  - *Fixed traction:* Pull applied against a fixed point of counter pressure, e.g. Thomas splint.
  - *Sliding/balanced traction:* Pull is counter balanced by patient's own body weight after giving a head low position, e.g. Bohler-Braun (BB) frame.

SKIN TRACTION

In skin traction, the traction force is applied over a large area of skin, distal to the affected area. This spreads the load and is more comfortable and efficient. Adhesive or non-adhesive strappings can be used.

Maximum weight: 10% of body weight.

Technique and Care of Patient with Skin Traction
(Fig. 39.1)

- After shaving and cleaning the skin, adhesive straps are applied in two strips on medial and lateral sides of the fractured limb below the level of injury.
- The encircling bandage must be firmly applied from below upward but must not compromise the circulation.
- The malleoli must be checked regularly for evidence of friction from skin traction.
- The spreader bar to which traction cords are attached should lie 4–6 inches beyond the ankle/wrist to allow free movement of the foot/hand
- If the skin becomes sore, discontinue skin traction.

Contraindications

- *Poor skin condition:* Abrasion, laceration, dermatitis
- *Impairment of circulation:* Varicose ulcer, impending gangrene
- When traction weight required is greater than can be applied through skin, e.g. marked shortening of bony fragments.

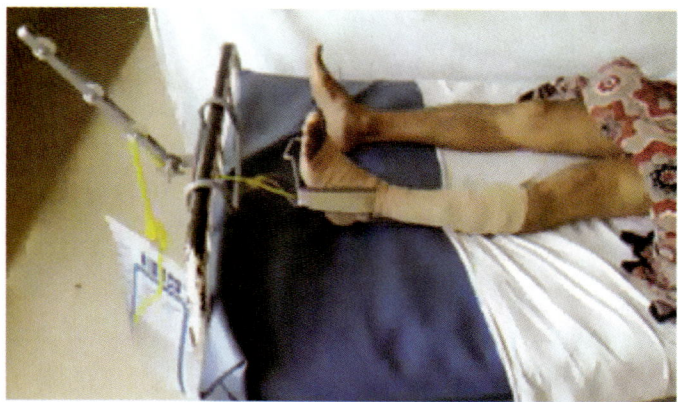

Fig. 39.1: Skin traction for lower limb

Complications of Skin Traction

- Allergic reactions to the adhesive
- Excoriation of the skin from slipping of the adhesive strapping
- Pressure sores around the malleoli and over tendo achilles.
- Common peroneal nerve palsy due to external rotation of the limb or sliding down of loose traction and pressure on nerve.

SKELETAL TRACTION

Introduction

When more traction force is necessary, it is applied directly to the skeleton by passing a metal pin or wire. This type of traction is called skeletal traction.

Indications

- Management of lower limb fractures: For reduction of fractures, for maintenance of reduction, and for preoperative immobilization.
- When skin traction is contraindicated.

Requirements

- **Steinmann pin:** Rigid stainless steel pin of varying length 4 to 6 mm diameter, named after Fritz Steinmann, who described it in 1916 (Fig. 39.2).
- **Denham pin:** Similar to Steinmann pin, but with short raised threaded middle portion, designed for use in cancellous bone like calcaneum and in osteoporotic bone.
- **Kirschner wire:** It is of small diameter and is insufficiently rigid until pulled taut in a special stirrup. Used mainly in children and in upper limb.

Bohler stirrup: Attached to the pin, for varying the direction of traction without turning the pin in the bone (Fig. 39.3).

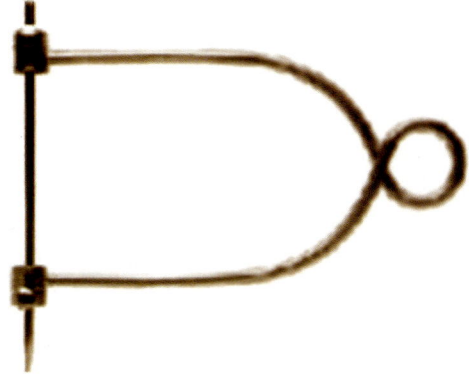

Fig. 39.3: Bohler stirrup

Common Sites for Application of Skeletal Traction

Lower limb
- Upper end of tibia (commonest): 2 cm behind the crest, just below the level of the tibial tubercle.
- Distal femur
- Lower end of tibia
- Upper end of femur—greater trochanter
- *Calcaneum:* 2.5 cm below and behind lateral malleolus

Upper limb
- *Olecranon:* 3 cm distal to olecranon tip just deep to the subcutaneous border of upper end of ulna. Care should be taken to avoid ulnar nerve
- 2nd/3rd metacarpal

Skull
- Traction for cervical spine fracture/dislocation
- Gardner well's/Crutchfield tongs are used
- Weight is applied according to the level of the fracture/dislocation

Principles and Technique (Fig. 39.4)

- Pin is inserted under local anaesthesia with strict aseptic precautions.

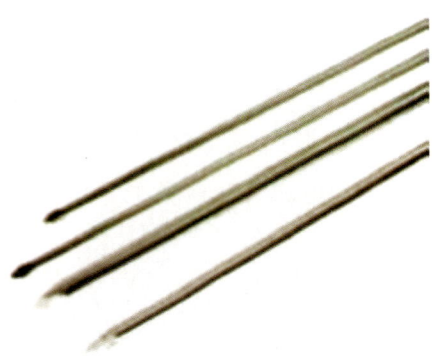

Fig. 39.2: Steinmann pins

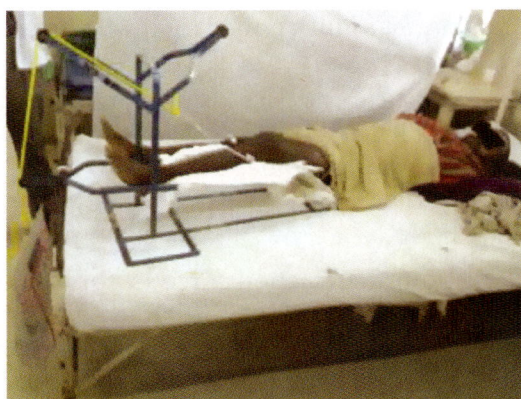

Fig. 39.4: Patient with skeletal traction of lower limb on a Bohler-Braun frame

- Avoid physis/epiphysis and be away from the neurovascular structures.
- Pin is passed in an axis at 90 degrees to the long axis of fractured bone.
- Skin is stretched and incised at points of entry and exit.
- Pin should be cleaned daily to avoid infection.

Complications

- Introduction of infection into the bone
- Incorrect placement of the pin or wire, leading to
  - Cutting out of bone
  - Difficulty in control of rotation of the limb
  - Neurovascular injury
- Distraction at fracture site if very large traction force is applied
- Damage to the growth plate in children
- Depressed scars
- Loosening of pins

Some Common Traction Methods

- *Gallow's traction/Bryant's traction:* Fracture shaft femur in children below 2 years.
- *Russell's traction:* Trochanter fracture
- *Perkin's traction:* Fracture shaft femur in adults
- *Buck's traction:* Conventional skin traction
- *Dunlop traction:* Supracondylar fracture of humerus
- *Crutchfield traction/Gardner Well's traction:* Cervical spine injury
- *Halo pelvic traction:* Scoliosis.

PLASTER OF PARIS

Introduction

Plaster of Paris bandages were first used by Matthysen, a Dutch military surgeon in 1852. They became commercially available since 1931 (Fig. 39.5).

Constitution

Chemically, POP is calcium sulphate hemihydrate. Plaster of Paris (POP) is made from gypsum by heating it to drive off water. When water is added to the resulting powder, the original mineral reforms and heat is released.

$$2\ CaSO_4.2H_2O + Heat \rightarrow 2CaSO_4.1/2H_2O + 3H_2O$$

Calcium sulphate dihydrate + heat $\rightarrow$ calcium sulphate hemihydrate + Water

POP can be used in two ways:

Slabs (only applied on one side of the limb and covered with bandage) and casts (circular cover of the limb)

Indications

- To support fractured bones.
- To stabilize and rest joints where there has been ligamentous injury.
- To ensure rest to infected tissues.
- For postoperative immobilization of joints and limbs.
- To correct a deformity by serial casts/wedging of cast.

Principles of Application

- Apply adequate layer of cotton padding over the skin
- The joints of the limb, immobilized by POP should be in functional position.
- The extent of POP cast should be from one joint above to one joint below the fracture.
- Encourage active mobilization of free joints, beyond the extent of POP.
- Regular check for development of complications is essential.

Complications

Impairment of circulation

- This may be due to swelling within POP cast because of haemorrhage or reactionary tissue oedema
- It is indicated by severe pain
- If circulatory impairment is suspected, split the cast immediately throughout its length or remove completely.

Pressure sores

They develop due to irregularity of the inner surface of the cast, insufficient padding especially over bony prominences or presence of foreign bodies like coins, match sticks between the cast and skin.

Instructions to an Out-patient Wearing a Plaster Cast

- Report back to the hospital immediately at any time of the day or night if
  - Increased pain or pins and needles sensation in fingers/toes

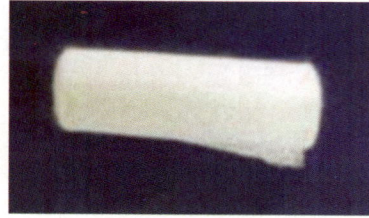

Fig. 39.5: Plaster of Paris

- Fingers/toes turn blue/white or grossly swollen and numb
- Inability to move fingers/toes
- Plaster loose, cracked, or soft
- Keep the plaster cast dry
- Do not rest the plaster cast on a firm surface and don't hang the splinted limb down
- Actively mobilize the free joints.

Removal of Plaster Cast

Use of electric saw, plaster cutter, scissor is helpful.

Common POP Casts

- *Upper limb:* Shoulder spica/above elbow/below elbow/Colles' cast/scaphoid cast/metacarpal cast.
- *Lower limb:* Hip spica/above knee/below knee cast/patellar tendon bearing cast.

THOMAS' SPLINT

Introduction

Thomas' splint was originally described by Hugh Owen Thomas (1876) as a knee appliance for use in the ambulant management of chronic or subacute inflammation of the knee joint (Fig. 39.6).

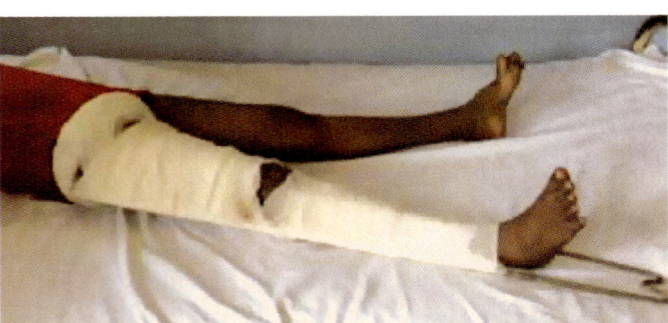

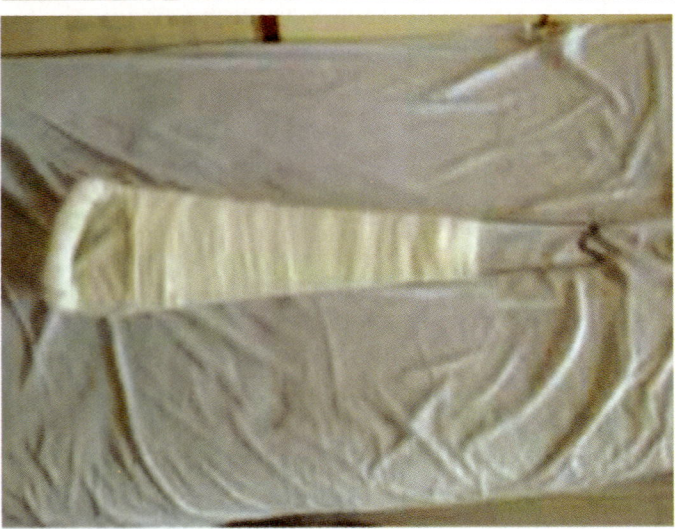

Fig. 39.6: Thomas splint

Description/Parts of the Splint

- Padded oval metal ring covered with soft leather, attached at 120° to inner and outer side bars. The side bars bisect the ring and are of unequal length. They are joined together at the distal end in the form of a 'W'
- Outer side bar angled out 2 inches (5 cm) below the ring to accommodate greater trochanter.

Ideal size of a Thomas' Splint

Size of the ring: Measure the oblique circumference of the normal thigh just below the gluteal fold and ischial tuberosity, add 2 inches and this should be the internal circumference of the padded ring.

Length of the inner side bar: Add 6 to 9 inches to the distance from the crotch to the heel.

Preparing a Thomas' Splint

- Fashion slings, between the side bars, on which the limb can rest. The distal sling must end around 6 cm above the heel, in order to avoid pressure sores over tendo achilles.
- Line the slings with Gamzee tissue
- After fitting the splint, bandage the limb into the splint.

Indications

Fixed traction in a Thomas' splint

- For maintenance of reduction of a fracture (ideally suited for a transverse femur shaft fracture).
- For preoperative immobilization of the limb.

The traction cords are tied over the end of the Thomas' splint. The outer cord passes above and inner cord below its respective side bar, to hold the limb in internal rotation. Counter thrust (traction) passes up the side bars, to the root of the limb. Windlass may be used to compensate for any stretching of the cords or sliding downward of adhesive strapping.

Thomas' splint along with above knee cast is known as *Tobruk splint.*

WALKING AIDS

Introduction

Walking aids are the devices used to increase the mobility of a patient, by enabling part of the body weight to be supported by upper limbs.

Selection of Correct Walking Aid

Based on
- Stability of the patient
- Co-ordination of upper and lower limbs

- Strength of upper and lower limbs
- Degree of relief from weight bearing required

Examples of Walking Aids
- Parallel bars
- Walking frames/walkers
- Axillary crutches
- Walking sticks

WALKER

Useful in the initial period when a patient is unstable or fearful of falling.

Types
1. Standard walking frame
2. *Reciprocal walking frame:* Used for elderly patients.
3. *Rollator:* For patients suffering from neurological conditions like disseminated sclerosis.

The standard walking frame consists of a rectangle and joined together on three sides by upper and lower horizontal tubes (Fig. 39.7).

The height of the vertical tubes are arranged in such a way that a patient can hold it with 30° elbow flexion.

The reciprocal walking frame is identical with a standard frame, except that each side of the frame can be moved forward alternatively. Due to presence of swivel joint, this frame gives better stability to the patient.

Rollator has two small wheels at front and two short legs at the back, protected by rubber tips.

AXILLARY CRUTCHES

Introduction

Crutches are a type of walking aids used for relieving weight to varying degree. There are 3 main types of

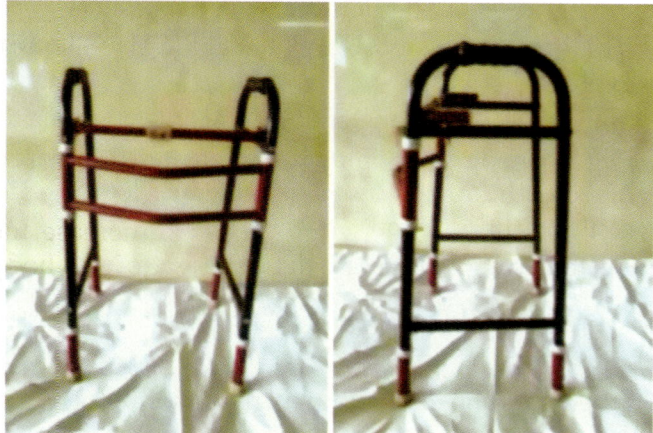

Fig. 39.7: Walker

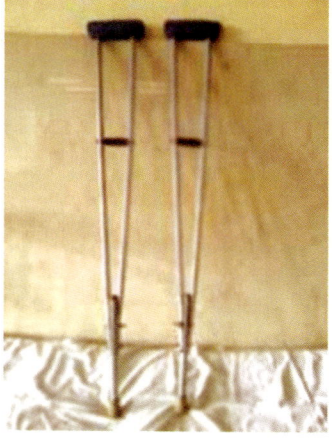

Fig. 39.8: Axillary crutches

crutches: Axillary or underarm crutches (Fig. 39.8), elbow crutches and gutter crutches.

Parts of Axillary Crutches
- Padded axillary portion
- Double upright joined at the height of the top to axillary portion
- A handgrip
- Rubber tip covering the lower end

Ideal Length of Axillary Crutches

Beckwith's method of measurement:
- Subtract 16 inches from the height of the patient.
- Distance from anterior axillary fold to the bottom edge of the heel of the shoe, in supine patient.

Length and position of the handgrip must be adjusted such that with the patient standing up straight, the axillary crutches extend from a point 2 inches below the anterior axillary fold to a point on the ground 6 inches in front and lateral to the tips of the toes. The shoulder should be depressed and the palms of the hands rest on top of the handgrips with the elbow in 30° flexion.

Crutch Walking Patterns of Gait

Four different patterns:
1. Swinging crutch gait
2. Four point crutch gait
3. Three point crutch gait
4. Two point crutch gait

The different patterns vary in the combination of crutches and feet movements used in taking steps and in the sequence of such combination.

The two point and three point partial weight bearing gaits require 33% more energy than normal walking whereas 3 point non weight bearing or swing through gait require 78% more energy.

Amputations

Latin word 'Amputare' means 'cutting around'.

Definition

Amputation means removal of diseased, protruding, functioning unit of the body (removal of limb through one or more bones) (Fig. 40.1). It is different from disarticulation which means removal of limb through a joint.

Epidemiology

Age: Any age can be affected, most common in 50–70 yrs.
Sex: M:F = 3:1
Lower limb > upper limb

Indications

- Lack of circulation (irreparable loss of blood supply to a diseased/injured limb).
- *Infection:* Acute fulminating infection with death of tissues.
- Chronic osteomyelitis/infected gap non-union resistant to treatment.
- Malignant tumours.
- Congenital anomalies where prosthetic fitting likely to improve function.

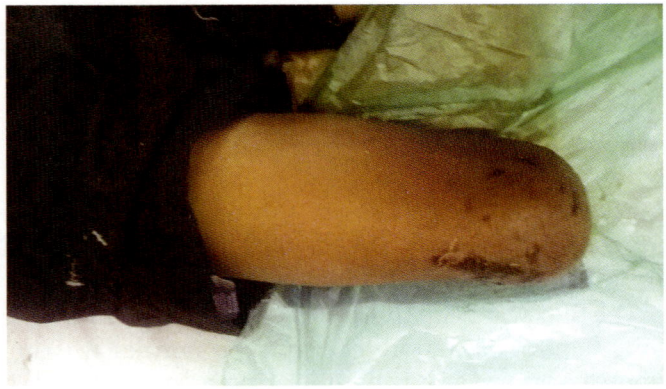

Fig. 40.1: Amputation stump

Types

- *Open:* Guillotine—all tissues from skin to bone are cut at the same level and wound is left open for further management. Usually it is done in emergency to save life of the patients, e.g. gangrene, crushed limb.
- *Closed:* Flaps fashioned and closed primarily.
- *Revision:* For guillotine amputation or for stumps with problems, revision amputation is done to create an ideal amputation stump.

Level of Amputations

Level	Ideal stump length
Above knee	23–28 cm from greater trochanter
Below knee	13 cm from tibial articular surface
Above elbow	10 cm above elbow
Below elbow	17 cm from olecranon

General Principles

- Conservation of every possible dynamic structure to preserve maximum sensations, proprioception and muscle power.
- Preservation of knee joint whenever possible.
- Amputation just above and just below a joint to be avoided.
- Stump should be long enough.
- Higher the level of amputation, greater the energy of expenditure and less available muscle power to control artificial limb.
- In children, growth plate to be preserved.

Basics of Surgical Technique

- *Use of tourniquet:* Avoid in ischaemic and atherosclerotic limb and malignant tumour.
- *Skin flaps:* Either equal anterior and posterior flaps or posterior longer. Dog ears to be avoided.

- *Muscle:* To be sectioned 5 cm distal to the bone section. Opposing muscles are sutured over the end of bone (myoplasty) or attached to the end of bone (myodesis).
- *Blood vessels:* Major ones to be isolated and ligated doubly individually with non-absorbable sutures.
- *Nerve:* Gently pull down and cut with a sharp knife, so that they retract into muscle mass and prevent formation of painful neuroma.
- *Bone:* Avoid periosteal stripping to avoid ring sequestrum.
- Suture periosteal flaps over the medullary canal.

Postoperative Protocol

- Drain for 48 hrs.
- Rigid dressing (plaster of Paris cast) preferred.
- Metal pylon prosthesis to allow early mobilization
- Use of elastic stump shrinkers/stump socket
- Stump exercise important for prevention of contractures and muscle strengthening.

Complications

- Hematoma
- Infection especially in diabetics, ischaemia
- Painful neuroma
- Phantom limb: Feeling by the patient of presence of amputation limb.

  If painful, treatment by analgesics, sedatives, exercise, local nerve block, TENS (transcutaneous electrical nerve stimulation).
- Contractures: Flexion contracture in below knee and flexion/abduction contracture in above knee amputation.

Characteristics of Ideal Stump

- Ideal length and shape
- Muscular and not flabby, with good muscle power
- No fixed deformity, full and free movement at joint above.
- Free of infection
- Nonadherent incision scar
- Absence of neuroma
- Bone ends well covered by muscles.

Special Amputations in Lower Limb

- Boyd's/Pirogoff's: Talus excised, anterior calcaneum cut, superior surface fixed to tibia.
- Syme's: Talus and calcaneum removed.
- Hindquarter amputation: Anterior cut at pubic symphysis. Posterior cut 2–3 inches lateral to sacro-iliac joint.

Special Amputation in Upper Limb

Forequarter amputation: Whole of upper limb, scapula and part of clavicle removed.

ORTHOSIS

Definition

Orthoses are appliance added to a patient to enable better use of the part of body to which they are fitted.

Aims

- To provide stability
- To overcome weakness
- To relieve pain
- To control deformities

Important Characteristics of Orthotic and Prosthetic Materials

- Strength
- Stiffness
- Durability
- Density
- Corrosion resistance
- Ease of fabrication
- Cost and availability

Various Materials Used for Orthoses and Prostheses

- *Metals:* Steel, alloy of titanium aluminium. Aluminium is lighter, therefore, used in children/upper limb,
- Plastics: Low temperature thermoplastic
- Foams: Rigid/flexible
- Wood
- Leather
- Rubber

Care of Orthoses

- Examine skin every night for evidence of undue pressure from orthosis.
- Open all locks and clean
- Oil each joint
- Inspect all moving parts for wear and all leather parts to keep them in good condition.

Varieties of Orthoses (*refer* to Chapter 51)

Spinal Braces

Lumbosacral frame/belt (PID, listhesis).

Taylor's brace with/without axillary support (thoracolumbar fracture).

Milwaukee brace (scoliosis).

Total contact spinal orthosis.

SOMI: Sterno-occipital-mandibular immobilizer (C_1–C_2 injury).

Four post collar/cervical collar (cervical trauma).

Halo body orthosis (scoliosis).

Lower Limb

KAFO, HKAFO, AFO
(H-hip, K-knee, A-ankle, F-foot, O-orthosis)

Footwear modifications:
- CTEV shoes
- Medial arch support
- Heel pad
- Medial/lateral raise
- Metatarsal bar/pad
- Thomas heel

Upper Limb

- Cockup splint
- Knuckle bender splint
- Volkmann's ischaemic contracture splint.

PROSTHESIS

Definition

Prosthesis in Greek means 'in addition'. It is defined as a replacement or substitution of a missing or diseased part of body.

Classification

Endoprosthesis: Implants used in surgery to replace joints, e.g. total hip prosthesis, AMP (Austin Moore prosthesis).

Exoprosthesis: Used externally to replace a lost part of a limb.

Types

- *Temporary/pylon:* Used following an amputation till definite permanent prosthesis is fitted.
- *Permanent:* Used when stump heals well with good soft tissue cover.

Examples of Common Lower Limb Prostheses
(Fig. 40.2)

- Quadrilateral socket prosthesis for AK amputation.
- PTB prosthesis for BK amputation
- Syme's prosthesis for Syme's amputation
- SACH (solid ankle cushioned heel) foot (Fig. 40.3).
- Shoe fillers for foot amputation.

Jaipur Foot (Fig. 40.3)

- Designed by Dr. PK Sethi and Mr. Ram Chander Sharma of Jaipur.
- Made using rubber and aluminium
- Best suited for Indian activities like sitting on the floor, squatting.

Examples of Common Upper Limb Prostheses

- Cosmetic sleeve fitter prosthesis: For forequarter amputations.
- Suction sockets/figure of 8 harness for above elbow amputations.
- Split hook prosthesis with harness for below elbow amputations
- Myoelectric prosthesis: Battery operated devices for carrying out fine activities of hand and upper limb (very expensive) (Fig. 40.4)
- Silicone finger prosthesis

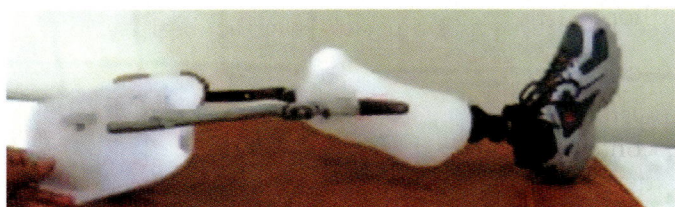

Fig. 40.2: Lower limb prosthesis

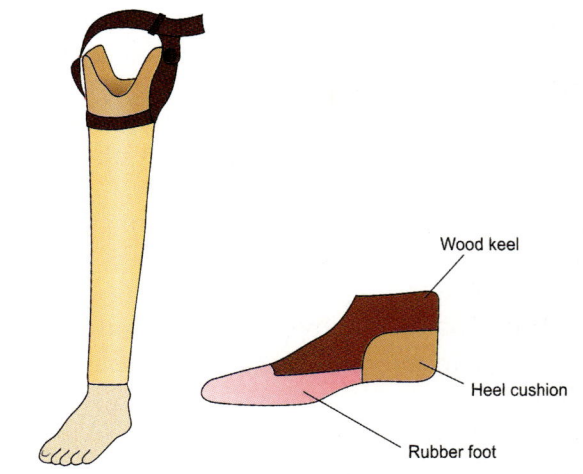

Fig. 40.3: Jaipur foot and SACH (solid ankle cushioned heel) foot

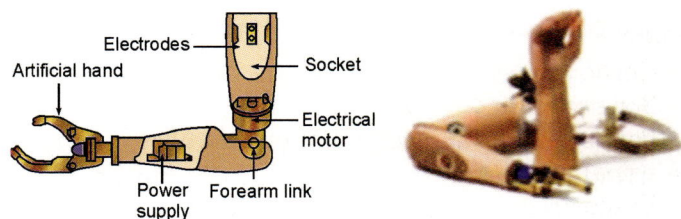

Fig. 40.4: Advanced myoelectric upper limb prosthesis

Special Orthopaedic Techniques

BONE GRAFTING

Introduction

Bone grafting is a procedure of transplanting bone from a donor area to a recipient area, often used in orthopaedic practice.

Mechanism of Action

1. *Osteoinduction:* Placing live bone pieces in close contact with a healthy raw bone surface stimulates new bone formation.
2. *Osteoconduction:* The grafted bone acts as a scaffold around which new bone tissue is laid by creeping substitution by vascular invasion from the surrounding tissue.

Indications

- For filling up cavities in bone (post-infection/tumour)
- For treatment of delayed union/nonunion and pseudoarthrosis
- For bridging gaps and increasing contact area in fractures, along with internal fixation.
- For arthrodesis (surgical fusion) of joints.

Types

According to origin

1. Autograft

Graft taken from the same person. It has the best chance of incorporation.

Sources
- Corticocancellous: Iliac crest, fibula, ulna (Fig. 41.1)
- Bone marrow
- Periosteal and perichondral, e.g. for articular defects, spinal fusion, etc.
- Vascularized bone (fibula, rib) and osteocutaneous flap

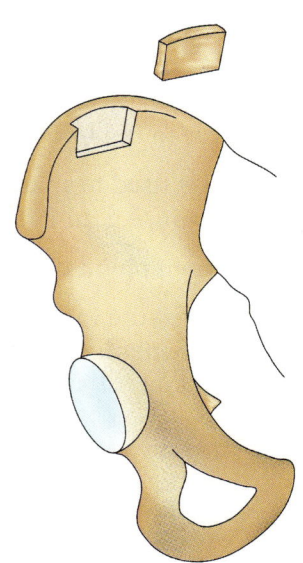

Fig. 41.1: Iliac crest bone graft

2. Allograft/Homogeneous Graft

- Graft taken from same species but different individual.
- Antigenicity may be decreased by freezing/irradiation/demineralization. The graft can be stored in bone bank.
- In children, maternal graft can be used.
- Cadaveric bone also used as graft.

3. Xenograft/Heterogeneous Graft

- Graft from different species, e.g. pig/calf
- Antigenicity high, so seldom used.

According to nutrition of graft

- Free graft: By diffusion from surrounding bone in host bed.
- Vascular pedicle
- Vascularized: Microanastomosis to reconnect vessels of supply.

Anatomical types
- Cortical: Provides better stability
- Cancellous: More osteogenic

Technique

Onlay graft: Strong cortical bone fixed to recipient bone with screws, graft functions as a splint and a framework for growth of new bone.

Sliver graft: Cancellous bone strips (e.g. iliac crest) laid about fracture site deep to periosteum and held in place by suturing soft issue over them. Also called phemister technique.

Chip grafts: Cancellous bone in the form of small pieces firmly packed into and around the recipient bone.

Nicoll's technique: Cancellous bone graft + plating

Sliding graft: From lower to upper bone.

Strut graft: Rib or fibula is used to span entire vertebral body/bodies after excision, e.g. in Pott's spine .

'H' graft: In posterior interspinous fusion.

Bone bank: In order to meet the increasing demand for bone grafts, special bone banks have been set up to store bone with special technique of storage in sterile and viable conditions.

ARTHROSCOPY

Introduction

Arthroscopy is a technique wherein a thin endoscope (arthroscope) is introduced aseptically into a joint through a small stab wound to visualize the interior of a joint for diagnostic and therapeutic purpose. It first started in Japan.

Parts of Arthroscope

- Sheath
- Sharp and blunt trocar
- Scope-lens system (for magnification)
- Eyepiece for direct view or connected to TV camera
- Fibreoptic cable
- Light source
- Probe (diameter 2 mm for small joint and 4–5 mm for large joint).

Sterilization

By ethylene dioxide.

Almost any joint can be reached, but mostly used in knee, shoulder, wrist, ankle and hip.

Indications

Diagnostic

Knee
- Synovial biopsy for Koch's, rheumatoid arthritis, synovial chondromatosis.
- Suspected meniscal/cruciate ligament tear.
- Osteochondritis dissecans.
- Chondromalacia patella.

Shoulder
- Suspected rotator cuff tear
- Shoulder impingement/instability

Therapeutic

- Lavage and debridement
- Scraping/removal of loose bodies.
- Osteochondritis dissecans: Removal of separated fragment and fixation of partially detached fragment.
- Repair of meniscal injury/ACL tear/meniscectomy
- Repair of rotator cuff tear.
- Breaking of intra-articular adhesions and capsular contracture.

Contraindications

- Ankylosed joint
- Active infection

Portals (for knee arthroscopy) (Fig. 41.2)

1. Standard portals
   - Anterolateral: Arthroscope/viewing portal
   - Anteromedial: Instrument/operating portal, for better access and visualization
2. Accessory portals
   - Superolateral/superomedial
   - Posteromedial/posterolateral

'Triangulation' is a technique where surgeon forms the base with instrument and the scope forming the

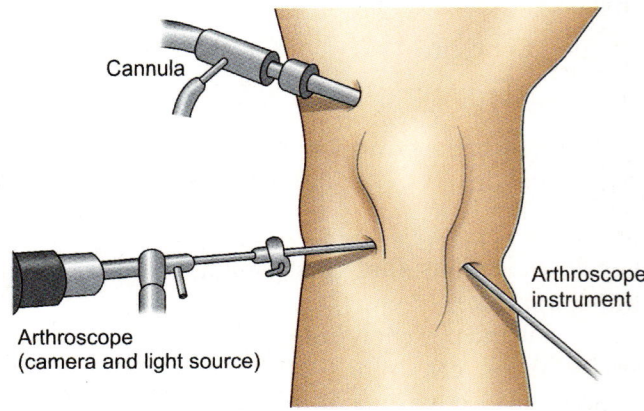

Fig. 41.2: Knee arthroscopy

sides of the triangle. Procedures are done by synchronous movement between the three sides of the triangle.

Advantages
- Quick method
- Minimally invasive day care procedure
- Cosmetic, as no big surgical scar
- Minimal blood loss
- Rapid rehabilitation and mobilization

Disadvantages
- Costly
- Special skills requirement

Complications

- Damage to articular cartilage, cruciate ligament, menisci, fat pad, vessels
- Infection
- Reactive joint effusion and haemarthrosis
- Thrombophlebitis
- Breaking of scope within the joint.

ARTHROPLASTY

Introduction

Arthroplasty is a surgical procedure of repairing and refashioning an arthritic or diseased joint to obtain a painless and mobile joint.

Indications

- Advanced osteoarthritis/rheumatoid arthritis with disabling pain.
- Quiescent destroyed Koch's arthritis especially hip and elbow.
- Correction of deformity of joint
- Nonunion of femur neck fracture.

Types of Arthroplasty

- Excision
- Interpositional
- Resurfacing
- *Replacement:* Hemi or total

Excision Arthroplasty

One or more articular surfaces of the bone are excised and gap in between gets filled with fibrous tissue, allowing flexibility of joint, but it is not very stable, e.g. Girdlestone arthroplasty for Koch's hip (Fig. 41.3).

Interpositional Arthroplasty

Tissues like muscle, tendon, skin are interposed between the articular surfaces of inflammatory joint to

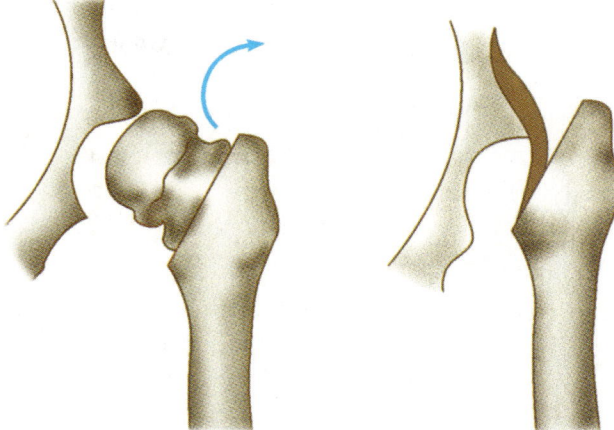
Fig. 41.3: Girdlestone arthroplasty

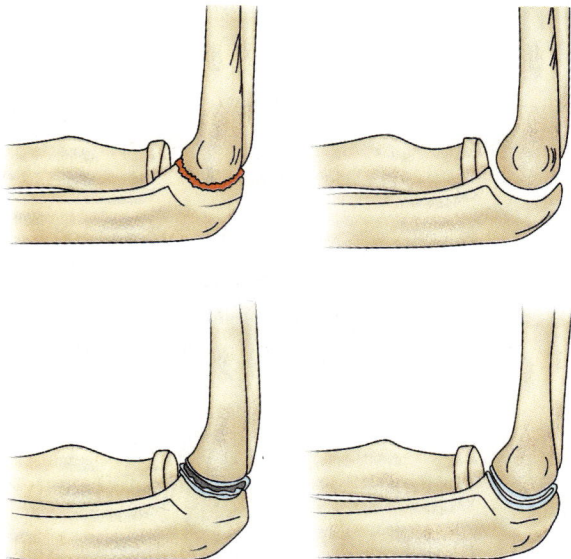
Fig. 41.4: Interpositional arthroplasty

keep them apart, thereby reducing pain and improving range of motion (Fig. 41.4).

Resurfacing Arthroplasty

Type of arthroplasty where the diseased articular surface alone is replaced with a prosthesis, e.g. early AVN hip, shoulder (Fig. 41.5).

Replacement Arthroplasty

One or both articular surfaces of bone are replaced with artificial prosthesis.

A. *Hemiarthroplasty hip:*
  1. Austin Moore prosthesis (Fig. 41.6).
  2. Thompson prosthesis (Fig. 41.7).
  3. Bipolar prosthesis (Fig. 41.8).

Most common indication: Fracture neck femur in elderly or pathological fracture/non-union/excision of tumour head/neck.

Used with/without bone cement.

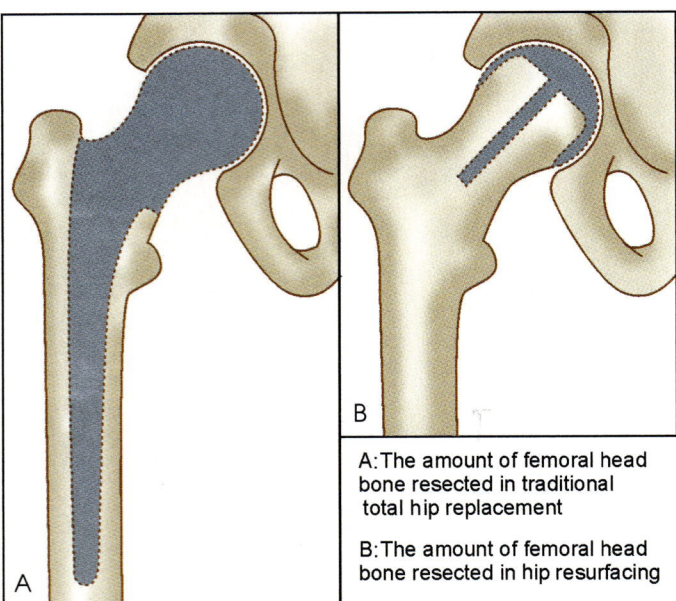

A: The amount of femoral head bone resected in traditional total hip replacement

B: The amount of femoral head bone resected in hip resurfacing

Fig. 41.5: Resurfacing arthroplasty of hip

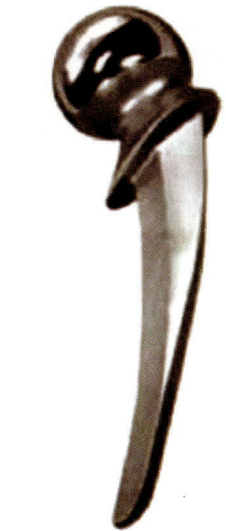

Fig. 41.7: Thompson prosthesis

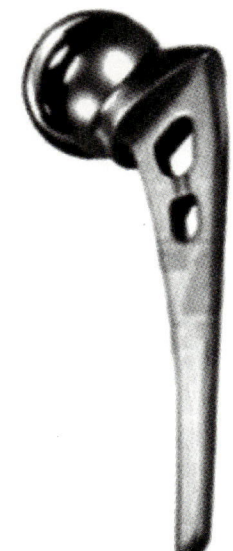

Fig. 41.6: Austin Moore prosthesis

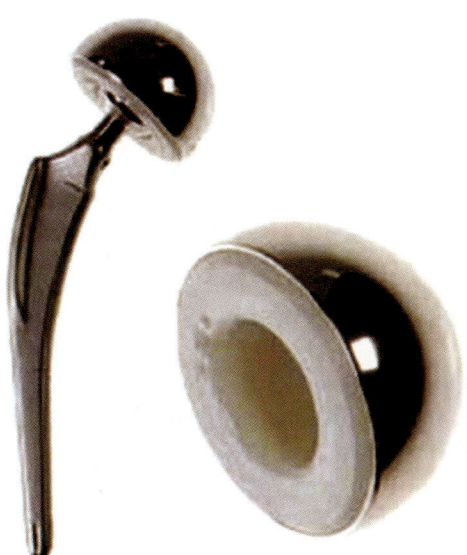

Fig. 41.8: Bipolar prosthesis

B. *Hemiarthroplasty shoulder:* Neer's prosthesis.
   Most common indication: Four parts proximal humerus fracture/nonunion/avascular necrosis
C. *Total hip replacement:*
   Femoral component: Metal (stainless steel, titanium, cobalt chromium alloy) or ceramic.
   Acetabular component: Cup of UHMWPE (ultra high molecular weight poly ethylene) backed by metal ring or cup.
   Can be cemented/uncemented/hybrid (especially in porotic bone).

Complications
- Sciatic nerve injury
- Periprosthetic fracture
- Dislocation of prosthesis
- Infection
- Deep vein thrombosis
- Aseptic loosening
- Heterotopic bone formation
D. *Total knee replacement:*
   - Femoral and tibial component made of metal alloy and spacer made of UHMWPE.
   - Patellar component also of UHMWPE, called patellar button.
Other common joints replaced are shoulder and elbow.

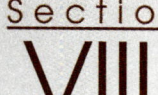

Orthopaedic Clinical Examinations

Shoulder

HISTORY

1. Pain

- True shoulder pain is felt anterolaterally over the deltoid muscle and radiates up to the deltoid tuberosity.
- Pain localised to the top of the shoulder usually arises from the acromioclavicular joint.
- Pain in the supraclavicular region is usually referred from the cervical spine.
- Cardiac ischaemia may cause referred pain in either shoulder.
- Pain in overhead activities only (flexion, abduction, internal rotation-typical of painting/cleaning wall), is suggestive of rotator cuff impingement.

2. Stiffness

- Denotes a decrease in the normal range of shoulder movements, may result in loss of function, such as inability to reach the back/comb hair.
- Aetiology may be idiopathic, post-traumatic, post-operative or secondary to glenohumeral/rotator cuff pathology.
- Progressive, severe stiffness of idiopathic aetiology is termed "frozen shoulder".

3. Deformity

- Prominence of acromioclavicular joint.
- Winging of scapula.

4. Instability

History of recurrent dislocations/subluxations.

5. Swelling

Localised or diffuse.

CLINICAL EXAMINATION

1. Attitude

If the arm is held internally rotated, suspect a posterior dislocation of shoulder.

2. Inspection

- Shoulder asymmetry, scapular winging, deltoid wasting, acromioclavicular dislocation observed from posterior.
- Swelling, pectoral wasting observed from anterior.
- Deltoid wasting suggests a nerve lesion or chronic joint disease.
- Supraspinatus wasting suggests a chronic rotator cuff tear or a suprascapular nerve lesion.
- Local skin condition, including sinuses and surgical scars.

3. Palpation

- Sternoclavicular joint.
- Acromioclavicular joint.
- Anterior glenohumeral joint line.
- Bicipital groove and biceps tendon.
- Posterior glenohumeral joint line.

4. Movements

- Normal range of shoulder movements are flexion 0–140 degrees, extension 0–45 degrees, abduction 0–180 degrees, adduction 0–180 degrees, external rotation 0–70 degrees, internal rotation 0–80 degrees, circumduction 360 degrees.
- Always compare flexion, extension, abduction, adduction and rotations with the opposite limb.
- Always check both active and passive movements.
- Whether associated with pain, crepitus, clicks, thuds, snapping.

- During the early phase of abduction, most of the movement takes place at the glenohumeral joint; as the arm rises, the scapula begins to rotate on the thorax; in terminal abduction, the movement is almost entirely scapulothoracic.
- Smooth scapulo-humeral rhythm is disturbed by glenohumeral disorders; or by dysfunction of glenohumeral stabilisers.
- To check true glenohumeral movements, the scapula is anchored with one hand by pressing firmly down on the scapula.
- Difficulty in initiating abduction indicates a supraspinatus tear.
- Painful movement in the mid-arc range indicates a 'painful arc syndrome' suggestive of subacromial impingement due to supraspinatus tendonitis, subacromial bursitis, calcific tendonitis of supraspinatus, or partial rotator cuff tear.
- Pain at terminal abduction is caused by acromioclavicular arthritis.

5. Muscle Power

- Deltoid is examined for bulk and tautness while the patient abducts against resistance.
- To test serratus anterior (long thoracic nerve of Bell), the patient is asked to push forcefully against a wall with both hands; if the muscle is weak, the scapula stands out prominently (winged scapula).
- Pectoralis major is tested by having the patient thrust both hands firmly into the waist.

6. Neurovascular Deficit

Anterior glenohumeral dislocation may be associated with axillary nerve palsy.

7. Special Tests

- Tests for subacromial impingement.
- Tests for rotator cuff tear.
- Tests for glenohumeral instability.

NEER'S SIGN FOR SUBACROMIAL IMPINGEMENT (Fig. 42.1)

The examiner stands behind the patient and passively abducts the normal shoulder from 0 to 180 degrees. This should not be painful. He thereafter passively abducts the affected shoulder. If there is pain in a certain arc of abduction movement (usually 60 to 120 degrees), then the sign is positive and a diagnosis of painful arc syndrome is made. The causes for this painful subacromial impingement include: Supraspinatus tendonitis, subacromial bursitis, calcific tendonitis of rotator cuff, partial rotator cuff tear.

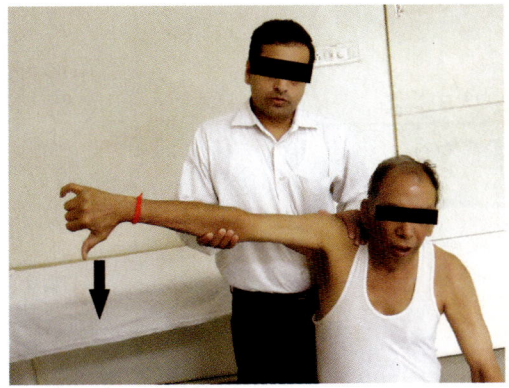

Fig. 42.1: Positive Neer's impingement sign

JOBE'S TEST FOR SUBACROMIAL IMPINGEMENT (Fig. 42.2)

The examiner stands behind the patient and resists forced abduction of the shoulder at 90 degrees abduction and shoulder being in external rotation. Thereafter, he resists forced abduction of the shoulder at 90 degrees abduction and shoulder being in internal rotation. At this position the greater tuberosity of the humerus is obstructed by the acromial arch. If there is no pain during external rotation, but pain during internal rotation, then a diagnosis of subacromial impingement is confirmed.

HAWKIN'S IMPINGEMENT REINFORCEMENT TEST (Fig. 42.3)

The shoulder is placed at 90 degrees of flexion and full external rotation. It is thereafter, passively internally rotated at this position. If this manoeuvre, which forcibly brings the greater tuberosity to rub against the subacromial arch, is painful, then subacromial impingement is confirmed.

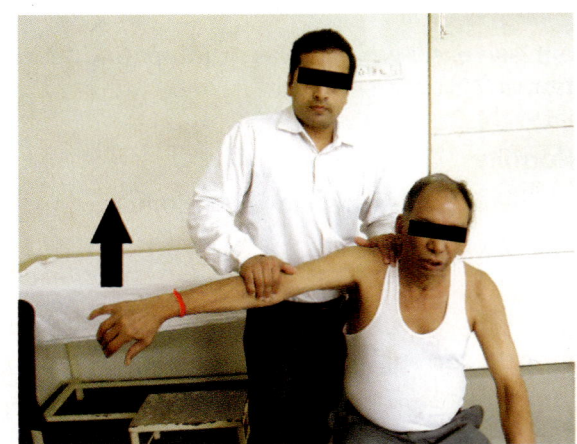

Fig. 42.2: Jobe's test for subacromial impingement

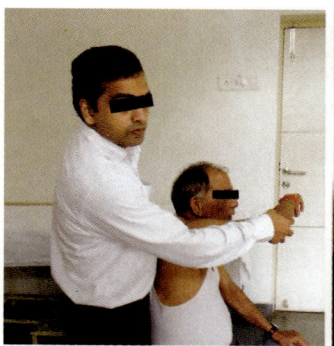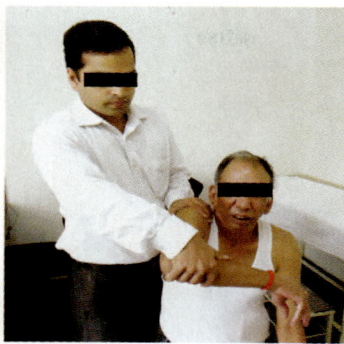

Fig. 42.3: Positive Hawkin's impingement reinforcement test

NEER'S IMPINGEMENT TEST

This test is performed to conclusively differentiate subacromial impingement from other painful problems around the shoulder. In a patient in whom Neer's impingement sign is positive, 10 ml of l% lignocaine is injected in the subacromial space. If the sign is now eliminated, then subacromial impingement is confirmed. If pain is still persistent, then the diagnosis cannot be subacromial impingement.

TESTS FOR COMPLETE ROTATOR CUFF TEAR

In massive rotator cuff tears in a thin patient, there will be deltoid wasting associated with a tender gap felt beneath the acromion. The patient will be unable to initiate active abduction of the glenohumeral joint if the supraspinatus has a full thickness tear. Strength of internal rotation is decreased if there is an associated subscapularis tear. Strength of external rotation is decreased if there is an infraspinatus tear. Incomplete tears of the rotator cuff can be diagnosed by infiltrating local anaesthetic in the subacromial space. This would abolish the pain and spasm arising from a partial thickness tear allowing the patient to abduct the shoulder and easily initiate abduction.

YERGASON'S TEST FOR BICIPITAL TENDONITIS

In Yergason's test, the patient flexes the elbow and then supinates the forearm against resistance. The forceful biceps contraction causes distal movement of the tendon and pain in the region of the bicipital groove.

HAMILTON'S RULER TEST FOR ANTERIOR DISLOCATION OF SHOULDER

In a normal shoulder the deltoid bulge prevents a straight ruler from touching the acromion process and lateral epicondyle of humerus at the same time. In anterior dislocation of shoulder, the humeral head support for the deltoid is lost, the deltoid contour is no

longer bulging, and a straight ruler can touch both the acromion process and lateral epicondyle of humerus at the same time.

CALLAWAY'S TEST FOR DISLOCATION OF SHOULDER

The girth from axillary base to shoulder top are symmetrical and same on both sides. If the humeral head occupies an abnormal position, the girth increases on the affected side.

DUGA'S TEST FOR ANTERIOR DISLOCATION OF SHOULDER

Normally it is possible to bring the hand to the top of the opposite shoulder. In shoulder dislocation, full flexion of the shoulder cannot be achieved and the hand cannot be taken to the opposite shoulder.

APPREHENSION TEST

It is performed to detect any instability of the shoulder (e.g. in recurrent subluxation/dislocation of shoulder).

The suspected shoulder is gradually abducted and externally rotated pressing the shoulder along the long axis of the arm. In case of instability, the patient becomes gradually apprehensive and tries to resist any further movement by his other hand and making the shoulder stiff.

COMMON CASES

1. Recurrent Anterior Dislocations of Shoulder

- History of first traumatic shoulder dislocation followed by subsequent episodes of instability caused by minor trauma or during sleep.
- Apprehension test positive.
- Reduction of apprehension in response to relocation test.
- Increased anterior laxity to passive testing (anterior drawer test).
- Signs of axillary nerve palsy (deltoid weakness, 'regimental patch' hypoaesthesia over lateral aspect of shoulder).

2. Multidirectional Instability

- Sulcus sign positive (Fig. 42.4) indicating inferior laxity.
- Increased anterior and posterior laxity to passive testing (anterior and posterior drawer tests).
- Occasionally ability to voluntarily dislocate.

3. Old Unreduced Shoulder Dislocation (Fig. 42.5)

- History of significant injury followed by pain and restricted shoulder range.

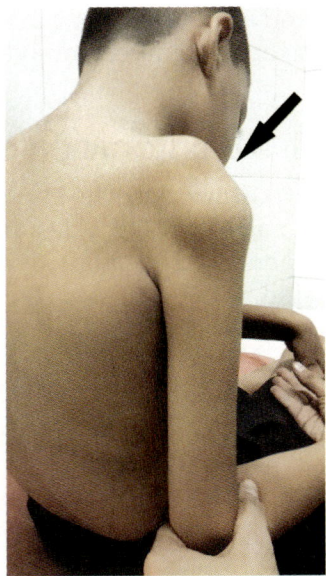

Fig. 42.4: Positive sulcus sign

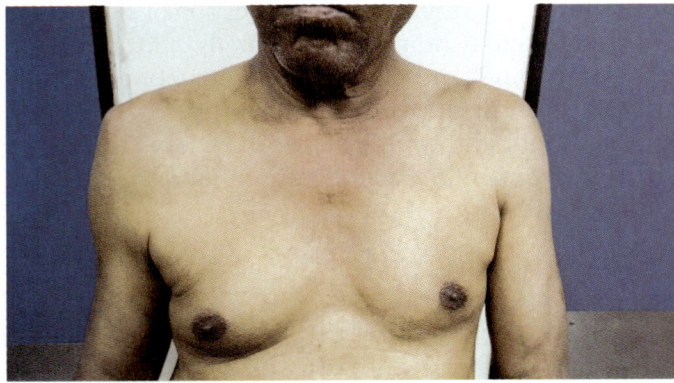

Fig. 42.5: Old unreduced anterior dislocation of shoulder showing loss of shoulder contour with presence of humeral head in subcoracoid region

- Loss of normal shoulder contour.
- Humeral head palpable in subcoracoid region.
- Shoulder range often restricted significantly.
- In anterior dislocation Duga's, Callaway's Hamilton's ruler test positive.

4. Frozen Shoulder/Adhesive Capsulitis (Fig. 42.6)

- Generalised decrease in both active and passive range of motion, including forward flexion, abduction, internal rotation and external rotation.
- Pain elicited by passive range of motion or any passive manipulation that stresses the limits of the patient's reduced motion.
- Generalised weakness or atrophy.

5. Painful Arc Syndrome

- Neer's impingement sign positive.

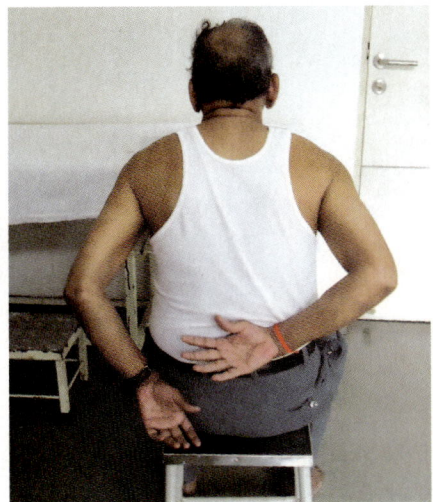

Fig. 42.6: Left frozen shoulder showing decreased shoulder movements with atrophy

- Hawkin's impingement reinforcement test positive.
- Jobe's supraspinatus resistance test positive and painful.
- Painful arc of abduction present (45 degrees to 160 degrees).
- Subacromial tenderness may be present.

6. Rotator Cuff Tear

- Neer's impingement sign positive.
- Hawkin's impingement reinforcement test positive.
- Painful arc of abduction present (60° to 120°).
- Supraspinatus resistance test painful and weak.
- Supraspinatus/infraspinatus atrophy in chronic tears.
- Loss of active abduction, however passive movements often normal (Fig. 42.7).
- Drop-arm sign' may be present in large tears (the passively abducted arm cannot be actively maintained in that position by the patient)
- Weakness/loss of active external rotation in large tears (involving infraspinatus).

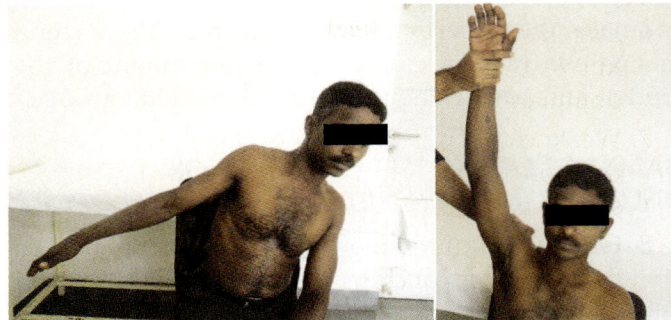

Fig. 42.7: Rotator cuff tear with loss of active abduction however passive movements full

Elbow

HISTORY

1. *Age:* Supracondylar and lateral condyle fractures common in children.

2. *Mode of injury:* Many of the upper limb injuries are caused by fall on the outstretched hand.

3. Time since injury

4. *First aid received:* Inappropriate primary management by bone setters.

   History of massage, application of splints especially if tight can cause compartment syndrome and sequelae. Massage around the elbow region can promote formation of heterotopic ossification (The word "Myositis ossificans" to be avoided if possible).

5. What made the patient seek the treatment (in the chronic setting)

   a. *Cosmetic appearance:* Prominent bump/ugly deformity/progressive deformity (in a growing child)

   b. *Functional disability:* Limitation of the range of movements necessary to carry out ADL (activities of daily living): Hand to mouth for feeding on the right side; combing hairs, to use the hand for ablution purposes (toilet activities) on the left side.

6. *Dominance of the hand (right/left):* Important to know as the treatment sometimes differs for dominant/non-dominant hand

7. Weakness of the elbow to lift heavy weights/for throwing a ball during the sport for the athlete: suggestive of instability of the elbow (subtle/overt)

8. Gradual onset neurological symptoms like paraesthesia, weakness of the ulnar two fingers, with/without clawing: Tardy ulnar nerve symptoms in a case of long standing deformity of cubitus valgus.

9. Pain, swelling, deformity:
   • Following trauma or infective aetiology like tuberculosis in synovitis or arthritic stage.
   • Occasionally swelling around the region of the elbow may be due to any tumour arising from the bones around the elbow.

10. *History suggestive of aetiology in pathological joints:* like Koch's, RA

CLINICAL EXAMINATION

Inspection

1. *Alignment of the Elbow and Forearm* (Fig. 43.1) (Carrying angle)
   • Excessive carrying angle: Cubitus valgus
   • Carrying angle 0°: Cubitus rectus
   • Carrying angle reversed: Cubitus varus
     Normal carrying angle = average 13° for females, 10° for males.

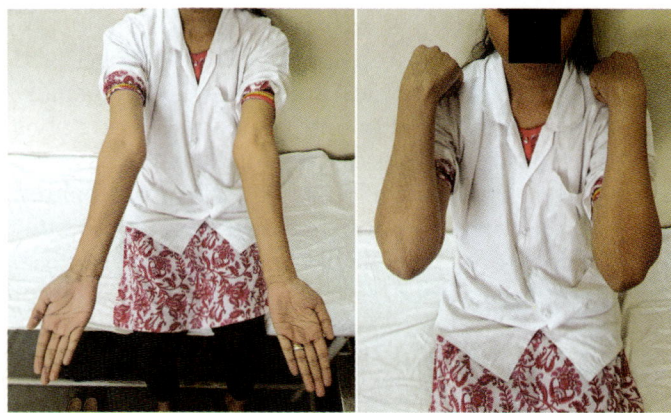

Fig. 43.1: Carrying angle is the normal outward deviation of the extended and supinated forearm from the axis of the arm. It disappears on pronation or on full flexion of the forearm

2. Swellings around the Elbow

- *Paratendinous:* Besides the triceps tendon on either sides due to effusion in the elbow or synovitis.
- Cold abscesses
- *Lymph nodes:* Supratrochlear/epitrochlear
  In elbow 80° flexion, lymph nodes are palpated on the anterior surface of the medial intermuscular septum 1 cm above the base of the medial epicondyle
- Over olecranon process in Olecranon bursitis
- In front/antecubital fossa in large effusions/ bicipitoradial bursitis

3. Scars around the Elbow

- Branding marks
  (Quack treatment with the seeds-seeds are heated and are used for hot fomentation)
- Scars of injury/healed cold abscesses, etc.

4. Muscular Wasting

Especially in Koch's elbow.

Palpation

1. *Warmth/tenderness/confirmation of inspection findings:* Localised tenderness on the particular point of attachment of the tendon is diagnostic of any type of tendonitis, e.g.
   - Lateral epicondyle attachment of the extensor muscles of the forearm—Tennis elbow.
   - Medial epicondyle/attachment of the flexor muscles of the forearm—Golfer's elbow.
2. *Examination of the 3 bony points.*
   - Medial epicondyle, lateral epicondyle and the tip of olecranon form a scalene triangle. Three sides of the triangle are of unequal length with the shortest side being the distance between the olecranon and the medial epicondyle. In fractures or dislocations around the elbow, these 3 bony point relationships are often altered.
   - Three bony point relationships are best observed with elbows in identical amount of flexion (usually to 90, if feasible) with both hands rested on pelvis so as to eliminate the discrepancies in the distances on both the sides. Elbows are seen from behind and the corresponding distances on both the sides are compared (Fig. 43.2).
   - Many times, after trauma there is obliteration of these clinical landmarks as a result of the response to trauma and new bone formation later on. The landmarks which are described, as points are not points in reality and even an astute examiner can make mistakes.
   - In extended elbow, these 3 bony points lie on a straight horizontal line.

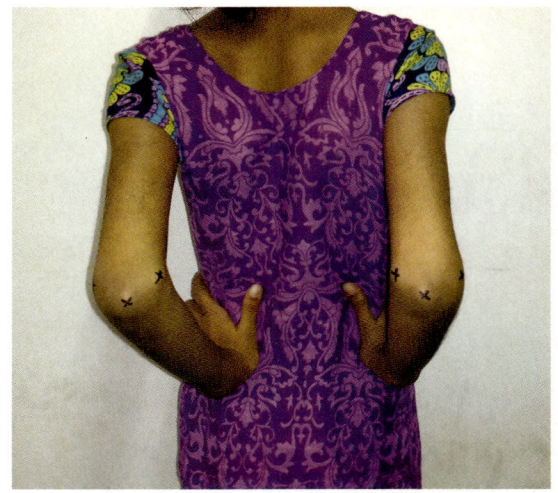

Fig. 43.2: 3-point relationship around elbow: Photograph with points marked

- Always compare the relative positions of the three bony points with those of the sound side
3. *Head of the radius:* Best palpated in the lower part of the dimple just below the lateral condyle of the humerus, when the forearm is pronated and supinated, with the elbow flexed.
   Direction of dislocation of the head of the radius can be noted in c/o old Monteggia fracture.
4. *Thickening/irregularity:* The lower part of humerus and the upper parts of the ulna and radius are palpated-thickening suggests previous osteomyelitis or malunited fracture.

Range of Movements

The reference plane for the measurement of the range is from the fully extended elbow (i.e. anatomical position). Thus fully extended elbow is at 0°.

- Note the range of motion active as well as passive.
- Deformity if any.
- *Block to further range:*
  - *Springy (elastic) feel:* Suggestive of soft tissue causes of the block like contractures, adhesions (periarticular/intra-articular).
  - *Bony block to further motion:* Note if there is any change of arc., e.g. in malunited supracondylar fractures, which have united in extension, there is hyperextension at the expense of flexion range.
- Supination/pronation at the proximal radioulnar joint is checked as well, with the elbow flexed to 90° (in extended elbow, rotation of the humerus gives a false impression of pronation-supination).
- *Normal flexion-extension range:* 0–130° (humero-ulnar joint) (Fig. 43.3).
- *Normal range of supination–pronation:* Supination: 80–85°, pronation: 70–80°.

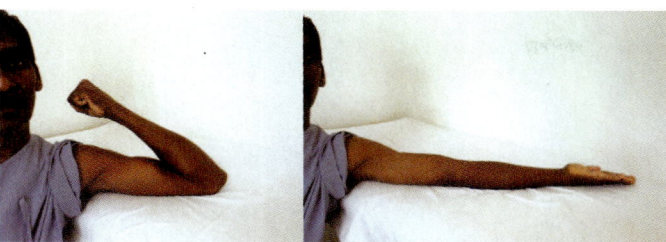

Fig. 43.3: Elbow range of motion

Measurements

1. Though 3 point bony relationships have been described, in practice localisation of these points can have interobserver and intraobserver variability.
   These points are localised as follows:
   - Most distal and prominent point on the medial supracondylar pillar: Medial epicondyle.
   - Most prominent and proximal point when one palpates proximally along the crest of ulna: Olecranon.
   - First most prominent point, which is proximal to the radial head. OR distal most point along the lateral supracondylar pillar: Lateral epicondyle.
2. Measurement of the arm length and forearm length:
   - Arm length is measured from the angle of the acromion (deltoid tubercle) to the lateral epicondyle.
   - Forearm length is measured from the lateral epicondyle to the radial styloid process with elbow in 90° flexion and forearm in neutral position as regards pronation and supination.
   - Arm length is altered in cases where there is proximal migration of the lateral condyle (fractures of the lateral condyle). Forearm length is altered (shortened) in cases of forearm fractures, Monteggia fracture dislocations, etc.
3. Measurement of range of motion:
   Functional arc of movement is between 30° and 130°. Most of the activities of the daily living (ADL) are carried out in this range. This includes taking hand to mouth for feeding (dominant hand) and using the hand for the toilet and hygiene purposes.

Examination of the Lymph Nodes

Epitrochlear group of lymph nodes as well as axillary group of lymph nodes.

Examination of other Joints in the same Extremity

- Wrist
- Hand
- Shoulder

Examination of the neurological function of the extremity and distal vascular status.

COMMON CASES

1. *Tennis elbow*
   - C/o pain on the lateral aspect of the elbow, accentuated by dorsiflexion of the wrist, e.g. pouring out tea in a cup, turning a door handle
   - On palpation, tenderness over the lateral epicondyle of humerus
   - *Cozen's test:* Ask the patient to extend his clenched fist against resistance. Considerable pain is experienced at the lateral epicondyle.
   - *Mill's manoeuvre:* The patient's wrist is passively flexed when his forearm is pronated. This causes tremendous pain on the attachment of the common extensor tendons.
2. *Malunited supracondylar humerus* (Fig. 43.4)
   - H/o fall
   - ? H/o massage—treatment by a quack.
   - Duration between the time of injury and time of seeking treatment.
   - H/o splinting
   - *On examination:* Gunstock deformity/cubitus varus deformity
   - Reversal of the normal carrying angle.
   - Normal 3 bony point relationship between the olecranon, medial and lateral epicondyles.

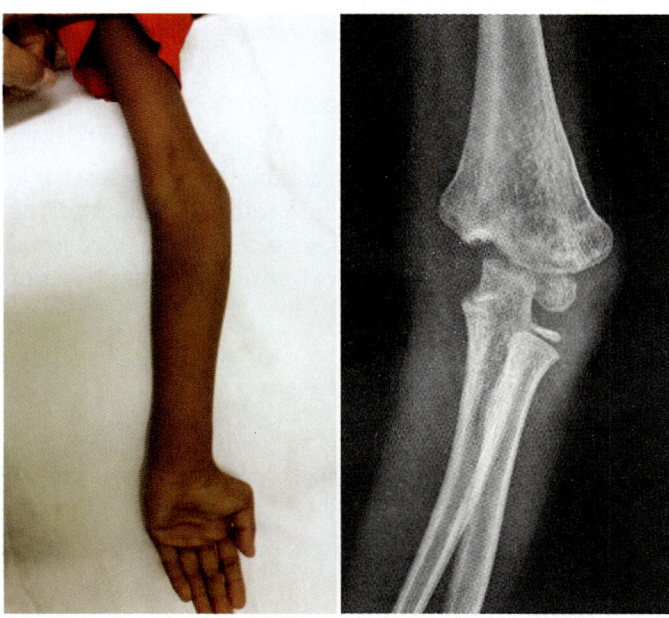

Fig. 43.4: Child with left malunited supracondylar humerus fracture showing cubitus varus deformity—clinical picture and X-ray

- Thickening of the medial and lateral supracondylar pillars (columns).
- Altered arc of motion (often hyper-extension at the cost of flexion. Decreased flexion due to change of arc of motion in the usual extension type of supracondylar fractures united in hyper-extension. Decreased flexion may also be due to the anterior bony block.)
- Note if the block to flexion is bony (because of the anterior bony bump) or springy (extra-articular/intra-articular fibrous adhesions).
- Increased internal rotation of the shoulder when tested with shoulder in neutral position as well as in with shoulder in 90° abduction and elbow placed in 90° flexion (*Yamamoto's test*). This is due to malunited distal fragment in more internal rotation. The change in arc is more apparent than real (Fig. 43.5).

3. *Nonunion of the lateral condyle with cubitus valgus deformity* (Fig. 43.6)
- H/o trauma
- Treatment history
- Deformity static/progressive
- Symptoms of ulnar nerve deficit (paraesthesia in ulnar 2 digits, clawing of these 2 fingers, ulcer over the pulps of little/ring fingers.
- Abnormal prominence near lateral condyle/epicondyle.
- Abnormal mobility may be elicited.
- Cubitus valgus (increased carrying angle).
- Increased distance between the tip of olecranon and lateral epicondyle.
- Thickening of the lateral pillar/supracondylar column.
- Decreased arm length (distance between the angle of the acromion or the deltoid tubercle and the lateral epicondyle. This is because of the proximal migration of the lateral condyle which is not united).

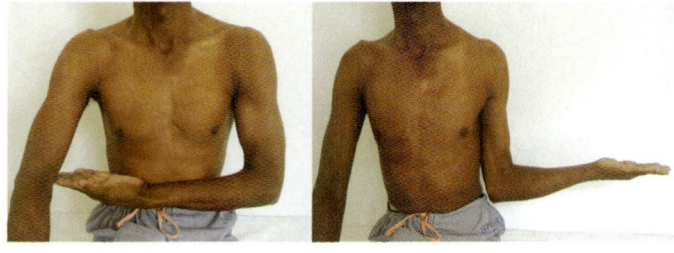

Fig. 43.5: Shoulder rotations can be checked with arm by the side and elbow flexed in 90° flexion as shown in the adjacent figure in a patient with different pathology

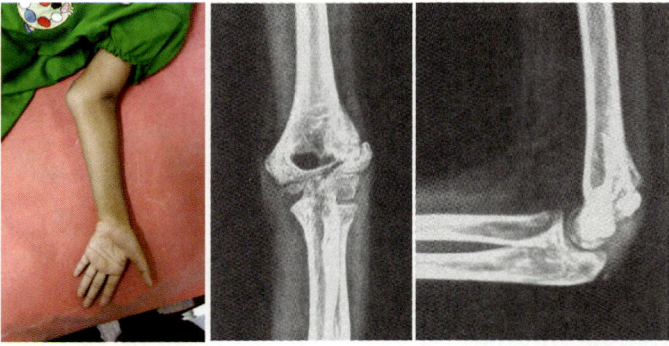

Fig. 43.6: X-ray and clinical photograph of a child with left non-union of the lateral condyle fracture with cubitus valgus

- Elbow range may be normal/restricted.
- In case of long standing/progressive cubitus valgus deformity: Symptoms of tardy ulnar nerve palsy.

4. *Unreduced (neglected) posterior dislocation of elbow*
- H/o trauma
- H/o treatment at home, by quacks
- H/o massage/splinting
- Deformity of the elbow: Note the attitude of the elbow.
- Prominent triceps tendon ("heel cord" sign) (Fig. 43.7)
- Tip of olecranon riding higher than the line joining both the epicondyles (reversal of the triangle)
- Restricted elbow range. Flexion deformity is often present with bony block to further flexion. Pronation-supination also may be restricted.
- Decreased forearm length with normal arm length measurements.

This is because there is no alteration of relationship between the lateral epicondyle and the angle of acromion (arm length) however, the distance between the lateral epicondyle and the radial styloid process is relatively shortened due to the dislocation. This holds true in cases of pure posterior dislocations of the elbow without any fractures. In cases of fracture-dislocations, it may not be possible to locate the exact landmarks of the epicondyles since they are also displaced.

5. *Old malunited Monteggia fracture dislocation*
- History of trauma
- Decreased forearm length with normal arm length.
- Abnormal prominence of the radial head with bony block to flexion when dislocation of the radial head is anterior. By rotating the forearm it is felt as a globular bony structure, which moves

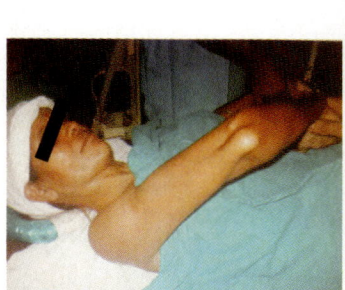 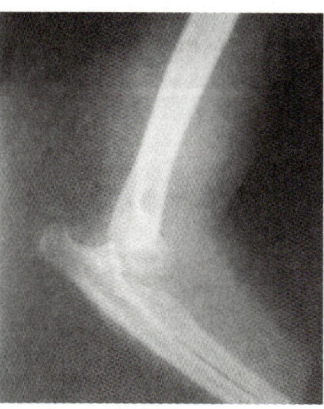 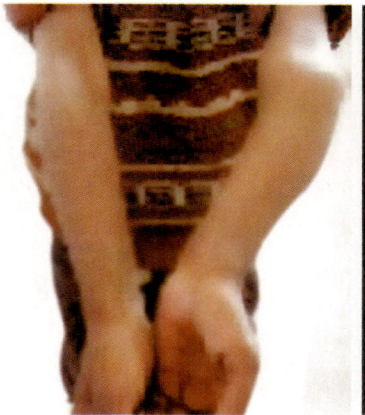 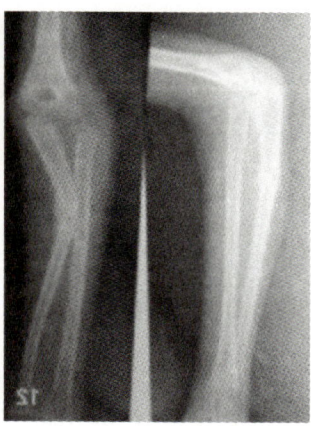

Fig. 43.7: Clinical photograph of a neglected posterior dislocation of the elbow showing "heel cord" sign (prominent triceps tendon), reversal of 3 bony points relationship with inversion of the triangle formed by them. X-ray of the case is attached below it

Fig. 43.8: X-ray of a patient with left malunited Monteggia fracture dislocation type III, with lateral dislocation of radial head and lateral angulation of ulna fracture

in unison with the radius and is immediately distal to the lateral epicondyle. Radial head is not in its usual position articulating with ulna.

- Pronation-supination may be restricted due to bowing of the ulna with loss of normal interosseous space (Fig. 43.8).

Wrist, Forearm and Hand

As in other parts of the body, examination proceeds in the sequence of inspection, palpation, identifying the bony landmarks and their relationship with each other, measurements of the lengths of the arm, forearm as well as measurement of individual length of the radius as well as ulna and the range of movement at the joint. It is important to examine the hand's prehensile function (especially, tip-to-tip opposition, key grip, precision grip, power grip in Fig. 44.1).

HISTORY

a. Pain

- Site of pain
  1. Over radial styloid and along the tendon sheaths of abductor pollicis longus and extensor pollicis brevis.
  2. Over the metacarpal heads (i.e. over the site of A1 flexor pulley).
  3. Over the inferior radio-ulnar joint.

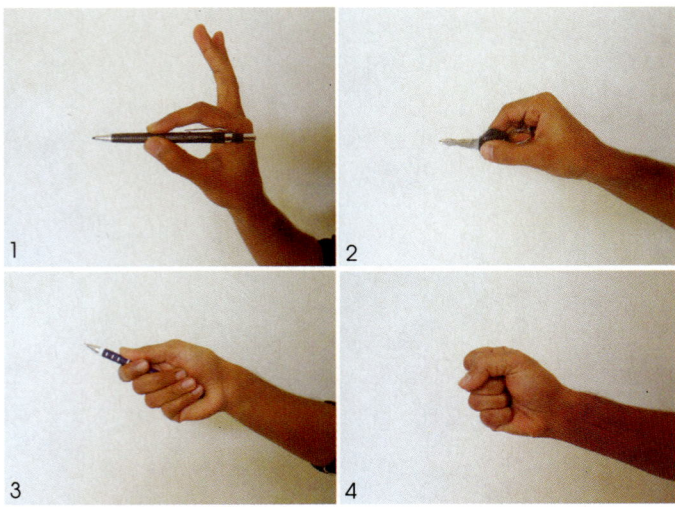

Fig. 44.1: (1) tip-to-tip opposition, (2) key pinch, (3) precision grip, (4) power grip.

4. Over the site of lunate along the joint line of the wrist dorsally.
- Duration of pain.
- Activity aggravating the pain.
- Occupation related factors causing exacerbation.
- Radiation of pain.
- Accompanying swelling, if any.
- Associated neurological symptoms, if any (like tingling, numbness-pins and needles, etc.).
- Associated with the stiffness.

Examples
- Pain long after a trauma associated with increasing stiffness of the fingers.
- Pain typically awakening the patient in the late night with the feeling of pins and needles in the distribution of the median nerve (radial 3½ fingers).
- Pain aggravated during lifting a cup of tea, squeezing clothes during washing.

b. Swelling

- Location
- Duration
- Onset-whether it was following a trauma or was insidious.
- Whether it was associated with pain.
- Did the swelling appear before or after pain.
- Waxing and waning of the swelling.

c. Deformity

- Static or progressive.
- *Duration:* Whether since birth or recently developed.
- Whether following a trauma.

d. Functional Disability

One must enquire about the limitations of activities of daily living faced by the patient due to the ailment.

CLINICAL EXAMINATION

Inspection

- Attitude of wrist and fingers
  - Flexion of the wrist: In majority of the wrist pathologies
  - Ulnar deviation of finger joints (RA)
  - Thumb-clawing
  - Pointing index
  - Simian thumb (ape thumb)—thumb in the same plane as the palm
- Swelling/swellings
  - Number, extent, location
  - Size
  - Shape—dumbbell shape might signify communication between two swellings
  - Edge and surface of the swelling
  - Relationship of the swelling with the joint, joint capsule, tendon, and tendon sheaths—engulfing/surrounding the tendons and tendon sheaths or eccentric arising only from one side of the tendon sheath
  - Sessile/pedunculated
- Skin and nails
  - Presence of dry skin with anhidrosis
  - Lackluster nails with ridges
  - Loss of pulp of the fingers
  - Trophic ulcers, if any
- *Muscles:* Wasting of the thenar, hypothenar, dorsal interossei (especially in the 1st web space dorsally), flattening of arches of the palm.
- *Digits:* Presence of extra digit, absence of digit, and abnormal digits as well as abnormal cleft between the digits or fused digits.
- Deformity
  - Manus varus/valgus (occurring at the wrist)
  - Dinner fork deformity.
  - Swan neck/buttonniere deformities of the fingers.
  - Flexion contractures of the wrist.
- *Sinus:* In Koch's wrist

Palpation

- Radial and ulnar styloid processes.
  Note the radioulnar variance (difference between the levels of these 2 processes).
  Usually the radial styloid process is distal to the ulnar styloid process by around ½ inch.
- Swelling
  - Consistency
  - Fluctuation: Positive in wrist effusion, ganglion and compound palmar ganglion

1. Wrist effusion—crossed fluctuation elicited both on the anterior and the posterior aspect of the wrist.
2. Compound palmar ganglion—crossed fluctuation elicited above and below the flexor retinaculum
3. Ganglion—usually so tense that no elicitable fluctuation, occasionally feels hard as a bone and fixed
- Tenderness
  - On the joint line—s/o arthritis
  - Along the tendon sheaths—s/o tenosynovitis

Measurement

Forearm length as well as the lengths of individual bones (radius, ulna). Forearm length is measured from the lateral epicondyle to the radial styloid process with the elbow in 90° flexion and forearm in neutral position as regards pronation and supination.

Range of Movement

1. *Supination/pronation*
   Checked in 90° flexion of the elbow to eliminate the rotations occurring at the shoulder level. With arms and elbow stabilised by holding them adjacent to the body, range is measured from the neutral rotation taken as 0° rotation (Fig. 44.2).
   - To measure the exact angles of pronation and supination, patient is asked to hold a pen in each hand as shown and the angles that the pens sustain with the vertical are measured with the goniometer.
   - Normal supination: 85°
   - Normal pronation: 70–80°.
   - Functional range of supination–pronation: 50° supination and 50° pronation. This is the range in which most of the activities of daily living are performed.
2. *Dorsiflexion and palmar flexion (at the wrist)*
   It can be compared on both the sides as follows:
   - Indian namaste gesture compares dorsiflexion on both the sides as shown in the figure above. Asking the patient to keep dorsum of both the hands in contact with each other and lowering the elbows can compare palmar flexion (Fig. 44.3).
   - Quantitatively, exact angles can be measured by goniometer (Fig. 44.4).
   - *Normal range:* Palmar flexion: 60–80°. Dorsiflexion: 60–70°.
3. *Finger flexion*
   - Finger flexion can be expressed as the distance remaining between the fingertips and the palmar crease.
   - Normally when the fingers are flexed to make a

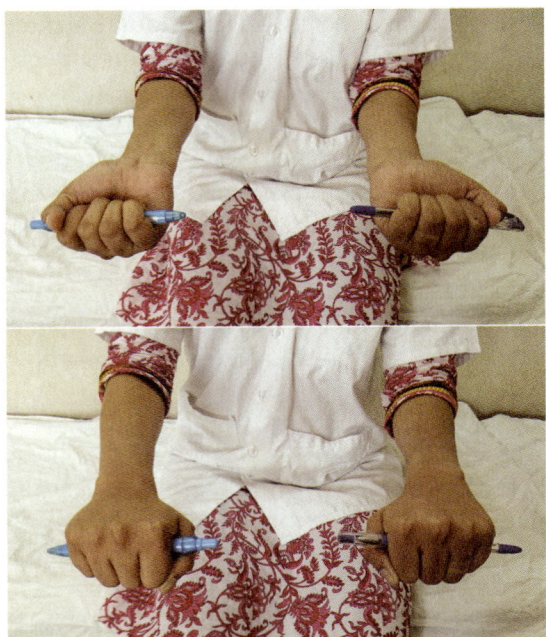

Fig. 44.2: Correct method of checking supination and pronation

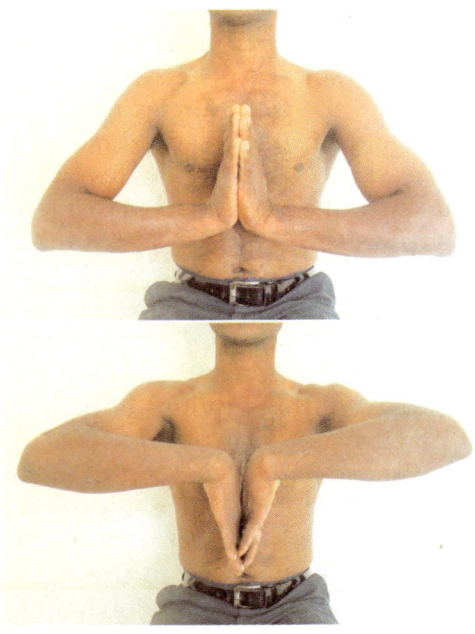

Fig. 44.3: Method of checking active dorsiflexion and palmar flexion at the wrist

fist, the nails of all the fingers point towards the scaphoid. In cases of rotational malalignment following phalangeal fractures, this alignment is lost.

4. *Radial deviation:* 20°, ulnar deviation: 30–40°
5. *Fingers and thumb*
6. *Finger opposition*

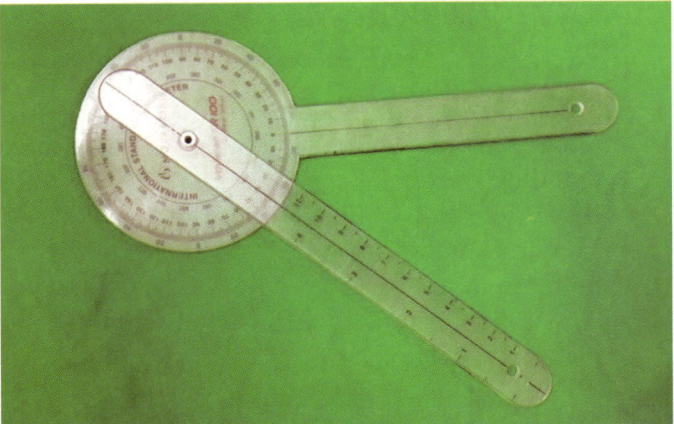

Fig. 44.4: Goniometer

Fingers except thumb	Flexion	Extension
MCP joint	90°	30–45°
PIP joint	100°	0°
DIP joint	90°'	20°
Thumb		
MCP joint	50°	0°
IP joint	90°	20°

Special Tests

- *Finkelstein's test:* In case of de Quervain's disease, ulnar deviation with the thumb in the clenched fist elicits pain over the tendons of extensor pollicis brevis and abductor pollicis longus (Fig. 44.5).
- *Phalen's test:* In cases of carpal tunnel syndrome, palmar flexion of the wrist for one minute starts tingling and numbness symptoms of carpal tunnel syndrome due to pressure over the median nerve. This test is augmented by elevating the forearm and holding it up till the symptoms start.

COMMON CASES

1. Malunited Colles' Fracture

- Especially in an elderly postmenopausal woman with osteoporosis
- H/o fall on the outstretched hand

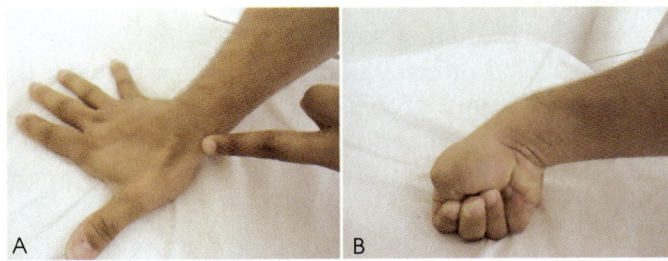

Fig. 44.5: de Quervain's disease: (A) Site of tenderness, (B) Finkelstein's test elicits pain

- ? H/o similar fall in the past (H/o trivial trauma-fragility fractures—vertebral body fracture.)
- H/o treatment taken (e.g. plastering under anaesthesia).

Present Complaints

- Pain
- Inability to make a fist/to do day-to-day activities.
- Shoulder stiffness (in shoulder-hand syndrome)
- Cosmetic deformity only

Examination

- Dinner-fork deformity (Fig. 44.6).
- Loss of normal radio-ulnar variance.
- Restricted ulnar deviation and palmar flexion due to the deformity.
- In classical Colles' fracture radial deviation as well as dorsiflexion may be exaggerated.
- Tender inferior radio-ulnar joint.
- 'Piano key' sign present → Ballotment of the ulnar head against lower end radius elicits tenderness as well an abnormal mobility as compared to the opposite side.
- Decrease in the forearm length.

Complications

- Finger flexion may be restricted, especially at the metacarpophalangeal joint level.
- In shoulder hand syndrome, shoulder movements may also be restricted similar to that in periarthritis of shoulder.

- Features suggestive of Sudeck's dystrophy, causalgia should be looked for.
- Features suggestive of ruptured tendon of EPL (extensor pollicis longus).

2. Nonunion Radius or Ulna (Fig. 44.7)

Loss of radio-ulnar variance in case of nonunion of radius or ulna.
- Palpable gap in the continuity of bone.
- Restricted supination/pronation.
- Deformity due to dorsal dislocation of inferior radio-ulnar joint.

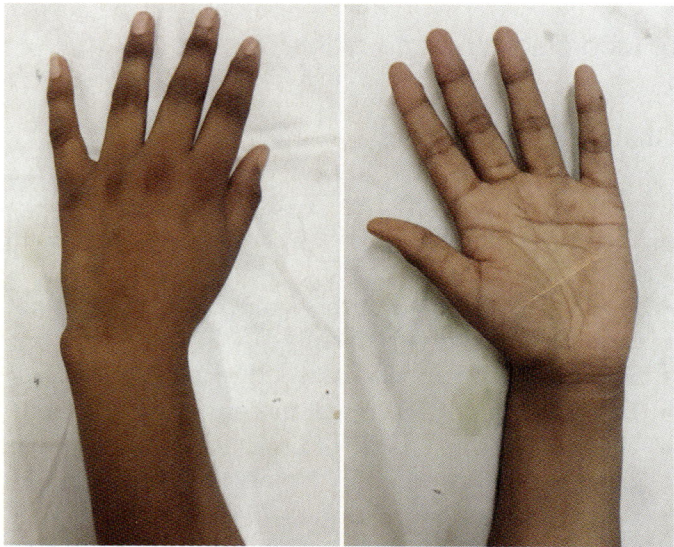

Fig. 44.7: Nonunion radius with loss of normal radio-ulnar variance and deformity

3. Malunited Phalangeal Fractures

- Deformity of the finger (Fg. 44.8)
- Restricted range of motion

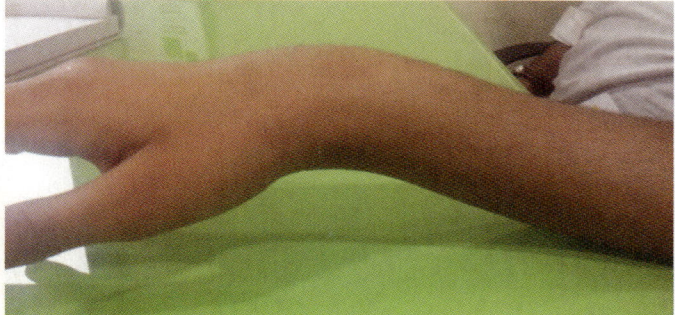

Fig. 44.6: Malunited Colles' fracture showing classical dinner fork deformity

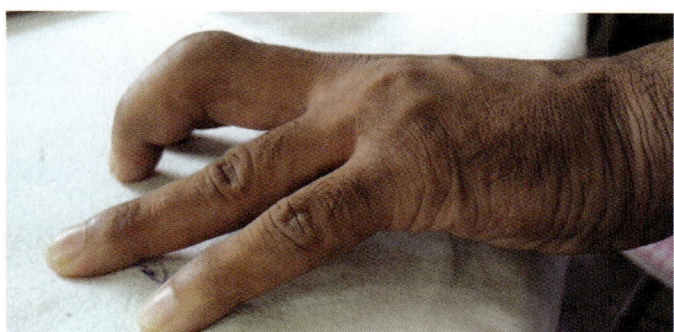

Fig. 44.8: Malaligned middle finger deformity

4. Tuberculous Dactylitis

- Bony tenderness and swelling (usually fusiform with uniform thickening).

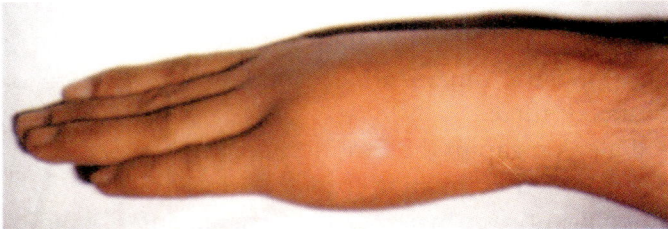

Fig. 44.9: 5th metacarpal Koch's involvement with cold abscess presenting superficially

5. Tuberculous Arthritis of the Wrist (Fig. 44.10)

History

Gradual aching, stiffness.

Examination

- Diffuse swelling along the wrist joint, especially on the dorsal side.
- Swelling is confined to the wrist joint and does not extend proximally or distally.
- Soft to firm, boggy elastic feel due to synovitis.
- Tenderness-joint line as well as bony may be present.
- There may be instability of DRUJ (distal radio-ulnar joint) as demonstrated by a piano key sign.
- Epitrochlear lymph node enlargement may be present.
- Cold abscess and sinus formation may be present.

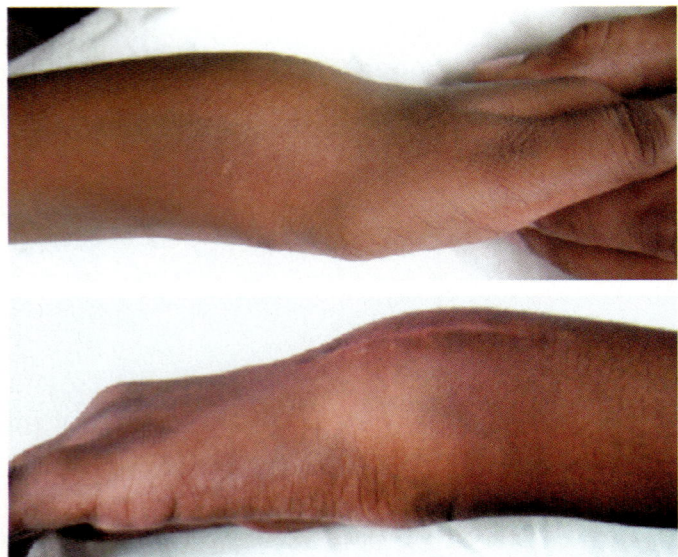

Fig. 44.10: Swelling of wrist in a case of tuberculous arthrtitis in early stage

6. Ganglion

Young adults.

History

Painless lump may be associated with dull ache and weakness.

Examination

- Soft cystic swelling usually on the dorsal aspect arising from the wrist.
- It becomes more prominent on palmar flexion of the wrist and disappears on dorsiflexion.
- Usually sessile (non pedunculated) and cannot be moved in the longitudinal direction.
- It may occasionally be moved side to side
- Differentiate it from the extensor tenosynovitis.

7. Extensor Tenosynovitis (Fig. 44.11)

Examination

- Swelling longitudinally along the extensor tendons of the wrist.
- Dumbbell-shaped due to extensor retinaculum creating central depression.
- Moves with the contraction of the extensor tendons on dorsiflexion of the wrist and fingers.
- Cannot be moved longitudinally but can be moved transversely perpendicular to the direction of the tendons when they are not taut.
- Cross fluctuation may be present (pseudo-cross fluctuation since there is no fluid in it).
- Boggy elastic feel typical of synovitis may be present.

8. Rheumatoid Hand (Fig. 44.12)

- Metacarpophalangeal flexion deformity.
- Multiple swan neck/buttonniere deformities in the fingers
- Ulnar deviation of fingers
- Thumb deformity.

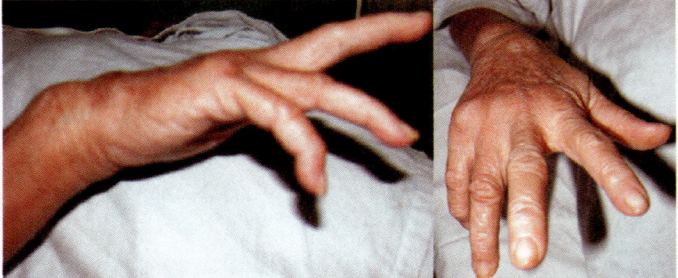

Dumbbell-shaped swelling

Fig. 44.11: Extensor tenosynovitis in a rheumatoid wrist with rupture of extensors to ring and little finger

9. Volkmann's Ischaemic Contracture

- History of trauma to the supracondylar region of humerus
- ? Tight bandaging and H/o intense pain in the forearm with burning in the forearm.
  Examination: Detail neurological examination essential.
- Attitude of flexion at the wrist with flexion at the fingers.
- Fixed length phenomenon or Volkmann's sign: With wrist in flexion, it is possible to extend the fingers but with wrist in maximal possible extension, fingers cannot be extended.

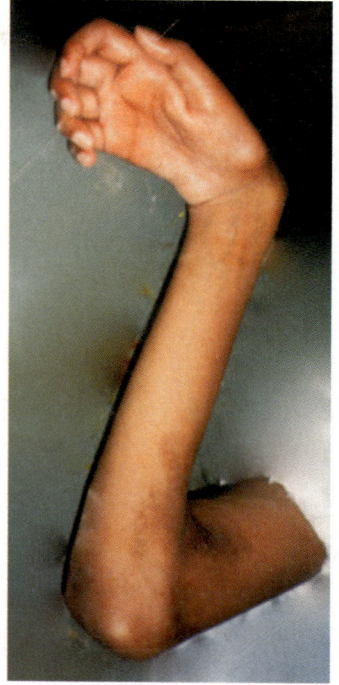

Fig. 44.13: Illustration shows the attitude of hand and wrist in Volkmann's ischaemic contracture (VIC) as well as median and ulnar nerve involvement evident from wasting of thenar and hypothenar eminences. There is a simian (ape) thumb deformity

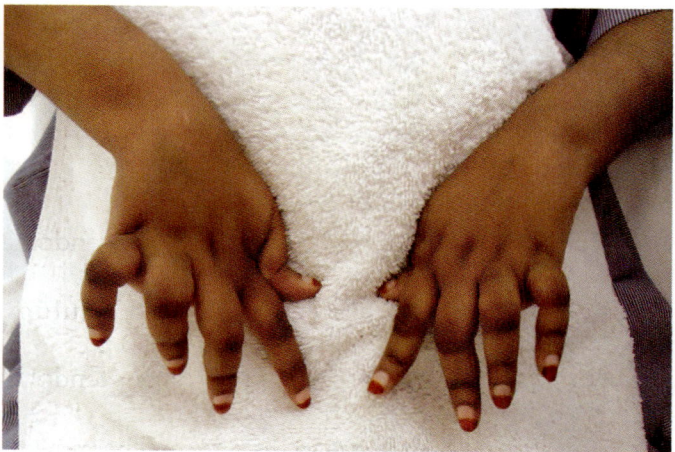

Fig. 44.12: Rheumatoid hand: bilateral affection

10. Carpal Tunnel Syndrome

- Women 40–60 years.

History

- C/O pain, tingling, numbness, progressive weakness and impairment of fine movements especially of the radial three and half fingers.
- Pain may get aggravated at night, relieved by vigorous shaking of the wrist.

Examination

- Sensory changes and motor impairment corresponds to median nerve distribution.
- Phalen's sign positive.
- Tinel's sign—tapping at the wrist causes reproduction of tingling pain in the distribution of the median nerve.
- Atrophy of the thenar muscles in long standing cases.

11. de Quervain's Disease

- Middle aged women
- C/o pain on the radial styloid process
- Aggravated by extension of thumb against resistance
- Localised tenderness
- Swelling
- Finkelstein's test positive

12. Trigger Finger

- Pain, swelling, tenderness over distal palmar crease
- Palpable nodule opposite metacarpal head
- Palpable and audible snapping on flexion and extension of the finger
- In severe cases, finger after flexing may remain locked in flexion. Patient has to manually extend the finger with other hand and it extends with a snap.

CHAPTER
45

Spine

HISTORY

Personal Information

1. Age
   - Spondylosis, degenerative disc disease, spondylolisthesis > 40 yrs.
   - Ankylosing spondylitis—young adults: 15–35 yrs.
   - Tuberculosis of spine—any age, but common in children and adolescents.
2. Sex
   - Ankylosing spondylitis common in males.
3. Occupation
   - *Heavy manual workers:* Early spondylosis.
   - *Computer operators with wrong height of chair:* Cervical spondylosis.
   - *Students and jobs involving prolonged sitting:* Postural pain.
4. Sleeping habits
   Use of thick pillow or very soft mattress can be contributory to neck and back pain.

Chief Complaints

1. Pain

- Onset—sudden after trauma or lifting weights in fracture/acute disc prolapse
- Duration
- Progress—gradually increasing in Koch's, degenerative disc disease
- Site—indicates the level of spine involvement
- Nature—dull, continuous pain in inflammatory conditions. Only on movements in degenerative disc disease. Night pain in infective or certain neoplastic conditions.
- May be associated with giddiness in cervical spondylosis
- Severity—whether interferes with normal activities and function

- *Aggravating and relieving factors:*
  - Pain arising from mechanical causes/bad posture/disc/degenerative causes is aggravated on activity, bending, lifting weights, jerky movements, maintaining one posture over a period of time and relieved on rest, lying down.
  - Lumbar disc pain is maximum in sitting, decreased in standing and relieved in lying down position.
  - Pain arising from non-mechanical causes is present even at rest.
  - Pain shooting down the leg as a result of coughing, sneezing is highly suggestive of root compression.
- *Any radiation:* Disc compressing on a nerve root will give rise to pain radiating down the upper/lower limb along the course of the specific nerve.
- Referred pain:
  - Pain arising from cervical causes can be referred to the occipital region, periscapular area.
  - Pain arising from lumbar causes can be referred to buttocks, paraspinal region, back of the thigh. (Referred pain is rarely felt below the knee, whereas pain due to root irritation may spread to calf or even into the foot and may be associated with paraesthesia/numbness).
  - Pain arising from thoracic causes can be referred to the chest-girdle pain
- Diurnal variation
  - Morning stiffness in ankylosing spondylitis and rheumatoid arthritis
  - Night cries in Koch's

2. Deformity

- Time of onset
- Correctibility
- Progression

3. Swelling

- Site
  - Paraspinal in cold abscess
  - Central in myelomeningocoele
- Painful/painless

4. Neurological Symptoms

- Numbness, tingling in a particular area
- Ground feeling like cottonwool
- Weakness (lower limb)
  - Chappals slipping out
  - Frequent falls
  - Unsteady gait
- Weakness (upper limb)
  - Poor grip
  - Inability to hold objects
  - Difficulty in fine movements, e.g. buttoning, feeding
- Bladder/bowel complaints
  - Incontinence
  - Inability to feel full bladder
  - Inability to void
- H/o claudication
  - Vascular/neurogenic
  - Claudication distance

H/S/O Aetiology

1. *Trauma*
   - Nature
   - Any associated onset of weakness
2. *Koch's*
   - Loss of weight and appetite
   - Evening rise of temperature
   - Past/family h/o Koch's
3. *Ankylosing spondylitis*
   - Morning stiffness
   - Associated chest discomfort
   - Associated hip/major joint pain
   - H/o urethritis/iritis
4. *Osteoporosis*
   - Multiple bone and joint pain
5. *Metastasis*
   - History suggestive of primary tumour, e.g. thyroid, breast, prostate
6. *Rheumatoid arthritis*
   - Morning stiffness
   - Other joint pain including hand

Past History

Similar episodes of neck/back pain.

H/O Treatment

- Medication
- Traction
- Physiotherapy
- Surgery
- Brace
- Bedrest
- Weight reduction
- Job modification

Referred Back Pain History

- *Abdominal disorders*
  - Pancreatitis (very imp.)
  - Cholecystitis
  - Peptic ulcer
- *Pelvic*
  - Inflammatory conditions of ovaries and tubes
  - Intrapelvic tumour
- *Genitourinary*
  - Renal infection/calculus
  - Prostate
- *Vascular*
  Ischaemic pain from occlusion of aorta/ iliac artery

CLINICAL EXAMINATION

Examination of Cervical Spine

Instruction: All spine cases, especially the traumatic ones with neurological deficit or instability have to be handled with utmost care, avoiding any jerky movements.

1. Inspection

- Attitude and posture of the head
  - *Normal:* The head is erect, perpendicular to the floor
  - *Abnormal:* The head is tilted to one side/ supported by hands under the chin to protect or splint an area of pain, e.g. torticollis, acute exacerbation of cervical spondylosis, cervical fracture or dislocation
- Attitude of the limbs and body need to be checked in cases of spinal cord injury to judge the level of affection
- Deformity
  Kyphosis, e.g. in cases of tuberculosis
- Abrasion/ bruise
  Indicate the level of injury
- Scars
  Irregular, pitted scars are likely evidence of previous Koch's adenitis

- Swelling
  Cold abscess/haematoma
- Taut paraspinal muscles preventing the normal movements.

2. *Palpation*

- The spinous processes are to be palpated along the posterior midline starting at the base of the skull.
  - C1 spinous process—small deep tubercle, so cannot be palpated
  - C2 spinous process the first one that is palpable.
  - While palpating from C2 to T1, note the normal lordosis of the cervical spine.
  - C3 to C5—may be bifid
  - C7 and T1—larger
- Look for tenderness, abnormal prominence or gap in the spinous process
- *Facet joints:* Laterally, about 1 inch from midline, with deep palpation, one can identify the facet joints. They may be tender in cases of facetal arthritis.
- Paraspinal muscle spasm/prominence
  - Supraclavicular fossa: Cervical rib
  - Swelling/lump due to trauma, lymph node

3. *Movements*

- 50% of flexion/extension occurs between the occiput and C1.
- 50% of rotation takes place between C1 and C2.
- Lateral bending is a function of all the cervical vertebrae and it occurs in conjunction with elements of rotation.
- In Klippel-Feil deformity, the range of movements is restricted because of fusion of 2 or more vertebral bodies.
- During movements, check for
  - Associated pain
  - Muscle spasm
  - Clicking
  - Crepitus

- *Active range of motion:*
  a. Flexion and extension:
    - Ask the patient to nod his head forward in a 'yes' movement.
    - He should be able to touch his chin to the chest.
    - Then ask the patient to look up directly at the ceiling above him.
    - Normal range—130°.
  b. Rotation:
    - Ask the patient to shake his head from side to side in a 'no' motion.
    - Normal range—80°.
  c. Lateral bending:
    - Ask the patient to touch his ear to his shoulder.
    - Normal range: 45° tilting towards each shoulder.

4. *Neurological Examination*

There are 8 nerves exiting the cervical spine, but only 7 cervical vertebrae.

The first through 7th nerves exit above the corresponding vertebrae, whereas the 8th nerve exits between C7 and T1 vertebrae. Individual nerve roots need to be tested to know the level of the pathology, e.g. degenerative disc.

5. *Special Tests*

Adson's test: To know the compression of the subclavian artery, e.g. by cervical rib or tightened scalenus medius muscle.

Feel for the radial pulse of the patient at the wrist on the affected side. Now ask the patient to take deep breath and turn the head towards the arm being tested. If there is compression of the subclavian artery, there will be a marked diminution or absence of the radial pulse.

EXAMINATION OF LUMBAR SPINE

Back pain is a very common orthopaedic problem in day-to-day practice. So thorough evaluation of lumbar spine is essential to correctly diagnose the pathologies

Disc	Nerve root	Motor	Sensory	Reflex
C4-5	C5	• Deltoid	Lateral arm (axillary nerve)	Biceps
C5-6	C6	• Wrist extensors • Biceps	Lateral forearm (Musculocutaneous nerve)	Brachioradialis
C6-7	C7	• Wrist flexors • Finger extensors • Triceps	Middle finger	Triceps
C7-T1	C8	• Finger flexors	• Medial forearm (Medial anterior cutaneous nerve)	
T1-2	T1	• Hand intrinsics	• Medial arm (Medial brachial cutaneous nerve)	

of lumbar spine like fracture, degenerative disc disease, lumbar canal stenosis, tuberculosis, trauma, etc. Adequate exposure of the entire spine is essential for proper examination.

1. Inspection

- *Gait:* Types of gait
  - Antalgic: Hip/knee problem
  - Shuffling: Neurological disorder of rigidity/ spasticity
  - Walking slightly flexed/stooped: Lumbar canal stenosis

Examination in Prone Position with Patient lying Down

- Curvature of the spine
  - In coronal plane (lateral)—scoliosis
    a. Structural
    b. Functional
  - In sagittal plane—kyphosis
  - Curvature can be better appreciated in standing position.
- Obvious step—listhesis
- *Swelling:*
  - Lump in the area of the low back—possibility of spina bifida
  - Accompanied by cafe au lait spots—possibility of neurofibromatosis
- *Skin:*
  - Hairy patch/café au lait spots/birth marks/ excessive port wine marks—may suggest underlying bony pathology (spina bifida/ diastematomyelia).
  - Patchy, reddened discolouration—infection/ long term use of heating elements to relieve pain.

Examination in Standing Position from Front, Back and Side

- *Posture*
  - List towards one side may indicate underlying paraspinal muscle spasm
- Level of shoulder, scapula, pelvis (Fig. 45.1):
  - In scoliosis, these levels are higher on the side of convexity
- *Loss of lordosis*
  - Due to paraspinal muscle spasm
- Exaggerated lordosis/step: Listhesis
- Kyphosis/Gibbus:
  - Post-traumatic
  - Post-TB
- Chest deformity with prominent one side/sternum: In scoliosis/kyphosis

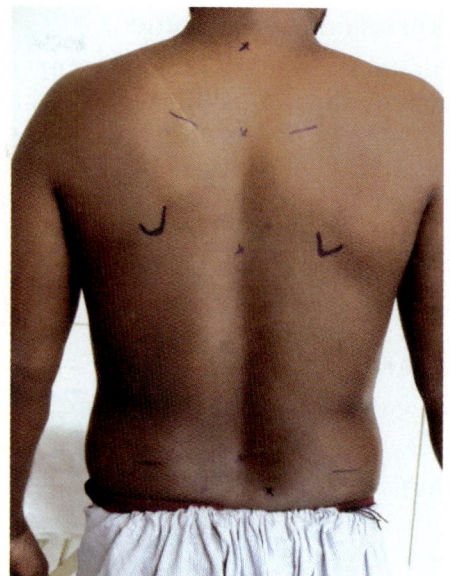

Fig. 45.1: Examination of the spine in standing position showing the levels of the shoulder, scapula, iliac crest

2. Palpation

Posterior aspect

- Superficial palpation
  - Gently roll the finger down the spinous process. Any tender point suggests underlying soft tissue pathology, e.g. supraspinous/interspinous ligaments, muscular pathology
- Deep palpation
  - Tenderness on deep palpation suggests bony pathology.
  - One can actually rotate the vertebral body between thumb and index finger and find out anterior vertebral pathologies.
  - Tenderness may be elicited by pressing upon the side of spinous process to rotate the vertebra or by gentle blows on either side of spine.
  - Tenderness of the facet joints can be checked at approximately 3 cm lateral to the midline.
  - Also check for tenderness on both sacroiliac joints.
  - One can also judge the exact level of the pathology by counting the spinous processes by certain landmarks—the highest point of iliac crest corresponds to L4–L5 interspace and the sacral dimple or the line joining the PSIS corresponds to S2 spinous process
  - Any step-off from one spinous process to another can be palpated, suggestive of listhesis.
  - Tip of the coccyx can be palpated posteriorly, though the best method is rectal examination.

3. PA Examination (Per abdomen)

The lumbar spine examination is incomplete without abdominal examination. With both hips and knees flexed, palpate the abdomen to look for any psoas swelling or any other mass. Poor abdominal muscle tone can be contributing to back pain. So the muscle tone should be examined by asking the patient to raise the straight legs or raise head and neck without support.

4. Range of Motion

The movements of the lumbar spine are:

1. Flexion
2. Extension
3. Lateral bending
4. Rotation

Since there are no restraining ribs in the lumbar spine, more movements occur in the lumbar spine compared to the thoracic spine.

Flexion

Ask the patient to bend forward with his knees straight and try to touch the toes. Determine the degrees of flexion by noting the distance between the fingertips and the floor. Normal is within 7 cm. Flexion will be restricted in cases of painful pathologies of the lumbar spine, associated with paraspinal muscle spasm.

Range: 105°

Extension

Standing by the side of the patient and placing one hand over his back at the level of PSIS (posterior superior iliac spine), thus providing fulcrum, ask the patient to bend backwards as far as he can and then record the range.

In case of lumbar canal stenosis or spondylolisthesis, the back pain increases on extension and is relieved to some extent in flexion.

Range: 30°.

Lateral Bending

Not a pure motion and occurs in conjunction with rotation. Stabilise the iliac crest and ask the patient to bend to the left and to the right, as far as he can (Fig. 45.2).

Normal range: 30°

Rotation

Again stabilising the pelvis by placing one hand on the iliac crest and the other on his opposite shoulder, turn the trunk by rotating the pelvis and the shoulder

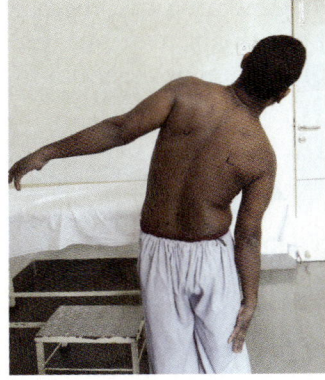
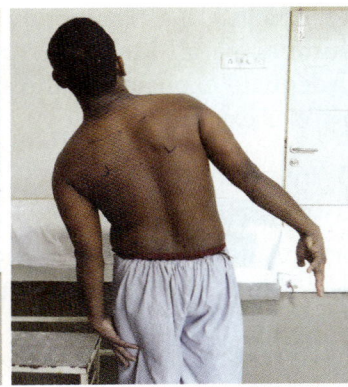

Fig. 45.2: Method of checking the movements of the spine

posteriorly. It can also be checked by making the patient sit so as to fix the pelvis.

Normal range: 40°–45°

5. Neurological Examination

Superficial Reflexes

These are mediated through the central nervous system and require skin stimulation.

The absence of superficial reflex, especially if associated with exaggerated deep tendon reflexes, is indicative of upper motor neuron pathology.

1. Superficial abdominal reflex: With patient supine, stroke each quadrant of the abdomen and note whether the umbilicus moves towards the portion being stroked.
Root value:
T7–T10 Upper muscle
T10–L1 Lower muscles

2. Superficial cremasteric reflex: Stroke the inner side of the upper thigh and look for the scrotal sac on that side being pulled upwards. Root value: T12
3. Superficial anal reflex: On touching the perianal skin, the external anal sphincter muscle contracts.

Pathological Reflexes

Their presence indicates upper motor neuron lesion.
1. Babinski test: Stroke the plantar surface of the foot from the calcaneus along the lateral border of the forefoot.
   • Normal/negative: The toes do not move or bunch up uniformly.
   • Positive: the great toe extends while the other toes plantar flex and splay.
   • In infants, Babinski test is often positive.
2. Oppenheim test: Run your fingernail along the crest of the tibia, normally there is no reaction at all or the patient complains of pain.
   Abnormal response is the same as for Babinski.

Disc	Root	Motor	Sensory	Reflex
L3–4	L4	Tibialis anterior	Medial leg	Knee
			Medial foot	
L4–5	L5	Extensor hallucis longus	Lateral leg	
			Dorsum of foot	
L5–S1	S1	Peroneus longus, peroneus brevis, gastrosoleus	Lateral foot, Sole	Ankle

6. Special Tests

a. Tests to Stretch the Spinal Cord or Sciatic Nerve

SLR (Straight leg raising) test (Fig. 45.3): The patient lies supine. Rule out any lordosis by placing your hand beneath the lumbar spine. Lift his leg upwards by supporting his foot around the calcaneus and keeping the knee straight. Normally the leg can be raised without any discomfort or pain up to 80 degrees (angle between the leg and the table).

- The patient may complain of low back pain radiating down the same leg at lower angle. At the point where the patient experiences pain, lower the leg slightly and dorsiflex the ankle. If this does not reproduce the pain, the earlier pain is probably due to hamstring tightness which often manifests only as the posterior thigh pain.

- However if the pain is reproduced, it indicates positive SLR and suggests pathology in the lumbar spine or along the course of the sciatic nerve, e.g. disc lateral to nerve root. The pathology is again confirmed if the patient admits relief of pain on bending the knee.

Well leg SLR: On raising the normal leg, if back and leg pain is produced on the involved side, it is further presumptive evidence of compression on the sciatic nerve, e.g. due to a herniated axillary disc in the lumbar region or huge central disc prolapse.

Bowstring sign: It is the most reliable test of root tension. SLR is done till pain is reproduced. At this level,

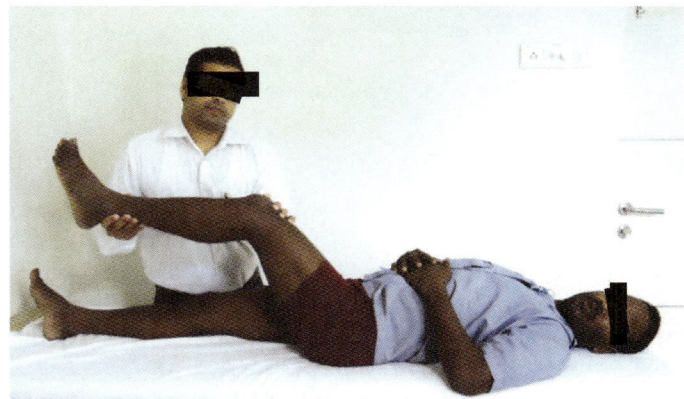
Fig. 45.4: Bowstring sign

the knee is slightly flexed till pain abates. Place the thumb in the popliteal fossa over the sciatic nerve. If sudden firm pressure on the nerve causes pain in the back or leg, it is highly suggestive of root tension (Fig. 45.4).

Hoover test: This test helps to know whether the patient is malingering when he states that he cannot raise his leg and it should be performed in conjunction with SLR test. As the patient tries to raise his leg, keep one hand under the calcaneum of the opposite foot. If the patient is genuinely trying to raise his leg, he puts pressure on the calcaneus of his opposite leg to gain leverage, so you will feel downward pressure on your hand. If the patient is malingering, no pressure will be felt.

Femoral stretch test: For L3 and L4 nerve roots.

In prone position, the hip is extended with the knee maintained in a slightly flexed position. If pain is produced radiating down the front of the thigh, the test is considered positive (Fig. 45.5).

b. Kernig Test

With the patient supine and both his hands placed behind the head, ask him to forcibly raise and flex his head onto the chest. If he experiences pain in the cervical spine, low back or leg, it suggests meningeal irritation, nerve root involvement or irritation of dural covering of the nerve root.

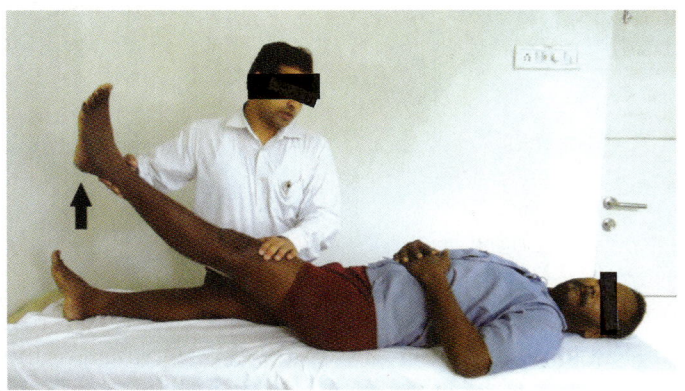
Fig. 45.3: Straight leg raising test

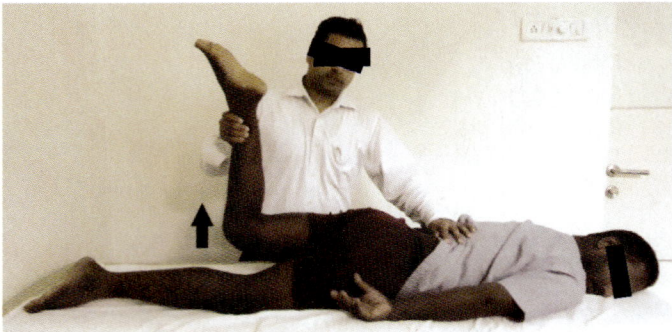

Fig. 45.5: Femoral stretch test

c. Schober's Test (Fig. 45.6)

Mark S2 level. Mark two points, 5 cm below and 10 cm above S2 and measure the distance between them. Now ask the patient to bend forward and again measure the distance between the two points. Normally, the distance should increase by at least 5–8 cm indicating flexion occurring in lumbar spine.

d. Tests for Sacroiliac Joint

1. *Pelvic rock test:* In supine patient, place your thumb on the anterior superior iliac spine and palm on the iliac tubercles. Now forcibly compress the pelvis towards the midline of the body. If there is increased pain around the sacroiliac joint, it suggests SI joint pathology.
2. *Gaenslen's test:* The hip and the knee joint of the affected side are flexed to fix the pelvis, and hip of the unaffected side is hyperextended over the edge of the examination table. This exerts a rotational strain on the sacroiliac joint. The test is considered positive, if pain is produced on this manoeuvre.
3. *Patrick or FABER test* (Fig 45.7)

   In supine patient, place the foot of the affected side on the opposite knee. The hip is now flexed, abducted and externally rotated (F AB ER) to stress the SI joint. Now increase the above ranges by placing one hand on the flexed knee joint and the

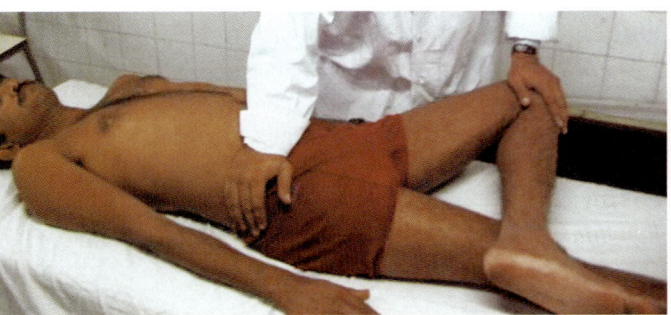

Fig. 45.7: FABER test

other on the opposite anterior superior iliac spine. Press down on each of these points. If the patient c/o increased pain, it suggests SI joint pathology (Fig. 45.7).

4. SLR—active and passive

7. Associated Examination

- Abdominal
- PR/PV
- *Chest:* Normal chest expansion is around 5 cm. at the level of 4th rib. In cases of ankylosing spondylitis, it is decreased to less than 2 cm.
- For search of primary in cases of metastasis
  - Thyroid
  - Breast
  - Kidney
  - Prostate
  - Lung
- Examination in case of scoliosis (as given in case 9) (Fig. 45.8)

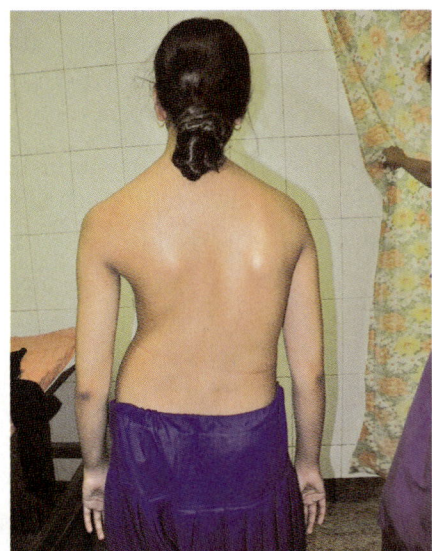

Fig. 45.8: Figure showing dorsolumbar scoliosis with convexity to right. Note the different levels of the inferior ends of scapulae on two sides

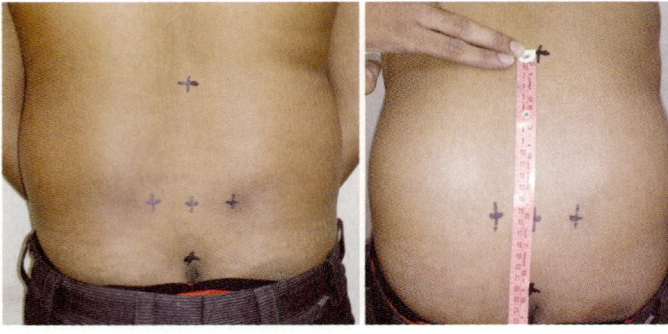

Fig. 45.6: Schober's test

COMMON CASES

Cervical Spine

1. Cervical Spondylosis with/without Myelopathy/Radiculopathy

History
Personal
- Age—usually elderly/more than 40 years
- Occupation—involving prolonged bending of neck/carrying load on the head
- Use of thick pillows

Clinical symptoms
- Pain in the neck aggravated on movements and relieved on rest
- May radiate to occipital region/periscapular region/along the arm, radiating pain exacerbated by axial compression test.
- Neck may be bent/stooped/tilted towards one side due to paraspinal muscle spasm
- Neurological: Numbness/weakness in a nerve root territory/associated lower limb weakness with unsteady gait
- Difference in fine movements of hand/fingers.
  - Poor grip

Past history: Similar attacks of severe pain, relieved after traction and/or analgesics, physiotherapy

Examination
- Rigid posture/torticollis.
- Paraspinal muscle spasm.
- Tenderness on deep palpation at the affected level.
- Painful restricted range of motion.
- *Neurological:* Motor, sensory and/or reflex deficit in the distribution of the involved nerve root.
- In case of cervical myelopathy, upper motor neuron signs in the lower limb.

2. Cervical Strain (Whiplash Injury/Mechanical Cervical Pain)
- Diffuse tenderness of the posterior neck muscles.
- Restricted range of motion.
- Normal neurological examination.

3. Cervical Spine Fracture/Dislocation
- History suggestive of significant trauma.
- Point tenderness at the level of the injury.
- Palpable defect, such as step-off or break in the normal alignment or spacing of the spinous processes.

- Neurological deficit (may vary from no or partial spinal cord injury syndrome to complete spinal cord injury).
- Partial spinal cord injury syndrome include anterior/central/posterior cord syndrome/Brown-Sequard syndrome.

Lumbar Spine

1. Lumbar Spondylosis

On similar grounds as cervical spondylosis.

2. Degenerative Disc Disease
- Age > 40 years
- Occupation: Involving prolonged sitting/bending/lifting weights
- Symptoms: Back pain aggravated by bending/lifting/prolonged sitting, relieved by rest.

3. Acute Disc Prolapse
- Age > 40 years
- H/o sudden onset severe back pain, usually while lifting weights from bent position/coughing/sneezing
  The pain may radiate down one/both lower limbs and may be associated with numbness, weakness in lower limbs
  The pain may be severe enough to cause list/stooped position
- Past history of similar episodes of back pain with symptoms subsiding in a few days/weeks after rest/analgesics/traction
- O/E: Patient stands with a characteristic attitude-lumbar scoliosis with convexity to the affected side, kyphosis and slight flexion of hips and knees
  - Localised tenderness at the affected site
  - Paraspinal muscle spasm
  - SLR: Positive
  - Range of motion: Extremely painful flexion/extension/lateral flexion on the side of the lesion
  - Neurological abnormality according to the nerve root affected

4. Cauda Equina Syndrome
- History suggestive of degenerative disc disease
- Sudden onset severe back pain followed by neurological deficit in both lower limbs, may involve bladder/bowel also
- O/E
  - Localised tenderness
  - Flaccid paraparesis
  - Areflexia
  - Hypoaesthesia below a particular sensory level (as well as perianally in saddle shape region)

5. Lumbar Canal Stenosis

- Age : > 40 years
- H/o neurological claudication, more compared to back pain
- Claudication distance important.

6. Spondylolisthesis

- Any age, but degenerative variety > 40 years
- Back pain, more obvious after exercise/strain
- The pain may radiate down to the legs and there may be weakness of lower limbs if nerve root compression is present
- *O/E:*
  - The height of the trunk may be reduced
  - Buttocks look flat
  - Visible and palpable step/transverse furrow encircling the body between the ribs and iliac crest
  - Nerve root compression signs +/−

7. Koch's Spine

- Children and adolescents more affected than adults
- General symptoms:
  - Easy fatiguability
  - Evening rise of temperature
  - Loss of weight and appetite
- *Back pain:* Dull ache in the early stage, becoming worse on walking/jolting. In later stage increased pain, even at rest and night
  May radiate along the nerve root
  May be referred to back of head/arm, chest/abdomen/girdle pain, lateral thigh (Fig. 45.9)
- Swelling—due to paraspinal abscess
- Deformity—angular kyphosis/hunchback

O/E
- Tenderness at the affected site
- Paraspinal muscle spasm
- *Swelling:* Paraspinal/fluctuant cold abscess
- Discharging sinus may be present
- *Deformity:* Kyphosis/gibbus/kyphoscoliosis
- *Range of motion:* Painful, restricted
- *Neurological S/S:* Depending on the level of affection.

8. Ankylosing Spondylitis

- Young males 15–35 years
- Pain and stiffness in the low back and buttocks especially in the morning on rising from bed. Gradually entire back/neck may get involved
- Other major joints like shoulder, hip, knee may be involved

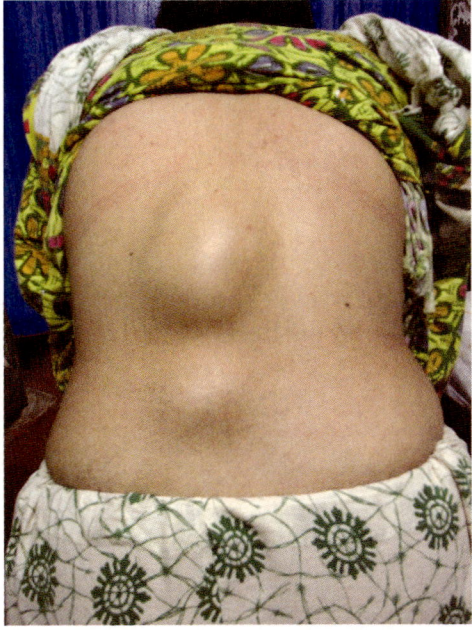

Fig. 45.9: Koch's spine showing paraspinal abscess

- Pain at the tendon insertion sites—enthesopathy, e.g. heel pain
- Tightness in the chest in late stages

O/E
Tenderness over SI joints/lumbar spine
- SI joint stress test positive
- SLR+/−
- Schober's test positive
- Chest expansion decreased (Fig. 45.10)
- *Range of motion:* Restricted

9. Scoliosis (Fig. 45.8)

- Usually children/adolescents
- Presence of deformity
- Late cases of kyphoscoliosis may have neurological problems

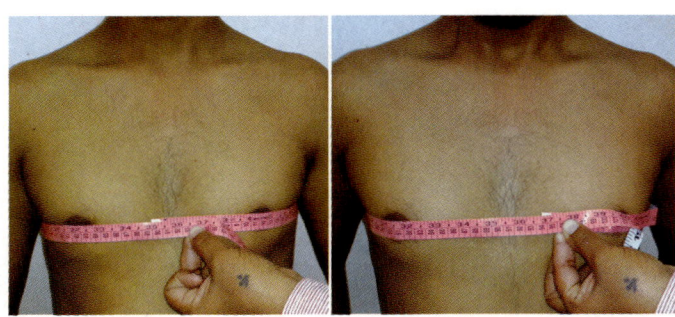

Fig. 45.10: Measurement of chest expansion in a case of ankylosing spondylitis

O/E

Site of curve

- Side of convexity
- Primary/secondary
- Balanced/compensated
- *Correctability:*
  - Adam's forward bending test
  - Suspension or on traction
  - Lateral flexion

- Levels of shoulder/scapula/PSIS
- Limb length discrepancy/pelvic obliquity
  - Plumb line in sagittal as well as coronal plane
- Rib hump
- Stigmata of congenital variety: Naevi/angioma/tuft of hair/dimple/lipoma
- Neurological examination
- Also check for other associated congenital anomalies

Hip

HISTORY

A. Personal Data

1. *Age:* Common hip disorders in different age group
   - 0–2 years: Septic hip and its sequelae, DDH (developmental dysplasia of the hip)
   - 2–5 years: Tuberculosis of hip
   - 4–12 years: Perthes' disease
   - 20–50 years: AVN (avascular necrosis)
2. *Sex*
   - DDH more common in females
   - Perthes' disease more common in males
3. Occupation

B. Complaints

1. Pain
   - True hip pain is felt mainly in the groin, front or inner aspect of the thigh
   - Hip pathology may present with pain referred to the inner aspect of the knee
   - Spinal pathology resulting in referred hip pain is felt in the gluteal region
   - Origin
   - Duration
   - Progress
   - Character of pain
   - Relation of pain with joint movements
   - Relation of symptoms with time of day and weather
   - Associated with fever
2. Deformity/stiffness/restricted movements: Functional problems such as squatting, sitting cross-legged, walking.
3. Swelling

4. Limp
   - Painless
   - Painful
5. Instability

C. Past History

- Similar episodes in the past with waxing and waning of symptoms suggest an inflammatory hip disease such as rheumatoid arthritis.
- Other joint involvement in past suggests polyarticular problem such as rheumatoid arthritis.

D. History Suggestive of Aetiology

- Trauma
- Congenital
- Developmental
- Inflammatory
- Infective
- Degenerative
- History of excessive alcohol intake, steroid medication, sickle cell anaemia in avascular necrosis of head of femur.

E. History of Treatment

Nature, duration, effect of treatment.

F. Family History

- Contact with tuberculosis
- Family history of gout, rheumatoid arthritis, haemophilia

CLINICAL EXAMINATION

Performed in standing, supine and lateral positions.

A. Inspection

1. Presence of increased lumbar lordosis
   a. Observed as lifting off of the lumbar spine from the bed in supine position.

b. Indicates FFD of the hip compensated (masked) by increased pelvic tilt and lumbar lordosis.

2. Attitude of limb
   a. Flexion/extension and abduction/adduction deformities of the hip are compensated by the pelvis and lumbar spine; however rotational deformities cannot be compensated (Fig. 46.1).
   b. Hip synovitis: Flexion, abduction, external rotation
   c. Hip arthritis: Flexion, adduction
   d. Posterior dislocation of hip: Flexion, adduction, internal rotation
   e. Anterior dislocation of hip: Flexion, abduction, external rotation

3. Levels of ASIS, patellae, malleoli
   a. Normally, both ASIS should be at the same horizontal level and should be perpendicular to the spine: This is termed as a 'squared pelvis'
   b. In adduction deformity the ipsilateral ASIS is at a higher level, in abduction deformity the ipsilateral ASIS is at a lower level.

4. Swelling
   a. DD (differential diagnosis) of swelling in the gluteal region: Cold abscess (soft), posteriorly dislocated femoral head (hard)
   b. DD of swelling in the Scarpa's triangle: Cold abscess (soft), inguinal lymphadenopathy (firm), anteriorly dislocated femoral head (hard)
   c. DD of swelling in the trochanteric region: Trochanteric bursitis, malunited trochanteric fracture, neoplasm arising from greater trochanter

5. Ulcers, sinus: Suggestive of active/healed tuberculosis or chronic osteomyelitis.

6. Skin over the joint
   a. Old surgical scars
   b. Whether healed by primary intention

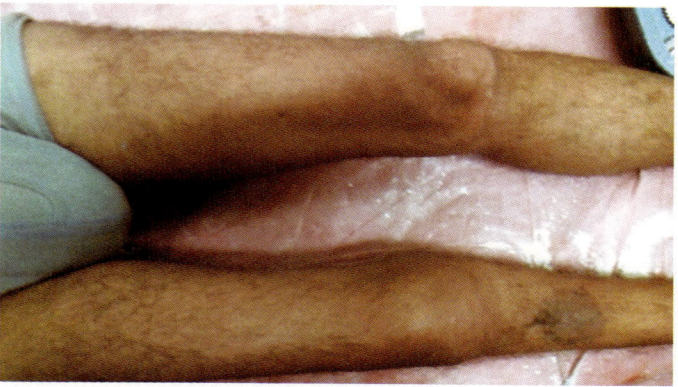

Fig. 46.2: Wasting of the thigh suggesting chronic hip joint pathology

7. Muscle wasting (Fig. 46.2)
   a. Denotes chronicity
   b. Seen in gluteal, thigh and hamstring muscles

B. Palpation

1. Temperature
2. Tenderness
   a. Anterior joint line
   b. Posterior joint line
3. Trochanteric palpation
   a. Superficial trochanteric tenderness
   b. Deep trochanteric tenderness
   c. Transtrochanteric tenderness
   d. Trochanteric thickening
   e. Trochanteric irregularity
4. Palpable swelling
   a. Hard: Femoral head, bony neoplasm
   b. Firm: Soft tissue neoplasm
   c. Soft: Cold abscess
5. Vascular sign of Narath
   In posterior dislocation of the hip, there is no femoral head to palpate the femoral artery pulsation against, and the femoral artery pulsation is weak.

C. Deformity Evaluation

1. *Thomas' test for fixed flexion deformity:* Hyperlordosis of the lumbar spine gives a clue to the possibility of flexion deformity of the hip (Fig. 46.3).
   Hugh Owen Thomas described the test in 1876. Thomas' test unmasks the flexion deformity and assesses the true range occurring at the hip joint. Patient lies supine on a hard mattress. Exaggerated lumbar lordosis if any is looked for. The examiner holds the contralateral knee tightly against the chest till exaggerated lumbar lordosis is obliterated. The hip joint to be examined is allowed to extend as much

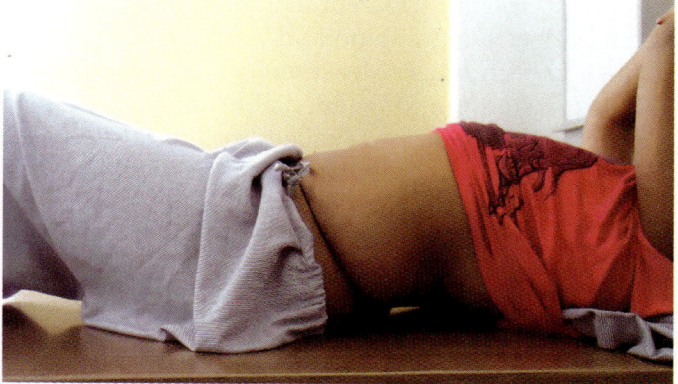

Fig. 46.1: Fixed flexion deformity of the hip, manifesting as hyperlordosis of spine

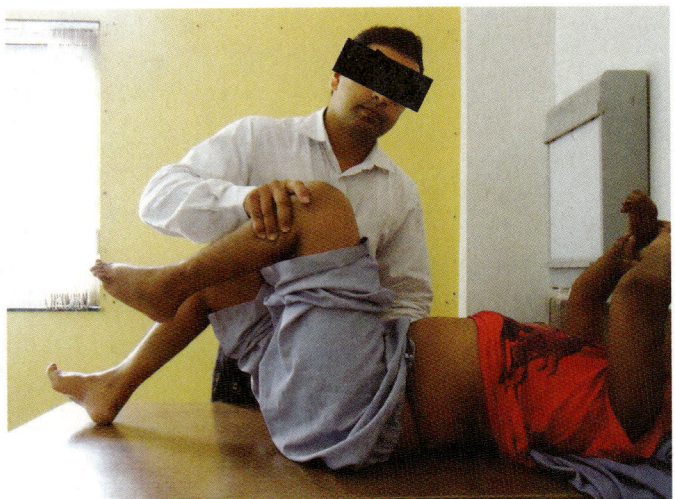

Fig. 46.3: Thomas' test to check FFD hip

as possible. The angle the long axis of the thigh subtends to the plane of the examination couch is the amount of flexion deformity. Normally the hip should be able to extend fully to touch the examination table. One also checks the normal flexion of the hip while testing the flexion deformity on the other side. Normal flexion is ~110°.

2. *Determination of abduction/adduction deformity*
   - Coronal plane deformities of the hip such as these are compensated at the pelvis by tilting it up or down.
   - With both the limbs lying parallel (or close to each other), pelvis on the side of the adduction deformity would be tilted up whereas pelvis on the abduction deformity side would be tilted down. This compensation at the pelvis level enables the limb to lie straight even in the presence of the adduction or abduction deformities. Ascertaining the level of the anterior superior iliac spines (ASIS) on the symptomatic side would help to detect the deformity.
   - The method of noting the amount of deformity is to unmask the deformity by eliminating the compensation made by the pelvis. This is done by placing the affected hip in adduction or abduction (depending upon the type of deformity that exists in the hip) till the pelvis tilts back into a horizontal position. An angle the long axis of the affected limb subtends with the long axis of the body is the amount of deformity. The range of movement beyond the deformity is calculated by further moving the hip in the same direction. (e.g. adduction deformity of x° and further adduction till y).
   - Normal abduction is 45° whereas normal adduction is ~30°.

Rotational deformity
- As opposed to flexion or abduction–adduction deformities, tilting the pelvis cannot usually mask rotational deformity. It is noted by observing the direction in which the patella points while the patient is lying supine. Normally due to the weight of the thigh the resting position of the limbs is up to 30° external rotation. Anterior surface of the patella points outwards towards the ceiling. If the patella points straight upwards or inwards there exists an internal rotation deformity.
- Rotation can be checked in supine position with hip and knee flexed to 90°.
- Rotational deformity in extension can also be observed in prone position. With patient in prone position and knees flexed to 90°, rotations can be tested in either direction. Normal external rotation is ~45° while internal rotation is ~ 35°. In the prone position, long axis of the leg (tibia) can be used to indicate the amount of rotation.

D. Movements

1. Range of active movements
2. Range of passive movements
   - Check whether associated with pain, spasm, crepitus
   - Besides the extension, flexion, abduction, adduction in extension we need to examine the combination of the movements. Abduction in flexion is one of the earlier movements to be lost. Hip rotations should be tested in full extension as well as in 90° flexion. These are called differential rotations. Improved rotations especially the internal rotation in flexion is found whenever there is a sectoral involvement of the femoral head (as in avascular necrosis of the femoral head).

E. Measurements

1. *Apparent length:* Apparent length is measured with the patient lying supine and both the limbs lying close to each other. Measurements are made from the xiphisternum to the medial malleolus on either side. The discrepancy is called apparent/functional limb length discrepancy. This is because the discrepancy is largely due to deformities at the hip or knee joints or pelvic obliquity besides being due to actual bony shortening. This should be considered while giving the shoe raises to the patient if deformity is not going to be corrected.
2. *True length:* True lengths try to estimate the limb length discrepancies caused by true affection of the bones or joints per se. It tries to eliminate the

discrepancies due to deformities. This is done by placing the affected hip in the position of deformity. This step corrects the pelvic obliquity (also known as "squaring the pelvis"). Next step is to keep the unaffected hip also in the identical position. This is necessary because one cannot make the actual bony length measurements from the centre of the femoral head. Measurement is then taken from the ASIS (anterior superior iliac spines) to the medial malleoli on either side. These represent true bony lengths. These are subdivided into:

a. Supratrochanteric

b. Infratrochanteric segmental lengths.

Supratrochanteric limb length discrepancy is due to segment of the bone proximal to the greater trochanter. Valgus neck can present as supratrochanteric lengthening whereas varus neck as supratrochanteric shortening.

3. Bryant's triangle is formed by 3 lines. (i) Line joining the ASIS and greater trochanter. (ii) Perpendicular dropped from the ASIS to the ground (examination table). (iii) Line joining the greater trochanter to the 2nd line (Fig. 46.4). Bryant's triangles on either side are compared. The length of the line joining the greater trochanter to perpendicular line from the ASIS gives the supratrochanteric segment length. When compared with the opposite side it gives an idea about supratrochanteric shortening.

4. *Nelaton's line:* While Bryant's triangle is a comparative measurement, Nelaton's line detects the supratrochanteric shortening without having to compare with the opposite side. It is the line joining the ASIS to the most prominent part of the ischial tuberosity. Normally the tip of greater trochanter is at the level of the line. Any upward migration of the tip above this line suggests supratrochanteric shortening.

5. *Shoemaker's line:* It is the line joining the tip of the greater trochanter to ASIS drawn over anterior abdominal wall. It is drawn forwards towards the opposite side to cross similar line on the opposite side. Normally it crosses the corresponding line on the opposite side at or above the level of the umbilicus. If it crosses below the umbilicus it suggests supratrochanteric shortening.

Infratrochanteric limb length: This can be measured directly from the tip of the greater trochanter to the lateral knee joint line. It is the length of the femoral diaphyseal segment below the level of greater trochanter.

3. *Thigh girth:* This is measured at a fixed distance from the knee joint line (10 cms from the joint line on either side).

F. Instability Assessment

1. *Telescoping sign:* Push and pull the thigh with the hip and knee in 90° flexion. Proximal-distal movement of the greater trochanter with it suggests instability at the hip joint.

2. Piston sign in neutral position

Special Tests

Trendelenburg's test: The examiner stands behind the patient and marks both the posterior superior iliac spines (PSIS). Normally in a unilateral stance (patient standing on one leg), the opposite PSIS rises up. This is due to the action of the abductor muscle on the side on which the patient is standing. It helps the patient clear the ground during walking. It also indicates the intactness of the abductor, body weight lever arms, and fulcrum as well as adequate strength of the abductors on the side being tested (Fig. 46.5B).

Abnormal response would be failure to raise or drooping down of the PSIS on the opposite side (Fig. 46.5A). A patient with positive Trendelenburg's test would also have Trendelenburg gait. In a bilateral pathology, the patient has a duck waddle/pelvic waddle (bilateral Trendelenburg gait).

G. Gait

1. *Trendelenburg gait:* Side-to-side lurch due to failure of abductor mechanism of hip seen commonly in congenital dislocation of hip, Perthes' disease, nonunion of transcervical fractures of hip, coxa vara, gluteus medius weakness due to poliomyelitis. Pelvis drops on the opposite side. However, in order to clear the ground during walking the person tries to sway the trunk to the affected side.

2. *Short limb gait:* The affected side is tilted so as to bring the foot to the ground.

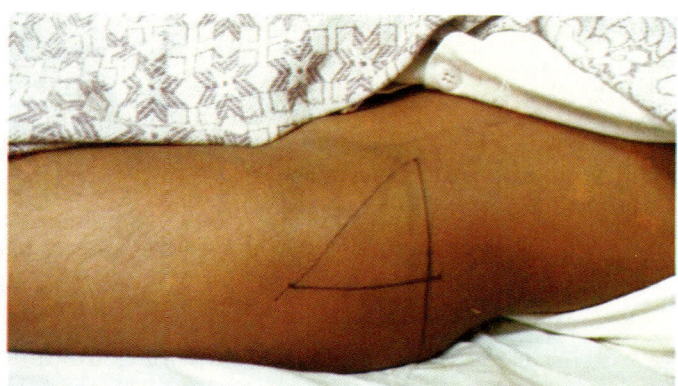

Fig. 46.4: The bony landmarks for Bryant's triangle

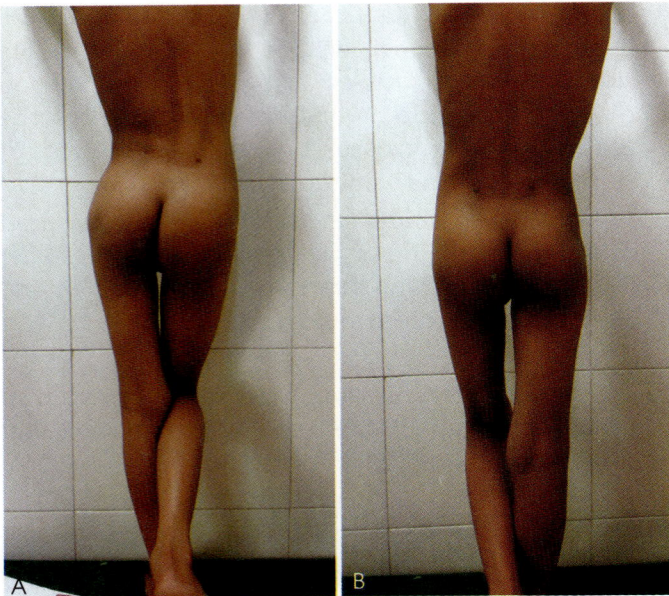

Fig. 46.5: Trendelenburg's test: positive (A) and, (B) normal

3. *Antalgic gait:* Shortened stance phase so as to avoid weight bearing on the affected side.
4. *Gluteal lurch:* Backward lurch on the affected side during stance phase to compensate for gluteus maximus weakness.
5. *In-toeing gait:* The foot is turned inwards due to excessive femoral anteversion.
6. *Circumduction gait:* With apparent lengthening of the limb in fixed abduction deformity of hip, the patient takes affected limb in a round-about fashion while stepping forward.

Examination of Adjoining Joints

1. S-I joint
2. Knee joint

General Examination

1. Draining lymph nodes (external iliac group).
2. Per-abdominal examination for psoas abscess.

COMMON CASES

1. *Non-union of transcervical femur neck fracture*
   • H/o fall: Significant/trivial in old age. Inability to walk and bear weight on the affected limb
   • H/o treatment +/–
   O/E
   • Limb lies in external rotation
   • Tenderness +/– in Scarpa's triangle

   – Greater trochnter—High riding, with normal contour and thickness
   – Telescoping test positive with bony crepitus felt due to friction between the fractured neck fragments.
   – True supratrochanteric shortening
   – *Gait:* Trendelenburg (if the patient is able to walk)
   – Active SLR not possible

2. *Malunited intertrochanteric fracture*
   • H/o fall with significant trauma to hip
   • H/o treatment taken in the form of traction and immobilisation
   • *O/E:*
     – Limb may/may not be in external rotation
     – High riding, thickened, irregular greater trochanter
     – True supratrochanteric shortening
     – Trendelenburg test and gait positive
     – Telescoping sign: Negative

3. *Koch's hip*
   • H/o constitutional symptoms (evening rise of temperature, loss of weight and appetite) may/ may not be present.
   • Past H/o pulmonary/abdominal Koch's/ lymphadenopathy
   • H/o AKT (anti Koch's treatment): Duration/ dosage of different drugs
   O/E
   • *Attitude:* Flexion, adduction/abduction, internal/ external rotation (depending on the stages of Koch's hip)
     – Stage of synovitis: Flexion, abduction, external rotation
     – Stage of early arthritis: Flexion, adduction, internal rotation
     – Stage of late arthritis: Abduction/adduction, internal/external rotation
     – Stage of joint destruction/deformity: Variable
   • Tenderness present in Scarpa's triangle
   • Greater trochanter: Tenderness +/–
   • Transtrochanteric tenderness present
   • Range of motion: Painful and restricted.
   • Apparent shortening/lengthening depending on the stage
   • True supratrochanteric shortening
   • Trendelenburg test and gait: Positive
   • *Telescoping test:* +/– (depending on the destruction of femoral head)

4. *Avascular necrosis of hip (unilateral or bilateral)*
   - *Age:* Any, more common in middle age
   - H/o gradually progressive pain and difficulty in walking/squatting/sitting cross legged
   - History suggestive of aetiology
     - Past trauma
     - Heavy alcohol consumption/smoking
     - Prolonged steroid intake

O/E
   - Attitude: Flexion, abduction/adduction, external rotation +/−
   - Tenderness present in Scarpa's triangle
   - Greater trochanter: Normal
   - Range of motion: Restricted, painful abduction and internal rotation, differential rotation present
   - True supratrochanteric shortening +/−

Knee

HISTORY

1. Pain

- Diffuse with degenerative and inflammatory disorders.
- Localised with mechanical and post-traumatic disorders.

2. Swelling

- Localised or diffuse.
- Post-traumatic swelling appearing immediately suggests haemarthrosis (e.g. ACL—anterior cruciate ligament tear, osteochondral fracture).
- Post-traumatic swelling appearing after some hours suggests sympathetic/reactive effusion.

3. Stiffness

Denotes a decrease in the normal range of knee movements.

4. Deformity

- Knock knees
- Bow legs
- Flexion/external rotation/valgus at knee (triple deformity)

5. Locking

- Defined as a sudden episodic inability to straighten the knee fully, although further flexion is possible.
- Denotes an unstable meniscal tear, loose body, or torn ACL stump getting caught between the articular surfaces.
- Patients often learn to unlock their knee by complete flexion and rotatory movements.

6. Giving Way/Buckling

- Symptom of instability

- Commonly suggests a mechanical disorder (e.g. ACL tear, unstable meniscal tear)
- May also result from patellofemoral instability, muscle imbalance around the knee, axial malalignment of lower extremity.

In post-traumatic conditions, if the patient can describe the mechanism of injury, this can be very useful:

- A significant direct blunt force at the lateral aspect of the knee while walking results in flexion - abduction-external rotation of the tibia over the femur causing "O' Donoghue's unhappy triad" of ACL tear, MCL (medial collateral ligament) tear and medial meniscus tear.
- A direct force to the proximal anterior tibia while seated (90 degrees knee flexion) results in a "dashboard injury" causing either a PCL tear, or posterior knee dislocation, or posterior dislocation of the hip.
- An extreme hyper-extension injury to the knee would result in tears of both the ACL and PCL.

CLINICAL EXAMINATION

1. Alignment

Valgus or varus deformity is best seen with the patient standing and bearing weight.

2. Attitude

The position of rest for a painful, swollen knee is 30 degrees of flexion.

3. Inspection

- Swelling
- Contours/abnormal shifts/prominence
- Wasting (quadriceps wasting is a sure sign of chronic knee disorder)

- Surgical scars
- Local skin condition
- Patellar shape/size/position

4. Palpation

- Increased warmth
- Soft tissue (muscles, synovium, tendons, ligaments) thickening and tenderness
  1. Morant Baker cyst in popliteal fossa is located in the midline just below the joint line
  2. Semimembranosus bursa is usually located just above the joint line towards the medial aspect
- Bony irregularity and tenderness (patellar grate, retropatellar tenderness, fibular head, femoral and tibial condyles, tibial tuberosity)
- Effusion
  1. Patellar tap (enough fluid without being in much tension): The suprapatellar pouch is compressed with the left hand, while the right index finger pushes the patella posteriorly; with a positive test the patella can be felt striking the femur and bouncing off again.
  2. Cross fluctuation (moderate amount of fluid): The left hand compresses and empties the suprapatellar pouch while the right hand straddles the front of the joint below the patella; by squeezing with each hand alternately, a fluid impulse is transmitted across the joint.
- Apprehension test for patellar subluxation (laterally directed force on the medial border of patella in an extended knee results in severe apprehension of patellar dislocation in a patient with patellofemoral joint instability)

5. Movements

Normal range of knee movements are: Flexion 0 to 130°, i.e. till the thigh touches the back of the leg; extension 0 to 5°; at 90° knee flexion some minimal rotations may be normally present

- Always compare with the opposite limb
- Deformity/lag/critical arc
- Abnormal movements
- Associated with pain, crepitus, clicks, thuds, snapping

6. Measurements

Linear and circumferential (thigh girth).

7. Neurovascular Deficit

- Peroneal nerve palsy may be associated with dislocation of the knee or severe varus stress injuries.
- Popliteal artery disruption is seen in 50% of dislocated knees.

8. Tests for Meniscal Integrity

i. *McMurray's test:* Based on the fact that a torn meniscal fragment can be trapped between the articular surfaces and then induced to snap free with a palpable and audible click. The knee is taken from a position of complete flexion to extension with medial or lateral rotation, stressed in varus or valgus (for a medial meniscus tear the knee is kept in external rotation and valgus). The other hand is placed at the joint line so as to appreciate a click when the torn meniscal fragment displaces.

ii. *Apley's grinding test:* The knee is flexed to 90 degrees and rotated while in compression. This grinding reproduces symptoms, if a meniscus is torn.

9. Tests for Ligament Integrity and Stability

i. ACL (anterior cruciate ligament)
  1. Anterior drawer test (Fig. 47.1)
  2. Lachman test (Fig. 47.3)

ii. PCL (posterior cruciate ligament)
  1. Posterior drawer test
  2. Sag sign (Fig. 47.2)

iii. MCL(medial collateral ligament) and LCL (lateral collateral ligament)
  - Valgus and varus stress test at 30° (Fig. 47.4)

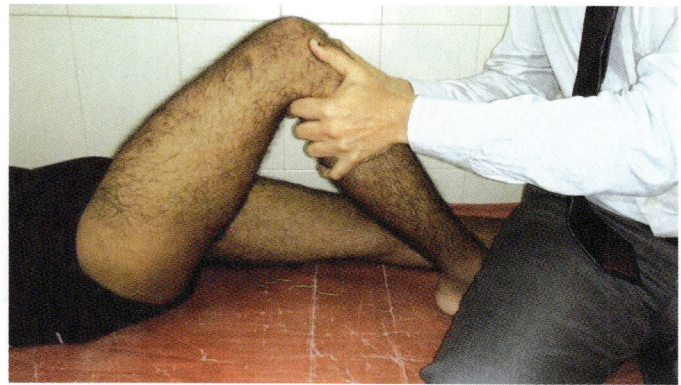

Fig. 47.1: The Drawer test: With the knee placed at 90 degrees the foot is anchored on the couch by the examiner sitting on it. Then, using both hands, the upper end of the tibia is grasped firmly and rocked forwards and backwards to see if there is any anteroposterior glide. The fingers should ensure that the hamstrings are relaxed. Excessive anterior movement as compared to the opposite normal knee (positive anterior drawer sign) denotes anterior cruciate laxity, excessive posterior movement (positive posterior drawer sign) denotes posterior cruciate laxity

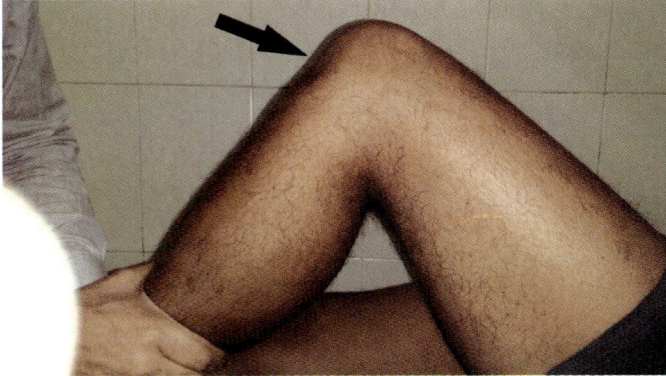

Fig. 47.2: The sag sign in a PCL tear. With the knee flexed 90 degrees, the proximal tibia is inspected from the side; if its upper end has dropped back or can be gently pushed back, this indicates a PCL tear

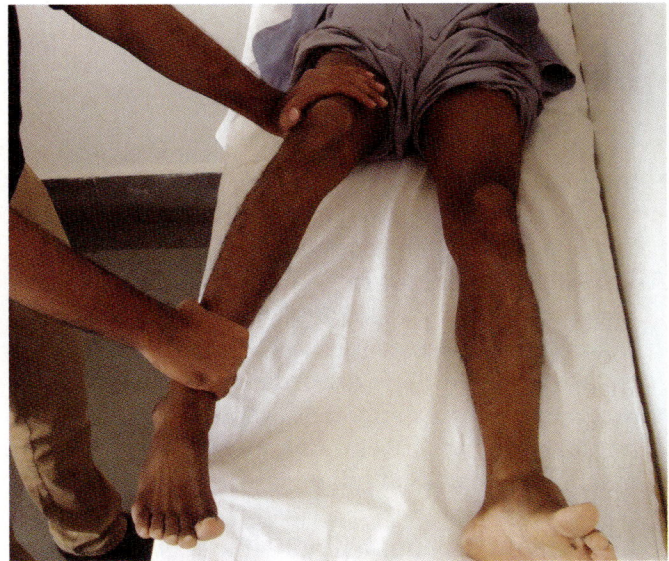

Fig. 47.4: Valgus stress test at 30 degrees knee flexion for MCL laxity: The knee is flexed to 30 degrees so as to make the cruciate ligaments lax and a valgus force is applied to the knee so as to check the laxity of the MCL. An opening of the medial joint space more than that of the opposite side is taken as indicative of an MCL injury, similarly, a varus stress test at 30 degrees knee flexion assesses the structural and functional integrity of the lateral collateral ligament

- Synovial effusion
- Varying flexion deformity
- Relatively free movements, however painful at extremes
- Sometimes warm and tender
- Wasting of thigh and calf muscles
- Triple deformity in advanced cases of tuberculous knee
- Inguinal lymphadenopathy
- Differential diagnosis—tuberculosis of knee, rheumatoid arthritis (usually polyarticular affection), haemophilic synovitis (commonest joints affected are knee and elbow since these joints are most prone to subtle trauma), post-traumatic chronic synovitis, nonspecific synovitis, reactive synovitis, pigmented villonodular synovitis.

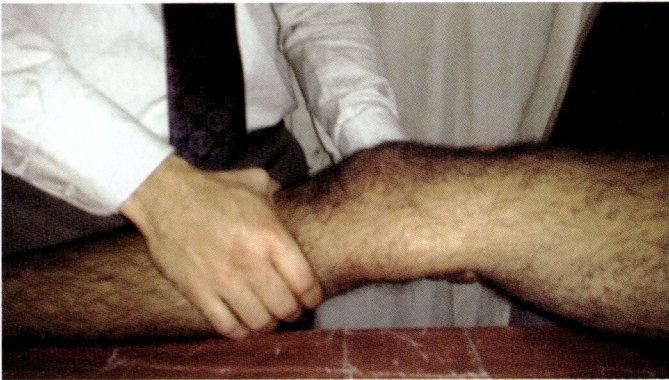

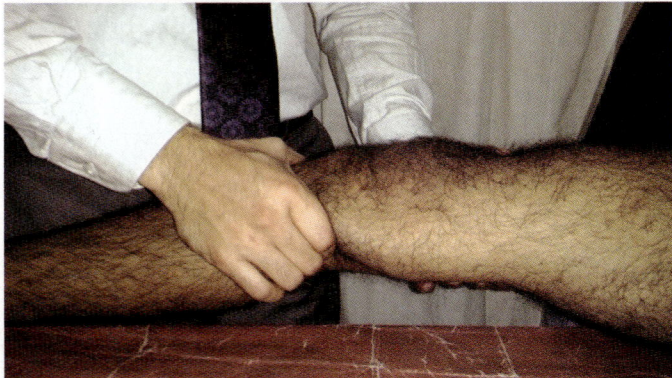

Fig. 47.3: The Lachman test for ACL and PCL integrity. With the knee flexed to 30 degrees, the leg and thigh are grasped firmly and moved in opposite directions. The extent of anteroposterior translation and the nature of end-point (firm or soft) is noted. This is then compared to the contralateral normal knee.

COMMON CASES

Chronic Synovitis of Knee

- Synovial thickening palpable on superomedial aspect of knee

Osteoarthritis

- Chronic history of knee pain.
- Initially symptoms start after rest, i.e. pain with inactivity ("cinema sign"), relieved after mild activity
- Later pain is caused by prolonged activity
- Coarse crepitations felt over the knee joint with movements
- Varus and flexion deformity
- Occasionally acute exacerbations of synovitis with painful swellings of the knee

- Sometimes painless popliteal swellings of synovitis and effusion called Morant-Baker cysts (become prominent with extension and disappear on knee flexion)
- In later stages limitations of knee movements and joint deformities.
- Patellofemoral joint tenderness and crepitus

ACL Tear

- History of twisting injury to knee associated with a 'pop' sensation and immediate painful knee swelling (haemarthrosis)
- Tenderness and painful movements in acute cases
- Complaints of knee instability (sensation of buckling on jumping or while taking turns/cutting activities)
- Anterior drawer test and Lachman test positive.

Medial Meniscus Tear

- Twisting injury (rotational strain) in weight bearing partially flexed knee
- Immediate pain and inability to extend knee
- Mild swelling

- Movements possible but extreme flexion painful
- Medial joint line tenderness
- Rotational stress tests including McMurray's test, Apley's grinding test, sqatting painful and positive

Recurrent Dislocation of Patella

- Common in adolescent females
- History of multiple episodes of patellar instability including frank dislocations
- Often self-reduction of dislocation possible
- May be associated with genu valgum
- Often associated with tight lateral soft tissue structures and lax medial musculature
- Patellar apprehension test positive

Osgood-Schlatter's Disease

- Complaints of tibial tuberosity pain in adolescents, often bilateral
- Pain increases with activity and jumping
- Prominence of tibial tuberosity
- Tenderness of tibial tuberosity
- Resisted quadriceps contraction causes pain

Foot and Ankle

HISTORY

Chief complaints:
Deformity:
  i. Onset
   • Since birth: Congenital
   • Following an attack suggestive of poliomyelitis
   • Following trauma
  ii. Associated with polyarticular symptoms
  iii. Progressive/static
  iv. Associated pain
  v. Reason for seeking treatment:
   • Cannot wear footwear
   • Cosmetic appearance
   • Footwear wears off too early on one side

Pain
  i. Duration
  ii. Onset: Acute/insidious
  iii. Nature: Continuous/intermittent
  iv. Associated with morning stiffness
  v. Associated with swelling
  vi. Episodic/continuous: Episodic—in attacks wakening the patient in the middle of the night or early hours of morning
  vii. Character of pain
  viii. Aggravating, relieving factors
  ix. Pain after standing for long hours

CLINICAL EXAMINATION

Inspection

Ankle

• Swelling
  – Doughnut shaped for ankle synovitis/effusion
  – Horseshoe shaped in cases of subtalar synovitis or arthritis
  – An effusion of the tendon sheath will produce a swelling that extends along the long axis of the leg and foot far beyond the joint level
• Redness/scars/sinuses/ulcerations
• Broadening of the ankle
• Deformities, if any
  – Equinus, calcaneus at the ankle.
  – Heel varus/valgus (inspected from behind). Varus/valgus occurs at the subtalar joint.
• Varicosities, hyperpigmentation (especially surrounding an ulcer).

Foot

• Deformity
  – Pes cavus (also called midfoot equinus)
  – Pes planus/flatfoot
  – Splay foot, metatarsus adductus (adduction of first metatarsal bone)
  – Hallux valgus (abnormal lateral deviation of great toe)
  – Bunion (bursa over 1st metatarsophalangeal joint), bunionnete (bursa over 5th metatarsophalangeal joint)
• Callosities over lateral aspect of foot
• Abnormal skin creases or absence of them
• Deformities of toes (claw/hammer toes)
  – Claw toe: Like that in hand, there is flexion deformity at both proximal as well as distal interphalangeal joints.
  – Hammer toe: Hyperextension at metatarsophalangeal and distal interphalangeal joints with hyperflexion of proximal interphalangeal joint.
• Ulcerations, if any.
  – Classical sites of trophic ulcers are over the pressure points (normal/abnormal due to collapsed arch of the foot), over plantar aspect of 1st and 5th metatarsal heads, calcaneum.

Calf

- Any associated wasting—especially in Koch's ankle
- Any gap seen in the continuity of tendon Achilles
- Knee alignment
- Genu varum/valgum (genu valgum is often associated with the flat feet).

Palpation

- Warmth
- Tenderness over bone
- Tenderness along the joint line (ankle, subtalar joint)
- Palpation of bony prominences
  - Medial and lateral malleoli: Their relationship with each other. Normally lateral malleolus is behind the medial malleolus (in the coronal plane by ~20°) and 1 cm lower.
- Observe if there is any intorsion (intoeing) or any out toeing, by change of this relationship while patient sitting on the bed with legs hanging by the side of the bed. This may also be confirmed during gait examination by foot-progression angle (whether the foot falls inwards/outwards while walking).
- Distance between the medial and the lateral malleolus as compared to the opposite (normal) side
  - Measurement may be done by a caliper. Widening of the distance can occur in the disruption of the ankle or in cases of bimalleolar fracture.
- Distance between the heel/ground and the tip of the medial malleolus: This also suggests heel height.
  - Decreased distance occurs in cases of calcaneal fractures.
- Palpation of tendo achillis to find out if there is any gap/tenderness at its attachment with the os calcis.
- Palpation of the lymph nodes: Popliteal and inguinal.

Range of Movements

- Determine if there is any deformity and if there is any further range possible at that particular joint.
  - If not, is the joint fused (ankylosed)? Which position?
  - Is the position the joint ankylosed in, compatible with activities of daily living (functional position)?
  - If joint is ankylosed in a nonfunctional position and is associated with pain and tenderness, it is called unsound ankylosis. (It also suggests that it is a fibrous ankylosis rather than a bony ankylosis. In a fibrous ankylosis there may be just a jog of movement rather than a complete absence of movement at the joint.)

- Pain
  - Pain at the extreme range with relatively painless overall possible range may suggest synovitis. It is often associated with the effusion. Effusion places the joint in the position of ease. (Position in which maximum fluid can be accommodated in the joint.)
  - Pain throughout the range suggests arthritis; this is often associated with crepitus throughout the range and deformity.
- Range of movements (active and passive) should be checked.
  - For eliciting the range of movements, one holds proximal and distal ends of the joint as close to the joint as possible so that passive range of movement being elicited is across only one joint rather than the two or more joints.
- Ankle range
  - Examiner's one hand holds the ankle mortise, close to the joint while the other hand holds the talus at the neck or beyond.
- Subtalar joint
  - Examiner holds the talar neck with one hand stabilising it within the ankle mortise in dorsiflexion while the other hand holds the heel trying to move it in inversion and eversion.
- Midfoot/midtarsal joints
  - Adduction and abduction take place. To demonstrate it, one holds the forefoot with one hand and hindfoot with the other and applies adduction and abduction force to the foot.
  - Movements at the ankle, subtalar and midfoot (midtarsal) joint are usually coupled movements rather than the isolated ones.
  - Ankle dorsiflexion, subtalar eversion as well as midfoot abduction are coupled and are called "Pronation".
  - Ankle plantar flexion, subtalar inversion and midfoot adduction are coupled and called "supination".
- Normal range of movements across the joints
  - Ankle: Dorsiflexion: 25°
    Plantar flexion: 35°
  - Subtalar inversion: 20°
    Eversion: 20°

COMMON CASES

1. CTEV (congenital talipes equinovarus deformity)

History

- Presence since birth
- May be present in the siblings/parents.

- Racial predisposition (1 in 1000 live births)
- H/o previous treatment taken.
a. Recurrent clubfoot
   If recurrence after completed previous treatment, the foot is labeled recurrent/relapsed clubfoot.
b. Resistant clubfoot
   If in spite of adequate attempts of conservative treatment (manipulation and plastering), foot fails to yeild/correct, it is labeled resistant clubfoot.

Clinical Features (Fig. 48.1)

- Short foot which is plantar flexed, inverted and adducted.
- Small heel
- Extra creases on the medial border of the foot as well as on the heel near tendo Achillis insertion
- Callosities on the lateral aspect of the foot in a child who is ambulatory.
- Equinus at ankle, varus at subtalar joint and midfoot adduction may be associated with the midfoot cavus.
- Find out the correctibility/flexibility of the deformities with the passive stretch.
   This helps in classifying the deformities into mild, moderate and severe (rigid) depending upon the correctibility of the forefoot and the hindfoot.
- Find out whether dorsum of the foot can be brought to touch the shin as on the normal side in a newborn.
- Neurovascular condition of the foot:
   – Palpate for the anterior tibial, dorsalis pedis pulsation.
   – Look for any neurological abnormality or neuromuscular imbalance.

- Spine examination to rule out any spinal dysraphism.
- Other joints for any anomalies

2. Malunited Calcaneal Fractures

History

- H/o trauma-usually fall from height.
- Associated spine, occasionally pelvic fractures.
- Swelling, deformity of the hindfoot.
- H/o appearance of blisters on the foot.
- Gradual amelioration of symptoms of pain and swelling.
- Pain in the heel/awkward gait/inability to run/ inability to walk on the rough surface.

Examination findings (Fig. 48.2)

- Broadened heel.
- Loss of heel valgus as compared to opposite side (if it is normal).
- Decreased distance between the medial malleolus and the ground (due to loss of heel height).
- Flat foot/loss of the longitudinal arch.
- Too many toes sign (one can see more toes from behind than usual due to pes planus).
- Horseshoe swelling around the heel in case of subtalar synovitis/arthritis.
- Inability to stand on the tiptoes.
- Calcaneus/apropulsive gait with loss of heel push off during the early swing phase.
- Decreased subtalar movements (inversion, eversion).
- Occasionally findings suggestive of tarsal tunnel syndrome (due to impingement of bony fragments against plantar nerves within the tarsal tunnel).

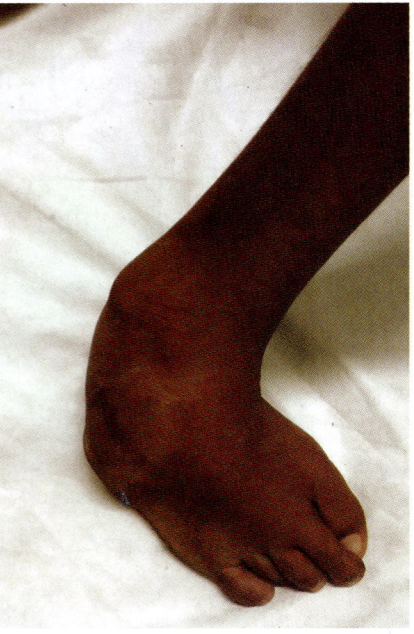

Fig. 48.1: Rigid CTEV in an infant

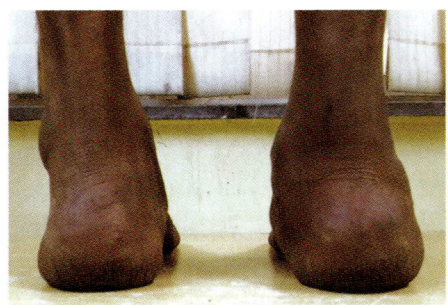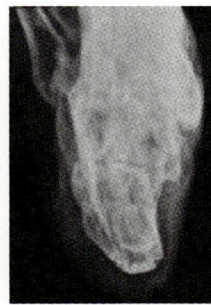

Fig. 48.2: (Right) malunited fracture calcaneum showing broadened heel, subtalar region swelling

3. Synovitis of the Ankle (due to RA, Koch's)

- Swelling, pain in the ankle.

– Swelling, pain: Progressive, gradually increasing in size in cases of Koch's aetiology.

– Waxing and waning, associated morning stiffness, with involvement of other joints in the body, especially the small joints like fingers, toes in cases of RA aetiology. Symmetrical involvement. If long standing, note if it occurs in particular weather (Barometer joints).

– Doughnut shaped swelling, both anteriorly as well as posteriorly around the ankle and confined to the ankle region. (This differentiates it from the other conditions like extensor tenosynovitis, tibialis posterior tenosynovitis or peroneal tenosynovitis. In these cases the swelling extends along the tendon sheaths well proximal and distal to the joints.)

- Usually some amount of equinus deformity in the presence of fluid in the joint (position of ease for the joint)
- Further plantar flexion usually possible and the range is pain free except in the terminal few degrees of motion.
- Lymph nodes: Significant palpable vertical chain of inguinal lymph nodes in cases of Koch's aetiology.

4. Old Neglected Rupture of Tendo Achilles

History
- H/o trauma may be present.
- H/o pain in the region of tendon prior to rupture. (When rupture occurs in the absence of any significant trauma, predisposing factors such as previous degeneration, tendo Achilles tendinosis, diabetes, are to be kept in mind).
- Difficult to run or walk briskly.
- Difficulty in activities like jumping, ascending and descending the stairs.

Examination
- Visible/palpable defect in the continuity of tendo Achilles.
- Thompson's "squeeze test" positive: On squeezing the calf, there is a plantar flexion of the ankle due to the intactness of the tendo Achilles. In case of ruptured tendo Achilles, there is no plantar flexion on squeezing the tendon.
- Active plantar flexion of the ankle may however be present due to the action of long flexors of the toes.
- Occasionally one may find increased dorsiflexion range at the ankle due to healing of the neglected tear with lengthening.
- Inability to stand on tiptoes.
- *Gait:* Push off affected (calcaneus gait).

5. Hallux Valgus

- Associated with wearing of shoes with narrow toe-box (unphysiologically designed footwear).
- Familial.
- Site of pain.
- Whether progressive
- Unilateral/bilateral, involvement of other joints
- Bunion.
- Forefoot examination, examination of corns, calluses, interdigital neuromas, bunionettes, hammer toes, claw toes.
- Flexibility of the deformity (severity)
- Range of movements at metatarsophalangeal joint (if painful, it suggests arthritis).

6. Peroneal Spastic Flat Foot (rigid flat foot in adults)

Clinical symptoms
- Pain in the area of dorsolateral aspect of the foot.
- Difficulty in walking on uneven surfaces.
- Adolescent (cause tarsal coalition, inflammatory aetiology like RA, etc.)
- Painful limp.

Examination
- Heel valgus, flattening of plantar arches.
- Tenderness in the region of sinus tarsi (dorsolateral aspect of the foot).
- Prominent/taut peroneal tendons.
- Loss of subtalar motion

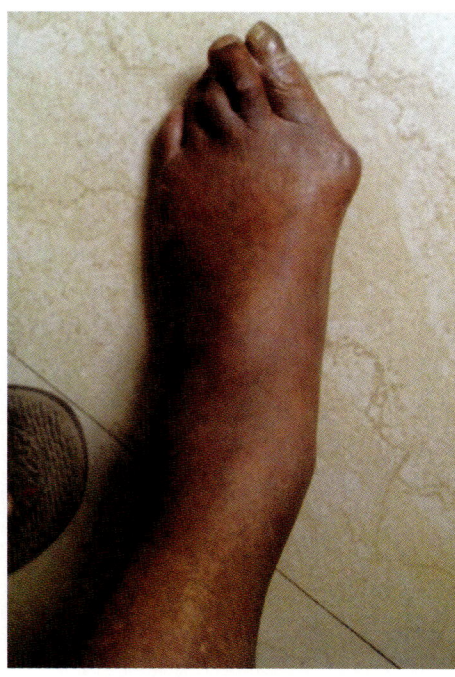

Fig. 48.3: Hallux valgus

7. Midtarsal Synovitis/Arthritis (Fig. 48.4)

History
- Monoarticular affection, insidious onset, progressive.
- Painful on activity as well as rest (night pain)... tuberculous origin.
- Polyarticular affection, associated with morning stiffness with multiple fingers, toes joint affection. Often waxing and waning of the symptoms... rheumatoid in origin.

Sign
- Swelling in the region of midtarsal joint.
- Warmth, tenderness
- *Range:* Passive abduction, adduction painful throughout the range in cases of arthritis; at the extremes of the range in cases of synovitis.

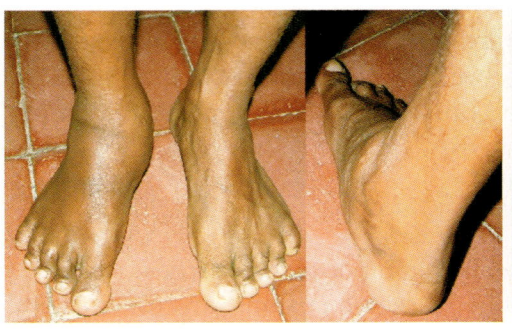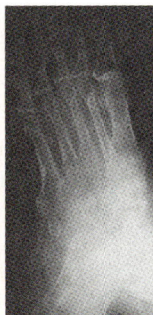

Fig. 48.4: Midtarsal synovitis

8. Post-polio Residual Paralysis

- History of childhood high-grade fever, followed by weakness in the limbs and deformities.
- Nonprogressive.
- Shortening.
- Limp
- History of using walking aids (cane, crutch, forearm/ elbow crutch)
- Ambulatory status.
- Any treatment in the past-surgery, splints, physiotherapy

Foot examination (Fig. 48.5)
- Deformities in the lower limb, shortening.
- Foot deformities: Equinus/calcaneus; varus/valgus, cavus.
- Gait:
  – Hand to knee suggests quadriceps weakness.
  – Short limb gait.
- Check power in the muscle groups.
- Tight structures, e.g. iliotibial band.

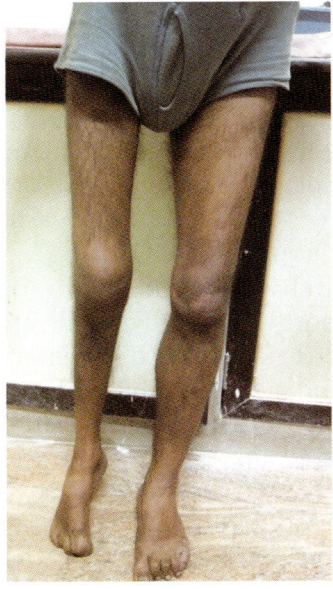

Fig. 48.5: Post-polio residual paralysis of right lower limb showing wasting, shortening and equinus deformity of the ankle. (Note: Unlike in other cases, deformities in the polio can be dynamic (flexible/correctible)

- Stability of the joints (whether unstable/subluxated/ dislocated).
- Drop of the first metatarsal head (in cases of tibialis anterior insufficiency).

9. Malunited Fractures around the Ankle (e.g. bimalleolar fracture)

- History of fall (twisting, fall in the ditch/missing a step while climbing down the staircase).
- History of treatment taken.

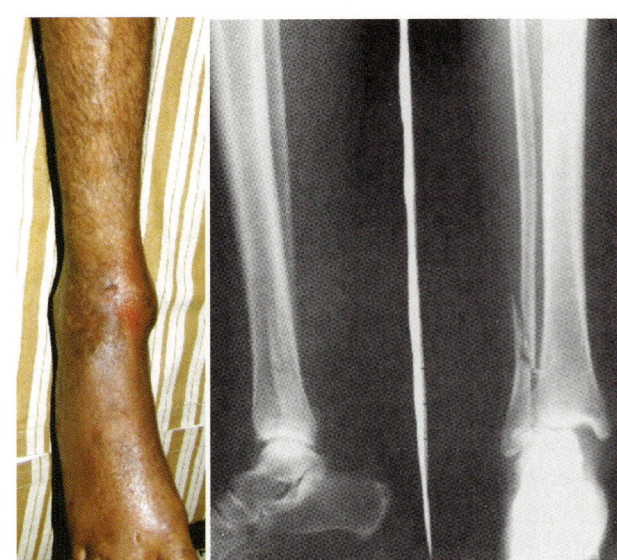

Fig. 48.6: Clinical photograph and X-ray of Right malunited Pott's fracture. Note the increase in medial joint space due to lateral subluxation of talus

Examination

- Loss of the usual contour of the ankle.
- Increased distance between the medial malleolus and lateral malleolus.
- Anterior drawer of the talus within the ankle mortise positive in cases of severe grades of ruptures of lateral ligament of the ankle.

10. Accessory Navicular Bone with Flexible Flat Feet (tibialis posterior tendon insufficiency)

- Flat foot flexible at the subtalar joint (Fig. 48.7).
- Occasionally symptomatic due to bursa over accessory navicular, direct pressure.

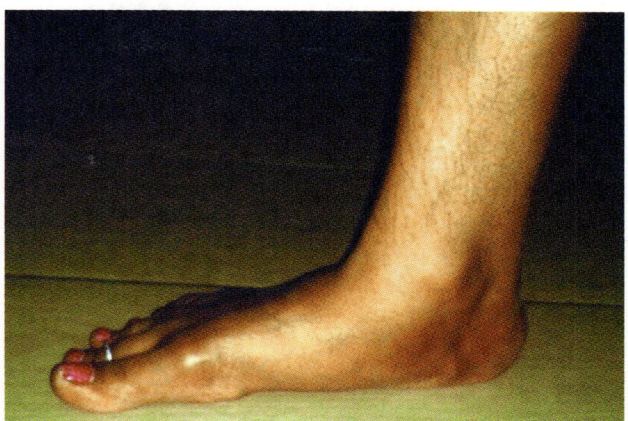

Fig. 48.7: Flat foot

Orthopaedic Implants, Radiology and Orthotics

Orthopaedic Implants

Majority of the orthopaedic implants are made up of 316-L stainless steel. For each implant, the following features are to be described.

1. Identification, i.e. name
2. Use
3. Size
4. Method of insertion
5. Special feature, if any

1. Hip Replacement Prosthesis (Austin Moore prosthesis) (Fig. 49.1)

1. Acetabular cup used for total hip replacement (retrieved at the time of revision hip replacement with the cement).
2. Austin Moore hemireplacement prosthesis, available in various head sizes from 39 to 53 mm.
3. Original Muller prosthesis femoral component (part of total hip replacement).
4. Charnley round back prosthesis with 22 mm head. (part of total hip replacement)

2. Richard's Screw/Dynamic Hip Screw (Fig. 49.2)

Use: Intertrochanteric fracture
Subtrochanteric fracture
Supracondylar femur fracture

Size: 50–100 mm (50, 55, 60, etc.)

Method: Triple reamer over guide wire in acceptable position (central-central or posterior-inferior)

↓

Richard's tap

↓

Insertion with screw driver

- 135° Richard's plate available as 4 hole plate, 5 hole plate, etc.
- 95° Richard'splate

3. Nails (Fig. 49.3)

1. 'V' nail
2. 'K' (Kuntscher nail)

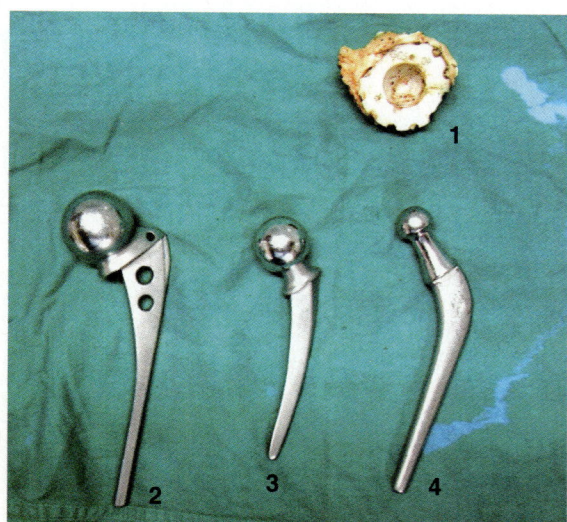

Fig. 49.1: Hip replacement prosthesis

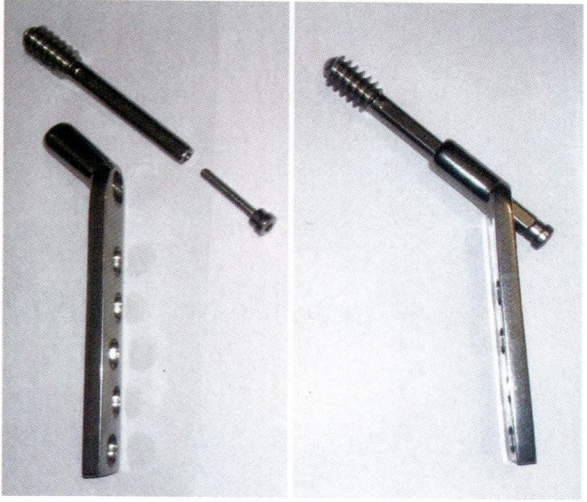

Fig. 49.2: Dynamic hip screw

3. Rush nail
4. Ulna nail
5. Radius nail
6. Ender's nail

1. *Tibia nail*

Name	'V' nail
Use	For tibial shaft fracture
Size	Variable length and diameter
Method of insertion	From just above tibial tuberosity-antegrade
Special features	11° 'Herzog's bend' at U/3–M/3 junction

2. *Femur nail*
   - 'K'—Kuntscher nail
   - Used for femur shaft fracture
   - Available in variable length and diameter (usually 8–12 mm)
   - Can be inserted antegrade or retrograde
   - Clover—leaf shaped. Eyes at either ends.

3. *Rush nail*
   - For humerus shaft fracture, children fracture
   - Solid nail available in variable length and diameter
   - Antegrade insertion
   - Proximal end is hook shaped, that prevents sinking in of the nail.

4. *Ulna nail*
   - For ulna shaft fracture
   - Variable length and diameter (2–4 mm diameter and 17–30 cm length)
   - Insertion from olecranon process

   - Square shape, threaded at one end and pointed at the tip (threads for extraction, to get a grip of the nail)

5. *Radius nail*
   - For radius shaft fracture
   - *Diameter:* 2–4 mm
     Length: 17–30 cm
   - Insertion from lower end of the radius around Lister's tubercle or through the styloid process.
   - Square shape (prevents rotation).
     Theaded at one end and bevelled tip with a notch (for smooth insertion).

6. *Ender's nail*
   - For long bone shaft fracture, osteoporotic bones.
   - Variable length and diameter
   - Can be used antegrade/retrograde
   - Multiple Ender's nails can be used to improve the stability.
     Broad at one end and pointed at the other.
   - In paediatric age group, femur fractures can be stabilised with these.

4. Plates (Fig. 49.4)

1. Narrow dynamic compression plate (DCP)
2. Broad DCP
3. Limited contact DCP (LC DCP)
4,5,6. Buttress plates for proximal tibia

1. *Dynamic compression plate:* 3.5 mm
   - Used for radius, ulna shaft (diaphyseal) fracture, T-Y fracture distal humerus, fibula
   - Available as variable number of holes plate (4 holes, 5 holes, etc)

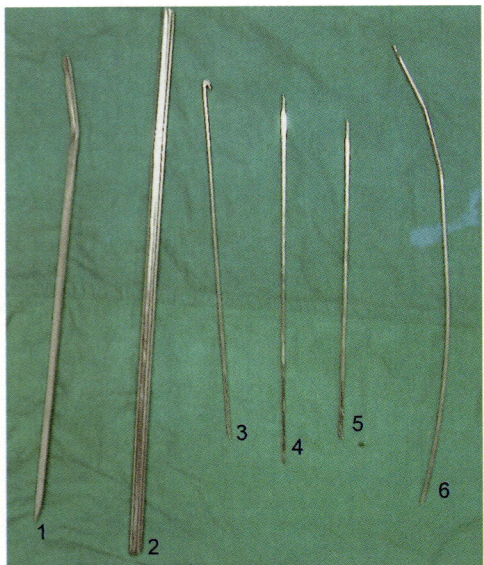

Fig. 49.3: Nails

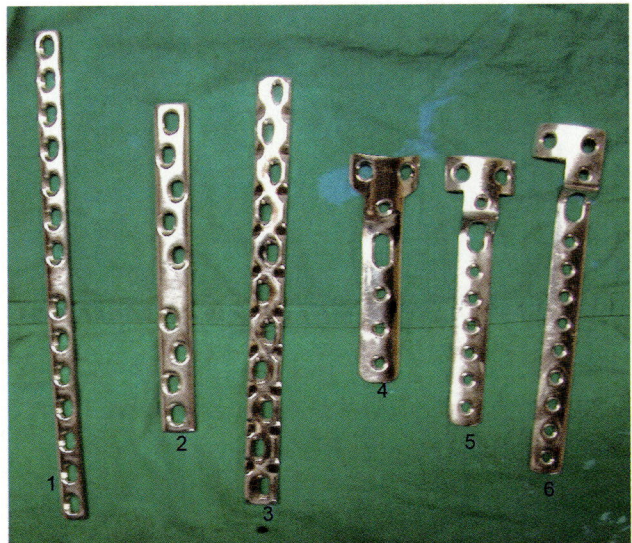

Fig. 49.4: Plates

- Fixed to the bone with 3.5 mm cortical screws using 'spherical gliding hole principle' to achieve compression at the fracture site

2. *Dynamic compression plate:* 4.5 mm
   - Used for humerus (narrow 4.5 DCP) and for femur (broad 4.5 mm DCP): Staggered holes arrangement to prevent linear cracking of the shaft.

3. *LCDCP:* Limited contact dynamic compression plate: The undersurface of the plate that comes in contact with the bone is grooved, thereby limiting its contact with the bone.
   The advantage is that it preserves the vascularity of the bone

4. *T-plate:* For upper humerus fracture
5. *T-buttress plate:* For tibial condyle fracture
6. *L-buttress plate:* For tibial condyle fracture

5. Screws (Fig. 49.5)

1. Cortical screw (4.5 mm)
2. 4 mm cancellous screw
3. 6.5 mm cancellous screw
4. Malleolar screw

1. *4.5 mm cortical screw*
   - Used with the plate for the fractures of femur, tibia, humerus, radius, ulna diaphyses.
   - Available in various diameters (1.5 mm, 2.5 mm etc.) and lengths
   - *Method of insertion for any screw:*
   - Drill the bone with appropriate drill bit
     - Measure the size of the screw with a depth gauge.
     - Tap the bone with appropriate tap (to cut the threads in the path created by drill bit)
     - Pass the screw with the screw driver
     - Head is hexagonal (older screws-slotted head)
     - Threaded throughout
     - Smaller pitch (distance between the threads)

   They are the types of machine screws—usually nonself tapping variety.

2. *4 mm cancellous screw*
   - Used in metaphyseal fractures of small bones, intercondylar fracture of humerus, medial malleolus
   - Cannulated screws can be used with a guide wire
   - Partially threaded.

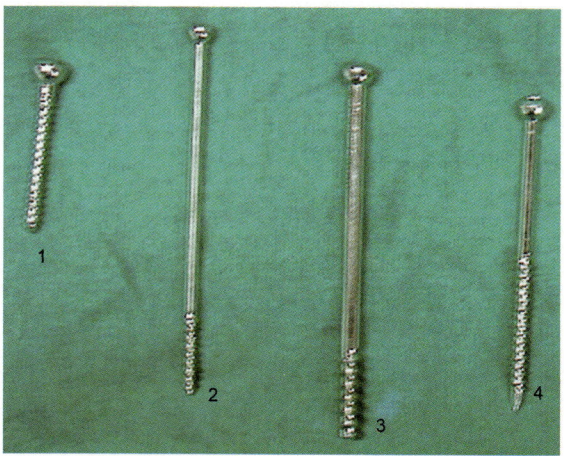

Fig. 49.5: Types of screws

3. *6.5 mm cancellous screws*
   - Can be fully/partially threaded
   - Used for transcervical neck femur fracture, metaphyseal fracture, tibial condyle, supracondylar femur fracture
   - Cancellous screws are the types of wood screws. They act by crushing the trabeculae while advancing. They have coarse (large) threads and larger pitch.

4. *Malleolar screws*
   - Used in medial malleolus
   - Pointed tip
   - Their thread characteristic matches that of cortical screw. However, they are self-tapping.

6. Spine Implants (Fig. 49.6)

Posterior instrumentation of the spine
1. Harrington distraction rod with ratchets with a hook attached in this figure
2. Variable screw placement plate (like Steffi plate)
3. Pedicular screws used along with the plates.
4. Drummond wire with button
5. Hartshill rectangle used with (4)

1. *Harrington distraction rod and hook*
   - Used for scoliosis, fracture spine
   - Hooks: Different types of hooks are available →
     Adult/child
     Laminar/Facetal
   - *Rods:* Variable sizes (½ inch difference)
     One end has ratchets

Screw-Drill bit-Tap					
Screw	3.5 mm cortical	4.5 mm cortical	4 mm cancellous	6.5 mm cancellous	Malleolar
Drill bit size	2.5 mm	3.2 mm	2.5 mm	3.2 mm	3.2 mm
Tap	3.5 mm cortical	4.5 mm	3.5 mm cancellous	6.5 mm	4.5 mm

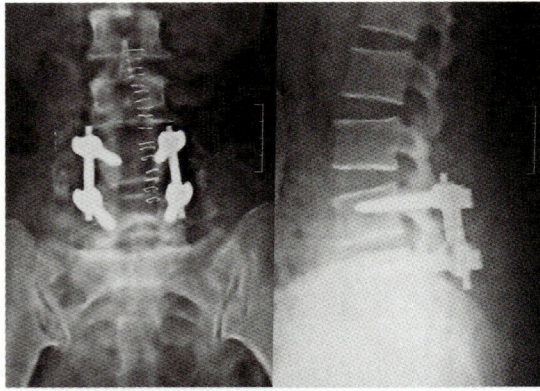

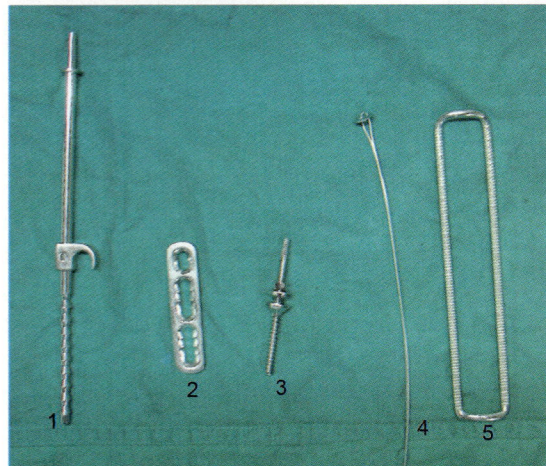

Fig. 49.6: Spine implants

- Specialised instruments available for rod and hook insertion
2. *Steffi plate* and
3. *Steffi screw*
   - For posterior fixation of dorsal and lumbosacral spine, e.g. in fracture spine, deformity correction
   - *Plates:* Variable length with different number of holes (2 hole, 2½ hole, etc.)
   - *Screws:* –4.5 mm, 5.5 mm diameter
   - Variable length
   - Screws are inserted with special spanners in the holes of Steffi plates
   - Screws engage the pedicle and body of the vertebrae.
4. *Drummond wire*
   - Used with Hartshill ring for posterior fixation
   - Passed below the lamina (sublaminar wires) or through the spinous processes.
   - 16 G/18 G
   - Button (8 mm diameter) at one end
5. *Hartshill ring*
   - For posterior fixation of cervical and dorsal spine.

- Hartshill ring:
  - Rectangular
  - Plain/serrated
  - Variable length and width

7. Steinmann Pin/Denham Pin (Fig. 49.7)

1. *Steinmann pin*
   Use: For skeletal traction in limb bone fracture
   Size: Width—4 mm/4.5 mm ... 6 mm.
   Method of insertion: With T-handle using local anaesthesia.
2. *Denham pin:* Denham pin has central threaded portion for better stability
   ↓
   Useful in elderly osteoporotic fractures

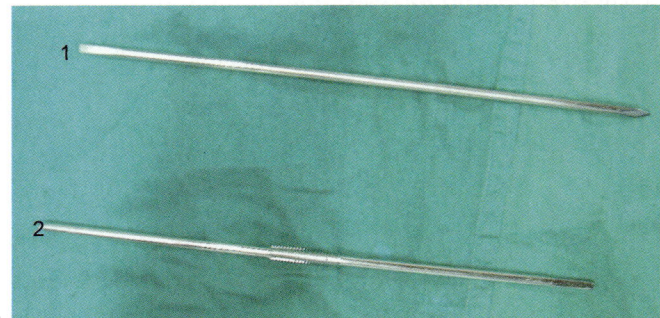

Fig. 49.7: Steinmann and Denham pin

8. Miscellaneous

1. Spool of stainless steel wire (Fig. 49.8)
2. Kirschner ('K') wire
3. Drill bit
4. Staple

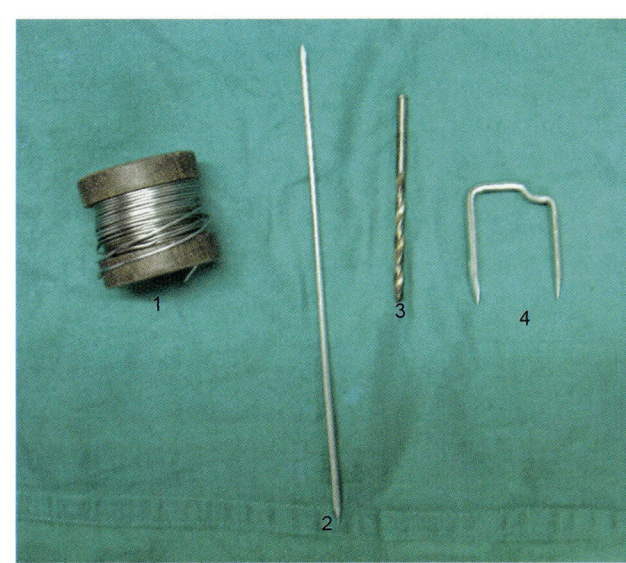

Fig. 49.8: Miscellaneous implants

1. *Tension band wire + 2) K wire (Kirschner)*
   Use: For fracture fixation of small bones like patella, medial malleolus, greater tuberosity of humerus
   Size: TBW: Variable thickness – 16G, 18G, 20G, etc.
       K wire: Variable thickness – 1 mm, 1.5 mm, etc., 6 inches in length
       Pointed at both ends

2. *Drill bit*
   Use: For drilling the bone before insertion of a screw.
   Size: 2.5 mm, 3.2 mm, etc. depending on the screw size.
   Method of insertion: Using a drill machine.
   Usually made up of carbon or stainless steel

3. *Staple*
   Use: For arthrodesis of a joint/closure of osteotomy, epiphysiodesis
   Size: Variable width
   Method of insertion: Using a hammer
   2 varieties: Coventry/plain

NEWER IMPLANTS

1. Nails (Fig. 49.9)

1. 2. *TENS: Titanium Elastic Nail System*

- Available in 2 to 4 mm diameter and variable length
- Used in paediatric long bone fractures like femur, tibia, radius-ulna

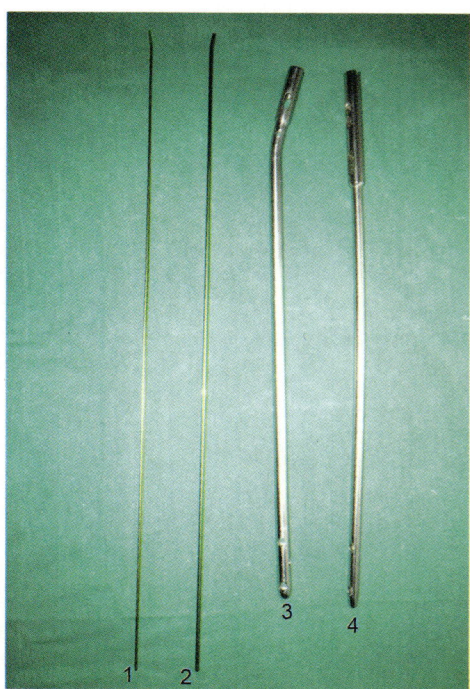

Fig. 49.9: Nails

3.4. *Interlocking Nails*

- Nails with proximal and distal holes for screw insertion, in order to provide rotational stability
- Special jigs are available for inserting locking screws.

3. *Tibial Interlocking Nail*

- *Diameter:* 8–13 mm
- *Length:* Variable

4. *Femur Interlocking Nail*

- *Diameter:* 9–14 mm
- *Length:* Variable
- Due to anatomical design separate nails for right and left

2. Plates (Fig. 49.10)

1,2,3. *Distal Radius Plates*

- For fixation of fractures and osteotomies involving distal radius
- Dorsal and volar plates available in righ and left designs.
- Low profile, precontoured for anatomical fit
- Broader distal part for multiple screw insertion option in distal radius metaphysis

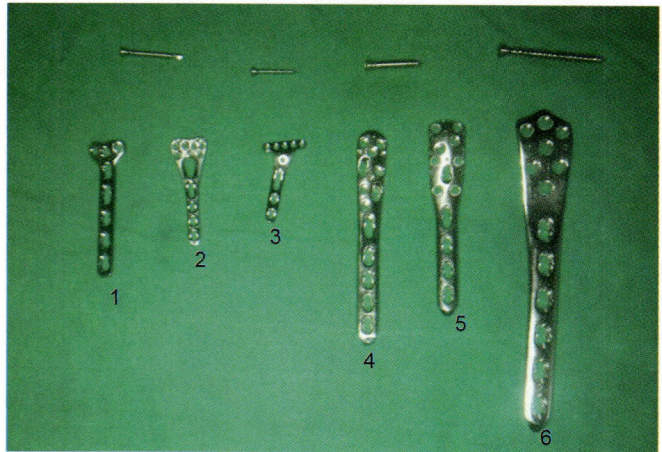

Fig. 49.10: Plates

4,5,6. *Locking Plates*

- As the screws are tightened, they "lock" to the plate, thus stabilising the segment without the need to compress the bone to the plate.
- The screws are unlikely to loosen from the plate
- Provide more stable fixation than conventional plates
- Plates have threaded holes for screws which are also threaded
- Some plates have 'combi' holes for both conventional and locking screw option.

3. 8 Plate/Guided Growth Plate and Screws (Fig. 49.11)

- Figure 8 shaped device about the size of a paper clip
- Used for hemiepiphyseodesis in angular deformity correction like genu varum/valgum in skeletally immature child
- 8 plate holds one side of the growth plate. As the opposite side of the physis continues to expand and grow, the screws diverge within the plate, effectively serving as a hinge.

4. Moss-Miami Pedicle Screw System (Fig. 49.12)

- Polyaxial pedicle screws of variable diameter (5 to 8.5 mm) and length (30–60 mm)
- For lumbar, thoracic and sacral vertebrae
- The screws are placed at 2–3 consecutive spine segments and then a short rod is usded to connect the screws
- The screw-rod construct prevents motion at the segment that are being fused

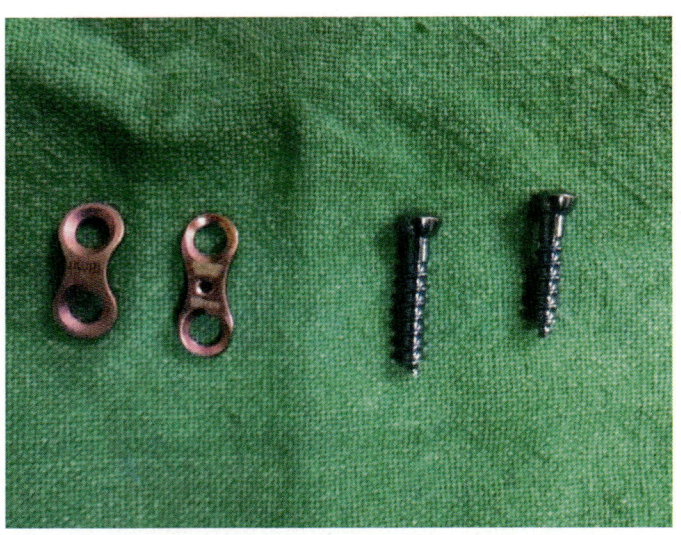

Fig. 49.11: 8 plate and screws

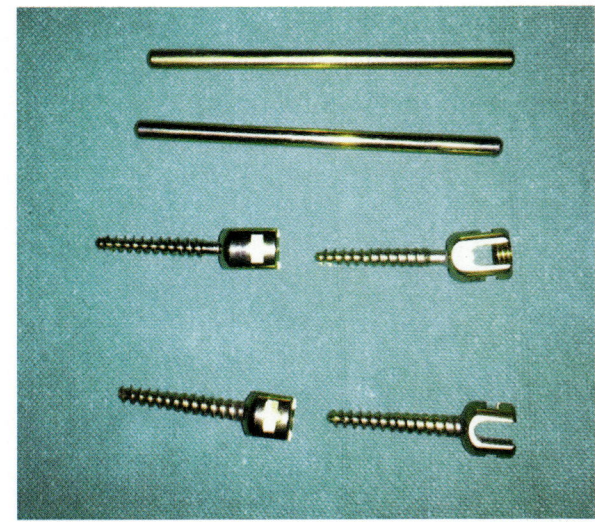

Fig. 49.12: Moss-Miami

Orthopaedic Radiology

X-ray reading is an art. In order to get complete and accurate diagnosis of any condition, the following features are to be mentioned while reading any X-ray.

1. *View of the X-ray*
   - Anteroposterior (AP)
   - Lateral
   - Oblique
   - Special view
2. *Anatomical region visualised in a given X-ray:* For example, X-ray radius and ulna/forearm with elbow and wrist joint
3. *Child or adult X-ray:* Depending upon whether the physes are open/closed.
4. *Soft tissue appearance:* For example, soft tissue swelling in c/o fracture/tumour
5. *Appearance of bone*
   - Density   Osteopenia
                   Osteoporosis
                   Sclerosis
   - Periosteum   Periosteal reaction in fractures, tumours, osteomyelitis
   - Cortex   Thinning
                   Break s/o fracture
   - Medulla   Any lytic lesion
6. *Appearance of the joint*
   - Any decrease in joint space
   - Osteophytes
   - Alignment
   - Deformity
7. *Details of the pathological features and diagnosis.*
a. Fractures:
   - Site of fracture
   - Direction of displacement of fracture fragments
   - Amount of displacement
   - Type of fracture: Transverse/oblique/spiral/comminuted

b. Tumours:
   - Site: Diaphysis/metaphysis/epiphysis
   - Central/eccentric
   - Lytic/sclerotic
   - Well/ill-defined
   - Periosteal reaction

RADIOLOGY—GENERAL

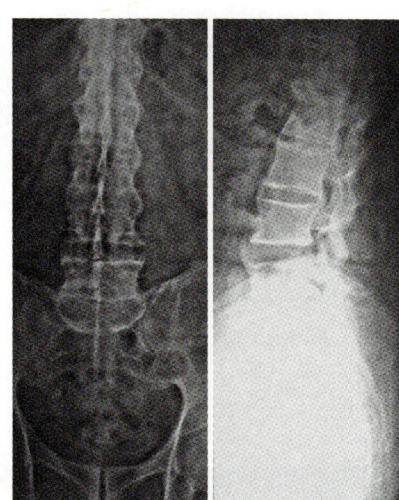

Fig. 50.1: Ankylosing spondylitis showing fusion of both the sacroiliac joints and 'bamboo spine'

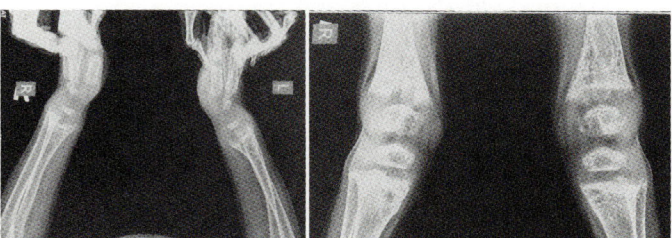

Fig. 50.2: Rickets showing cupping, fraying, splaying of the metaphysis and generalised osteopenia

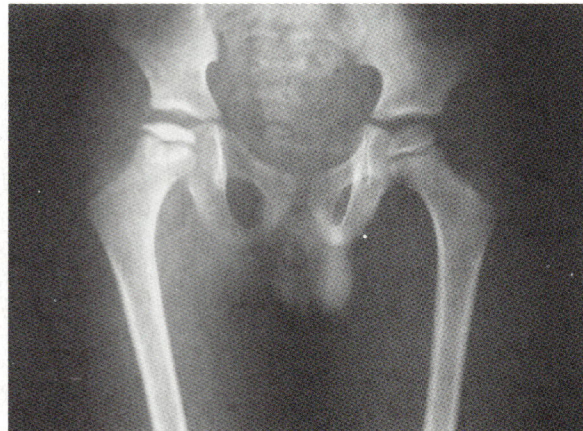

Fig. 50.3: Perthes' disease showing flattening, sclerosis and early extrusion of femoral head

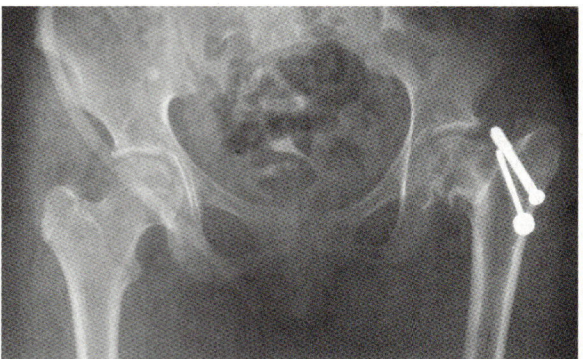

Fig. 50.4: Failed transcervical neck femur fracture fixed with 4 mm cancellous screws, showing collapsed head with cystic, sclerotic changes and irregularity of joint margin F/S/O avascular necrosis and osteoarthritis

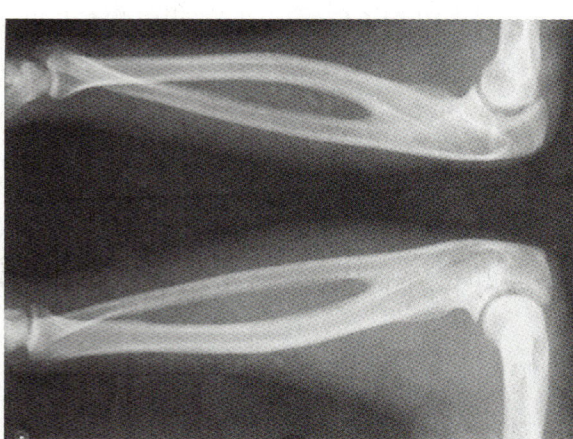

Fig. 50.5: Congenital radio-ulnar synostosis showing fusion of the proximal radius and ulna with bowing of the radius

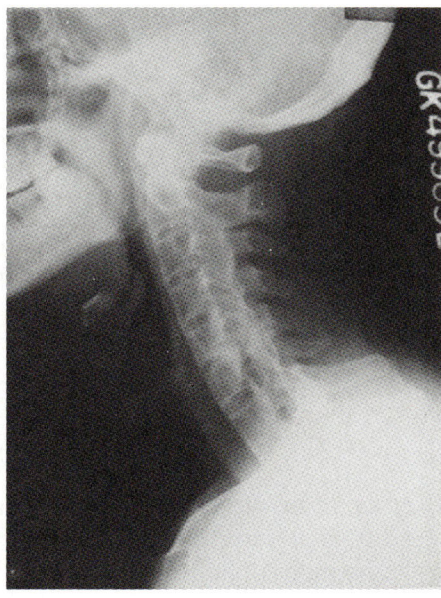

Fig. 50.6: Ankylosing spondylitis showing loss of lordosis and fusion of the facet joints

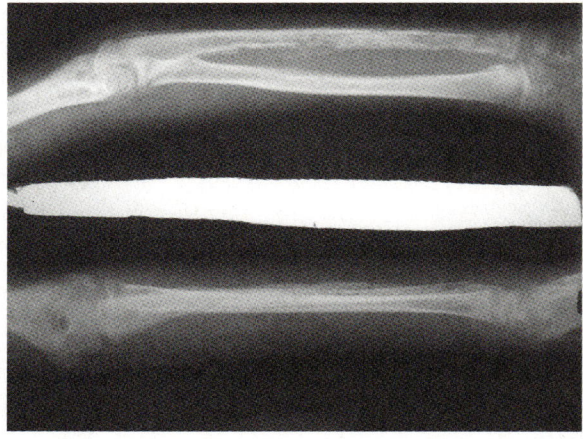

Fig. 50.7: Acute diaphyseal osteomyelitis of ulna

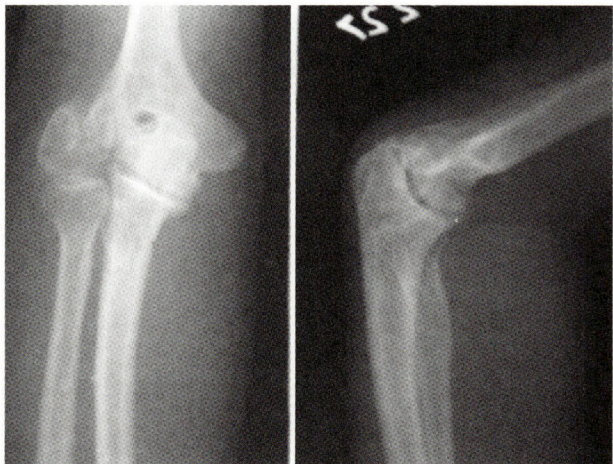

Fig. 50.8: Non-union of the lateral condyle of humerus

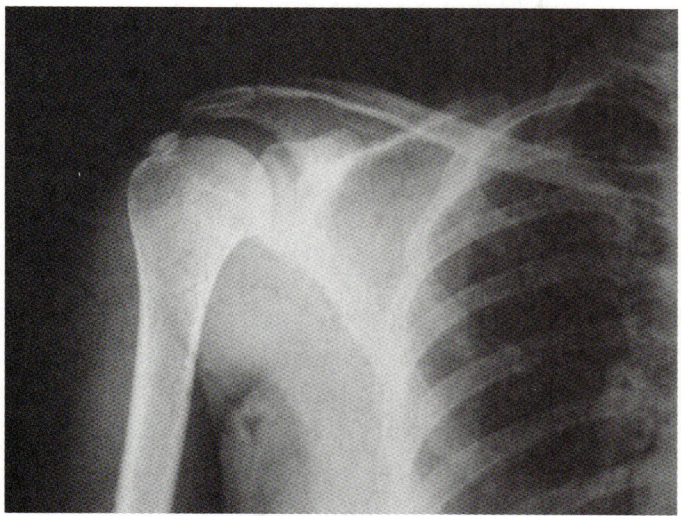

Fig. 50.9: Calcific supraspinatus tendinitis

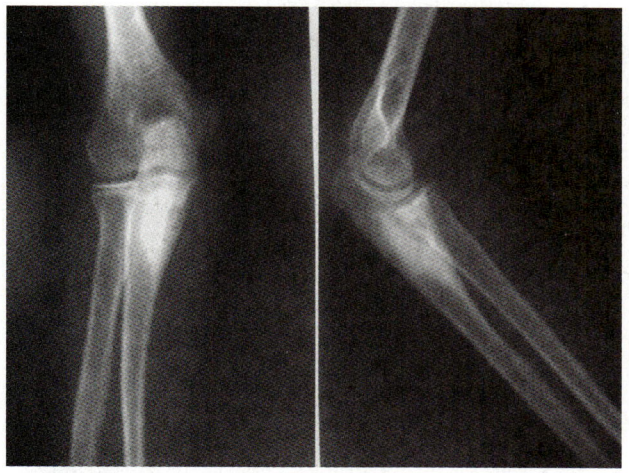

Fig. 50.10: Proximal ulna showing radiolucent nidus surrounded by sclerosis differential diagnosis: Osteoid osteoma/sequestrum

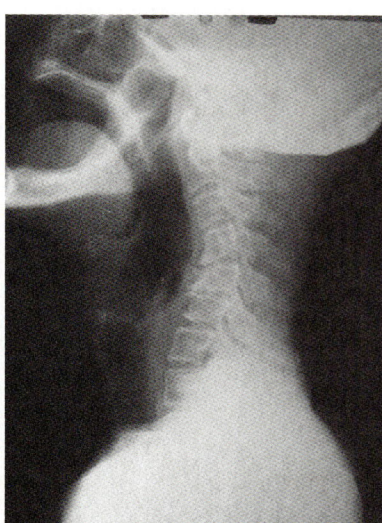

Fig. 50.11: C5–6 spondylosis showing osteophytes, disc space reduction and localised kyphosis

RADIOLOGY—TRAUMA

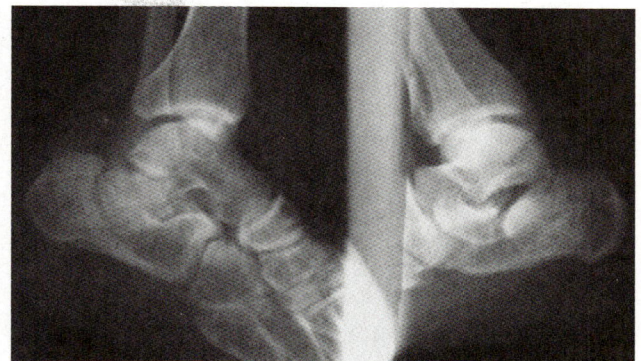

Fig. 50.12: Joint depression type fracture of calcaneum

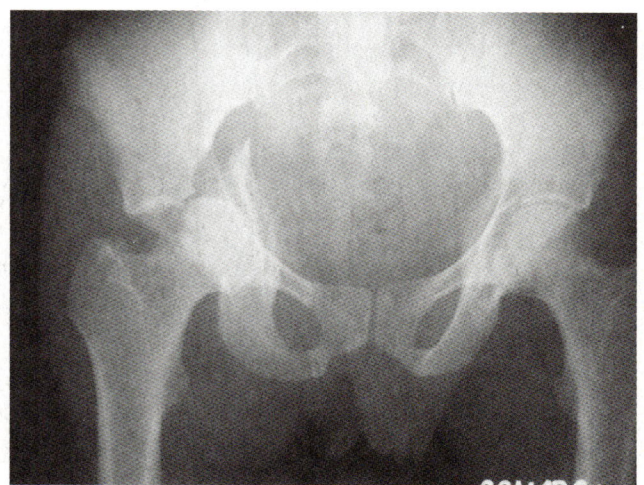

Fig. 50.13: Fracture acetabulum with central disclocation of the femoral head

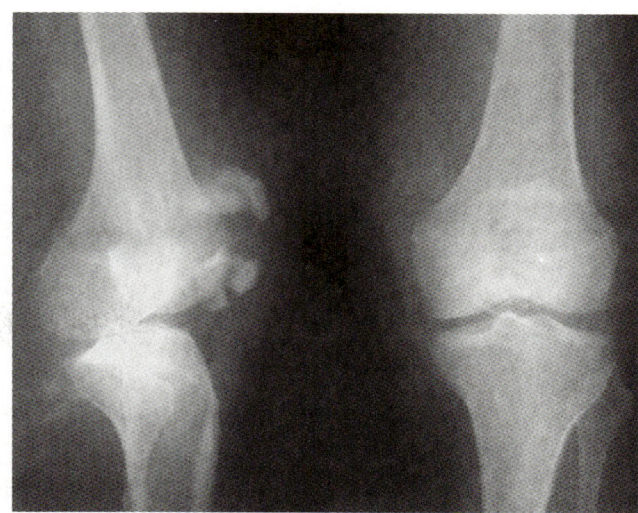

Fig. 50.14: Comminuted fracture of the patella

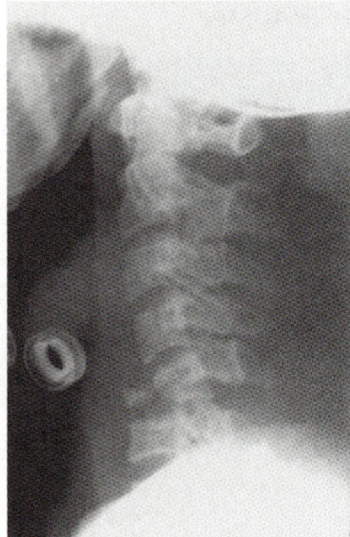

Fig. 50.15: Compression flexion type injury of C5 vertebral body. Note the increase in the interspinous distance between C5 and C6 and canal compromise

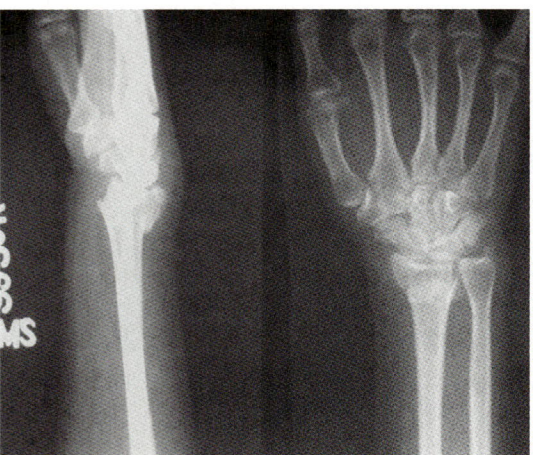

Fig. 50.16: Colle's fracture showing dorsal and lateral displacement and tilt, with loss of normal radio-ulnar variance and shortening

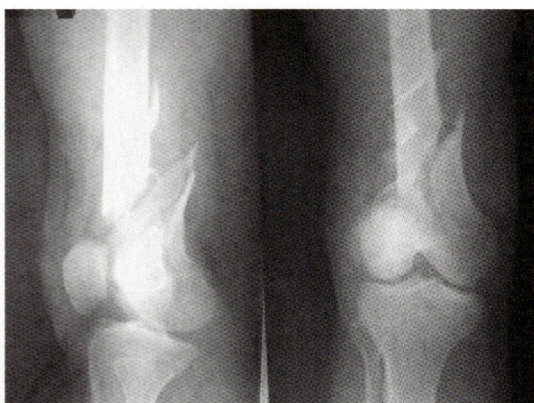

Fig. 50.17: Intra-articular, comminuted distal femur fracture (T-Y type)

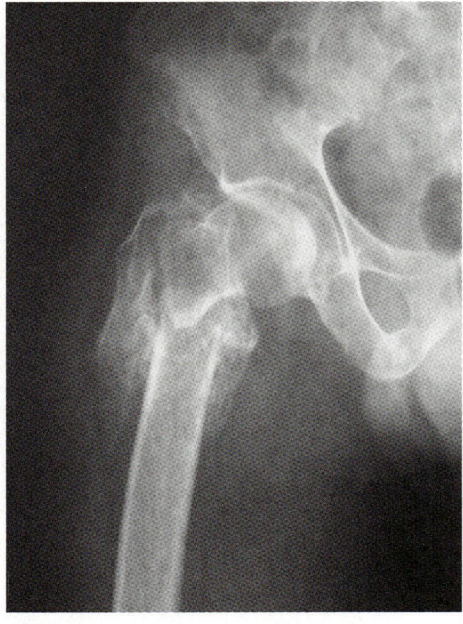

Fig. 50.18: Malunited intertrochanteric fracture with varus. Note the callus formation

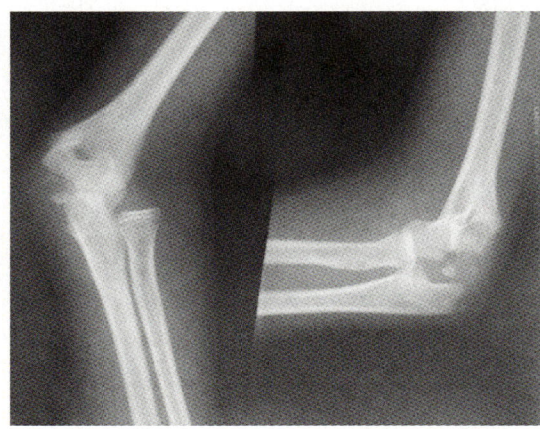

Fig. 50.19: Fracture-dislocation of the elbow with incarcerated medial epicondyle fracture fragment

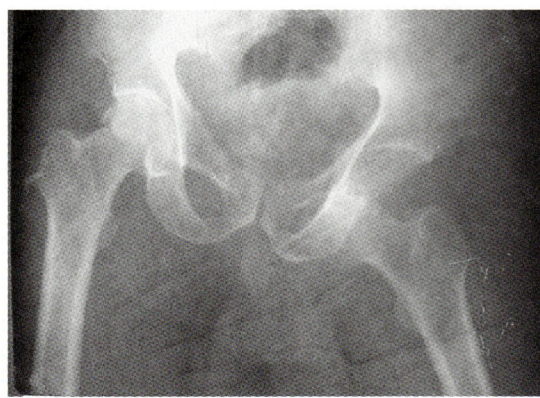

Fig. 50.20: Antero-inferior dislocation of the hip

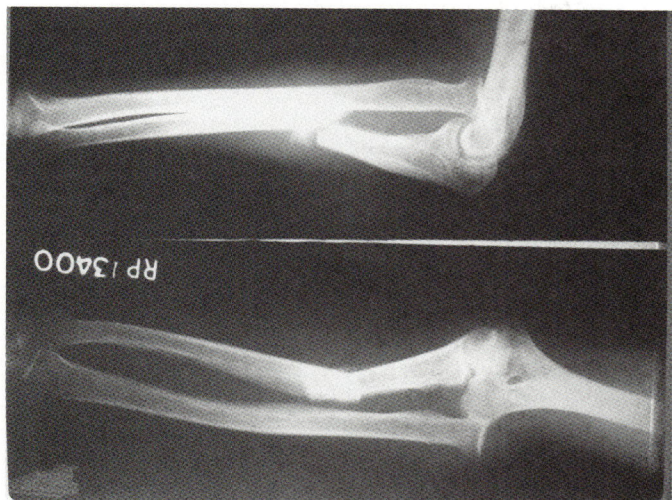

Fig. 50.21: Type III Monteggia fracture—dislocation with lateral angulation of ulna and lateral dislocation of radial head

RADIOLOGY—TUMOURS

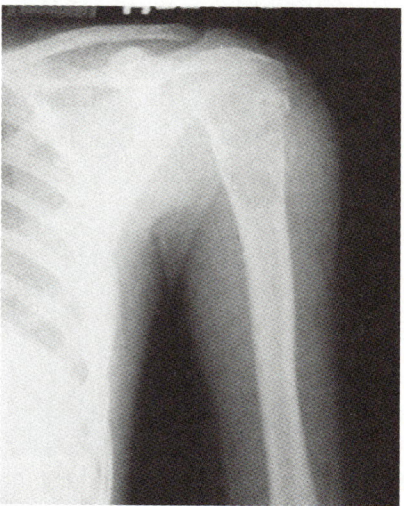

Fig. 50.23: Osteolytic tumour in upper humerus metaphysis—unicameral bone cyst

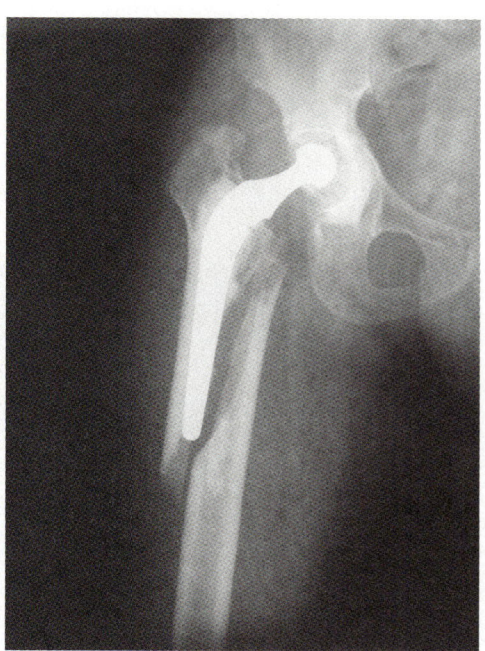

Fig. 50.22: Peri-prosthetic fracture in a c/o total hip replacement

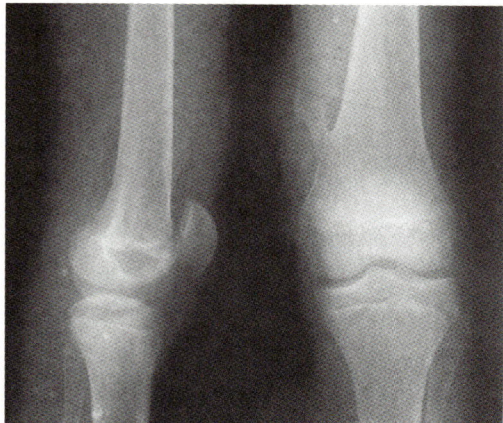

Fig. 50.24: Pedunculated outgrowth from medial lower femoral metaphysis—osteochondroma

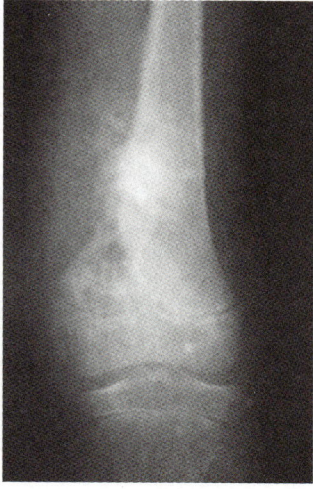

Fig. 50.25: Osteogenic sarcoma distal femur showing sun-ray apperance

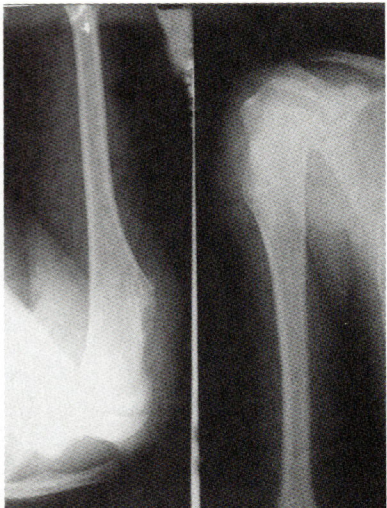

Fig. 50.26: Sessile osteochondroma arising from proximal humerus metaphysis

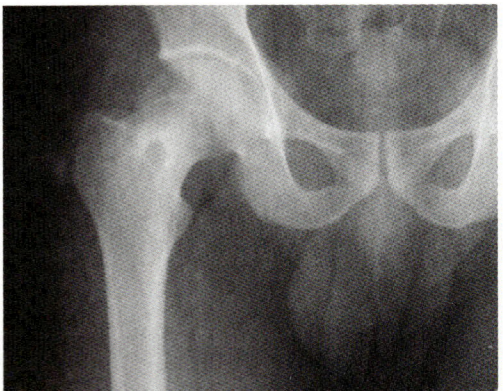

Fig. 50.27: Osteolytic lesion surrounded by sclerotic margin in the neck of femur—osteoid osteoma

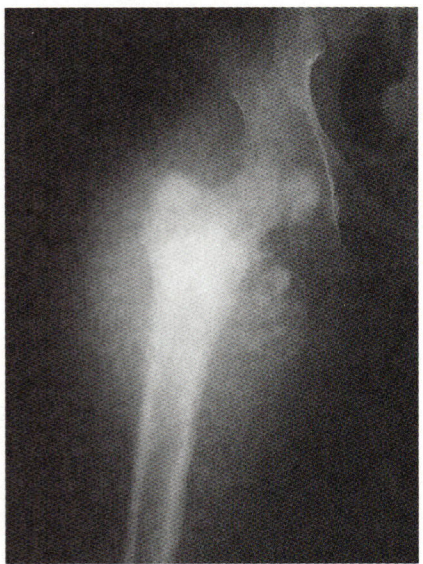

Fig. 50.28: Malignant tumour involving proximal femur, showing increased osteoblastic activity—osteogenic sarcoma

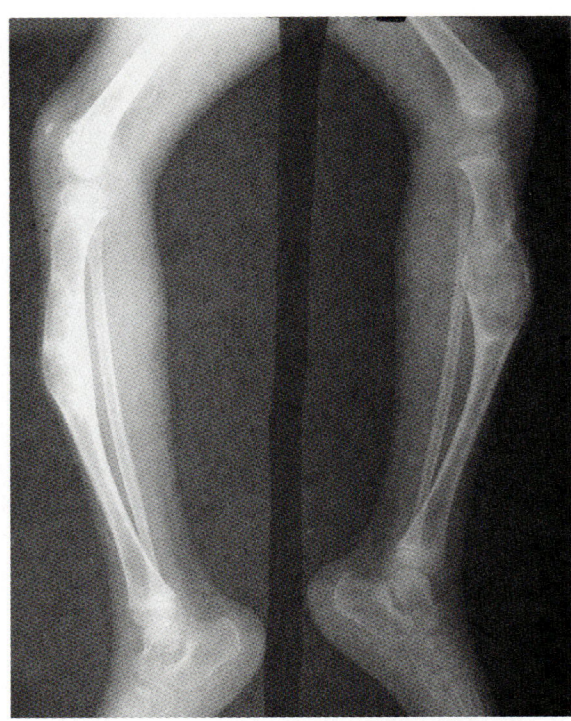

Fig. 50.29: Explansile, osteolytic tumour involving proximal diaphysis of tibia in a child differential diagnosis: Adamantinoma/fibrous dysplasia

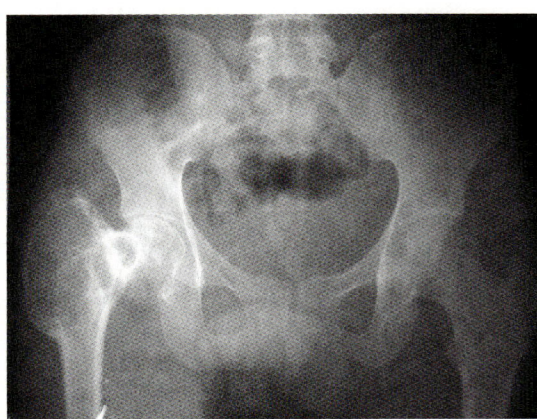

Fig. 50.30: Giant cell tumour involving proximal femur showing irregular destruction with remnants of heavily trabeculated original bone-soap bubble apperance

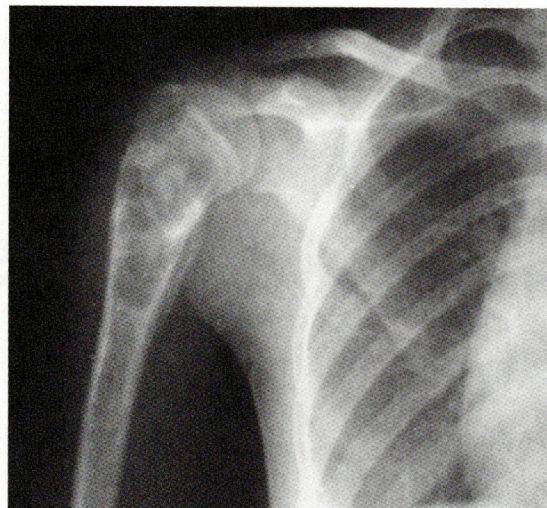

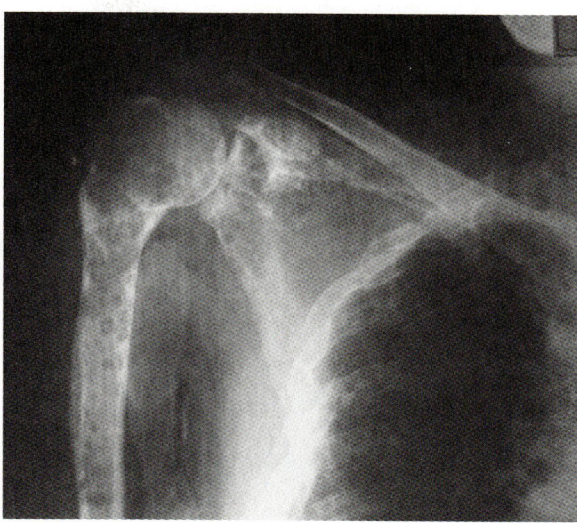

Fig. 50.31: Unicameral bone cyst with pathological fracture showing healing, involving proximal humeral metaphysis

Fig. 50.32: Multiple osteolytic lesions involving humerus, scapula, ribs: Differential diagnosis: Metastasis/multiple myeloma

Orthopaedic Orthotics

Orthoses are mechanical devices to promote stability, relieve pain, control deformity and restrict movements.

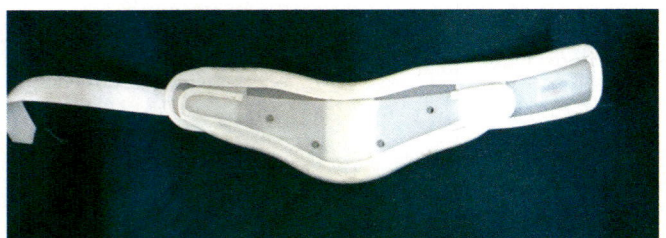

Fig. 51.1: Cervical collar (hard): For rigid immobilisation of cervical spine

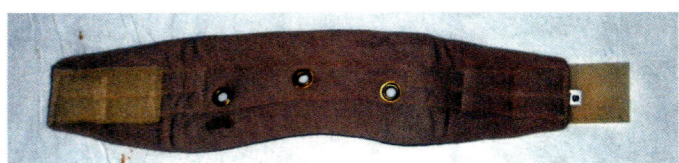

Fig. 51.2: Cervical collar (soft): For immobilisation of cervical spine

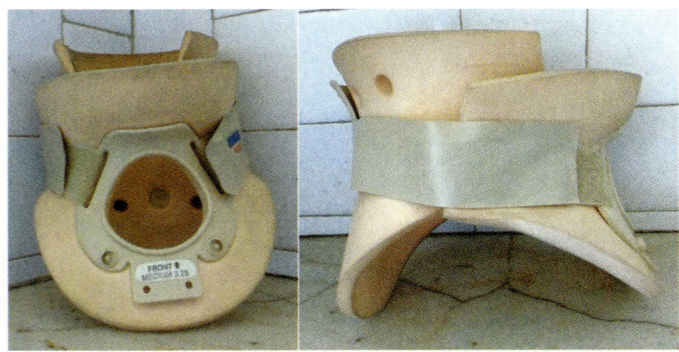

Fig. 51.3: Philadelphia collar: For immobilisation of upper cervical spine, especially C1–C2

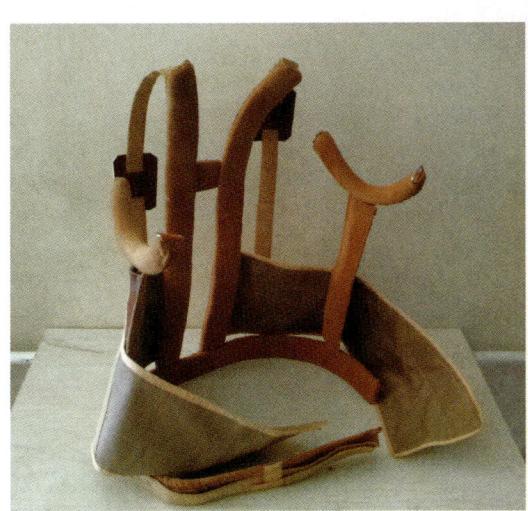

Fig. 51.4: Taylor's brace with axillary support: For supporting the dorsal spine

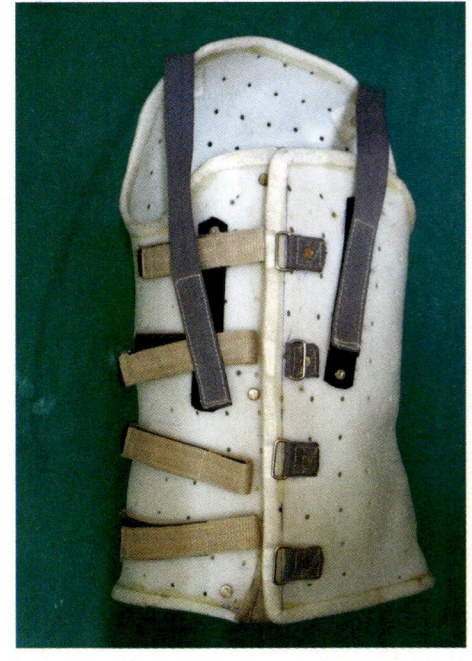

Fig. 51.5: Total contact brace: It is used in children, in scoliosis

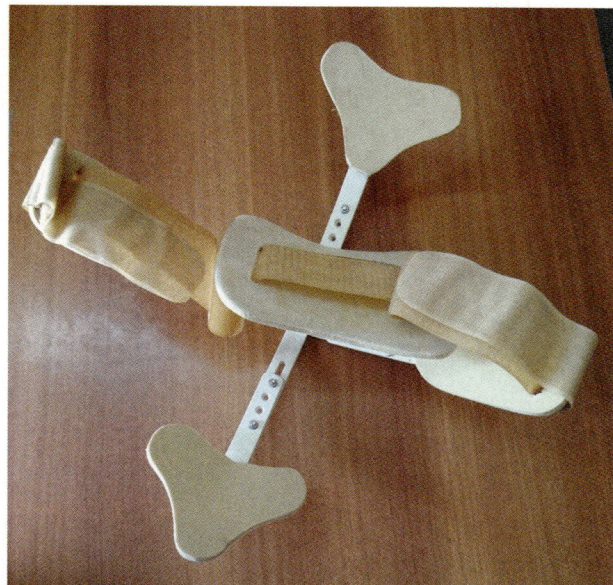

Fig. 51.6: ASH (anterior spinal hyperextension) brace: For compression fracture in osteoporotic dorsolumbar spine

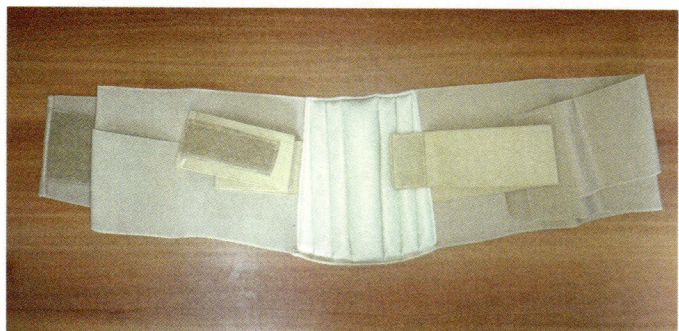

Fig. 51.7: Lumbosacral belt: For immobilisation of lumbar spine

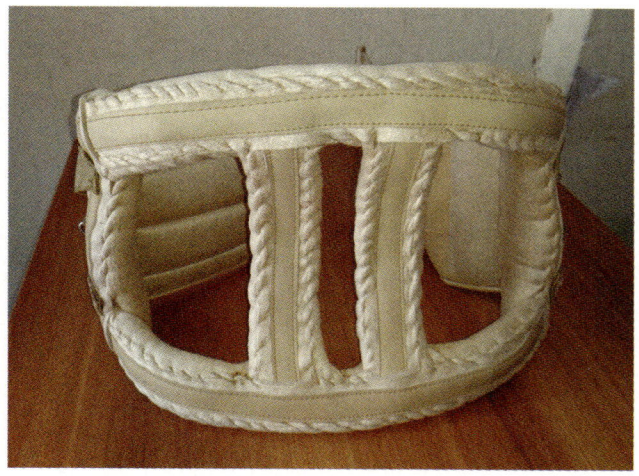

Fig. 51.8: Lumbosacral frame: For rigid immobilisation of lumbar spine

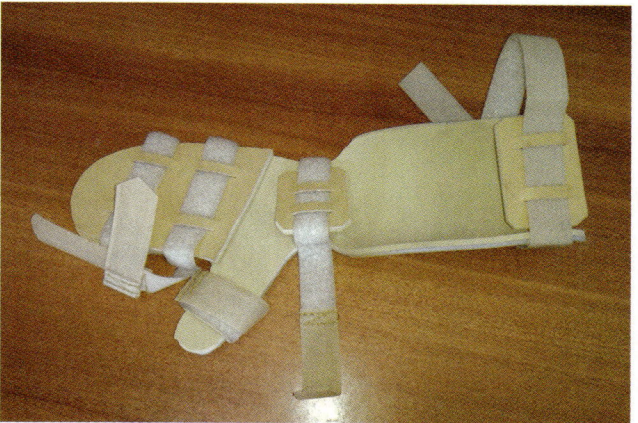

Fig. 51.9: Wrist hand orthosis (WHO): For immobilisation of wrist/hand in correct resting position, allowing healing of injured structures and minimising joint contractures

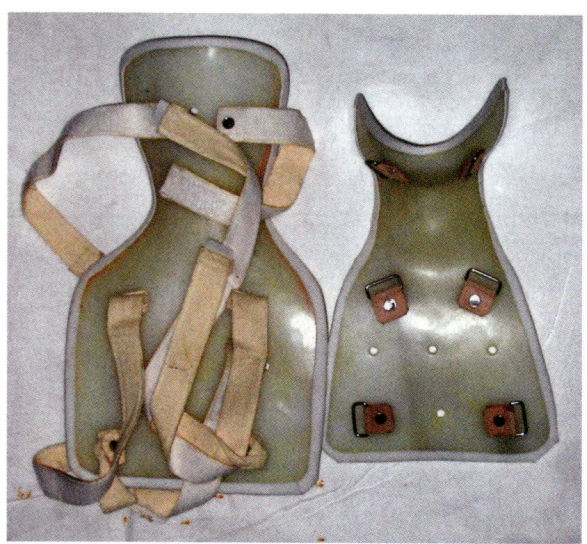

Fig. 51.10: SOMI (sternal–occipital–mandibular immobiliser) brace: For atlanto-axial instability and C2 fracture

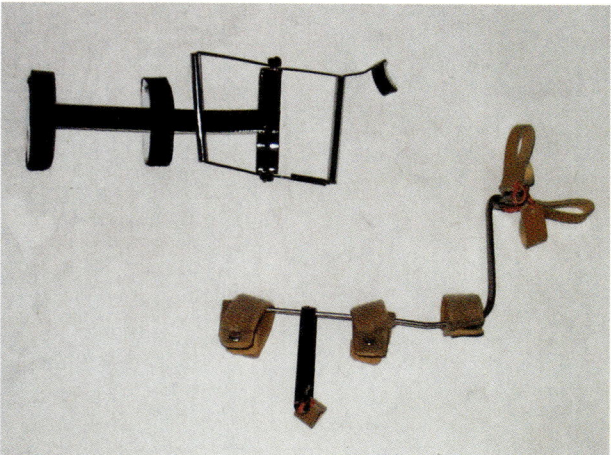

Fig. 51.11: Knuckle bender splint in ulnar nerve palsy with clawhand (top) and dynamic cock up splint in radial nerve palsy with wrist drop (bottom)

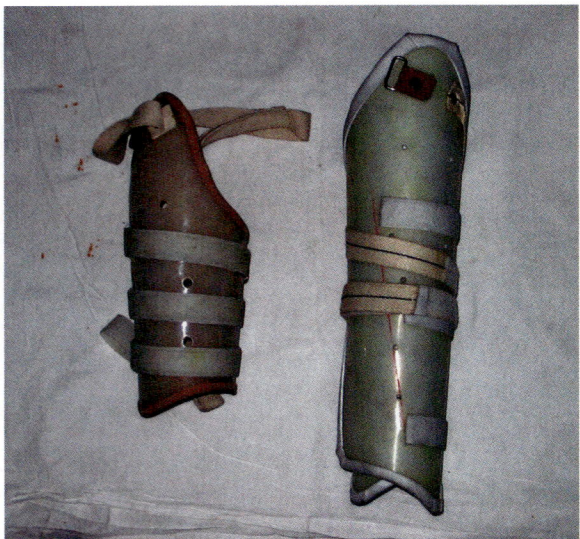

Fig. 51.12: Functional humeral brace and functional femoral brace for protection of recently united humerus and femur shaft fracture, allowing adjacent joints mobilisation

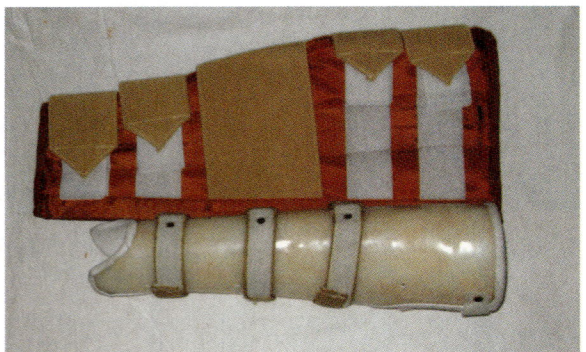

Fig. 51.13: Knee immobiliser for immobilisation of knee (top) and patellar tendon bearing (PTB) brace for recently united tibia fracture, allowing knee mobilisation (bottom)

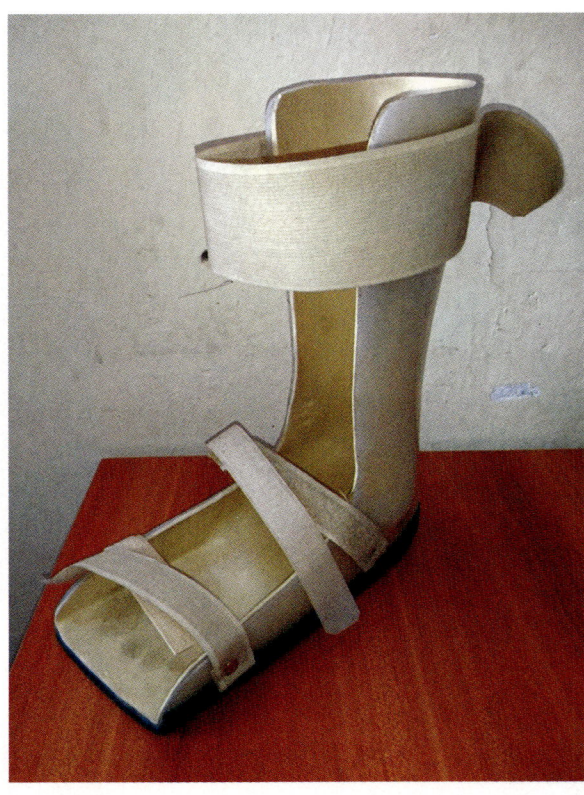

Fig. 51.14: Ankle foot orthosis (AFO) for maintaining the ankle in neutral position

Index